The Vulnerable Plaque

The Vulnerable Plaque

Second Edition

Edited by

Ron Waksman MD

Chairman, Cardiovascular Research Institute
Division of Cardiology
Washington, DC
USA

Patrick W Serruys MD PhD

Thoraxcenter, Erasmus Medical Center
Rotterdam
The Netherlands

Johannes Schaar MD

Thoraxcenter, Erasmus Medical Center
Rotterdam
The Netherlands

informa
healthcare

First published in the United Kingdom in 2004 by Taylor & Francis.

This edition published in 2010 by Informa Healthcare, Telephone House, 69-77 Paul Street, London EC2A 4LQ, UK.

Simultaneously published in the USA by Informa Healthcare, 52 Vanderbilt Avenue, 7th Floor, New York, NY 10017, USA.

Informa Healthcare is a trading division of Informa UK Ltd. Registered Office: 37–41 Mortimer Street, London W1T 3JH, UK. Registered in England and Wales number 1072954.

A CIP record for this book is available from the British Library.

Library of Congress Cataloging-in-Publication Data available on application

ISBN-13: 9781841846217

Orders may be sent to: Informa Healthcare, Sheepen Place, Colchester, Essex CO3 3LP, UK
Telephone: +44 (0)20 7017 5540
Email: CSDhealthcarebooks@informa.com
Website: http://informahealthcarebooks.com/

For corporate sales please contact: CorporateBooksIHC@informa.com
For foreign rights please contact: RightsIHC@informa.com
For reprint permissions please contact: PermissionsIHC@informa.com

Printed and bound by CPI Group (UK) Ltd, Croydon, CR0 4YY

Transferred to Digital Print 2012

Contents

List of Contributors   ix

Foreword   xvii

Preface   xix

Acknowledgments   xxi

Section I Background epidemiology and pathology

1. Definition and terminology of the vulnerable plaque   3
   James E Muller, Pedro R Moreno, and Pavan K Cheruvu

2. Pathology of the vulnerable plaque   13
   Renu Virmani, Allen Burke, Andrew Farb, Frank D Kolodgie,
   Aloke V Finn, and Herman K Gold

3. The molecular basics of vulnerable plaque   29
   Esther Lutgens, Tim Leiner, Robert-Jan van Suylen, and Mat JAP Daemen

4. Platelets and the vulnerable plaque   39
   Marc Sirol, Juan F Viles-Gonzalez, and Juan J Badimon

5. Role of metalloproteinases in the vulnerable plaque   53
   Jason L Johnson and Andrew C Newby

6. Oxidative stress and the vulnerable plaque   67
   Donald D Heistad and Yi Chu

7. Carotid vulnerable plaque   75
   Erica CS Camargo and Karen L Furie

8. Psychological triggers for plaque rupture   87
   Geoffrey H Tofler and Thomas Buckley

9. Animal models of vulnerable plaque   103
   Juan F Granada and Robert S Schwartz

Section II Biomarkers

10. Endothelial biomarkers of vulnerable plaque progression   121
    Victoria LM Herrera

11. Biomarkers   141
    Michael Weber and Christian W Hamm

12. Epidemiology of lipoprotein-associated phospholipase A_2 153
    Isabella Kardys and Jacqueline CM Witteman

Section III Invasive imaging

13. Angiography and the vulnerable plaque   169
    John A Ambrose and Cezar S Staniloae

14. Imaging the vulnerable plaque by ultrasound   179
    Ehtisham Mahmud and Anthony N DeMaria

15. Intravascular palpography for vulnerable plaque assessment   191
    Johannes A Schaar, Anton FW van der Steen, Frits Mastik,
    and Patrick W Serruys

16. Diffuse reflectance near-infrared spectroscopy as a clinical technique
    to detect high-risk atherosclerotic plaques   199
    Pavan K Cheruvu, Pedro R Moreno, Barbara J Marshik,
    and James E Muller

17. Optical coherence tomography   211
    Evelyn Regar and Ik-Kyung Jang

18. Virtual histology   223
    Hector M Garcia-Garcia, Neville Kukreja, and Patrick W Serruys

19. Shear stress and the vulnerable plaque   233
    Jolanda J Wentzel, Frank JH Gijsen, Rob Krams, Rini de Crom,
    Caroline Cheng, Harald C Groen, Alina G van der Giessen,
    Anton FW van der Steen, and Patrick W Serruys

20. Vasa vasorum and vulnerable plaques   245
    Mario Gössl and Amir Lerman

21. Intravascular magnetic resonance imaging   255
    Robert L Wilensky and David A Halon

22. Intracoronary thermography: basic principles   267
    Anna G ten Have, Frank JH Gijsen, Joland J Wentzel, Cornelis J Slager,
    Patrick W Serruys, and Anton FW van der Steen

23. Intracoronary thermography   279
    Christodoulos Stefanadis and Konstantinos Toutouzas

Section IV Non-invasive imaging

24. Targeted nanoparticle contrast agents for vascular molecular imaging and therapy   289
    Samuel A Wickline, Anne M Neubauer, Patrick Winter, Shelton Caruthers, and Gregory Lanza

25. Nuclear imaging of the vulnerable plaque   303
    Sotirios Tsimikas and Jagat Narula

26. Nanoparticle-based targeted delivery of therapeutics and non-invasive imaging of unstable endothelium   313
    Thomas R Porter, Feng Xie, SJ Adelman, and Nicholas Kipshidze

27. Multislice computed tomography coronary plaque imaging   327
    Pim J de Feyter, A Weustink, WB Meijboom, Nico Mollet, and Filippo Cademartiri

28. Magnetic resonance imaging   335
    Chun Yuan, William S Kerwin, Vasily L Yarnykh, Jianming Cai, Marina S Ferguson, Baocheng Chu, Tobias Saam, Norihide Takaya, Hunter R Underhill, Fei Liu, Dongxiang Xu, and Thomas S Hatsukami

Section V Systemic therapy

29. Influenza vaccination as a strategy to prevent cardiovascular events   353
    Mohammad Madjid and S Ward Casscells III

30. Vaccination: bedside   361
    Enrique P Gurfinkel and Veronica S Lernoud

31. Immunomodulation of atherosclerosis   371
    Jan Nilsson, Gunilla Nordin Fredrikson, Alexandru Schiopu, Isabel Gonçalves, Kuang-Yuh Chyu, and Prediman K Shah

32. Multifocal coronary plaque instability: evidence for a systemic inflammatory process   383
    James A Goldstein

33. Stem cell therapy in heart disease   399
    Emerson C Perin, Guilherme V Silva, and James T Willerson

Section VI Local therapy

34. Photodynamic therapy   427
    Ron Waksman

35. Stenting the vulnerable plaque   437
    Probal Roy and Ron Waksman

Section VII Clinical management

36. PREVAIL study   447
     Heidar Arjomand, Roxana Mehran, George Dangas, and Sheldon Goldberg

37. Regulatory issues of the Food and Drug Administration   461
     Felipe Aguel, Andrew Farb, and Elias Mallis

38. Investing in vulnerable plaque   471
     Jan David Wald

     Index   483

Contributors

SJ Adelman
Cardiovascular and Metabolic Diseases
Wyeth Research
Collegeville, PA
USA

Felipe Aguel PhD
Food and Drug Administration
Center for Devices and Radiological Health
Rockville, MD
USA

John A Ambrose MD
Professor of Medicine, UCSF
Chief of Cardiology, UCSF Fresno
CA
USA

Heidar Arjomand MD FACC
Director, Endovascular Intervention
Seacoast Cardiology Associates
Dover, NH
USA

Juan J Badimon PhD
Professor of Medicine
Cardiovascular Biology Research Laboratory
Zena and Michael A. Wiener Cardiovascular
    Institute
Mount Sinai School of Medicine
New York, NY
USA

Thomas Buckley BSc
Cardiology Department
Royal North Shore Hospital
St Leonards, NSW
Australia

Allen Burke MD
Department of Cardiovascular Pathology
Armed Forces Institute of Pathology
Washington, DC
USA

Jianming Cai
Department of Radiology
University of Washington
Seattle, WA
USA

Filippo Cademartiri MD
Department of Radiology
Erasmus Medical Center
Rotterdam
The Netherlands

Erica CS Camargo MD PhD
Research Fellow, Neurology
Massachusetts General Hospital
Stroke Service
Boston, MA
USA

Shelton Caruthers
Philips Medical Systems
Best
The Netherlands

S Ward Casscells III MD
John E Tyson Distinguished Professor of
    Medicine (Cardiology and Public Health)
Vice President for Biotechnology
School of Medicine
University of Texas – Houston Health
    Science Center and
Director, Cardiology Research
Texas Heart Institute/St. Luke's Episcopal
    Hospital
Houston, TX
USA

Caroline Cheng
Biomedical Engineering, Thoraxcenter
Erasmus Medical Center
Rotterdam
The Netherlands

Pavan K Cheruvu
Massachusetts General Hospital
Boston, MA
USA

Pavan K Cheruvu
Infraredx Inc.
Cambridge, MA
USA

Baocheng Chu
Department of Radiology
University of Washington
Seattle, WA
USA

Yi Chu MD
Department of Internal Medicine
University of Iowa College of Medicine and
   VA Medical Center
Iowa City, IA
USA

Kuang-Yuh Chuy MD PhD
Staff Cardiologist
Division of Cardiology
Cedars-Sinai Medical Center
David Geffen School of Medicine, UCLA
Los Angeles, CA
USA

Rini de Crom
Biomedical Engineering, Thoraxcenter
Erasmus Medical Center
Rotterdam
The Netherlands

Mat JAP Daemen
Cardiovascular Research Institute
   Maastricht
University of Maastricht
Maastricht
The Netherlands

George Dangas MD FACC
Director, Academic Affairs and
   Investigational Pharmacology
Cardiovascular Research Foundation
New York, NY
USA

Pim J de Feyter MD PhD
Departments of Radiology and Cardiology
Erasmus Medical Center
Rotterdam
The Netherlands

Anthony N DeMaria MD
Division of Cardiovascular Medicine
UCSD Medical Center
San Diego, CA
USA

Alina G van der Giessen
Biomedical Engineering, Thoraxcenter
Erasmus Medical Center
Rotterdam
The Netherlands

Andrew Farb MD
Food and Drug Administration
Center for Devices and Radiological
   Health
Rockville, MD
USA

Marina S Ferguson
Department of Radiology
University of Washington
Seattle, WA
USA

Aloke V Finn MD
Department of Cardiovascular Pathology
Armed Forces Institute of Pathology
Washington, DC
USA

Gunilla Nordin Fredrikson PhD
Professor of Experimental Cardiovascular
    Research
Department of Clinical Sciences
Malmö University Hospital
Lund University
Malmö
Sweden

Karen L Furie MD MPH
Associate Professor of Neurology
Harvard Medical School
and
Director, Stroke Prevention Clinic
Massachusetts General Hospital
Boston, MA
USA

Hector M Garcia-Garcia MD
Professor of Interventional Cardiology
Thoraxcenter
Erasmus Medical Center
Rotterdam
The Netherlands

Frank J Gijsen PhD
Biomedical Engineering, Thoraxcenter
Erasmus Medical Center
DR Rotterdam
The Netherlands

Frank J Gijsen PhD
Hemodynamics
Biomedical Engineering, Thoraxcenter
Erasmus Medical Center
Rotterdam
The Netherlands

Herman K Gold MD
Department of Cardiovascular Pathology
Armed Forces Institute of Pathology
Washington, DC
USA

Sheldon Goldberg MD FACC
Director, Interventional Cardiovascular
    Medicine
Hahnemann University Hospital
Drexel University College of Medicine
Philadelphia, PA
USA

James A Goldstein MD
Director of Cardiovascular Research and
    Education
William Beaumont Hospital
Royal Oak, MI
USA

Isabel Gonçalves MD PhD
Department of Clinical Sciences
Malmö University Hospital
Lund University
Malmö
Sweden

Mario Gössl MD
Division of Cardiovascular Diseases
Mayo Clinic College of Medicine
Rochester, MN
USA

Juan F Granada
The Methodist DeBakey Heart Center
Pearland, TX
USA

Harald C Groen
Biomedical Engineering, Thoraxcenter
Erasmus Medical Center
Rotterdam
The Netherlands

Enrique P Gurfinkel MD PhD
Chief of Coronary Care Unit
Cardiology and Cardiovascular Surgery
    Institute
Buenos Aires
Argentina

David A Halon MB ChB
Lady Davis Carmel Medical Center
Haifa
Israel

Christian W Hamm MD
Department of Cardiology
Kerckhoff Heart Center
Bad Nauheim
Germany

Thomas S Hatsukami
Department of Radiology
University of Washington
Seattle, WA
USA

Anna G ten Have MSc
Biomedical Engineering, Thoraxcenter
Erasmus Medical Center
Rotterdam
The Netherlands

Donald D Heistad MD
Department of Internal Medicine
University of Iowa College of Medicine and
    VA Medical Center
Iowa City, IA
USA

Victoria LM Herrera MD
Molecular Genetics, Whitaker
    Cardiovascular Institute
Section of Molecular Medicine,
    Department of Medicine
Boston University School of Medicine
Boston, MA
USA

Ik-Kyung Jang MD
Massachusetts General Hospital and
    Harvard Medical School
Boston
Massachusetts
USA

Jason L Johnson
Bristol Heart Institute
Bristol Royal Infirmary
Bristol
UK

Isabella Kardys MD
Department of Epidemiology and
    Biostatistics
Erasmus Medical Center
Rotterdam
The Netherlands

William S Kerwin
Department of Radiology
University of Washington
Seattle, WA
USA

Nicholas Kipshidze MD
Lennox Hill Heart and Vascular Institute
New York
USA

Frank D Kolodgie PhD
Department of Cardiovascular Pathology
Armed Forces Institute of Pathology
Washington, DC
USA

Rob Krams
Biomedical Engineering, Thoraxcenter
Erasmus Medical Center
Rotterdam
The Netherlands

Neville Kukreja MRCP
Professor of Interventional Cardiology
Thoraxcenter
Erasmus Medical Center
Rotterdam
The Netherlands

Gregory Lanza
Departments of Medicine and Biomedical
    Engineering
Washington University
St Louis, MO
USA

Tim Leiner
Departments of Pathology and Radiology
University of Maastricht
Maastricht
The Netherlands

Amir Lerman MD
Division of Cardiovascular Diseases
Mayo Clinic College of Medicine
Rochester, MN
USA

Veronica S Lernoud MD
Cardiology and Cardiovascular Surgery
    Institute
Buenos Aires
Argentina

Fei Liu
Department of Radiology
University of Washington
Seattle, WA
USA

Esther Lutgens
Cardiovascular Research Institute
Maastricht
University of Maastricht
Maastricht
The Netherlands

Mohammad Madjid MD
Assistant Professor of Medicine
Department of Internal Medicine/Division of
    Cardiology
School of Medicine
University of Texas – Houston Health
    Science Center
and
Senior Research Scientist
Texas Heart Institute
Houston, TX
USA

Ehtisham Mahmud MD FACC
Division of Cardiovascular Medicine
UCSD Medical Center
San Diego, CA
USA

Elias Mallis MD
Food and Drug Administration
Center for Devices and Radiological Health
Rockville, MD
USA

Barbara J Marshik PhD
Infraredx Inc.
Cambridge, MA
USA

Frits Mastik
Experimental Echocardiography
Erasmus Medical Center
Rotterdam
The Netherlands

Nico Mollet MD
Department of Cardiology and Radiology
Thoraxcenter
Erasmus Medical Center
Rotterdam
The Netherlands

Roxana Mehran MD FACC
Director, Clinical Research and the Data
    Coordinating and Analysis Center
Cardiovascular Research Foundation
New York, NY
USA

Pedro R Moreno MD
Zena and Michael Wiener Cardiovascular
    Institute
Mount Sinai School of Medicine
New York, NY
USA

James E Muller MD
Director of Clinical Research
Co-director of CIMIT Vulnerable Plaque
    Research Program
Massachusetts General Hospital
Harvard Medical School
Boston, MA
USA

James E Muller MD
Director of Clinical Research in Cardiology,
Massachusetts General Hospital
Boston, MA
USA

Jagat Narula MD
UCI Medical Center
Orange, CA
USA

Anne M Neubauer
Department of Biomedical Engineering
Washington University
St Louis, MO
USA

Andrew C Newby
Bristol Heart Institute
Bristol Royal Infirmary
Bristol
UK

Jan Nilsson MD PhD
Professor of Medicine
Department of Clinical Sciences
Malmö University Hospital
Lund University
Malmö
Sweden

Emerson C Perin MD PhD
Department of Adult Cardiology
Texas Heart Institute at St. Luke's
    Episcopal Hospital
Houston, TX
USA

Thomas R Porter
University of Nebraska Medical Center
Section of Cardiology
Department of Internal Medicine
Omaha, NE
USA

Evelyn Regar MD PhD
Department of Cardiology
Thoraxcenter
Erasmus Medical Center
Rotterdam
The Netherlands

Probal Roy MD
Division of Cardiology
Washington Hospital Center
Washington, DC
USA

Tobias Saam
Department of Radiology
University of Washington
Seattle, WA
USA

Johannes A Schaar MD
Experimental Echocardiography
Erasmus Medical Center
Rotterdam
The Netherlands

Alexandru Schiopu MD
Department of Clinical Sciences
Malmö University Hospital
Lund University
Malmö
Sweden

Robert S Schwartz MD FACC
Minneapolis Heart Institute
    and Foundation
Minneapolis, MN
USA

Patrick W Serruys MD PhD
Experimental Echocardiography
Erasmus Medical Center
Rotterdam
The Netherlands

Patrick W Serruys MD PhD
Professor of Interventional Cardiology
Thoraxcenter
Erasmus Medical Center
Rotterdam
The Netherlands

Prediman K Shah MD
Director, Division of Cardiology and
    Atherosclerosis Research Center
Staff Cardiologist
Division of Cardiology
Cedars-Sinai Medical Center
David Geffen School of Medicine, UCLA
Los Angeles, CA
USA

Guilherme V Silva MD
Department of Adult Cardiology
Texas Heart Institute at St. Luke's Episcopal
  Hospital
Houston, TX
USA

Marc Sirol MD PhD
Service de Cardiologie Hôpital Lariboisière
Paris
France

Cornelis J Slager PhD
Biomedical Engineering, Thoraxcenter
Erasmus Medical Center
DR Rotterdam
The Netherlands

Cezar S Staniloae MD
Assistant Professor of Medicine
NY Medical College
and
Director of Cardiovascular Research
Saint Vincent's Hospital
New York
USA

Christodoulos Stefanadis
First Department of Cardiology
Medical School of Athens University
Hippokration Hospital
Athens
Greece

Robert-Jan Van Suylen
Cardiovascular Research Institute Maastricht
University of Maastricht
Maastricht
The Netherlands

Norihide Takaya
Department of Radiology
University of Washington
Seattle, WA
USA

Geoffrey H Tofler MD
Professor of Preventive Cardiology
Cardiology Department
Royal North Shore Hospital
St Leonards, NSW
Australia

Konstantinos Toutouzas
First Department of Cardiology
Medical School of Athens University
Hippokration Hospital
Athens
Greece

Sotirios Tsimikas MD
Division of Cardiovascular Diseases
Department of Medicine
UCSD Cardiology La Jolla
Perlman Ambulatory Center
La Jolla, CA
USA

Hunter R Underhill
Department of Radiology
University of Washington
Seattle, WA
USA

Anton FW van der Steen PhD
Experimental Echocardiography
Erasmus Medical Center
Rotterdam
The Netherlands

Anton FW van der Steen
Biomedical Engineering, Thoraxcenter
Erasmus Medical Center
Rotterdam
The Netherlands

Juan F Viles-Gonzalez MD
Cardiovascular Institute
Mount Sinai School of Medicine
New York, NY
USA

Renu Virmani MD
Department of Cardiovascular Pathology
Armed Forces Institute of Pathology
Washington, DC
USA

Ron Waksman MD
Division of Cardiology
Washington Hospital Center
Washington, DC
USA

Jan David Wald PhD
AG Edwards & Sons, Inc.
St Louis, MO
USA

Michael Weber
Department of Cardiology
Kerckhoff Heart Center
Bad Nauheim
Germany

WB Weijboom
Department of Cardiology and Radiology
Thoraxcenter
Erasmus Medical Center
Rotterdam
The Netherlands

Jolanda J Wentzel PhD
Biomedical Engineering, Thoraxcenter
Erasmus Medical Center
Rotterdam
The Netherlands

Jolanda J Wentzel PhD
Biomedical Engineering, Thoraxcenter
Erasmus Medical Center
DR Rotterdam
The Netherlands

A Weustink
Department of Cardiology and Radiology
Thoraxcenter
Erasmus Medical Center
Rotterdam
The Netherlands

Samuel A Wickline
Departments of Medicine and Biomedical
    Engineering
Washington University
St Louis, MO
USA

Robert L Wilensky MD
Hospital of the University of Pennsylvania
Philadelphia, PA
USA

James T Willerson MD
Department of Adult Cardiology
Texas Heart Institute at St. Luke's
    Episcopal Hospital
Houston, TX
USA

Patrick Winter
Department of Medicine
Washington University
St Louis, MO
USA

Jacqueline CM Witteman PhD
Department of Epidemiology and
    Biostatistics
Erasmus Medical Center
Rotterdam
The Netherlands

Feng Xie
University of Nebraska Medical Center
Section of Cardiology
Department of Internal Medicine
Omaha, NE
USA

Dongxiang Xu
Department of Radiology
University of Washington
Seattle, WA
USA

Vasily L Yarnykh
Department of Radiology
University of Washington
Seattle, WA
USA

Chun Yuan
Department of Radiology
University of Washington
Seattle, WA
USA

Foreword

Although pathologic evidence for coronary thrombosis as a manifestation of coronary artery disease was recognized in the mid-nineteenth century, debate about its pathogenetic role in myocardial infarction persisted well into the 1970s. One group held that a coronary thrombus on a markedly narrowed vessel was the *coup de grace* responsible for myocardial infarction and/or sudden cardiac death. Others argued that the thrombus was not the cause but rather the result of myocardial infarction.

A paradigm shift occurred in the mid-seventies, when it was observed that after successful coronary fibrinolytic therapy of acute myocardial infarction, the culprit artery usually showed only mild to moderate obstruction rather than the critical obstruction that was expected. This was followed in the early eighties by observations that patients who had coronary angiograms before and after myocardial infarction usually showed only mild or moderate obstruction in the culprit artery before the event and total occlusion, presumably secondary to the thrombus, afterwards. Pathologists, always the final arbiters of such disputes, pointed out that at post mortem examination, thrombotic occlusion usually occurred on ruptured, thin walled or eroded plaques. By the late eighties, the cardiovascular community agreed that acute coronary syndromes resulted from thrombotic obstruction of such plaques, named *vulnerable plaques* by Muller et al, in 1989.

The term caught on and spread like wildfire. Cardiovascular investigators – immunologists, platelet biologists, pathologists, lipidologists, imagers, interventionalists, clinical trialists, and epidemiologists all focused attention on such plaques as the cause of one of mankind's most frequent life-threatening conditions. Since then, research on these plaques has grown exponentially.

This second edition of *The Vulnerable Plaque* builds on the first edition and provides an excellent summary of this important field. It is well written and illustrated. The editors and authors are authoritative contributors to the subject. The book is both broad and deep and displays how much progress has been made on the pathologic characteristics of these plaques, the use of biomarkers in diagnosis and risk stratification, both invasive and non-invasive imaging, as well as developing modes of local and systemic therapy.

There is now a large army of basic and clinical investigators in this field. All will benefit from this elegant presentation of research on the vulnerable plaque, as will clinicians, imagers, interventionalists and their trainees, who are now or soon will be responsible for the care of the millions of patients with acute coronary syndromes.

Eugene Braunwald
Boston, MA

Preface

It has been three years since our first edition of the *Handbook of the Vulnerable Plaque* and yet in 2007 atherosclerotic cardiovascular disease continues to account for nearly 20 million deaths annually, and coronary heart disease accounts for the majority of this toll. It is well known that the rupture of vulnerable plaque is responsible for most coronary events; while inflammation has also been recognized as playing a major role in plaque disruption. These insights have helped us to move beyond the stress test and coronary angiogram when attempting to diagnose and treat vulnerable/high-risk plaques. New diagnostic methods for the assessment of plaque are becoming available, especially in the areas of blood sampling, noninvasive imaging, and intracoronary diagnostic devices. Research is also being conducted on multiple invasive coronary artery diagnostic devices to improve plaque characterization. These methods include intravascular MRI, near infrared spectroscopy, nuclear methods, optical coherence tomography, palpography, thermography, and molecular strategies to target delivery of imaging and therapeutic agents. Novel therapeutic approaches are emerging as well, creating the hope that these new agents, which can raise high-density lipoprotein or reduce inflammation, offer additional promise for improved systemic treatment of vulnerable plaques.

The recognition of the vulnerability of plaques as a major cause for heart attacks and sudden cardiac death has been established; yet over the past three years the vulnerable plaque field has evolved and advanced in the understanding of the pathophysiology, mechanisms, and diagnosis of the disease. These advances, together with the understanding of the role of vulnerable plaque in the causation of coronary events, have mandated this second edition of *The Vulnerable Plaque*. As the field has progressed so has this book. It is no longer a handbook, but a comprehensive, inclusive textbook with the latest developments in the field. This second edition provides new insights into the vulnerable plaque world — including mechanism and pathological findings with an emphasis on diagnostic tools such as biomarkers and noninvasive imaging, and new invasive imaging modalities, some of which have recently completed the first round of clinical testing.

Further, as natural history observational studies are being conducted, interventional cardiologists will find in this book the information it takes to understand the state of the field and the potential diagnostic and therapeutic modalities available to identify and treat the vulnerable patient. Included is information on drug-eluting stents, photodynamic therapy, and systemic therapy beyond statins, including cell therapy. Scientists and vascular biologists will find the latest information on genetics, immunology, and molecular biology.

It our hope that this book will provide insight into the progress made in the field, diagnostic capabilities, and new therapeutic approaches regarding the vulnerable plaque. When discussing the topic of vulnerable plaque with colleagues, it has been said that advances in these areas will create the opportunity for progress against acute coronary events. It is imperative that the medical community embrace these advances so that the new knowledge gained can be rapidly translated into the 'real world' care of our patients.

Ron Waksman, Patrick W Serruys
and Johannes Schaar

Acknowledgments

The editors wish to thank the contributing authors for their hard work and dedication. Recognized and respected worldwide for their work with vulnerable plaque, each has made a tremendous effort in helping to bring this book to fruition. Many thanks also to Mr Oliver Walter, our development editor at Informa Healthcare, and to Ms Kathryn Coons, our medical editor at Medstar Research Institute at Washington Hospital Center for their logistical and editing assistance throughout this endeavor.

SECTION I

Background epidemiology and pathology

Definition and terminology of the vulnerable plaque

1

James E Muller, Pedro R Moreno, and Pavan K Cheruvu

INTRODUCTION

Four years ago, when the first edition of this handbook on this novel topic was still being formulated, there was considerable controversy over the meaning of the term 'vulnerable plaque'. Fortunately, there is now widespread agreement on the definition of 'plaque vulnerability' and related terms.

This strong consensus on terminology was expressed in two reports published in 2003. The first appeared in the *European Heart Journal* and presented the opinions of a group of 12 investigators who attended a meeting on vulnerable plaque in Santorini, Greece.[1] The second publication, appeared as a 'Current Perspectives' report in *Circulation*, and presented the thoughts of 57 investigators active in the field.[2]

Both publications recommended that the term 'vulnerable plaque' be used to identify all *thrombosis-prone plaques that have a high probability of undergoing rapid progression*. It was noted that the terms 'vulnerable plaque', 'thrombosis-prone plaque', and 'high-risk plaque' can be used interchangeably.

In addition to this agreement on the functional definition of plaque vulnerability cited above, it was noted in both publications that there are different histologic types of plaques that are suspected to be vulnerable. These include an inflamed, thin-cap fibroatheroma (the type thought to be most common), a proteoglycan-rich site prone to erosion, and a calcified nodule.[1-3] Plaques with these features can be considered to be 'indicted but not yet convicted' suspects to be vulnerable plaques. Proof that such plaques are vulnerable will require prospective studies in which the suspected plaques are identified in advance, and follow-up studies document that they have a high-risk of progressing and thereby causing a cardiac event.

The Current Perspective article in *Circulation* also notes that 'vulnerable blood' and 'vulnerable myocardium' may contribute to the occurrence of a cardiac event. Construction of a 'vulnerability index', which would reflect the contributions of all types of vulnerability, was advocated as a means of identifying the 'vulnerable patient'.[2]

The agreement on general terminology is a welcome development which will assist the conduct of more detailed studies of the determinants, diagnosis, and treatment of vulnerability at all levels.

HISTORY OF THE RECOGNITION OF PLAQUE VULNERABILITY

Plaque rupture

In 1966, Dr Paris Constantinides provided the first convincing evidence that plaque rupture was the cause of onset of most acute cardiovascular disease.[4] Prior to his work, several authors had proposed that coronary thrombosis was caused by breaks in the atheroma surface, but data supporting such a mechanism were limited.[5-7]

Dr Constantinides examined the coronary arteries of 22 patients with coronary artery disease, 17 of whom had acute coronary thrombosis. In order to avoid missing a site of rupture, he studied a total of more than 40000 histologic sections, covering the entire segment of each artery containing a thrombus. All 17 of the acute thrombi were found to originate over cracks in the intimal surface of the plaque, confirming the hypothesis he had formulated based on the pre-existing literature, and his prior animal studies. This observation has been confirmed by many investigators, through data derived from autopsy studies, surgical exposure, angiography, and angioscopy, and is the basis of modern understanding of the atherosclerotic substrate causing thrombus formation in the arterial circulation.

Regional factors affecting the outcome of plaque rupture

In the decades since the work of Constantides, much has been learned about the multiple factors that influence the thrombotic process at the site of a ruptured atherosclerotic plaque. Whether a particular plaque rupture leads to an occlusive thrombus or causes only a mural thrombus is determined by a complex balance of factors in an individual patient.

In 1984 (and in a series of subsequent studies), Willerson et al advanced the concept that conversion of chronic to acute coronary disease occurs when such an anatomically altered plaque becomes a stimulus for platelet adhesion, aggregation, and mediator accumulation.[8] Studies have now documented that thromboxane A_2, tissue factor, and other mediators are generated, which may cause subsequent thrombosis and vasoconstriction.[9-11] The animal model of cyclic coronary artery flow reductions developed by Folts has been particularly useful in studying such mediators and their inhibitors.[12-14]

In addition, cellular responses can exacerbate a coronary artery flow limitation. Endothelial cells are the first cells to be damaged by high shear stress or serum factors (for example, oxidized cholesterol, chemical irritants, or catecholamines).

A dysfunctional endothelium cannot maintain its normal antithrombotic and vasodilatory properties. In addition, macrophages that reside in the plaque core are thought to secrete thrombogenic substances. Supporting this idea, a study of coronary atherectomy specimens in patients with unstable angina demonstrated co-localization of lipid-laden macrophages and tissue factor (TF).[15]

The multitude of local mediators, cellular elements, and plaque features influencing the outcome of plaque rupture (of which only a small sampling are reviewed here) explain why rupture of a vulnerable plaque may not lead to a clinical event, and complicate studies designed to test the linkage of plaque vulnerability to clinical outcomes.

DEFINITIONS OF PLAQUE VULNERABILITY

A functional definition

By 1994, there was widespread recognition of the importance of plaque rupture, thrombosis, and mediator generation in the onset of cardiovascular disease. On the basis of this knowledge, our studies on triggering of disease onset led us to propose that the term 'vulnerable' be used to describe a plaque that had a high likelihood of becoming disrupted and thereby starting an adverse cascade resulting in thrombosis.[13] This is an uncomplicated functional definition that does not (i) depend on the histologic features of the plaque and (ii) does not indicate how such a plaque might be identified prospectively, or stabilized before it caused the onset of disease.

A histologic definition

Following the introduction of the functional definition above, evidence continued to accumulate suggesting, but not proving, that plaques with a large necrotic core, thin cap, and inflammatory cell infiltrate were vulnerable plaques. Such plaques can be described as inflamed thin-cap fibroatheromas (TCFAs).[14–26] When Burke et al analyzed a morphometric series of 41 ruptured plaques in 113 men with coronary artery disease who died suddenly, they determined that 95% of ruptured caps measured less than 64 μm in thickness.[27] This finding led to widespread acceptance of cap thickness less than 65 μm as likely to be a sign of vulnerability. In addition, there is abundant evidence linking inflammation to vulnerability from autopsy studies, and studies in experimental animals. In recent years additional TCFA features have been associated with vulnerability, such as increased matrix metalloproteinase (MMP) activity, expansive remodeling, neovascularization, and hemorrhage.

Whereas inflamed TCFAs are strongly suspected of representing vulnerable plaques, there are, as yet, no replicated prospective studies proving that they are at increased risk of leading to thrombosis and lesion progression. However, just as an examination of the wreckage can yield information about an airplane's malfunction prior to a crash, the extensive pathologic studies have made it possible to describe the likely histologic features of the plaque prior to disruption. They strongly suggest that an inflamed TCFA is likely to be a vulnerable plaque, but proof is not yet available.

Not all inflamed TCFAs will cause acute coronary events. First, not all will rupture. It is known that plaques with a large necrotic core, thin cap, and increased inflammatory cell infiltrate, which are not ruptured, can be found at autopsy.[24,26] In addition, rupture may be asymptomatic or produce only stable angina.

There are additional types of plaque suspected to be vulnerable. Recent pathologic studies have revealed that a number of plaques causing thrombosis – and hence proved to have been vulnerable – were not TCFAs. Farb et al analyzed plaque

characteristics in 50 subjects with sudden cardiac death due to coronary thrombosis.[22] In 22 of the cases (44%) the thrombosis occurred at a site with erosion which did not occur over a thin cap and lipid pool. The plaque appeared to have large regions of denuded endothelium, where the underlying intima consisted primarily of smooth muscle cells (SMCs) and an increased proteoglycan content, and minimal evidence of inflammation. Hence, a non-inflamed plaque rich in proteoglycans might be a second histologic type of vulnerable or high-risk plaque. The process by which such a plaque causes thrombosis has been termed 'erosion'.

Furthermore, a calcified nodule has been identified as a potentially vulnerable plaque. In an autopsy study, Virmani et al discovered arterial thrombus at sites where the fibrous cap was interrupted by dense, eruptive calcium granules. More detailed description of this lesion type is limited at this time because of its rarity (<5% prevalence).

A prospective definition

The most useful definition of a vulnerable plaque is one that can be applied prospectively to individual lesions. Whereas routine coronary angiograms are often used to make inferences about plaque vulnerability, as recently noted by Little and Applegate, 'The shadows leave a doubt'.[28] In a 2005 review of non-invasive and invasive strategies, Fayad and Fuster stated that no method available at that time accurately identified plaques prone to rupture and thrombosis.[29] With the possible exception of angioscopy (see below), the situation remains the same in 2006. However, there is reason to believe that one, or more, of a broad array of new technologies will make it possible to identify vulnerable plaques prospectively in the coronary arteries of living patients.

In a study that has received much less attention than it deserves, Uchida and colleagues reported that angioscopy could identify vulnerable plaques prospectively in living patients.[30] A prospective angioscopic survey was done of all three coronary arteries of 157 patients with angina. Thirteen of these patients had a glistening yellow plaque, shown in a separate autopsy series to represent a lipid pool with a very thin cap. During a 1-year follow-up, 68% of the patients with the vulnerable glistening yellow plaque experienced an acute coronary syndrome; only 4% of those without such a plaque experienced an event.

This study, when replicated in a larger group, is likely to permit a vulnerable plaque to be defined prospectively as a glistening yellow plaque identified by angioscopy. While such an achievement is valuable for research purposes, it is unlikely to have clinical utility. Angioscopy requires coronary artery occlusion, the identification of a 'glistening yellow' appearance is subjective, and angioscopy would not be expected to identify the vulnerable plaques discussed above, which are not associated with a lipid pool and a thin fibrous cap.

While non-invasive detection of vulnerable coronary plaques must be the ultimate goal, such approaches face formidable obstacles of coronary artery motion, small size, and central location. Promising results have been obtained with MRA (magnetic resonance angiography) detection of presumably vulnerable plaques in the aorta and carotid arteries, which are larger and less mobile than the coronary arteries.[31,32] Black-blood MRA has been successfully employed to evaluate plaque burden in vivo, but evaluating plaque composition – necessary for vulnerable plaque detection – has not been possible.[29] In addition, long MR acquisition times will hinder clinical acceptance of the technology in the near future. Contrast-enhanced multidetector computed tomography (MDCT) has also been used to differentiate plaque components but presently suffers from limited contrast between signals from lipid and fibrotic tissue, spatial resolution issues, the need for beta-blockers to minimize cardiac motion, and the risk of contrast-induced nephropathy.[29]

It is likely that the initial prospective identification of vulnerable coronary plaques will first be achieved by one of several competing intracoronary technologies applied to patients already undergoing an intervention. In addition to angioscopy, diffuse reflectance near-infrared spectroscopy, Raman near-infrared spectroscopy, optical coherence tomography, thermography, intracoronary magnetic resonance imaging (MRI), intracoronary ultrasound, and quantitative angiography are all being advocated for vulnerable plaque detection.[33–41] Prospective clinical trials will identify the optimal intracoronary method, or methods, that will aid the subsequent development of non-invasive means of detection of vulnerable coronary plaques.

For each technique (invasive, and subsequently non-invasive) to be evaluated, prospective identification should start with mapping of the three main coronary arteries for the features the technique can detect. A group of approximately 1000 patients followed prospectively for 1 year would produce a number of coronary events (unstable angina, myocardial infarction, and sudden cardiac death) in which the plaque proved to be vulnerable could be localized by angiography or autopsy examination. Repeat angiography at 1 year in all patients could also identify plaques that showed major progression, but did not cause an event. Such rapid increases in stenosis have been shown to result from plaque rupture and thrombosis.

A combination of criteria for vulnerability that included clinical events and angiographic progression may provide sufficient statistical power for prospective analysis. If such a study validated the hypothesis that a certain signature of a plaque predicted a negative outcome, a great advance in the diagnostic capability of the catheterization laboratory would be achieved. By examining the baseline characteristics of coronary plaques that met the criteria for vulnerability, cardiologists would be able to identify vulnerable plaques in advance, a major challenge for contemporary medicine. It is likely that varying signatures would be associated with varying degrees of risk, i.e. plaques that appear softer by palpography, or more extreme spectroscopic score would be more vulnerable.

From such a study, the following prospective definition of a vulnerable plaque could then be formulated: a plaque, identified prospectively (by the technology tested), that is documented to have a high likelihood of forming a thrombogenic focus. The thrombus could produce immediate disease onset, or rapid, asymptomatic, angiographic progression. On the other hand, a plaque with a low likelihood of causing such an outcome would be termed 'non-vulnerable'.

Nonetheless, as discussed above, at the present time three histologic subtypes of plaque suspected to be vulnerable have been identified:

- a thin-capped fibroatheroma
- plaques with increased proteoglycan content leading to erosion and thrombosis
- a plaque with a calcified nodule.

Prospective studies are needed to confirm these hypotheses.

TREATMENT OF VULNERABLE PLAQUES

The ability to measure plaque vulnerability would open a vast field of study of plaque stabilization therapy.[42] Systemic pharmacologic approaches that have been advocated include intense lipid-lowering, HDL (high-density lipoprotein) raising agents, MMP inhibitors, ACE (angiotensin-converting enzyme) inhibitors, anti-inflammatory agents, and vaccination.[43–50] Local, intracoronary therapies that might stabilize vulnerable plaques include stenting of lesions with less than critical stenosis, radiation therapy, photodynamic therapy, cryotherapy, gene therapy, angioplasty, or coronary stenting to induce fibrosis.[51–55] Randomized trials are needed to evaluate the benefit and risk of such treatments.

DISRUPTED PLAQUES

The term 'disrupted' has been used in some cases to refer to a plaque that causes some degree of thrombosis, but in other cases to describe the nature of the lesion. As is clear from the prior discussion, in some cases thrombosis may result from rupture of a thin cap covering a lipid pool, while in others it may be caused by erosion of the surface of a plaque rich in proteoglycans, or one having a less distinctive histologic appearance. In any case, the plaque proved itself to have been vulnerable by its transformation into a 'thrombosed plaque'.

It seems best to avoid the use of the word 'disrupted' and refer instead to 'thrombosed plaques', the meaning of which is less ambiguous. The transition would then be from a vulnerable/high-risk/thrombosis-prone plaque to a 'thrombosed plaque'. Since plaques that have recently ruptured and thrombosed are suspected to be at high risk for growth of thrombus (in the absence of antithrombotic therapy), a thrombosed plaque could also be considered to be yet another form of 'vulnerable' plaque.

UNSTABLE PLAQUES

The term 'unstable' has received highly variable usage. In some cases, it has been used to describe vulnerable plaques, and in others to refer to disrupted plaques, as defined above. A symposium has been dedicated to the topic of 'potentially unstable plaques'. Because the term also has well-accepted clinical usage to describe unstable angina pectoris, confusion between the clinical syndrome and the plaque under discussion is inevitable. Given the difficulties with the term, and the adequacy of the terms 'vulnerable' and 'thrombosed plaque', we propose that the term 'unstable' be reserved for the clinical syndrome and not applied to the plaque.

RELATION TO THE AHA CLASSIFICATION OF ATHEROSCLEROTIC LESIONS

The usage of the terms 'vulnerable/high-risk plaque' and 'thrombosed plaque' proposed above complements the AHA (American Heart Association) classification of atherosclerotic lesions.[56,57] The AHA classification, which is based on histologic features rather than functional significance, divides plaques into six types with increasing complexity: type I (initial changes); type II (fatty streak); type III (pre-atheroma); type IV (atheroma); type V (fibroatheroma); and type VI (complicated plaque).

The relation of thrombosed plaques with this classification is quite simple – all thrombosed lesions would be included in type VI as complicated lesions. Differences between functional and histologic definitions are more marked for the vulnerable/high-risk plaque, because, as noted by the AHA committee, thrombosis may result from any of the six histologic types. In the extreme case, thrombosis may even occur due to endothelial dysfunction at a site with no detectable histologic abnormality. However, most vulnerable/high-risk plaques will exhibit a type IV (atheroma) or type V (fibroatheroma) histologic appearance. The advent of a prospective means of quantitating vulnerability will make it possible to assign vulnerability scores to the different AHA classification types.

Virmani et al have noted several deficiencies of the AHA histologic classification and proposed alternative categories.[58] Alteration of histologic categories would not affect the usage of 'vulnerable/high-risk plaque' and 'thrombosed plaque' proposed above.

FREQUENCY OF SUSPECTED VULNERABLE/HIGH-RISK PLAQUES IN INDIVIDUAL PATIENTS

There are several obstacles to answering the seemingly simple question of the frequency of vulnerable plaques in individual patients. While clinical events indicate how many vulnerable plaques might cause symptoms in a given group of patients – for instance, a 10% annual rate of cardiac events in a population of patients post stenting would signify that, at the least, 10% of the patients had one vulnerable plaque – as discussed above, the frequency of vulnerable plaques (thrombosi-prone) is higher than the event rate because not all vulnerable plaques thrombose and not all thromboses lead to symptoms. Even with a complete occlusion due to thrombosis, some patients may have collateral vessels that can provide an alternative source of blood flow. In other patients, the thrombosis may not be occlusive, and the residual flow may be sufficient to meet the needs of the myocardium downstream.

An additional obstacle to determining frequency of vulnerable plaques, or even thrombosed plaques, has been the lack of a method to easily identify either type of plaque in patients.

Finally, since, as stated earlier, there are no replicated prospective studies clearly establishing that any particular histologic type of plaque is indeed a vulnerable plaque, it is not possible, without the use of simplifying assumptions, to identify the frequency of vulnerable plaque. Efforts therefore shift to determination of the frequency of an inflamed TCFA, which is a suspected, but not proven, vulnerable plaque.

While autopsy-based studies have a certain selection bias, the best evidence about the frequency of various histologic types of plaques comes from postmortem specimens. It is, of course, easier to determine the incidence of thrombosed plaques, than vulnerable plaques. Falk identified 103 ruptured plaques in 47 patients dying from coronary atherosclerosis preceded by chest pain.[58] Forty of these were associated with occlusive thrombosis. The remaining 63 ruptured sites were associated with grossly discernible intimal hemorrhage without occlusive thrombosis but with a tiny mural thrombus sealing the ruptured site.[59] Davies and Thomas identified 115 thrombotic segments in 74 patients dying from sudden cardiac death. Of note, intraluminal thrombus was also found in eight out of 79 control patients dying from non-cardiac causes.[60] In addition, Frink identified 211 ruptured plaques in 83 patients dying from acute coronary events.[61] This number included many sites of chronic rupture, which no longer demonstrated any sign of intraluminal thrombosis. This supports the concept of atherosclerosis as a multifocal process in which multiple vulnerable plaques can develop and thrombose, with only a subset of thromboses leading to clinical events.[61]

Although the visualization of ruptured plaques in patients is not an easy task, intravascular ultrasound (IVUS) has provided some information about their frequency in patients with acute coronary events. Rioufol et al reported on IVUS evidence of ruptured plaques obtained in 24 patients with acute coronary events.[62] Many ruptured plaques (41/50) were identified at sites other than the site responsible for the clinical event. These additional ruptured lesions were less stenotic and less calcified than the culprit lesions.[62]

Angioscopy, which is more difficult to perform than IVUS but provides better information about endoluminal structures, has also been used to identify thrombosed plaques. Asakura et al performed three-vessel coronary angioscopy in 20 patients 1 month after acute myocardial infarction. The incidence of coronary thrombosis, as might be expected, was 81% on lesions responsible for the event.[63] In addition, 2% of lesions not associated with the clinical event also showed evidence of thrombosis.[63] This occurred despite the likelihood that such post-myocardial infarction patients were receiving antithrombotic therapy.

The deficiencies in information about the number of thrombosed plaques are minor compared with problems of identifying the number of vulnerable/high-risk plaques for the reasons stated above. If the assumption is made that an inflamed TCFA is a vulnerable plaque, some information is available.

Postmortem studies were performed by Burke et al in 113 individuals who died suddenly of severe coronary artery disease.[27] They identified an average of 1.2 TCFA per patient. TCFAs were more frequently found in white, hypercholesterolemic men and correlated directly with levels of blood cholesterol. Similar findings were found in women by the same group of investigators.[64]

Precise quantitation of the frequency of TCFAs in living patients is difficult due to limitations of the technology that is currently available. For instance, few instruments have the capability of determining that a cap is less than 65 µm in thickness. However, yellow appearance of a plaque has been taken as presumptive evidence of a thin cap covering a lipid pool. Asakura et al identified yellow plaques as a rather common angioscopic finding in living patients after acute myocardial infarction.[63] Yellow plaques were equally prevalent in the infarct-related and non-infarct-related coronary arteries (3.7 ± 1.6 and 3.4 ± 1.8 plaques/artery, respectively). However, detailed pathologic studies have found that yellow plaques often have a fibrous cap thickness greater than 65 μm and hence would not qualify as TCFAs.[20]

In the study cited earlier, Uchida et al[30] have reported that glistening yellow plaques have an average fibrous cap thickness of only 10 μm and hence could be considered to be TCFAs. Uchida identified 118 white and 39 yellow plaques in 186 consecutive patients with stable angina who underwent three-vessel angioscopy. Of the 39 yellow plaques identified, 13 were glistening and 26 non-glistening. Hence in this carefully studied group of patients with stable angina pectoris, there were 13 (7%) presumed TCFAs.

In the following chapters, many techniques are described that will provide improved characterization of plaques in living patients. Studies conducted with these new instruments will provide much better information about the incidence of vulnerable and thrombosed plaques than is currently available.

SUMMARY

A widespread consensus reached in 2003 now supports the definition of a 'vulnerable plaque' as one that has a high likelihood of becoming disrupted and thereby causing thrombosis, which in turn may lead to asymptomatic lesion progression or a clinical event. The terms 'high-risk' and 'thrombosis-prone' can also be used as synonyms for 'vulnerable plaque.'

While the histologic features of vulnerable plaques are not yet proven in a prospective study, it is widely suspected that inflamed TCFAs, proteoglycan-rich areas, and calcified nodules are three types of vulnerable plaque.

There is abundant evidence that more that one vulnerable plaque may be present in an individual patient, but the number is usually less than five, and hence local therapy remains an option.

In his classic 1966 publication, Dr Constantinides noted that 'it would appear rewarding to search not only for changes in the blood favouring coagulation, but also for factors increasing the fragility – or provoking the fracture – of atheroma surfaces in human victims of coronary thrombosis'.[4] A standardized nomenclature and novel devices are now aiding the efforts to find and treat such fragile plaques before they cause their catastrophic consequences.

REFERENCES

1. Schaar JA, Muller JE, Falk E et al. Terminology for high-risk and vulnerable coronary artery plaques. Eur Heart J 2004; 25:1077–82.
2. Naghavi M, Libby P, Falk E et al. From vulnerable plaque to vulnerable patient: a call for new definitions and risk assessment strategies: Part I. Circulation 2003; 108:1664–72.
3. Virmani R, Burke AP, Kolodgie FD, Farb A. Pathology of the thin-cap fibroatheroma: a type of vulnerable plaque. J Interv Cardiol 2003; 16:267–72.
4. Constantinides P. Plaque fissures in human coronary thrombosis. J Atheroscler Res 1966; 6:1–17.
5. Koch LKaW. Uber die Formen des Coronarerschlusses, die Anderungen im Coronarkreislauf und die Beziehungen zur Angina Pectoris. Alleg Pathol 1932; 90:21–84.
6. Drury R. The role of initmal haemorrhage in coronary occlusion. J Pathol Bacteriol 1954; 67:207–15.
7. Leary T. Atherosclerosis; special consideration of aortic lesions. Arch Pathol 1936; 21:419–52.
8. Willerson JT, Campbell WB, Winniford MD et al. Conversion from chronic to acute coronary artery disease: speculation regarding mechanisms. Am J Cardiol 1984; 54:1349–54.
9. Willerson JT, Hillis LD, Winniford M, Buja LM. Speculation regarding mechanisms responsible for acute ischemic heart disease syndromes. J Am Coll Cardiol 1986; 8:245–50.
10. Willerson JT, Golino P, Eidt J, Campbell WB, Buja LM. Specific platelet mediators and unstable coronary artery lesions. Experimental evidence and potential clinical implications. Circulation 1989; 80:198–205.
11. Willerson JT. Stable angina pectoris: recent advances in predicting prognosis and treatment. Adv Intern Med 1998; 43:175–202.
12. Maalej N, Folts JD. Increased shear stress overcomes the antithrombotic platelet inhibitory effect of aspirin in stenosed dog coronary arteries. Circulation 1996; 93:1201–5.
13. Muller JE, Abela GS, Nesto RW, Tofler GH. Triggers, acute risk factors and vulnerable plaques: the lexicon of a new frontier. J Am Coll Cardiol 1994; 23:809–13.

14. Kolodgie FD, Burke AP, Farb A et al. The thin-cap fibroatheroma: a type of vulnerable plaque: the major precursor lesion to acute coronary syndromes. Curr Opin Cardiol 2001; 16:285–92.

15. Moreno PR, Bernardi VH, Lopez-Cuellar J et al. Macrophages, smooth muscle cells, and tissue factor in unstable angina: implications for cell-mediated thrombogenicity in acute coronary syndromes. Circulation 1996; 94:3090–7.

16. Farb A, Tang AL, Burke AP et al. Sudden coronary death. Frequency of active coronary lesions, inactive coronary lesions, and myocardial infarction. Circulation 1995; 92:1701–9.

17. Davies MJ. Detecting vulnerable coronary plaques. Lancet 1996; 347:1422–3.

18. Moreno PR, Falk E, Palacios IF et al. Macrophage infiltration in acute coronary syndromes. Implications for plaque rupture. Circulation 1994; 90:775–8.

19. Falk E, Shah PK, Fuster V. Coronary plaque disruption. Circulation 1995; 92:657–71.

20. Libby P. Molecular bases of the acute coronary syndromes. Circulation 1995; 91:2844–50.

21. Davies MJ. Acute coronary thrombosis – the role of plaque disruption and its initiation and prevention. Eur Heart J 1995; 16 (Suppl L):3–7.

22. Farb A, Burke AP, Tang AL et al. Coronary plaque erosion without rupture into a lipid core. A frequent cause of coronary thrombosis in sudden coronary death. Circulation 1996; 93:1354–63.

23. Burke AP, Farb A, Malcom GT et al. Plaque rupture and sudden death related to exertion in men with coronary artery disease. JAMA 1999; 281:921–6.

24. Pasterkamp G, Schoneveld AH, van der Wal AC et al. Inflammation of the atherosclerotic cap and shoulder of the plaque is a common and locally observed feature in unruptured plaques of femoral and coronary arteries. Arterioscler Thromb Vasc Biol 1999; 19:54–8.

25. Shah PK, Falk E, Badimon JJ et al. Human monocyte-derived macrophages induce collagen breakdown in fibrous caps of atherosclerotic plaques. Potential role of matrix-degrading metalloproteinases and implications for plaque rupture. Circulation 1995; 92:1565–9.

26. van der Wal AC, Becker AE, Koch KT et al. Clinically stable angina pectoris is not necessarily associated with histologically stable atherosclerotic plaques. Heart 1996; 76:312–16.

27. Burke AP, Farb A, Malcom GT et al. Coronary risk factors and plaque morphology in men with coronary disease who died suddenly. N Engl J Med 1997; 336:1276–82.

28. Little WC, Applegate RJ. The shadows leave a doubt – the angiographic recognition of vulnerable coronary artery plaques. J Am Coll Cardiol 1999; 33:1362–4.

29. Kullo IJ, Edwards WD, Schwartz RS. Vulnerable plaque: pathobiology and clinical implications. Ann Intern Med 1998; 129:1050–60.

29. Fuster VF, Fayad ZA, Moreno PR et al. Atherothrombosis and high-risk plaque: Part II: approaches by noninvasive computed tomographic/magnetic resonance imaging. J Am Coll Cardiol 2005; 46:1209–18.

30. Uchida Y, Nakamura F, Tomaru T et al. Prediction of acute coronary syndromes by percutaneous coronary angioscopy in patients with stable angina. Am Heart J 1995; 130:195–203.

31. Fuster V. Mechanisms of arterial thrombosis: foundation for therapy. Am Heart J 1998; 135:S361–6.

32. Toussaint JF, Pachot-Clouard M, Bridal SL, Gouya H, Berger G. Non-invasive imaging of atherosclerosis by MRI and ultrasonography. Arch Mal Coeur Vaiss 1999; 92:349–54.

33. Cassis LA, Lodder RA. Near-IR imaging of atheromas in living arterial tissue. Anal Chem 1993; 65:1247–56.

34. Dempsey RJ, Cassis LA, Davis DG, Lodder RA. Near-infrared imaging and spectroscopy in stroke research: lipoprotein distribution and disease. Ann NY Acad Sci 1997; 820:149–69.

35. Moreno PR, Lodder RA, Purushothaman KR et al. Detection of lipid pool, thin fibrous cap and inflammatory cell infiltration in human aortic atherosclerotic plaques by near infrared spectroscopy. Circulation 2002; 105:923–7.

36. Moreno PR, Lodder R, O'Connor WN et al. Characterization of vulnerable plaques by near-infrared spectroscopy in an atherosclerotic rabbit model. J Am Coll Cardiol 1999; 33:66A.

37. Moreno PR, Eric Ryan S, Hopkins D et al. Identification of lipid-rich plaques in human coronary artery autopsy specimens by near-infrared spectroscopy. J Am Coll Cardiol 2001; 37:1219–90.

38. Brennan JF III, Romer TJ, Lees RS et al. Determination of human coronary artery composition by Raman spectroscopy. Circulation 1997; 96:99–105.

39. Brezinski ME, Tearney GJ, Weissman NJ et al. Assessing atherosclerotic plaque morphology: comparison of optical coherence tomography and high frequency intravascular ultrasound. Heart 1997; 77:397–403.

40. Casscells W, Hathorn B, David M et al. Thermal detection of cellular infiltrates in living atherosclerotic plaques: possible implications for plaque rupture and thrombosis. Lancet 1996; 347:1447–51.

41. Stefanadis C, Diamantopoulos L, Vlachopoulos C et al. Thermal heterogeneity within human atherosclerotic coronary arteries detected in vivo: a new method of detection by application of a special thermography catheter. Circulation 1999; 99:1965–71.

42. Moreno PR, Shah PK, Falk E. Triggering of acute coronary syndromes – implications for prevention. In: Determinants of Rupture of Atherosclerotic Coronary Lesions. The Netherlands: Kluwer Academic Publishers; 1996:268–83.

43. Bocan TM, Mueller SB, Brown EQ et al. HMG-CoA reductase and ACAT inhibitors act synergistically to

lower plasma cholesterol and limit atherosclerotic lesion development in the cholesterol-fed rabbit. Atherosclerosis 1998; 139:21–30.

44. MacIsaac AI, Thomas JD, Topol EJ. Toward the quiescent coronary plaque. J Am Coll Cardiol 1993; 22:1228–41.

45. Cheng JW, Ngo MN. Current perspective on the use of angiotensin-converting enzyme inhibitors in the management of coronary (atherosclerotic) artery disease. Ann Pharmacother 1997; 31:1499–506.

46. Gurfinkel E, Bozovich G, Daroca A, Beck E, Mautner B. Randomised trial of roxithromycin in non-Q-wave coronary syndromes: ROXIS Pilot Study. ROXIS Study Group. Lancet 1997; 350:404–7.

47. Gupta S, Leatham EW, Carrington D et al. Elevated Chlamydia pneumoniae antibodies, cardiovascular events, and azithromycin in male survivors of myocardial infarction. Circulation 1997; 96:404–7.

48. Anderson JL, Muhlestein JB, Carlquist J et al. Randomized secondary prevention trial of azithromycin in patients with coronary artery disease and serological evidence for Chlamydia pneumoniae infection: The Azithromycin in Coronary Artery Disease: Elimination of Myocardial Infection with Chlamydia study. Circulation 1999; 99:1540–7.

49. Stein O, Dabach Y, Hollander G et al. Dexamethasone impairs cholesterol egress from a localized lipoprotein depot in vivo. Atherosclerosis 1998; 137:303–10.

50. Stephens NG, Parsons A, Schofield PM et al. Randomised controlled trial of vitamin E in patients with coronary disease: Cambridge Heart Antioxidant Study (CHAOS). Lancet 1996; 347:781–6.

51. Isner JM, Walsh K, Symes J et al. Arterial gene therapy for therapeutic angiogenesis in patients with peripheral artery disease. Circulation 1995; 91:2687–92.

52. Teirstein PS, Massullo V, Jani S et al. Catheter-based radiotherapy to inhibit restenosis after coronary stenting. N Engl J Med 1997; 336:1697–703.

53. Condado JA, Waksman R, Gurdiel O et al. Long-term angiographic and clinical outcome after percutaneous transluminal coronary angioplasty and intracoronary radiation therapy in humans. Circulation 1997; 96:727–32.

54. Lafont A, Libby P. The smooth muscle cell: sinner or saint in restenosis and the acute coronary syndromes? J Am Coll Cardiol 1998; 32:283–5.

55. Moreno PR, Kilpatrick D, Purushothaman KR, Coleman L, O'Connor WN. Stenting vulnerable plaques improves fibrous cap thickness and reduces lipid content: understanding alternatives for plaque stabilization. Am J Cardiol 2002: 90:50H.

56. Stary HC, Chandler AB, Dinsmore RE et al. A definition of advanced types of atherosclerotic lesions and a histological classification of atherosclerosis. A report from the Committee on Vascular Lesions of the Council on Arteriosclerosis, American Heart Association. Circulation 1995; 92:1355–74.

57. Stary HC, Chandler AB, Glagov S et al. A definition of initial, fatty streak, and intermediate lesions of atherosclerosis. A report from the Committee on Vascular Lesions of the Council on Arteriosclerosis, American Heart Association. Arterioscler Thromb 1994; 14:840–56.

58. Virmani R, Farb A, Burke AP. Risk factors in the pathogenesis of coronary artery disease. Compr Ther 1998; 24:519–29.

59. Falk E. Plaque rupture with severe pre-existing stenosis precipitating coronary thrombosis. Characteristics of coronary atherosclerotic plaques underlying fatal occlusive thrombi. Br Heart J 1983; 50:127–34.

60. Davies MJ, Thomas A. Thrombosis and acute coronary-artery lesions in sudden cardiac ischemic death. N Engl J Med 1984; 310:1137–40.

61. Frink RJ. Chronic ulcerated plaques: new insights into the pathogenesis of acute coronary disease. J Invasive Cardiol 1994; 6:173–85.

62. Rioufol G, Finet G, Ginon I et al. Multiple atherosclerotic plaque rupture in acute coronary syndrome: a three-vessel intravascular ultrasound study. Circulation 2002; 106:804–8.

63. Asakura M, Ueda Y, Yamaguchi O et al. Extensive development of vulnerable plaques as a pan-coronary process in patients with myocardial infarction: an angioscopic study. J Am Coll Cardiol 2001; 37:1284–8.

64. Burke AP, Farb A, Malcom GT et al. Effect of risk factors on the mechanism of acute thrombosis and sudden coronary death in women. Circulation 1998; 97:2110–16.

Pathology of the vulnerable plaque

2

Renu Virmani, Allen Burke, Andrew Farb, Frank D Kolodgie,
Aloke V Finn, and Herman K Gold

INTRODUCTION

Atherosclerosis is an inflammatory disease that occurs preferentially in patients with risk factors and a genetic predisposition.[1] Depending on the definitions used for inclusion of early lesions of atherosclerosis, it is a disease that affects all populations from an early age. Because 70% of the morbidity and mortality from coronary disease is the result of plaque rupture, which generally does not occur until the third decade of life, it is important to establish definitions of terminologies that are used to describe the progression of atherosclerotic lesions from the early stages through to advanced, unstable, thrombosis-prone plaques.

ATHEROSCLEROTIC PLAQUE COMPOSITION

The cellular and acellular structures that participate in the establishment of atherosclerosis include elements found in the normal arterial wall, such as smooth muscle cells, collagen and proteoglycan matrix, and endothelial cells that line the lumen. Other cells are derived from the circulation and include monocyte-derived macrophages, T and B lymphocytes, mast cells, neutrophils, red blood cells, and platelets. The blood coagulation factors contribute through the potentially deleterious effects of thrombosis. Analogous to tumors, the atherosclerotic plaque requires its own vascular supply to grow and develop; the role of angiogenesis in plaque progression and thrombosis is currently under intensive study.[2,3]

The various phases of atherosclerosis have been divided into six stages by the American Heart Association (AHA). Stary et al separated the stages into early (stages I–III)[4] and late stages (stages IV–VI)[5] (Table 2.1). The early stages consist of adaptive intimal thickening, fatty streak, and pathologic intimal thickening; the late stages include the fibroatheroma, multilayered fibrotic and calcified fibroatheroma, and surface disruption hemorrhage and thrombosis. The limitations of the AHA classification have been generally appreciated, especially in reference to late-stage lesions.[6] We have modified this classification because of new knowledge regarding the lesion substrates that lead to coronary thrombosis. The early stages in both classifications are similar, although the term fatty streak has been renamed intimal xanthoma, because the lesion mimics xanthomas that occur outside the cardiovascular system. At a later stage of plaque progression there is the formation of extracellular necrotic core, which is the result of cellular breakdown elements, especially apoptotic foamy macrophages and dead red cell membranes. There is a distinct difference between lipid pool and necrotic core, although it is not easy for non-pathologists to appreciate this distinction. Lipid pools are collections of lipid in a proteoglycan matrix, and lack macrophage infiltration,

Table 2.1 Atherosclerotic plaque classifications

	Traditional classification	Stary et al	Virmani et al	
			Initial	Progression
Early plaques		Type I: microscopic detection of lipid droplets in intima and small groups of macrophage foam cells	Intimal thickening	None
	Fatty streak	Type II: fatty streaks visible on gross inspection, layers of foam cells, occasional lymphocytes and mast cells	Intimal xanthoma	None
		Type III (intermediate): extracellular lipid pools present among layers of smooth muscle cells	Pathologic intimal thickening	Thrombus (erosion)
Intermediate plaque	Atheroma	Type IV: well-defined lipid core; may develop surface disruption (fissure)	Fibrous cap atheroma	Thrombus (erosion)[c]
Late lesions			Thin fibrous cap atheroma	Thrombus (rupture); hemorrhage/fibrin[d]
		Type Va: new fibrous tissue overlying lipid core (multilayered fibroatheroma)[a]	Healed plaque rupture; erosion	Repeated rupture or erosion with or without total occlusion
		Type Vb: calcification[b]	Fibrocalcific plaque (with or without necrotic core)	
	Fibrous plaque	Type Vc: fibrotic lesion with minimal lipid (could be result of organized thrombi)		
Miscellaneous/ complicated features	Complicated/ advanced plaques	Type VIa: surface disruption		
		Type VIb: intraplaque hemorrhage		
		Type VIc: thrombosis		
			Calcified nodule	Thrombus (usually non-occlusive)

[a]May overlap with healed plaque ruptures.
[b]Occasionally referred to as type VII lesion.
[c]May further progress with healing (healed erosion).
[d]May further progress with healing (healed rupture).
Adapted from data published in references 5 and 7.

whereas necrotic cores have macrophage infiltrations, which are undergoing apoptotic cell death, and the matrix is no longer distinct. Sirius red stains show absence of type I and III collagen in the areas of necrotic core.

The late stages of atherosclerotic plaque, therefore, include fibrous cap atheroma, thin cap atheroma (a type of vulnerable plaque), plaque rupture or erosion, healed plaque rupture or erosion, fibrocalcific plaque with or without a necrotic core, and calcified nodule. There are some lesions that are almost purely fibrous and should be called fibrous plaques, as they possess no lipid or calcium and have a rich proteoglycan collagenous matrix. Why some atherosclerotic lesions progress to large relatively acellular lesions, and others develop large cores early in their development, is unknown, although the presence of local and systemic inflammatory processes and risk factors are probably critical in the development of lesions prone to rupture. The concept that expands local vulnerability of coronary plaques prone to rupture to include systemic inflammatory factors, implicating so-called 'vulnerable blood,' has recently been proposed.[7–9]

Lipid pool is a collection of lipid within a matrix rich in proteoglycans. The lipid pool is largely devoid of viable smooth muscle cells (SMCs) and there is an absence of macrophage infiltration.[4,10] The absence of SMCs is probably a result of apoptotic cell death, and lipid pools commonly show the presence of speckled calcification indicative of calcification of SMC organelles and mitochondria derived from SMC death. These are best appreciated with use of special stains that identify calcium (e.g. von Kossa). Furthermore, electron microscopy and PAS (periodic acid–Schiff) stains demonstrate heavy staining of SMC basement membranes and surrounding vesicular bodies with or without calcification representative of SMC remnants.[11,12] Macrophages, if present, are located at the periphery of the lipid pools, interspersed among SMCs. The lipid pool either lacks cholesterol clefts or, if present, they are sparse and small crystals, less than 20 μm in length.

Necrotic cores are regions of the fibroatheroma that are largely devoid of viable cells and consist of cellular debris and cholesterol clefts (free cholesterol crystals). The term 'cleft' derives from the empty space resulting from dissolution of the crystal, which occurs following the use of solvents prior to dehydration steps in standard histology processing. In contrast to lipid pool, the necrotic core contains cell membranes derived from apoptosis of foamy macrophages, as evidenced by CD68-positive immunohistochemical staining; the periphery of the necrotic core is infiltrated by varying numbers of presumably viable foamy macrophages. We have further classified necrotic core lesions into '*early*' and '*late*' by staining fibroatheromas with Sirius red stain for collagen, and stains for proteoglycans. Versican and hyaluronan are abundantly present in early fibroatheromas, whereas they are absent in late fibroatheromas. Similarly, Sirius red stain for collagen matrix is positive in early necrotic core (type III collagen) and absent in the late necrotic core, with a sharp demarcation of the late core from the surrounding collagen matrix.

Calcification may be present at all stages of plaque development; however, it is significantly greater in more advanced lesions. In lipid pools and early cores, it is limited to dying smooth muscle cells and macrophages and occurs as microcalcifications of matrix vesicles. With plaque enlargement, large calcific areas involve necrotic core and fibrous tissue, the latter appearing as sheets of calcium plates. When macrophages infiltrate lipid pools and there is conversion to necrotic core, macrophage death is associated with calcification of the macrophage remnants; these are more feathery in appearance in decalcified sections, and the calcific areas are irregular. By radiologic and ultrasonographic examination, these calcification patterns have been described as absent, speckled, fragmented, and diffuse.[13] However, calcification of lipid pools cannot be visualized by radiography.

Fibrous cap is the region of the plaque that separates the necrotic core from the lumen. The fibrous cap is rich in type I collagen, and is of variable thickness. When less than 65 μm, it has been described as a 'vulnerable' or the thin-cap variant of fibroatheroma;[14] it is discussed in greater detail below.

LESIONS THAT LEAD TO ACUTE CORONARY SYNDROMES

The earliest recognized form of plaque thrombosis is the plaque rupture, which was described in the late 1800s. It has been shown in both sudden death and acute myocardial infarction that the most common form of thrombotic plaque disruption occurs as a result of rupture of a thin fibrous cap. More recently, other mechanisms have been described that may result in luminal thrombosis without disruption of the fibrous cap. Although at least 65–70% of atherothrombi are caused by plaque rupture, 25–30% of thrombi occur from plaque erosion, and 2–5% of atherothrombi occur as a result of calcified nodules that extrude into the lumen[10](Figure 2.1).

Pathology of plaque rupture

Plaque rupture is defined as a necrotic core with a thin fibrous cap that is disrupted or ruptured, allowing the flowing blood to come in contact with the thrombogenic necrotic core. The exposure of tissue factor and other factors within the lipid-rich necrotic core is probably involved in the induction of thrombosis.[15–19] The disrupted cap is essentially devoid of SMCs and is made up of type I collagen and there is absence of proteoglycans.

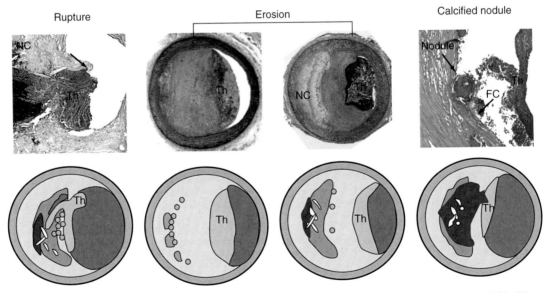

Figure 2.1 Lesions with thrombi. *Ruptured plaques* are thin fibrous cap atheromas with luminal thrombi (Th). These lesions usually have an extensive necrotic core (NC) containing large numbers of cholesterol crystals, and a thin fibrous cap (<65 μm) infiltrated by foamy macrophages and a paucity of T lymphocytes. The fibrous cap is thinnest at the site of rupture and consists of a few collagen bundles and rare smooth muscle cells. The luminal thrombus is in communication with the lipid-rich necrotic core. *Erosions* occur over lesions rich in smooth muscle cells and proteoglycans. Luminal thrombi overly areas lacking surface endothelium. The deep intima of the eroded plaque often shows extracellular lipid pools, but necrotic cores are uncommon; when present, the necrotic core does not communicate with the luminal thrombus. Inflammatory infiltrate is usually absent but, if present, is sparse and consists of macrophages and lymphocytes. *Calcified nodules* are plaques with luminal thrombi showing calcific nodules protruding into the lumen through a disrupted thin fibrous cap (FC). There is absence of endothelium at the site of the thrombus and inflammatory cells (macrophages, T lymphocytes) are absent. (Reproduced with permission from Virmani et al.[10])

The fibrous cap is heavily infiltrated by activated macrophages and T lymphocytes which show HLA-DR positivity.[20] The frequency of acute plaque rupture (platelet- and fibrin-rich thrombus) in a series of sudden death varies widely, and is dependent on the population studies and definition of the lesions. Davies[21-23] and Falk[24] believe this lesion is present in over 85% of patients dying suddenly. In our series, however, this lesion accounts for only 35% of cases of all sudden death. The differences in our study and those from Davies and Falk are related to age of the patients studied, defining chronic total occlusion as acute thrombus and plaque containing fibrin without a luminal thrombus with or without a plaque fissure as plaque rupture. Calcification is present in 80% of plaques that rupture but is usually speckled or fragmented and infrequently diffuse. We have reported that coronary plaques that rupture are equally concentric or eccentric and are more frequent in men and postmenopausal women.[25]

Mechanisms of plaque rupture

Inflammation–matrix interactions

T cells liberate proinflammatory cytokines such as γ-interferon, which inhibits collagen synthesis by smooth muscle cells.[26] Interstitial collagen fibrils, especially the triple helical collagen fibril, are susceptible to degradation by proteolytic enzymes. It is believed that the macrophages in the fibrous cap release matrix metalloproteinases (MMPs),[27] of which at least 23 have been described, which weaken the fibrous cap and result in rupture. Libby et al have demonstrated overexpression of all three important interstitial collagenases in atherosclerotic plaques (MMP-1, -8, and -13) that may be responsible for the breakdown of the fibrous cap.[28] More recent studies show increased MMP-12 expression in plaques of patients with symptomatic carotid disease as compared

with asymptomatic carotid stenosis.[29] In addition to MMP-1, -8, -12, and -13, there is evidence that MMP-2, -3, -9, and -14 may be up-regulated in atherosclerotic plaques. Transcriptional regulation of MMPs include several factors related to unstable atherosclerotic plaques, including oxidized low-density lipoprotein (oxLDL), interleukin-1, interleukin-1β, tumor necrosis factor-α (TNF-α), transforming growth factor-β, CD40 ligand, and thrombin.[30] Macrophage expression of MMPs, especially MMP-2 and MMP-9, occurs through a pathway depending on prostaglandin E_2 and cyclo-oxygenase 2, which is induced in response to inflammation.[31,32]

In contrast to interleukins and MMPs, transforming growth factor $β_1$ has been demonstrated to be a stabilizing factor in carotid plaques.[33]

Occlusive thrombi showed a greater density of CD68-positive macrophage and myeloperoxidase (MPO)-positive monocytes and neutrophils than non-occlusive thrombi.[34] Similarly, the length of the thrombus showed a positive correlation with the density of macrophages ($P = 0.004$) and MPO-positive cells ($P = 0.04$) within the thrombus. In the disrupted fibrous cap, the density of MPO-positive macrophages and neutrophils was greater in occlusive than non-occlusive thrombi. The precise role of MPO in triggering acute coronary thrombosis is unclear; in addition to providing a pro-oxidant milieu, the production of hypochlorous acid may cause breakdown of the fibrous cap.[35,36] Experimental studies suggest that hypochlorous acid promotes apoptotic EC death, partially via mitochondrial damage.[37]

Mechanical factors and shear stress

Two types of stress are implicated in plaque development and instability: shear stress and tensile stress.[38] At areas of low shear stress, blood flow is turbulent especially near branch points, develop atherosclerosis compared with high shear stress regions, flow dividers, which are protected from the development of atherosclerosis. The typical location of atherosclerotic lesions is at carotid bifurcation, coronary branch points, infrarenal abdominal aorta, and femoral arteries. The AHA type IV lesions called fibroatheromas consist of a necrotic core covered by a fibrous cap; they develop at locations of low shear on the outer wall of vessel bifurcation and are eccentric.[39,40]

Vascular remodeling initially preserves the lumen diameter while maintaining the low shear stress conditions that encourage plaque growth. However, once there is critical stenosis, particularly on its upstream site, eccentric plaques at preserved lumen locations experience increased tensile stress at the shoulders, making them prone to fissuring and thrombosis. Ultimately, increased tensile stress may be responsible for the occurrence of ruptures at the locations proximal to sites of severe narrowing.[38]

Evidence that circumferential tensile stress is involved in ultimate plaque rupture derives partly from pathologic studies. Rupture of the fibrous cap usually occurs in shoulder regions, the weakest portion where the stress is highest and MMP expression increased.[41] However, plaque rupture may not always occur at the region of highest stress, suggesting that local variations in plaque material properties contribute to rupture.[42]

When these plaques eventually start to intrude into the lumen, the shear stress in the area surrounding the plaque changes substantially, increasing tensile stress at the plaque shoulders and exacerbating fissuring and thrombosis. Wall stress has also been implicated in down-regulation of antithrombotic substances, such as thrombomodulin, in vein grafts.[43]

Plaque erosion

Plaque erosion is defined as a lesion with luminal thrombus with a base rich in SMCs and proteoglycan matrix.[44] At the site of thrombosis, there is absence of an endothelial layer. The underlying plaque in 50% of cases shows layering of the fibrin with interspersed SMCs and proteoglycans. The underlying plaque either shows pathologic intimal thickening or fibroatheroma with a thick fibrous cap that is rich in proteoglycans,[10] especially hyaluronan and versican along with type III collagen.[45] These lesions are usually not calcified, and when calcified the calcification is speckled.[46] Inflammatory cells are infrequently observed in the plaque underneath the thrombus. The majority of plaque erosions are eccentric, occur most frequently in young men and women <50 years of age, and are associated with smoking, especially in premenopausal women.[47] Luminal endothelial apoptosis,[37] possibly induced by vasospasm or secondary to low shear, has been implicated in the pathogenesis of plaque erosion.[48]

Calcified nodule

The third type of lesion is an infrequent cause of thrombosis in patients dying a sudden coronary death and its incidence in stable or unstable angina and acute myocardial infarction is unknown. The term refers to a lesion with fibrous cap disruption, absence of endothelium, and thrombus associated with eruptive, dense calcified nodule with bone formation. The origin of this lesion is unknown, but appears to be associated with healed plaque ruptures. Over one-half of these lesions are seen in the mid-right coronary artery, where coronary torsion stress is maximum. The underlying plaque is associated with calcified plates and it is proposed that the breakdown of the calcified plate results in release of certain growth factors that likely induce ossification and the fibrous cap wears down from physical forces exerted by the nodules themselves or from proteases released from the surrounding cellular infiltrates. This lesion is usually seen in elderly male patients with heavily calcified and tortuous arteries.[10]

Table 2.2   Morphologic characteristics of plaque rupture and thin-cap fibroatheroma

Plaque type	Necrotic core (%)	Fibrous cap thickness (μm)	Macrophage density (%)	Smooth muscle cells (%)	T lymphocytes/mm² × 1000	Calcification score
Rupture	34 ± 17	23 ± 19	26 ± 20	0.002 ± 0.004	4.9 ± 4.3	1.53 ± 1.03
Thin cap fibroatheroma	23 ± 17	< 65	14 ± 10	6.6 ± 10.4	6.6 ± 10.4	0.97 ± 1.1
P value	NS		0.005	NS	NS	0.014

Reproduced with permission from Kolodgie et al.[58]

THE THIN-CAP FIBROATHEROMA

'Vulnerable plaque,'[49] a term coined by Muller and colleagues[50,51] and Little,[52] refers to a lesion prone to thrombosis. Libby further defined the morphology of the 'vulnerable' plaque as a 'lesion composed of a lipid-rich core in an eccentric plaque'.[53] The central core contains 'many lipid-laden macrophage foam cells derived from blood monocytes' with a 'thin, friable fibrous cap'.[53]

Our laboratory has defined plaque vulnerability based on the actual cap thickness of fixed autopsy specimens (Table 2.2). The 'vulnerable' plaque, or thin-cap fibroatheroma (TCFA), was defined as a lesion with a fibrous cap <65 μm thick and infiltrated by macrophages (>25 cells per 0.3 mm diameter field).[14] A thickness of 65 μm was chosen as a criterion of instability because, in rupture, the mean cap thickness was 23 ± 19 μm; 95% of caps measured less than 64 μm within a limit of only 2 standard deviations. The plaque may or may not be eccentric and the necrotic core is well developed, although there is no correlation between the thickness of the fibrous cap and size of the necrotic core. However, the fibrous cap thickness correlates with macrophage infiltration: the thinner the cap, the greater the macrophage infiltration (Figure 2.2).

A detailed morphometric comparison of plaque variables between rupture and

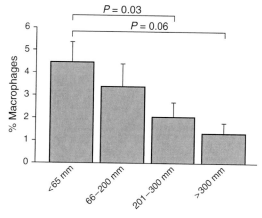

Figure 2.2   Correlation between fibrous cap thickness and macrophage density within the fibrous cap. As the thickness increases, the density of macrophages decreases. Data are derived from postmortem analysis of epicardial coronary artery sections from men and women dying suddenly from coronary artery disease.

TCFA is shown in Table 2.2. This analysis of culprit lesions[54] showed that the underlying necrotic core as a percent of plaque area was greatest in ruptured plaques (34 ± 17%) but was not significantly different (23 ± 17%) from TCFAs. In addition, we found that ruptures had a greater concentration of macrophages in the fibrous cap than TCFA (26 ± 20% vs 14 ± 10%, $P = 0.005$) and a marked reduction of SMCs at the rupture site (Table 2.3). No differences were noted in the number of T lymphocytes in areas of cap thinning.

The morphologic variants of the TCFA are detailed in Figures 2.3 and 2.4. These include lesions with insignificant plaque burden, large eccentric or concentric lipid cores, or previous healed ruptures. In a large series of 142 cases, only 11% of acute ruptures show rupture of a virgin plaque without evidence of prior rupture.[55]

Roberts and Jones have shown that at the site of rupture the necrotic core was the largest, as compared to plaques with intact fibroatheromas, supporting the concept that a large necrotic core is associated with plaque vulnerability.[56] We have corroborated these data in coronary arteries from patients dying suddenly, showing that mean necrotic core size, independent of cross-sectional area luminal narrowing, was greatest in plaque ruptures, followed by thin-cap atheromas and fibrous cap atheromas.[54] Ninety percent of ruptured plaques contain necrotic cores greater than 10% of plaque area; furthermore, 65% of plaque ruptures have >25% of plaque occupied by necrotic core. In contrast, only 75% of TCFAs have >10% of plaque area occupied by a core and only 35% of TCFAs have >25% of plaque occupied by the lipid core.[54,57] The length of the necrotic core in ruptures and TCFAs is similar, varying from 2 to 22 mm with a mean of 8 and 9 mm, respectively (Table 2.4). The mean percent cross-sectional area narrowing of TCFAs is 60%, compared with 73% for plaque rupture. Thus TCFAs are predominantly seen in arteries with <50% diameter stenosis. Over 50% of the plaque ruptures, healed plaque ruptures, and TCFAs occur in the proximal portions of the major coronary arteries, left anterior descending, right, left circumflex, and another third in the midportion of these arteries, and the rest are distributed in the distal segments.[58]

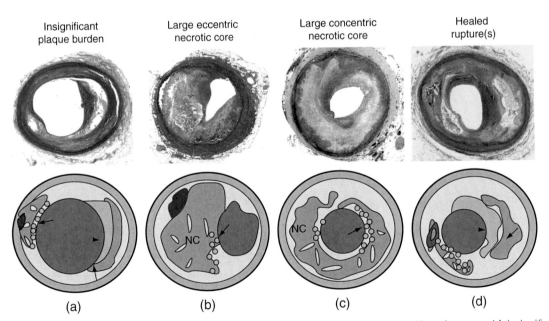

| Insignificant plaque burden | Large eccentric necrotic core | Large concentric necrotic core | Healed rupture(s) |
| (a) | (b) | (c) | (d) |

Figure 2.3 Morphologic variants of the thin-cap fibroatheroma. Thin caps may emerge in fibroatheromas with insignificant plaque burden and insignificant luminal narrowing, in fibroatheromas with large cores that are eccentric or eccentric, and frequently in plaques with evidence of prior rupture. (a) In this plaque with insignificant plaque burden, there is an area of proteoglycan-rich smooth muscle cells (arrowhead) suggestive of a prior rupture, and multiple areas of thin caps (arrows). (b) The necrotic core (NC) is large, with an area of thinned cap (arrow). (c) The necrotic core (NC) is concentric, with an extensive area of cap thinning (arrow). (d) There may be a healed rupture (arrow), with a proteoglycan-rich smooth muscle cell reparative layer (arrowhead).

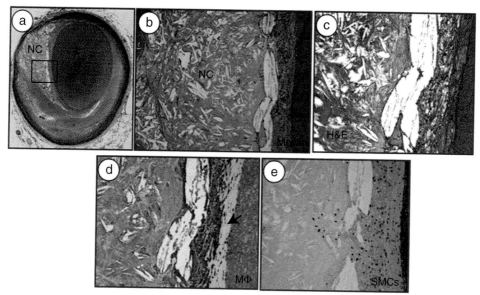

Figure 2.4 A non-hemodynamically limiting thin-cap fibroatheroma. (a) A thin-cap fibroatheroma having a necrotic core (NC) and an overlying thin fibrous cap (<65 μm). (b) A high-power view of the boxed area in (a); an advanced necrotic core (NC) with a large number of cholesterol clefts with surrounding loss of matrix and no cellular infiltration is seen. (c) The fibrous cap is infiltrated by macrophages, better appreciated when stained with hematoxylin and eosin (H&E). (d and e) Macrophage infiltration (CD 68 positive) (arrow in d) and rare staining of smooth muscle cells (SMCs; α-actin positive) in the fibrous cap.

ROLE OF APOPTOSIS

Apoptosis may be involved in many facets of the development of the atherosclerotic plaque. We have demonstrated that apoptotic macrophages are localized at the site of plaque rupture and may play a role in plaque instability.[59] Defective phagocytic clearance of apoptotic macrophages may lead to secondary necrosis of these cells and a proinflammatory response, contributing to the generation of the necrotic core.[60]

Table 2.3 Comparison of necrotic core size, number of cholesterol clefts, macrophage infiltration, mean number of vasa vasorum, and mean number of hemosiderin-laden macrophages in culprit plaques

Plaque type	Necrotic core (%)	No. of cholesterol clefts	Macrophage infiltration of fibrous cap (%)	Mean no. of vasa vasorum	Mean no. of hemosiderin-laden macrophages
Rupture	$34 \pm 17^{\Omega,\ni}$	$12 \pm 12^{*,\wedge}$	$26 \pm 20^{\psi,\tau,\varpi}$	$44 \pm 22^{\varphi,\perp,\partial}$	$18.9 \pm 11\delta,\lambda,\notin$
TCFA	24 ± 17	8 ± 9	$14 \pm 10^{\psi}$	$26 \pm 23^{\varphi}$	$4.4 \pm 3.6\delta$
Erosion	$14 \pm 14^{\Omega}$	$2 \pm 5^{*}$	$10 \pm 12^{\tau}$	$28 \pm 18^{\perp}$	$4.3 \pm 4.7\lambda$
Fibrocalcific	$12 \pm 25^{\ni}$	$4 \pm 6^{\wedge}$	$3 \pm 0.7^{\varpi}$	$13 \pm 9^{\partial}$	$5.0 \pm 9.3\notin$
P value	Ω 0.003 vs erosion	*0.002 vs erosion	ψ 0.005 vs TCFA	φ 0.07 vs TCFA	δ 0.001 vs erosion
	$\ni$ 0.01 vs fibrocalcific	$\wedge$0.04 vs fibrocalcific	τ <0.0001 vs erosion	$\perp$ 0.02 vs erosion	λ<0.0001,
			ϖ 0.0001 vs fibrocalcific	∂ 0.01 vs fibrocalcific	$\notin$ 0.03 vs fibrocalcific

Modified with permission from Virmani et al.[10]

Table 2.4   Approximate sizes of necrotic core, in fibroatheroma, thin-cap atheroma, and acute rupture

Dimension	Plaque type		
	Fibrous cap atheroma	Thin-cap atheroma	Acute plaque rupture
Length (mm; mean (range))	6 (1–18)	8 (2–17)	9 (2.5–22)
Necrotic core area (mm²)	1.2 ± 2.2	1.7 ± 1.1	3.8 ± 5.5
Necrotic core area (%)	15 ± 20%	23 ± 17%	34 ± 17%

Reproduced with permission from Virmani et al.[57]

In carotid plaques, the number of macrophages and SMCs in apoptosis has been shown to be higher in symptomatic plaque as compared with asymptomatic plaques.[61] The TNF-related apoptosis-inducing ligand/APO-2L, a member of the TNF superfamily, has a role in apoptosis induction TNF-related apoptosis-inducing ligand is present in stable atherosclerotic lesions, is increased in vulnerable plaques, and is found to colocalize with CD3 cells and oxLDL.[62]

ROLE OF HEMORRHAGE AND ANGIOGENESIS IN NECROTIC CORE EXPANSION IN PATIENTS WITH UNSTABLE CORONARY ATHEROSCLEROTIC PLAQUES

Macrophage infiltration has been shown to be the first step toward the formation of the fibroatheroma, as necrotic core formation has been attributed to the death of macrophages. The conversion of the macrophage to a foam cell requires the ingestion of lipid, which oxidizes and is recognized by the scavenger receptor. Felton et al showed that in human aortic atherosclerotic plaques, the progression from a non-disrupted to a disrupted lesion was associated with an increase in free cholesterol, cholesterol esters, and the ratio of free-to-esterified cholesterol.[63] Furthermore, the percentage of cholesterol clefts was greater in lesions that have ruptured than in fibrocalcific plaques. Many 20th century pathologists recognized

that intraplaque hemorrhage was a major contributor to the progression of coronary atherosclerosis. We have reported that patients with plaque rupture had twice as many sites of coronary plaque hemorrhage as patients dying with stable plaques.[10] We and others have reported that hemorrhages in non-vascular locations are associated with presence of free cholesterol, morphologically recognized by cholesterol crystals, and are surrounded by foamy macrophages, giant cells, and iron, with surrounding fibrosis lesions akin to atherosclerosis.[64] The cholesterol content of red cell membrane exceeds that of all other cells in the body, with lipid constituting 40% of the weight, and therefore the accumulation of free cholesterol in plaque may be in part derived from erythrocyte membrane. In addition, the red blood cell membrane cholesterol is elevated in patients with hypercholesterolemia and decreases with short-term treatment with statins. Using an antibody directed against glycophorin A, a protein specific to erythrocyte membranes, we have shown that the intensity and extent of glycophorin A staining correlates with larger necrotic cores and greater extent of macrophage infiltration.[64] Also, there were greater numbers of thin-wall leaky vasa vasorum in the vicinity, which showed diffuse staining by von Willebrand factor, suggesting that these vessels were leaky and may be contributing to the accumulation of the red cells within the plaques (Table 2.3).

These observations have been extended to postmortem studies of human aortic lesions, which have demonstrated an increase in vasa vasorum in rupture plaques than those without rupture.[65]

INCIDENCE OF THIN-CAP ATHEROMA IN ACUTE CORONARY SYNDROMES

By far the highest incidence of TCFAs occurs in patients dying with acute myocardial infarction (AMI) (3.1 ± 2.4 TCFAs per patient), less in sudden coronary death (1.8 ± 1.9) and least in incidental death (0.50 ± 1.1) or plaque erosion (0.50 ± 1.0).[54] The incidence of TCFAs is greater in men than women (AMI 3.1 vs 1.7; SD 1.8 vs 1.3, respectively). We have also observed in sudden coronary death that the highest incidence of TCFAs occurs in patients dying with acute rupture (1.3 ± 1.4 per heart) than patients dying from stable plaque (1.1 ± 1.3 per heart).[54] Similarly, the incidence of TCFAs was higher in coronary arteries of patients with evidence of healed plaque ruptures than in those without evidence of healed plaque (1.4 ± 1.4 vs 0.5 ± 0.8, respectively). TCFAs have not been characterized in patients dying with stable and unstable angina, as these patients usually do not die during the acute phase of the disease.

ROLE OF CALCIFICATION IN THE DETECTION OF A THIN-CAP ATHEROMA

Coronary calcification correlates with plaque burden and cardiovascular morbidity and mortality. As age advances, the mean percent calcified area increases both for plaques with moderate (≥50% and <75% area luminal narrowing) and severe (≥75% area luminal narrowing) coronary narrowing.[66,67] However, total occlusion may have less calcification and is duration dependent. It was previously thought that Framingham risk factor analysis only predicts up to 50% of coronary artery disease (CAD) mortality.[68,69] However, more recent data suggest that up to 90% of acute coronary events are predicted by conventional risk factors.[70] Kondos et al, using electron beam tomography (EBT) to image coronary arteries in self-referred men and women who did not have prior events and were followed for 37 ± 13 months, have shown that knowledge of coronary artery calcification provided incremental information beyond that defined by conventional CAD risk factor assessment.[71] However, pathologic analysis of coronary arteries from patients dying from sudden coronary death have shown that the maximum calcification area is seen in healed plaque ruptures, followed by fibroatheroma, thin-cap atheroma, plaque hemorrhage, fibrous plaque, plaque rupture, total occlusion, and plaque erosion.[12] These morphologic data suggest that calcification is not associated with plaque instability. In fact plaque ruptures and erosions showed mild calcification.

We have studied postmortem coronary radiographs and correlated the radiographs with histologic assessment of the type of atherosclerotic plaque. The radiographic calcification was typed according to Friedrich et al as absent, speckled, fragmented (linear or wide, single focus of calcium >2mm in diameter), or diffuse (>5mm segment of continuous calcification).[13] We classified plaques histologically as plaque rupture, plaque erosion, thin-cap atheroma, and healed plaque rupture. Plaque erosions had either no calcification or speckled calcification. Plaque ruptures showed speckled calcification in 70%, and the remaining 30% had a diffuse or fragmented calcification pattern. Fifty percent of TCFAs had absent or speckled calcification, and the remainder had a diffuse or fragmented calcification pattern. In contrast, 40% of healed plaque ruptures had diffuse calcification, 20% had a fragmented calcification pattern,

Figure 2.5 Relationship between plaque morphology and radiographic calcification. Plaque erosions (a) were exclusively present in areas with stippled or no calcification. Plaque ruptures (b) were most frequently seen in areas of speckled calcification, but were also present in blocked or diffuse calcification. Curiously, there were no ruptures in segments devoid of any calcification. Thin-capped atheroma were most frequently present in areas of speckled calcification (c), but were also seen in heavily calcified or uncalcified areas, suggesting that calcification pattern is not helpful in diagnosing these lesions. Healed ruptures are almost always seen in areas of calcification, and most frequently in diffusely calcified areas (d). (Reproduced with permission from Burke et al.[11])

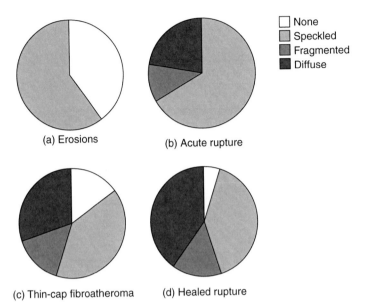

(a) Erosions   (b) Acute rupture

□ None
▨ Speckled
▨ Fragmented
■ Diffuse

(c) Thin-cap fibroatheroma   (d) Healed rupture

and the remainder had predominantly speckled calcification[46] (Figure 2.5).

VULNERABLE PLAQUE: THE FUTURE

Despite our progress in knowledge of episodic plaque progression, large gaps still remain in our understanding of factors that lead to acute coronary syndromes. Reliable methods of identifying, pathologically or by imaging, plaques that are likely to rupture are still elusive. Hypothetical pathologic factors that precipitate rupture have been identified largely by association with ruptured plaques, but etiology and causation have yet to be proven. The precursor lesion of plaque erosion is far from being identified. The precise mix of thrombotic, inflammatory, vasospastic, and systemic factors that precipitate an acute coronary event has thus far been elusive and we need better understanding to accurately predict based on plaque morphology alone. Only intensive risk factor modification and aggressive interventions that are increasingly tailored to individual types of lesions will together significantly

reduce the complications of coronary atherothrombosis.

REFERENCES

1. Libby P. Inflammation in atherosclerosis. Nature 2002; 420(19):868–74.
2. O'Brien ER, Garvin MR, Dev R et al. Angiogenesis in human coronary atherosclerotic plaques. Am J Pathol 1994; 145(4):883–94.
3. Depre C, Havaux X, Wijns W. Neovascularization in human coronary atherosclerotic lesions. Cathet Cardiovasc Diagn 1996; 39(3):215–20.
4. Stary HC, Chandler AB, Glagov S et al. A definition of initial, fatty streak, and intermediate lesions of atherosclerosis. A report from the Committee on Vascular Lesions of the Council on Arteriosclerosis, American Heart Association. Arterioscler Thromb 1994; 14(5):840–56.
5. Stary HC, Chandler AB, Dinsmore RE et al. A definition of advanced types of atherosclerotic lesions and a histological classification of atherosclerosis. A report from the Committee on Vascular Lesions of the Council on Arteriosclerosis, American Heart Association. Arterioscler Thromb Vasc Biol 1995; 15(9):1512–31.
6. Fuster V, Moreno PR, Fayad ZA, Corti R, Badimon JJ. Atherothrombosis and high-risk plaque: part I: evolving concepts. J Am Coll Cardiol 2005; 46(6):937–54.
7. Wasserman EJ, Shipley NM. Atherothrombosis in acute coronary syndromes: mechanisms, markers, and mediators of vulnerability. Mt Sinai J Med 2006; 73(1):431–9.

8. Lutgens E, van Suylen RJ, Faber BC et al. Atherosclerotic plaque rupture: local or systemic process? Arterioscler Thromb Vasc Biol 2003; 23(12):2123–30.

9. Schwartz RS, Bayes-Genis A, Lesser JR et al. Detecting vulnerable plaque using peripheral blood: inflammatory and cellular markers. J Interv Cardiol 2003; 16(3):231–42.

10. Virmani R, Kolodgie FD, Burke AP, Farb A, Schwartz SM. Lessons from sudden coronary death: a comprehensive morphological classification scheme for atherosclerotic lesions. Arterioscler Thromb Vasc Biol 2000; 20(5):1262–75.

11. Burke AP, Weber DK, Kolodgie FD et al. Pathophysiology of calcium deposition in coronary arteries. Herz 2001; 26(4):239–44.

12. Burke AP, Weber D, Farb A et al. Coronary calcification: insights from sudden coronary death victims. Z Kardiol 1999; 89(SII):49–53.

13. Friedrich GJ, Moes NY, Muhlberger VA et al. Detection of intralesional calcium by intracoronary ultrasound depends on the histologic pattern. Am Heart J 1994; 128(3):435–41.

14. Burke AP, Farb A, Malcom GT et al. Coronary risk factors and plaque morphology in men with coronary disease who died suddenly. N Engl J Med 1997; 336(18):1276–82.

15. Libby P, Geng YJ, Aikawa M et al. Macrophages and atherosclerotic plaque stability. Curr Opin Lipidol 1996; 7(5):330–5.

16. Zaman AG, Helft G, Worthley SG, Badimon JJ. The role of plaque rupture and thrombosis in coronary artery disease. Atherosclerosis 2000; 149(2):251–66.

17. Falk E, Shah PK, Fuster V. Coronary plaque disruption. Circulation 1995; 92(3):657–71.

18. Falk E, Fernandez-Ortiz A. Role of thrombosis in atherosclerosis and its complications. Am J Cardiol 1995; 75(6):3–11B.

19. Davies MJ. Acute coronary thrombosis – the role of plaque disruption and its initiation and prevention. Eur Heart J 1995; 16 (Suppl L):3–7.

20. Virmani R, Kolodgie F, Burke AP et al. Inflammation and coronary artery disease. In: Feuerstein GZ, Libby P, Mann DL, eds. Inflammation and Cardiac Diseases. Basel: Birkhäuser Verlag; 2003:21–53.

21. Davies MJ. Pathological view of sudden cardiac death. Br Heart J 1981; 45(1):88–96.

22. Davies MJ, Thomas A. Thrombosis and acute coronary-artery lesions in sudden cardiac ischemic death. N Engl J Med 1984; 310(18):1137–40.

23. Davies MJ, Thomas AC. Plaque fissuring – the cause of acute myocardial infarction, sudden ischaemic death, and crescendo angina. Br Heart J 1985; 53(4):363–73.

24. Falk E. Morphologic features of unstable atherothrombotic plaques underlying acute coronary syndromes. Am J Cardiol 1989; 63(10):114–20E.

25. Burke AP, Farb A, Malcom G, Virmani R. Effect of menopause on plaque morphologic characteristics in coronary atherosclerosis. Am Heart J 2001; 141 (2 Suppl):S58–62.

26. Schonbeck U, Mach F, Sukhova GK et al. Regulation of matrix metalloproteinase expression in human vascular smooth muscle cells by T lymphocytes: a role for CD40 signaling in plaque rupture? Circ Res 1997; 81(3):448–54.

27. Galis ZS, Sukhova GK, Kranzhofer R, Clark S, Libby P. Macrophage foam cells from experimental atheroma constitutively produce matrix-degrading proteinases. Proc Natl Acad Sci USA 1995; 92(2):402–6.

28. Sukhova GK, Schonbeck U, Rabkin E et al. Evidence for increased collagenolysis by interstitial collagenases-1 and -3 in vulnerable human atheromatous plaques. Circulation 1999; 99(19):2503–9.

29. Morgan AR, Rerkasem K, Gallagher PJ et al. Differences in matrix metalloproteinase-1 and matrix metalloproteinase-12 transcript levels among carotid atherosclerotic plaques with different histopathological characteristics. Stroke 2004; 35(6):1310–15.

30. Jones CB, Sane DC, Herrington DM. Matrix metalloproteinases: a review of their structure and role in acute coronary syndrome. Cardiovasc Res 2003; 59(4):812–23.

31. Cipollone F, Fazia M, Iezzi A et al. Balance between PGD synthase and PGE synthase is a major determinant of atherosclerotic plaque instability in humans. Arterioscler Thromb Vasc Biol 2004; 24(7):1259–65.

32. Cipollone F, Fazia M, Mezzetti A. Novel determinants of plaque instability. J Thromb Haemost 2005; 3(9):1962–75.

33. Cipollone F, Fazia M, Mincione G et al. Increased expression of transforming growth factor-beta1 as a stabilizing factor in human atherosclerotic plaques. Stroke 2004; 35(10):2253–7.

34. Virmani R, Burke AP, Kolodgie FD, Farb A. Pathology of the thin-cap fibroatheroma: a type of vulnerable plaque. J Interv Cardiol 2003; 16(3):267–72.

35. Woods AA, Davies MJ. Fragmentation of extracellular matrix by hypochlorous acid. Biochem J 2003; 376(Pt 1):219–27.

36. Woods AA, Linton SM, Davies MJ. Detection of HOCl-mediated protein oxidation products in the extracellular matrix of human atherosclerotic plaques. Biochem J 2003; 370(Pt 2):729–35.

37. Sugiyama S, Kugiyama K, Aikawa M et al. Hypochlorous acid, a macrophage product, induces endothelial apoptosis and tissue factor expression: involvement of myeloperoxidase-mediated oxidant in plaque erosion and thrombogenesis. Arterioscler Thromb Vasc Biol 2004; 24(7):1309–14.

38. Slager CJ, Wentzel JJ, Gijsen FJ et al. The role of shear stress in the destabilization of vulnerable plaques and related therapeutic implications. Nat Clin Pract Cardiovasc Med 2005; 2(9):456–64.

39. Wentzel JJ, Gijsen FJ, Schuurbiers JC et al. Geometry guided data averaging enables the interpretation of

shear stress related plaque development in human coronary arteries. J Biomech 2005; 38(7):1551–5.

40. Stone PH, Coskun AU, Yeghiazarians Y et al. Prediction of sites of coronary atherosclerosis progression: in vivo profiling of endothelial shear stress, lumen, and outer vessel wall characteristics to predict vascular behavior. Curr Opin Cardiol 2003; 18(6):458–70.

41. Galis ZS, Sukhova GK, Lark MW, Libby P. Increased expression of matrix metalloproteinases and matrix degrading activity in vulnerable regions of human atherosclerotic plaques. J Clin Invest 1994; 94(6):2493–503.

42. Cheng GC, Loree HM, Kamm RD, Fishbein MC, Lee RT. Distribution of circumferential stress in ruptured and stable atherosclerotic lesions. A structural analysis with histopathological correlation. Circulation 1993; 87(4):1179–87.

43. Sperry JL, Deming CB, Bian C et al. Wall tension is a potent negative regulator of in vivo thrombomodulin expression. Circ Res 2003; 92(1):41–7.

44. Farb A, Burke A, Tang A et al. Coronary plaque erosion without rupture into a lipid core: a frequent cause of coronary thrombosis in sudden coronary death. Circulation 1996; 93:1354–63.

45. Kolodgie FD, Burke AP, Farb A et al. Differential accumulation of proteoglycans and hyaluronan in culprit lesions: insights into plaque erosion. Arterioscler Thromb Vasc Biol 2002; 22(10):1642–8.

46. Burke AP, Taylor A, Farb A, Malcom GT, Virmani R. Coronary calcification: insights from sudden coronary death victims. Z Kardiol 2000; 89(Suppl 2):49–53.

47. Burke AP, Farb A, Malcom GT et al. Effect of risk factors on the mechanism of acute thrombosis and sudden coronary death in women. Circulation 1998; 97(21):2110–16.

48. Tedgui A, Mallat Z. Apoptosis as a determinant of atherothrombosis. Thromb Haemost 2001; 86(1):420–6.

49. Schroeder AP, Falk E. Vulnerable and dangerous coronary plaques. Atherosclerosis 1995; 118(Suppl): S141–9.

50. Muller JE, Tofler GH, Stone PH. Circadian variation and triggers of onset of acute cardiovascular disease. Circulation 1989; 79(4):733–43.

51. Muller JE, Tofler GH. Triggering and hourly variation of onset of arterial thrombosis. Ann Epidemiol 1992; 2(4):393–405.

52. Little WC. Angiographic assessment of the culprit coronary artery lesion before acute myocardial infarction. Am J Cardiol 1990; 66(16):44–47G.

53. Libby P. Coronary artery injury and the biology of atherosclerosis: inflammation, thrombosis, and stabilization. Am J Cardiol 2000; 86(8B):3–8J; discussion 8–9J.

54. Burke AP, Virmani R, Galis Z, Haudenschild CC, Muller JE. 34th Bethesda Conference: Task force #2 – What is the pathologic basis for new atherosclerosis imaging techniques? J Am Coll Cardiol 2003; 41(11):1874–86.

55. Burke AP, Kolodgie FD, Farb A et al. Healed plaque ruptures and sudden coronary death: evidence that subclinical rupture has a role in plaque progression. Circulation 2001; 103(7):934–40.

56. Roberts WC, Jones AA. Quantitation of coronary arterial narrowing at necropsy in sudden coronary death: analysis of 31 patients and comparison with 25 control subjects. Am J Cardiol 1979; 44(1):39–45.

57. Virmani R, Burke AP, Kolodgie F, Farb A. The pathology of unstable coronary lesions. J Intervent Cardiol 2002; 15(6):439–46.

58. Kolodgie FD, Burke AP, Farb A et al. The thin-cap fibroatheroma: a type of vulnerable plaque: the major precursor lesion to acute coronary syndromes. Curr Opin Cardiol 2001; 16(5):285–92.

59. Kolodgie FD, Narula J, Burke AP et al. Localization of apoptotic macrophages at the site of plaque rupture in sudden coronary death. Am J Pathol 2000; 157(4):1259–68.

60. Tabas I. Consequences and therapeutic implications of macrophage apoptosis in atherosclerosis: the importance of lesion stage and phagocytic efficiency. Arterioscler Thromb Vasc Biol 2005; 25(11):2255–64.

61. Artese L, Ucchino S, Piattelli A et al. Factors associated with apoptosis in symptomatic and asymptomatic carotid atherosclerotic plaques. Int J Immunopathol Pharmacol 2005; 18(4):645–53.

62. Michowitz Y, Goldstein E, Roth A et al. The involvement of tumor necrosis factor-related apoptosis-inducing ligand (TRAIL) in atherosclerosis. J Am Coll Cardiol 2005; 45(7):1018–24.

63. Felton CV, Crook D, Davies MJ, Oliver MF. Relation of plaque lipid composition and morphology to the stability of human aortic plaques. Arterioscler Thromb Vasc Biol 1997; 17(7):1337–45.

64. Kolodgie FD, Gold HK, Burke AP et al. Intraplaque hemorrhage and progression of coronary atheroma. N Engl J Med 2003; 349(24):2316–25.

65. Moreno PR, Purushothaman KR, Fuster V et al. Plaque neovascularization is increased in ruptured atherosclerotic lesions of human aorta: implications for plaque vulnerability. Circulation 2004; 110(14): 2032–8.

66. Kragel AH, Reddy SG, Wittes JT, Roberts WC. Morphometric analysis of the composition of atherosclerotic plaques in the four major epicardial coronary arteries in acute myocardial infarction and in sudden coronary death. Circulation 1989; 80(6): 1747–56.

67. Kragel AH, Reddy SG, Wittes JT, Roberts WC. Morphometric analysis of the composition of coronary arterial plaques in isolated unstable angina pectoris with pain at rest. Am J Cardiol 1990; 66(5):562–7.

68. Wilson PW, D'Agostino RB, Levy D et al. Prediction of coronary heart disease using risk factor categories. Circulation 1998; 97(18):1837–47.

69. Executive Summary of The Third Report of The National Cholesterol Education Program (NCEP)

Expert Panel on Detection, Evaluation, And Treatment of High Blood Cholesterol In Adults (Adult Treatment Panel III). JAMA 2001; 285(19):2486–97.

70. Greenland P, Knoll MD, Stamler J et al. Major risk factors as antecedents of fatal and nonfatal coronary heart disease events. JAMA 2003; 290(7):891–7.

71. Kondos GT, Hoff JA, Sevrukov A et al. Electron-beam tomography coronary artery calcium and cardiac events: a 37-month follow-up of 5635 initially asymptomatic low- to intermediate-risk adults. Circulation 2003; 107(20):2571–6.

The molecular basics of vulnerable plaque

3

Esther Lutgens, Tim Leiner, Robert-Jan van Suylen, and Mat JAP Daemen

INTRODUCTION

Complications of atherosclerotic plaque rupture such as myocardial infarction and stroke are the leading cause of death and disability in the developed world. Despite our familiarity with the clinical aspects of this disease, and the considerable insights into the microanatomic and histologic substrates underlying vulnerable and ruptured atherosclerotic plaques, precise molecular mechanisms are just beginning to be unraveled.

In the past few years, it has become clear that the transition from stable plaques to vulnerable plaques and subsequent plaque rupture involves a complex interplay between different pathways. To make things even more complex, pathways that are involved on the local 'plaque' level also contribute to destabilization of the plaque on a systemic level.

This chapter first focuses on the definition of a vulnerable plaque on a histologic basis and, subsequently, on the most important pathways known to induce plaque vulnerability. Their actions on both the plaque and systemic level will be discussed. These pathways comprise:

- the immune system
- extracellular matrix turnover
- coagulation.

MORPHOLOGIC AND HISTOLOGIC CHARACTERISTICS OF A VULNERABLE PLAQUE

During the last decades, it has become clear that the morphologic substrate of a vulnerable atherosclerotic plaque is not dependent on the degree of stenosis or the size of the plaque, but on plaque composition. It is mostly the modest stenotic plaques, angiographically interpreted as mild irregularities of the arterial wall, that are the anatomic substrates of clinical complications of atherosclerosis.[1]

Histologic characteristics of vulnerable plaques are (Figure 3.1a,b):[1]

1. A large lipid core.
2. A low number of plaque smooth muscle cells (SMCs) and a low collagen content of the fibrous cap.
3. The presence of enhanced inflammation within the shoulder region and fibrous cap region, characterized by an increased number of macrophages and T lymphocytes.
4. The presence of intraplaque capillaries and intraplaque hemorrhages.

Moreover, the likelihood of plaque rupture and subsequent clinical complications increases when the plaque surface is thrombogenic, because of flow disturbances due to stenosis and/or when the patient has a systemic thrombotic propensity.[2,3]

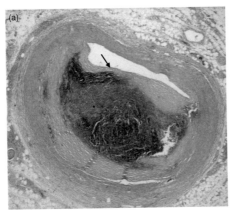
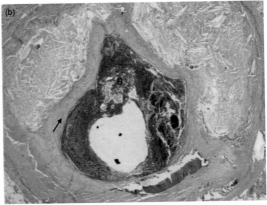

Figure 3.1   Left ascending coronary arteries containing vulnerable plaques. (a) The thin fibrous cap (arrow), as well as the large intraplaque hemorrhage (asterisk), can be appreciated. (b) The thin fibrous cap (arrow), as well as the large lipid core (asterisk), are shown. B is barium contrast reagent, which is used for postmortem angiography.

MOLECULAR MECHANISMS OF PLAQUE VULNERABILITY

Inflammation and the immune system

Inflammation and plaque vulnerability: general

Atherosclerosis is considered a chronic inflammatory disease. Even before the first histologic substrates of atherosclerosis become apparent, activation of the endothelium by shear stress or oxidative stress has already elicited the inflammatory process.[4] Endothelial cells express leukocyte adhesion molecules, and most cells present in the arterial wall are capable of secreting chemokines, thereby recruiting immune cells such as macrophages, dendritic cells, T and B lymphocytes, natural killer (NK) cells, mast cells, and polymorphonuclear cells (PMNs) into the vascular wall. Once trapped in the intima, both the acquired and innate immune systems start to work and recruit more and more immune cells to form the body of the plaque.[5] The chemokines and cytokines present in atherosclerotic plaques are especially important for regulating inflammatory and immune responses, and have crucial functions in controlling both innate and adaptive immunity.[6]

This continuous recruitment of cells and activation of immune cells make the plaque more vulnerable. A positive correlation between the presence of activated immune cells, and the occurrence of atherosclerotic plaque rupture,[7] was observed. Moreover, a broad spectrum of inflammatory mediators such as leukocyte adhesion molecules (P- and E-selectin, intercellular adhesion molecule [ICAM], vascular cell adhesion molecule [VCAM]), chemokines (monocyte chemoattractant protein-1 [MCP-1], chemokine (C-C motif) receptor-2 [CCR2], interleukin-8 [IL-8], CXCR3, CX3CR1), cytokines (granulocyte–macrophage colony-stimulating factor, interleukins IL-1, IL-6, and IL-18, tumor necrosis factor-α [TNF-α], interferon-γ [IFN-γ], CD40, CD40L), and C-reactive protein (CRP) are expressed in human atherosclerotic lesions,[4,5,8] and most of these show increased expression at sites of plaque rupture. Intervention-studies in atherosclerotic mouse models, in which one of these molecules, such as P-selectin,[9] ICAM-1,[9] GM-CSF,[10] or IL-1β,[11] was inhibited (genetically or pharmacologic), showed a decrease in plaque progression. Moreover, after inhibition of CD40L,[12–15] IFN-γ,[16] IL-18,[17] MCP-1,[18] CCR-2,[19] CXCR2,[20] and CX3CR1,[21] a change of plaque composition towards a collagen-rich, stable plaque phenotype with a relative paucity of inflammatory cells and lipids was observed.

Actions of the immune system in the induction of plaque vulnerability

The innate immune system in atherosclerosis
The first line of defense in the inflammatory response is formed by the innate immune system in which endothelial cells, SMCs, and macrophages are stimulated to produce a variety of chemokines, cytokines, and adhesion molecules that enhance the inflammatory response by recruiting immune cells into the vascular wall (Figure 3.2). The mechanism by which

they do that is largely unknown, but it is clear that pattern recognition receptors such as scavenger receptors and Toll-like receptors (TLRs) play a major role.[22] For example, oxidized low-density lipoprotein (oxLDL) is taken up by macrophages via scavenger receptors, thereby transforming macrophages into foam cells.[23] These macrophage foam cells are generally activated and proatherogenic in nature. Another example is the activation of Toll-like receptors by pathogen-associated molecular patterns (PAMPs). Different TLRs recognize a whole spectrum of antigens like lipopolysaccharide (LPS), oxLDL, flagellin, and peptidoglycan. After recognition, nuclear factor-kappa B (NF-κB) signaling is elicited, thereby

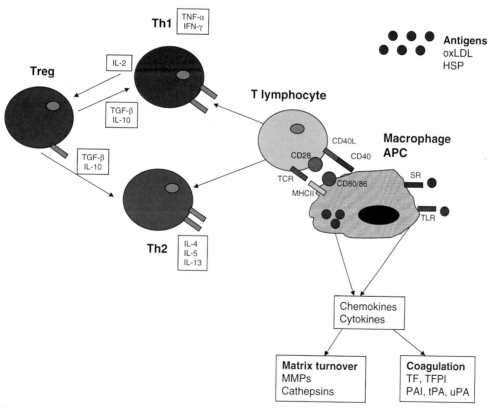

Figure 3.2 Both the innate and acquired immune system play a role in the activation of proatherogenic pathways. Antigens, like oxLDL and HSP, are able to activate macrophages by binding to scavenger receptors (SR) and Toll-like receptors (TLR). Moreover, interaction between macrophages and T lymphocytes fine-tunes the inflammatory response by generating a Th1-, Th2- or regulatory T-cell response.

initiating atherosclerosis.[24] In particular, TLR4, the receptor for LPS, is associated with atherosclerotic plaque progression.[25]

The acquired immune system

In atherosclerosis, the innate and acquired immune systems constantly interact with each other. Adaptive immunity develops when specific molecular epitopes on antigens are recognized by antigen receptors with high specificity and affinity, such as T- and B-cell receptors (TCRs and BCRs). Activation of the acquired immune system is accomplished through direct cell–cell interactions with elements of the innate immune system or indirectly by their secreted substances (see Figure 3.2). For example, macrophages that internalize oxLDL particles are capable of presenting the internalized antigens in major histocompatibility complex class II (MHCII) molecules to the acquired immune cells (T lymphocytes), thereby linking the innate immune response to the acquired immune response.[5] Moreover, chemokines, cytokines, and adhesion molecules that are expressed by cells of the innate immune system are able to recruit cells of the acquired immune system, such as T and B lymphocytes in the atherosclerotic lesion.[5]

An important role for the adaptive immune system in atherosclerosis has been shown in the last decade. In experimental animal models, it was shown that the adaptive immune system plays a role in atherosclerotic plaque initiation, but that it is even more important in atherosclerotic plaque progression, and consequently in the transition from stable to vulnerable atherosclerotic plaques. The first results were obtained in the spontaneous murine models for immunodeficiency: the SCID (scid/scid) mouse and the nude (nu/nu) mouse, which lack functional T and B lymphocytes or do not have a thymus, respectively. These mice were backcrossed to atherosclerotic ApoE−/− or LDLR−/− mice, and showed a hampered atherosclerotic lesion progression.[26,27] These results were confirmed in atherosclerotic mouse models that were backcrossed to RAG−/− mice, which lack a gene needed for the TCR or BCR rearrangement and therefore are deficient for mature T and B lymphocytes.[28]

T lymphocytes

Atherosclerotic plaques, especially vulnerable lesions, contain an extensive inflammatory infiltrate. This infiltrate consists predominantly of CD4+ T lymphocytes (Th lymphocytes). Activated Th lymphocytes are mainly found in the vicinity of macrophages or smooth muscle cells, which express MHCII molecules (HLA-DR) as well as co-stimulatory molecules (CD28 on Th lymphocytes, CD80/86 on the APC).[5,7] The interaction between MHCII and TCRs, and the subsequent activation of co-stimulatory molecules, lead to the generation of effector T lymphocytes that elicit either a Th1 or Th2 response.[6] Another system that, among many other functions, is important for the communication between T lymphocytes and other immune cells is the CD40–CD40L system. CD40–CD40L interactions have been shown to induce co-stimulatory molecules, direct the T-cell effector response towards a Th1 response and be responsible for T-lymphocyte-dependent B-lymphocyte activation.[29]

That Th cells play an important role in atherosclerotic plaque progression was shown by the observation that transfer of CD4+ cells in atherosclerotic mice aggravated atherosclerotic plaque progression.[30] Also, the co-stimulatory molecules, as well as the CD40–CD40L system, seem to be crucial in atherosclerosis development, progression, and the transition from stable to vulnerable plaques: inhibition of either CD80/86[31] or CD40L in experimental models reduces atherosclerosis and/or induces a more stable plaque phenotype.[12,13,15,32]

In atherosclerotic lesions, there is a delicate balance between actions of Th1 and Th2 response. The Th1 response, induced by IL-12 and characterized by the cytokines IFN-γ, IL-1, and TNF-α, is considered proatherogenic, whereas the Th2 response, characterized by the cytokines IL-4, IL-5, and IL-10, in general plays an antiatherogenic role. This has been confirmed by studies that show that inhibition of IFN-γ, TNF-α, or IL-12 reduces atherosclerosis and plaque vulnerability, whereas reduction of IL-10 enhances atherosclerotic plaque vulnerability.[33-36] However, deficiency in IL-4 decreases atherosclerotic lesion formation, and Th2 responses, when unbalanced, may also promote atherosclerosis.[34]

A more recently identified subset of T lymphocytes with regulatory activities, named regulatory T (Treg) cells, is believed to be central to the prevention of autoimmune and chronic inflammatory diseases, including atherosclerosis. Treg cells mediate their effects via immunosuppressive cytokines IL-10 and transforming growth factor-β (TGF-β), or by contact-dependent mechanisms, via IL-2 and CD25. Indeed, recently it has been shown that both subsets of regulatory T cells are crucial in preventing atherosclerotic lesion development and progression.[37]

Not only T lymphocytes but also B lymphocytes are involved in the progression of atherosclerosis. B lymphocytes are present in atherosclerotic plaques, and deficiency of B cells in atherosclerotic mouse models increases atherosclerotic lesion size, whereas B-cell transfer seems to protect against atherosclerosis.[38,39] However, it is still not clear how this protective effect is accomplished: whether it is by cell–cell interaction or by secreted inflammatory mediators or antibodies. Interestingly, there seems to be a positive correlation between the presence of circulating antibodies against oxLDL, heat-shock protein HSP60, and β2GPI and the risk for the development of cardiovascular

disease.[5,6] Moreover, vaccination of experimental animal models against these and other antigens showed a clear protective effect in the initiation and progression of atherosclerotic lesions.[5]

Systemic parameters of inflammation and cardiovascular risk

Although the levels of circulating cytokines do not necessarily reflect the actual activity of a cytokine, a variety of plasma inflammatory markers have been shown to predict future cardiovascular risk. Elevated levels of the inflammatory markers CRP, P-selectin, soluble ICAM-1 (sICAM-1), sVCAM, IL-6, TNF-α, IL-18, and sCD40L have been shown to predict future cardiovascular risk in a variety of clinical settings. Although most of these inflammatory markers are derived from the liver (CRP, IL-6), low levels may also be derived from other sources, including adipose tissue, activated endothelium, and the plaque itself.[40] Interestingly, patients already suffering from a chronic inflammatory (autoimmune) disease such as human immunodeficiency virus (HIV), systemic lupus erythematosus (SLE), and rheumatoid arthritis are more vulnerable to develop advanced, vulnerable atherosclerotic lesions, reflected by the increased risk for cardiovascular complications.[41-43]

Extracellular matrix turnover

In addition to immune cells, atherosclerotic plaques contain a significant amount of extracellular matrix. A high amount of extracellular matrix generally reflects a stable atherosclerotic plaque, whereas a reduced extracellular matrix content is associated with plaque vulnerability. The extracellular matrix of an atherosclerotic plaque is a highly active biologic structure. The fibrous cap, containing most of the extracellular matrix proteins, contains many connective tissue matrix proteins, particularly collagen I and III, but also elastin and proteoglycans.[1] These components are produced by vascular smooth muscle cells. Interactions between the immune system and SMCs and (myo)-fibroblasts regulate the synthesis and breakdown of the extracellular matrix components of the atherosclerotic plaque.[3,4]

The fibrous cap is the only structure separating the highly thrombogenic lipid core from the circulating blood with its thrombus-forming elements. Fibrous caps are believed to be important for the mechanical strength and stability of the plaque.[1]

Profibrotic molecules, such as TGF-β, contribute to formation of the fibrous cap, whereas proteolytic enzymes secreted by macrophages and other cells are capable of degrading the extracellular matrix.[4] Until now, two major families of enzymes are known to participate: matrix metalloproteinases (MMPs), and cysteine proteases such as cathepsins.

Matrix metalloproteinases

The MMPs are a family of proteinases that have a comparable structure but differ in their substrate preference. Interstitial collagenase (MMP-1) cleaves collagen, making the collagen fragments susceptible to further proteolysis by the gelatinases (MMP-2 and MMP-9). Stromelysins (MMP-3) are capable of digesting elastin and degrading core proteins of proteoglycans. MMP-1, -2, -3, -7, -8, -9, -12, -14 (MT-MMP1), and -16, as well as their specific inhibitors, such as the tissue inhibitors of MMPs (TIMPs), are all expressed in human atherosclerotic lesions, and mostly in the vulnerable shoulder region, suggesting an important role in inducing plaque vulnerability and rupture.[44] The MMPs are secreted in a latent zymogen form, lacking enzymatic activity and require extracellular activation to attain their enzymatic function. The activation of pro-MMPs can be produced by plasmin, tryptase, chymase,

oxidant stress, and oxLDL. The regulation of MMP gene expression is not fully understood, but it is known that proteolytic activity is driven by inflammatory activity and immunoregulation in the plaque.[44] Various cytokines, such as IFN-γ, TNF-α, IL-1, and macrophage colony-stimulating factor (M-CSF), as well as CD40 and CD40L, are known to enhance MMP expression in both macrophages and SMCs.[4,45]

Interestingly, polymorphisms in the MMP-1, -2, -7, -9, -12 and -13 genes are associated with an increased risk on cardiovascular events.[46] Moreover, elevated circulating MMP-3 levels also predict cardiovascular risk.[47]

Cathepsins

The lysosomal cysteine proteases or cathepsins recently received a lot of interest in the vascular field. Cathepsins were originally known to localize in endosomes and lysosomes where they degrade intracellular or endocytosed proteins. Now we know that they can function outside lysosomes and endosomes, and that they are strong elastases and collagenases.[48] Recently, large-scale gene expression studies indicated differential expression of cathepsin B, L, S, and H mRNA in atherosclerotic arteries. Moreover, cathepsin S, D, F, K, L, and V proteins were present in human atheromata. Interestingly, these cysteine proteases accounted for 40% of the total elastase activity of human atheroma extracts.[48] In particular, cathepsin S and cathepsin K are strongly expressed in atherosclerotic plaques.[49] Genetic disruption of cathepsin S and cathepsin K in atherosclerotic mouse models was able to reduce the extent and progression of atherosclerotic plaques,[50,51] whereas deficiency of cystatin C, the naturally occurring athepsin inhibitor, aggravated atherosclerotic disease.[52] ApoE−/− mice deficient in cathepsin K developed a fibrotic plaque phenotype, but also increased the scavenger-mediated oxLDL uptake, suggesting a dual role for cathepsin K in atherosclerosis development and progression.[51] Interestingly, as with many proteases, the activity of cathepsins is tightly regulated by cytokine and growth factor expression by macrophages and SMCs of the atherosclerotic plaque. Moreover, cathepsin S is also involved in antigen presentation by MHCII, thereby directly contributing to ongoing immune response in the atherosclerotic lesion.[53]

In patients suffering from cardiovascular disease, cathepsin S serum levels are elevated,[54] whereas cystatin C levels do not seem to correlate with atherosclerotic disease.[55]

Coagulation

The third major system responsible for inducing plaque vulnerability and plaque rupture is the coagulation system. Many factors of the coagulation cascade, such as tissue factor (TF) and the tissue factor pathway inhibitor, prothrombin, antithrombin III, tissue-type plasminogen activator (tPA), urokinase-type plasminogen activator (uPA), and plasminogen activator inhibitor (PAI) are highly expressed in advanced human atherosclerotic lesions and are abundant at sites of plaque rupture.[56] In particular, lipid cores in advanced atherosclerotic lesions, but also extracellular matrix constituents such as collagens and proteoglycans, are highly thrombogenic: i.e the lipid core is known to be rich in macrophage-derived tissue factor. TF is a key initiating factor in the coagulation cascade, promoting thrombosis through its ability to stimulate thrombin generation by augmenting factor VII (FVII) and factor Xa activity.[57] The expression of pro- and anticoagulant factors in the plaque is partly regulated by cytokines. For example, IL-1, TNF-α, and CD40L can induce TF expression in macrophages, endothelial cells (ECs), and

SMCs.[57] Furthermore, IL-1α and TNF-α can enhance the expression of PAI-1,[58] whereas IFN-γ has the opposite effect.[58]

Disruption of the fibrous cap occurs frequently during the development of atherosclerosis and in most cases does not cause a significant event such as myocardial infarction or death.[59] However, it is likely to be the main mechanism in sudden and rapid plaque progression, thereby inducing plaque vulnerability.[59] Fibrous cap disruption is followed by variable amounts of luminal thrombus and/or hemorrhage into the necrotic core, causing rapid growth of the lesion. In patients with coronary atheroma who died suddenly of non-cardiac causes, 14% had histologic evidence of previous rupture and thrombosis episodes based on finding healed hemorrhage in or thrombus on the plaque. This is supported by data demonstrating that more than 70% of stenotic plaques have had a subclinical episode of plaque rupture followed by healing.[1]

Although the phenomenon of intraplaque hemorrhage greatly contributes to plaque vulnerability, other less well-identified mechanisms elicited by the coagulation cascade contribute to initiation and progression of atherosclerotic plaques. Platelets are known to adhere already in the first stages of plaque development. Moreover, platelets are able to form platelet–leukocyte aggregates that trigger the inflammatory response, thereby probably contributing to atherosclerotic plaque progression. In ApoE−/− mice, repeated injection of activated platelets resulted in the formation of platelet–leukocyte aggregates, and in the exacerbation of atherosclerotic plaque progression.[60]

An interesting role for apoptosis in plaque thrombogenicity has recently been discovered. Shed membrane particles, rich in phosphatidylserine, are released in the serum as microparticles and are procoagulant; they are associated with an increased risk for cardiovascular complications.[61]

Interestingly, many serum markers that predict cardiovascular risk are associated with the coagulation cascade. Increased serum levels of fibrinogen, von Willebrand factor (vWF), PAI-1, TF and tPA indicate an increased risk of cardiovascular events.[3]

CONCLUSION

As described above, atherosclerosis has a complex etiology that involves interplay among major regulatory systems such as the immune system and inflammation, matrix turnover, and coagulation. Although many of these interactions have been unraveled in recent decades, precise mechanisms of many aspects of atherosclerosis, such as the transition of stable to vulnerable atherosclerotic lesions, are still unknown.

Until now, we only have a limited panel of serum markers that are correlated with an increased risk of (recurrent) cardiovascular disease (i.e. the presence of vulnerable or ruptured plaques). These serum makers are mostly members of the three major systems (immune system, matrix turnover, and coagulation), as described above. However, the increased relative risk for these serum markers is only modest, and it is impossible to identify individual risk profiles for each patient based on these serum markers. An interesting development is the search for novel biomarkers of plaque vulnerability by comparing antibody profiles in serum of patients with known stable atherosclerotic plaques vs serum of patients with known vulnerable plaques. In the future, this screening method will hopefully generate novel (combinations of) serum markers that give a high predictive value for an increased cardiovascular risk for the individual patient.

Also, the treatment options for patients with plaque vulnerability are rather limited. Besides 3-hydroxy-3-methylglutaryl coenzyme A (HMG-CoA) reductase inhibitors, platelet aggregation inhibitors, and several other classes of drugs, which have a broad-spectrum effect on the immune system, matrix turnover, and/or coagulation, no other therapy is available to prevent vulnerable plaques from rupturing. However, in the genomics and proteomics era, comparing plaque tissue representing several stages of atherosclerosis will generate novel insights into the pathogenesis of atherosclerosis, as well as more specific therapeutic targets, when the correct statistics and pathway-profiling tools are used.[62]

Another interesting development is the development of a novel screening tool: molecular imaging. By coupling known and novel markers of plaque vulnerability to imaging agents, vulnerable plaques can become visible and the patient can be identified and treated accordingly.[63]

REFERENCES

1. Virmani R, Kolodgie FD, Burke AP, Farb A, Schwartz SM. Lessons from sudden coronary death: a comprehensive morphological classification scheme for atherosclerotic lesions. Arterioscler Thromb Vasc Biol 2000; 20:1262–75.
2. Maseri A, Fuster V. Is there a vulnerable plaque? Circulation 2003; 107:2068–71.
3. Libby P, Theroux P. Pathophysiology of coronary artery disease. Circulation 2005; 111:3481–8.
4. Ross R. Atherosclerosis – an inflammatory disease. N Engl J Med 1999; 340:115–26.
5. Hansson GK. Inflammation, atherosclerosis, and coronary artery disease. N Engl J Med 2005; 352:1685–95.
6. Tedgui A, Mallat Z. Cytokines in atherosclerosis: pathogenic and regulatory pathways. Physiol Rev 2006; 86:515–81.
7. van der Wal AC, Becker AE, van der Loos CM, Das PK. Site of intimal rupture or erosion of thrombosed coronary atherosclerotic plaques is characterized by an inflammatory process irrespective of the dominant plaque morphology. Circulation 1994; 89:36–44.
8. Glass CK, Witztum JL. Atherosclerosis: the road ahead. Cell 2001; 104:503–16.
9. Collins RG, Velji R, Guevara NV et al. P-Selectin or intercellular adhesion molecule (ICAM)-1 deficiency substantially protects against atherosclerosis in apolipoprotein E-deficient mice. J Exp Med 2000; 191:189–94.

10. Qiao JH, Tripathi J, Mishra NK et al. Role of macrophage colony-stimulating factor in atherosclerosis: studies of osteopetrotic mice. Am J Pathol 1997; 150:1687–99.

11. Kirii H, Niwa T, Yamada Y et al. Lack of interleukin-1beta decreases the severity of atherosclerosis in ApoE-deficient mice. Arterioscler Thromb Vasc Biol 2003; 23:656–60.

12. Lutgens E, Gorelik L, Daemen MJ et al. Requirement for CD154 in the progression of atherosclerosis. Nat Med 1999; 5:1313–16.

13. Lutgens E, Cleutjens KB, Heeneman S et al. Both early and delayed anti-CD40L antibody treatment induces a stable plaque phenotype. Proc Natl Acad Sci USA 2000; 97:7464–9.

14. Mach F, Schonbeck U, Sukhova GK, Atkinson E, Libby P. Reduction of atherosclerosis in mice by inhibition of CD40 signalling. Nature 1998; 394:200–3.

15. Schonbeck U, Sukhova GK, Shimizu K, Mach F, Libby P. Inhibition of CD40 signaling limits evolution of established atherosclerosis in mice. Proc Natl Acad Sci USA 2000; 97:7458–63.

16. Buono C, Come CE, Stavrakis G et al. Influence of interferon-gamma on the extent and phenotype of diet-induced atherosclerosis in the LDLR-deficient mouse. Arterioscler Thromb Vasc Biol 2003; 23:454–60.

17. Mallat Z, Corbaz A, Scoazec A et al. Interleukin-18/interleukin-18 binding protein signaling modulates atherosclerotic lesion development and stability. Circ Res 2001; 89:E41–5.

18. Lutgens E, Faber B, Schapira K et al. Gene profiling in atherosclerosis reveals a key role for small inducible cytokines: validation using a novel monocyte chemoattractant protein monoclonal antibody. Circulation 2005; 111:3443–52.

19. Dawson TC, Kuziel WA, Osahar TA, Maeda N. Absence of CC chemokine receptor-2 reduces atherosclerosis in apolipoprotein E-deficient mice. Atherosclerosis 1999; 143:205–11.

20. Boisvert WA, Santiago R, Curtiss LK, Terkeltaub RA. A leukocyte homologue of the IL-8 receptor CXCR-2 mediates the accumulation of macrophages in atherosclerotic lesions of LDL receptor-deficient mice. J Clin Invest 1998; 101:353–63.

21. Lesnik P, Haskell CA, Charo IF. Decreased atherosclerosis in CX3CR1−/− mice reveals a role for fractalkine in atherogenesis. J Clin Invest 2003; 111:333–40.

22. Getz GS. Thematic review series: the immune system and atherogenesis. Immune function in atherogenesis. J Lipid Res 2005; 46:1–10.

23. de Winther MP, van Dijk KW, Havekes LM, Hofker MH. Macrophage scavenger receptor class A: a multifunctional receptor in atherosclerosis. Arterioscler Thromb Vasc Biol 2000; 20:290–7.

24. Michelsen KS, Doherty TM, Shah PK, Arditi M. Role of Toll-like receptors in atherosclerosis. Circ Res 2004; 95:e96–7.

25. Michelsen KS, Wong MH, Shah PK et al. Lack of Toll-like receptor 4 or myeloid differentiation factor 88 reduces atherosclerosis and alters plaque phenotype in mice deficient in apolipoprotein E. Proc Natl Acad Sci USA 2004; 101:10679–84.

26. Fyfe AI, Qiao JH, Lusis AJ. Immune-deficient mice develop typical atherosclerotic fatty streaks when fed an atherogenic diet. J Clin Invest 1994; 94:2516–20.

27. Emeson EE, Shen ML, Bell CG, Qureshi A. Inhibition of atherosclerosis in CD4 T-cell-ablated and nude (nu/nu) C57BL/6 hyperlipidemic mice. Am J Pathol 1996; 149:675–85.

28. Song L, Leung C, Schindler C. Lymphocytes are important in early atherosclerosis. J Clin Invest 2001; 108:251–9.

29. Foy TM, Aruffo A, Bajorath J, Buhlmann JE, Noelle RJ. Immune regulation by CD40 and its ligand GP39. Annu Rev Immunol 1996; 14:591–617.

30. Zhou X, Robertson AK, Hjerpe C, Hansson GK. Adoptive transfer of CD4+ T cells reactive to modified low-density lipoprotein aggravates atherosclerosis. Arterioscler Thromb Vasc Biol 2006; 26:864–70.

31. Buono C, Pang H, Uchida Y et al. B7–1/B7–2 costimulation regulates plaque antigen-specific T-cell responses and atherogenesis in low-density lipoprotein receptor-deficient mice. Circulation 2004; 109:2009–15.

32. Mach F, Schonbeck U, Libby P. CD40 signaling in vascular cells: a key role in atherosclerosis? Atherosclerosis 1998; 137 (Suppl):S89–95.

33. Gupta S, Pablo AM, Jiang X et al. IFN-gamma potentiates atherosclerosis in ApoE knock-out mice. J Clin Invest 1997; 99:2752–61.

34. Davenport P, Tipping PG. The role of interleukin-4 and interleukin-12 in the progression of atherosclerosis in apolipoprotein E-deficient mice. Am J Pathol 2003; 163:1117–25.

35. Ohta H, Wada H, Niwa T et al. Disruption of tumor necrosis factor-alpha gene diminishes the development of atherosclerosis in ApoE-deficient mice. Atherosclerosis 2005; 180:11–17.

36. Mallat Z, Besnard S, Duriez M et al. Protective role of interleukin-10 in atherosclerosis. Circ Res 1999; 85:e17–24.

37. Ait-Oufella H, Salomon BL, Potteaux S et al. Natural regulatory T cells control the development of atherosclerosis in mice. Nat Med 2006; 12:178–80.

38. Major AS, Fazio S, Linton MF. B-lymphocyte deficiency increases atherosclerosis in LDL receptor-null mice. Arterioscler Thromb Vasc Biol 2002; 22:1892–8.

39. Caligiuri G, Nicoletti A, Poirier B, Hansson GK. Protective immunity against atherosclerosis carried by B cells of hypercholesterolemic mice. J Clin Invest 2002; 109:745–53.

40. Willerson JT, Ridker PM. Inflammation as a cardiovascular risk factor. Circulation 2004; 109:II2–10.

41. de Saint Martin L, Vandhuick O, Guillo P et al. Premature atherosclerosis in HIV positive patients

and cumulated time of exposure to antiretroviral therapy (SHIVA study). Atherosclerosis 2006; 185: 361–7.

42. Ohlenschlaeger T, Garred P, Madsen HO, Jacobsen S. Mannose-binding lectin variant alleles and the risk of arterial thrombosis in systemic lupus erythematosus. N Engl J Med 2004; 351:260–7.

43. Roman MJ, Moeller E, Davis A et al. Preclinical carotid atherosclerosis in patients with rheumatoid arthritis. Ann Intern Med 2006; 144:249–56.

44. Newby AC, Pauschinger M, Spinale FG. From tadpole tails to transgenic mice: metalloproteinases have brought about a metamorphosis in our understanding of cardiovascular disease. Cardiovasc Res 2006; 69:559–61.

45. Libby P. Inflammation in atherosclerosis. Nature 2002; 420:868–74.

46. Ye S. Influence of matrix metalloproteinase genotype on cardiovascular disease susceptibility and outcome. Cardiovasc Res 2006; 69:636–45.

47. Wu TC, Leu HB, Lin WT et al. Plasma matrix metalloproteinase-3 level is an independent prognostic factor in stable coronary artery disease. Eur J Clin Invest 2005; 35:537–45.

48. Liu J, Sukhova GK, Sun JS et al. Lysosomal cysteine proteases in atherosclerosis. Arterioscler Thromb Vasc Biol 2004; 24:1359–66.

49. Sukhova GK, Shi GP, Simon DI, Chapman HA, Libby P. Expression of the elastolytic cathepsins S and K in human atheroma and regulation of their production in smooth muscle cells. J Clin Invest 1998; 102:576–83.

50. Sukhova GK, Zhang Y, Pan JH et al. Deficiency of cathepsin S reduces atherosclerosis in LDL receptor-deficient mice. J Clin Invest 2003; 111:897–906.

51. Lutgens E, Lutgens SP, Faber BC et al. Disruption of the cathepsin K gene reduces atherosclerosis progression and induces plaque fibrosis but accelerates macrophage foam cell formation. Circulation 2006; 113:98–107.

52. Sukhova GK, Wang B, Libby P et al. Cystatin C deficiency increases elastic lamina degradation and aortic dilatation in apolipoprotein E-null mice. Circ Res 2005; 96:368–75.

53. Kitamura H, Kamon H, Sawa S et al. IL-6-STAT3 controls intracellular MHC class II alphabeta dimer level through cathepsin S activity in dendritic cells. Immunity 2005; 23:491–502.

54. Liu J, Ma L, Yang J et al. Increased serum cathepsin S in patients with atherosclerosis and diabetes. Atherosclerosis 2006; 186:411–19.

55. Loew M, Hoffmann MM, Koenig W, Brenner H, Rothenbacher D. Genotype and plasma concentration of cystatin C in patients with coronary heart disease and risk for secondary cardiovascular events. Arterioscler Thromb Vasc Biol 2005; 25:1470–4.

56. Lutgens E, van Suylen RJ, Faber BC et al. Atherosclerotic plaque rupture: local or systemic process? Arterioscler Thromb Vasc Biol 2003; 23:2123–30.

57. Steffel J, Luscher TF, Tanner FC. Tissue factor in cardiovascular diseases: molecular mechanisms and clinical implications. Circulation 2006; 113:722–31.

58. Gallicchio M, Hufnagl P, Wojta J, Tipping P. IFN-gamma inhibits thrombin- and endotoxin-induced plasminogen activator inhibitor type 1 in human endothelial cells. J Immunol 1996; 157:2610–17.

59. Burke AP, Kolodgie FD, Farb A et al. Healed plaque ruptures and sudden coronary death: evidence that subclinical rupture has a role in plaque progression. Circulation 2001; 103:934–40.

60. Huo Y, Schober A, Forlow SB et al. Circulating activated platelets exacerbate atherosclerosis in mice deficient in apolipoprotein E. Nat Med 2003; 9:61–7.

61. Morel O, Hugel B, Jesel L et al. Circulating procoagulant microparticles and soluble GPV in myocardial infarction treated by primary percutaneous transluminal coronary angioplasty. A possible role for GPIIb-IIIa antagonists. J Thromb Haemost 2004; 2:1118–26.

62. Bijnens AP, Lutgens E, Ayoubi T et al. Genome-wide expression studies of atherosclerosis: critical issues in methodology, analysis, and interpretation of transcriptomics data. Arterioscler Thromb Vasc Biol 2006; 26:1226–35.

63. Raggi P, Taylor A, Fayad Z et al. Atherosclerotic plaque imaging: contemporary role in preventive cardiology. Arch Intern Med 2005; 165:2345–53.

Platelets and the vulnerable plaque

4

Marc Sirol, Juan F Viles-Gonzalez, and Juan J Badimon

INTRODUCTION

Platelets are blood cell fragments that originate from the cytoplasm of megakaryocytes in the bone marrow and circulate in blood. Although platelets were once considered to be merely passive participants in the coagulation cascade – just anucleate cells with a transient existence – they are now recognized as active synthesizers of humoral factors that potentiate both clot formation and inflammation. Platelets play a major role in the hemostatic process and in thrombus formation after an endothelial injury. Recent studies have provided insight into their functions in the onset of acute coronary syndromes (ACS), inflammation, and atherosclerosis. A range of molecules, present on the platelet surface and/or stored in platelet granules, contribute to the cross-talk of platelets with other inflammatory cells during the vascular inflammation involved in the development and progression of atherosclerosis. Platelets play a crucial role in plaque vulnerability. This chapter discusses the nature of these molecules and the mechanisms involved in the participation of platelets in atherosclerosis, with emphasis on vulnerable plaques and the role played by P-selectin, platelet–monocyte interactions, chemokines, and inflammatory cytokines.

ROLE OF PLATELETS

The normal function of platelets is to arrest bleeding from wounds, which requires adhesion to altered vascular surfaces and rapid cellular activation with the ensuing accumulation of additional platelets and fibrin into a growing thrombus. Platelets, with fibrin, are prominent components of the thrombi that occlude arteries, but may also participate in the development and progression of the atherosclerotic plaque.

Platelets are biologically active cells that play a critical role in homeostasis, thrombosis, the onset of ACS, inflammation, and atherosclerosis. The early phase of atherosclerosis starts with platelet activation. It may be attributed to reactive oxygen species generated by atherosclerosis risk factors, including superoxide, hydroxyl radical, and peroxynitrite. Reduction in endothelial antithrombotic properties such as production of nitric oxide, prostacyclin, and CD39, an ecto-ADPase that degrades ADP, have been also implicated. Additionally, an increase in prothrombotic and proinflammatory mediators, including tissue factor (TF) and chemokines in the circulation or immobilized on the endothelium, seems to play an important role. Interestingly, most risk factors of atherosclerosis – including hypercholesterolemia,[1] hypertension,[2] cigarette smoking, and diabetes[3] – are able to increase the number of activated platelets in circulation (Box 4.1). Furthermore, following formation of lesions on the vessel wall, platelet activation may be initiated by ligation of

---

Box 4.1   Factors modulating thrombus formation

Nature of the exposed substrate
- Degree of injury (mild vs severe arterial injury)
- Composition of atherosclerotic plaque
- Residual mural thrombus

Local fluid dynamics
- Shear stress
- Tensile stress

Systemic thrombogenic factors
- Hypercholesterolemia
- Catecholamines (smoking, cocaine, stress, etc.)
- Smoking
- Diabetes
- Homocysteine
- Lipoprotein(a)
- Infections (*Chlamydia pneumonia, Helicobacter pylori*, cytomegalovirus)
- Hypercoagulable state (*fibrogen, von Willebrand factor, tissue factor, factor VII*)
- Defective fibrinolytic state, etc.

---

glycoprotein (GP) Ib with the endothelial receptor P-selectin and endothelial von Willebrand factor (vWF) during platelet tethering on intact but dysfunctional endothelium.

The initiation of arterial thrombosis starts with platelet adhesion and activation. Platelet activation is defined by P-selectin surface expression, first described in peripheral blood of patients with unstable atherosclerotic disease. The presence of circulating activated platelets preceding massive thrombotic events such as myocardial infarction or stroke may be relevant to the development and progression of atherosclerosis.

THROMBOSIS AND ATHEROSCLEROSIS

Thrombosis is the acute complication that develops on the chronic lesions of atherosclerosis and is responsible for acute myocardial infarction (MI) and stroke. The term 'atherothrombosis' is therefore preferable since it describes the combination of acute thrombotic event

and atherosclerosis, a chronic disease that begins early in childhood and affects different vascular beds. Whereas arterial thrombi are predominantly formed by platelets, venous thrombi are intravascular deposits composed predominantly of fibrin and red cells, with a variable platelet and leukocyte component. Growing thrombi may locally occlude the lumen, or embolize and be washed away by the blood flow to occlude distal vessels. However, thrombi may be physiologically and spontaneously lysed by mechanisms that block thrombus propagation. Thrombus size, location, and composition are regulated by hemodynamic forces (mechanical effects), thrombogenicity of exposed substrate (local molecular effects), relative concentration of fluid phase and cellular blood components (local cellular effects), and the efficiency of the physiologic mechanisms of control of the system, mainly fibrinolysis.[4] An intact and healthy endothelium (Figure 4.1) possesses antiatherogenic activity and normally prevents platelet activation. Intimal injury associated with endothelial denudation and plaque rupture exposes subendothelial collagen and vWF, which support prompt platelet adhesion and activation. Circulating platelets can adhere either directly to collagen or indirectly, via the binding of vWF, to the GPIb/IX complex. The present consensus is that at high-shear rate conditions, both platelet GPIb and GPIIb-IIIa appear to be involved in the events of platelet adhesion, whereas GPIIb-IIIa may be involved predominantly in platelet–platelet interaction. Local platelet activation promotes thrombus formation and additional platelet recruitment by supporting cell surface thrombin formation and releasing potent platelet agonists, perpetuating the thrombotic process. The central role of platelet activation in ACS is supported by increased platelet-derived thromboxane and prostaglandin metabolites detected in patients with ACS and

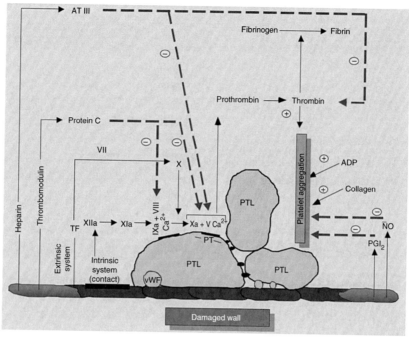

Figure 4.1   Diagram of platelet–vessel wall and platelet–platelet interaction with the participation of the coagulation and spontaneous fibrinolysis systems: continuous lines; pathways of activation; dashed lines, pathways of inhibition.

the clear clinical benefit of treatment with aspirin for prevention of acute coronary events.[5]

ATHEROTHROMBOSIS AND VULNERABLE PLAQUE

Atherosclerosis is a systemic disease involving the intima of large and medium-sized arteries, including the aorta, and the carotid, coronary, and peripheral arteries. Normal endothelium plays a pivotal role in vascular homeostasis, through the balanced production of potent vasodilators such as nitric oxide (NO) and vasoconstrictors such as endothelin-1 (ET-1), and limits the development of atherosclerosis (see Figure 4.1). Endothelial dysfunction is considered the earliest pathologic signal of atherosclerosis. Cardiovascular risk factors impair endothelial function and may trigger atherosclerosis without the need for physical endothelial injury.[6] These risk factors have been recognized

to induce endothelial dysfunction by reducing the bioavailability of NO, increasing tissue ET-1 content,[7] and activating proinflammatory signaling pathways such as nuclear factor kappa B (NF-κB).[8] The NF-κB signaling transduction pathway is an essential regulator of the transcription of a number of proinflammatory genes, such as those that lead to the expression of many cytokines, enzymes, and adhesion molecules (i.e. intercellular adhesion molecule-1, ICAM-1; vascular cell adhesion molecule-1, VCAM-1; and E-selectin).[9] In hypercholesterolemia, for example, endothelium-dependent relaxation is impaired, while contraction and adhesion of monocytes and platelets are enhanced. A recent study has demonstrated that the treatment with recombinant high-density lipoprotein (HDL) restores normal endothelial function in hypercholesterolemic patients, explaining the protective effect of HDL from ACS, and pointing out the potential role of the endothelium as a therapeutic target.[10]

Atherosclerosis is characterized by intimal thickening, owing to cellular and lipid accumulation that is due to an imbalance in lipid influx and efflux.[11,12] Secondary changes may occur in the underlying media and adventitia, particularly in advanced disease stages. Fatty streaks have been found in the intima of infants.[13] They progress to fibroatheroma by developing a cap of smooth muscle cells (SMCs) and collagen. These early atherosclerotic lesions can progress without compromising the lumen because of compensatory vascular enlargement (remodeling).[14] Importantly, the culprit lesions leading to ACS are often mildly stenotic and therefore not detectable by angiography.[15] These rupture-prone lesions usually have a large lipid core, a thin fibrous cap, and a high density of inflammatory cells, particularly at the

shoulder region, where disruptions most often occur.[16] Monocytes and macrophages are key to the development of vulnerable plaques. Macrophages produce growth, mitogenic, proinflammatory, and lytic factors that enhance the progression of atherosclerotic lesions.[17] Vulnerable plaques (type Va and VI), which are composed commonly of an abundant lipid core separated from the lumen by a thin fibrotic cap, are particularly soft and prone to disruption[12,15] (Figure 4.2). Platelets and inflammatory cells may be a source and target for inflammatory mediators.[17]

Three major factors determine the vulnerability of the fibrous cap: circumferential wall stress or cap 'fatigue,' lesion characteristics (location, size, and consistency), and blood flow characteristics.[18] Pathologic evidence suggests that a plaque must be considered vulnerable when the lipid core accounts for more than 40% of the whole. This may explain

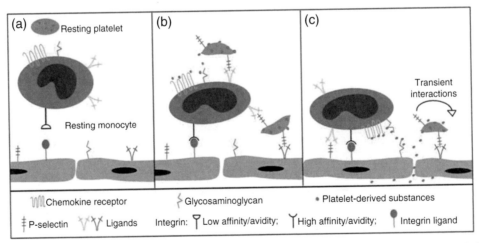

Figure 4.2 Mechanisms by which activated platelets participate in the development of atherosclerosis. (a) No interactions occur between resting platelets and monocytes. (b) Activated platelets promote monocyte recruitment via platelet–monocyte interactions. Activated platelets interacting with monocytes deliver their proinflammatory factors to monocytes. Consequently, affinity and/or avidity of monocyte integrins are up-regulated and monocytes arrest on endothelium. Additionally, monocyte–platelet aggregates may employ platelet P-selectin to mediate aggregates to interact with endothelium. (c) Activated platelets promote monocyte recruitment via platelet–endothelial interactions. Activated platelets transiently interacting with endothelium may deposit their proinflammatory factors on the surface of endothelium, causing subsequent rolling monocyte arrest. Also, platelet-derived proinflammatory factors may infiltrate into the vessel wall, triggering vascular cell proliferation, migration, and inflammation. (Adapted from Huo and Ley.[82])

the effects of lipid-lowering therapy in reducing coronary events.[12]

Plaque disruption, however, is not a purely mechanical process. Inflammation is also important.[19,20] Activated inflammatory cells have been detected in the disrupted areas of atherectomy specimens from patients with ACS.[21] These cells are capable of degrading extracellular matrix by secreting proteolytic enzymes, such as matrix metalloproteinases.[19] In addition, T cells isolated from rupture-prone sites can stimulate macrophages to produce metalloproteinases and may predispose disruption of lesions by weakening their fibrous cap.[22] Matrix metalloproteinases and their co-secreted tissue inhibitors affect vascular remodeling[19] and migration of SMCs across the basement membrane.[11,23]

Lesion thrombogenicity correlates with its TF content; furthermore, local TF inhibition reduces lesion thrombogenicity.[24] Cell apoptosis has been linked to inflammation and thrombosis via increased TF expression.[25,26] TF activity in the acellular lipid core was found mainly on apoptotic microparticles of monocytic and lymphocytic origin.[26] Recent studies have demonstrated an increased TF expression in the coronary arteries and in the plasma of patients with unstable angina or MI compared with patients with stable angina.[26] More recently, observations obtained from pathologic analysis of human coronary and carotid artery specimens showed that TF is often co-localized in macrophage apoptotic death and released microparticles rather than in biologically active macrophages. Specific inhibition of vascular TF by TF pathway inhibitor (TFPI) was associated with a significant reduction of acute thrombus formation in lipid-rich plaques.[24] Interestingly, in the pig model of arterial injury, TFPI administration during percutaneous coronary angioplasty prevented acute thrombus formation without increasing the bleeding complications, and it reduced intimal hyperplasia without affecting SMC growth.[27]

Plaque disruption and subsequent thrombus formation is responsible for the onset of ACS, the severity of which is modulated by the magnitude or stability of the thrombus.[25] In addition, successive events of plaque disruption and asymptomatic thrombus formation may be responsible for the progression of lesions.[28]

Once the plaque is disrupted, the highly thrombogenic lipid-rich core, abundant in macrophages and in TF, is exposed to the bloodstream, triggering the formation of a superimposed thrombus that leads to an acute coronary event. The disruption of lipid-rich plaques facilitates the interaction between TF and flowing blood, triggering activation of the coagulation cascade, thrombin generation, and platelet-rich thrombus formation.[29,30] The high level of thromboxane A_2 detected in coronary artery disease patients supports the role of platelets in atherothrombosis. An increase in platelet reactivity can be detected in coronary artery blood in the immediate vicinity of a disrupted plaque.[31] In addition, treatment with antiplatelet agents is beneficial among patients with ACS.[5,32]

One-third of ACS, particularly sudden death, occurs without plaque disruption but just superficial erosion of a markedly stenotic and fibrotic plaque.[25] Under such conditions, thrombus formation depends on the hyperthrombogenic state triggered by systemic factors. Indeed, systemic factors including elevated low-density lipoprotein (LDL) and decreased HDL cholesterol levels, cigarette smoking, diabetes, and hemostasis are associated with increased thrombotic complications.[28] High levels of circulating TF have been reported in patients with hyperlipidemia, diabetes, and ACS. Thus, TF is postulated as being responsible for the 'thrombogenic state'. Our group has reported an increased thrombogenicity associated with hyperlipemia as well as diabetes[33,34] that can be normalized with risk factor management.[34,35] Aside from apoptotic macrophages and microparticles from atherosclerotic plaques, activated monocytes in the circulating blood seem to be the source of TF microparticles and may represent the result of activation by the previously mentioned risk factors and others, thus contributing to thrombotic events. These observations emphasize the importance of not only the 'vulnerable' or 'high-risk' atherothrombotic lesions but also the relevance of 'hyperreactive' (vulnerable?) blood.

Platelets in atherogenesis

The pathogenesis of atherosclerosis is multifactorial, but the two aspects considered of greatest relevance are the deposition of lipids, which are then metabolized abnormally and oxidized in the vascular wall, and the local infiltration of leukocytes.[6] This creates an inflammatory environment[36] in which the function of endothelial cells (ECs) is also affected, and one of the manifestations of this alteration is an increase in the potential for interaction with other cells, including platelets.[37] A growing body of evidence highlights the interaction between platelets and ECs as a cornerstone in the initiation of atherogenesis.[38] P-selectin is considered pivotal in the interplay of platelets and ECs. If P-selectin is absent, fatty streak formation is delayed in mice lacking LDL receptor and fed a cholesterol-rich diet.[39] P-selectin also seems to play a role in the advanced lesions that develop in ApoE-knockout mice. In this model, absence of P-selectin results in smaller lesions with less macrophage recruitment and smooth muscle infiltrate.[40] Both endothelial and platelet P-selectin may be involved in macrophage recruitment.[41] The recruitment and adhesion of platelets to the endothelium of atherothrombosis-prone sites was recently demonstrated in two different animal models.[42–44] Interestingly, Tailor et al[45] established that hypercholesterolemia promotes platelet–EC interaction

in the postcapillary venules of mice fed a cholesterol-rich diet.

Understanding how platelets respond to alterations of the vessel wall that elicit hemostasis may explain the modalities of interaction with developing atherosclerotic plaques, where EC dysfunction may create the conditions for platelet adhesion. Enhanced secretion of vWF in response to inflammatory stimuli can lead to the local recruitment of platelets, and this process may be favored in hypercholesterolemia.[44,46] This may be one of the reasons why deficiency of vWF affords some level of protection from atherosclerosis.[46] Not all adhesion receptor–ligand pairs known to be important in thrombus formation may be equally relevant in mediating platelet interactions with developing atherosclerotic lesions, as shown by the fact that deficiency of integrin-aIIbβ3 is not associated with protection from atherosclerosis.[47]

Activated platelets attached to an atherosclerotic lesion may influence plaque progression in different ways. By releasing the content of their granules, by increasing the expression of adhesive ligands, such as P-selectin, or by binding molecules from the plasma milieu, such as fibrinogen, platelets may provide the reactive surface for the recruitment of monocytes and lymphocytes. These interactions may support the adhesion of leukocytes to the vessel wall even in conditions of high flow that would otherwise not permit this. Platelets also release growth factors; the involvement of platelet-derived growth factor (PDGF) in cellular proliferation has long been recognized.[48] Recent data emphasize the possible influence of platelets on the cellular metabolism of LDLs, indicating a more direct involvement in the early changes characteristic of the atherosclerotic lesion.[49] Along the same lines, processing of β-amyloid precursor protein derived from engulfed platelets contributes to macrophage activation in an atherosclerotic plaque.[50] These findings support the idea that platelets adherent to the vessel wall contribute directly to the development of the chronic lesions that precede, typically by many years, the acute onset of arterial thrombosis.

Evidence suggests that plaque rupture, subsequent thrombosis, and fibrous thrombus organization are also important in the progression of atherosclerosis in both asymptomatic patients and those with stable angina. Plaque disruption with subsequent change in plaque geometry and thrombosis results in a complicated lesion. Such a rapid change in atherosclerotic plaque geometry may result in acute occlusion or subocclusion, with clinical manifestations of unstable angina or other ACS. More frequently, however, the rapid changes seem to result in a mural thrombus, without evident clinical symptoms. This type of platelet-rich thrombus may be a main contributor to the rapid progression of atherosclerosis. A number of local and systemic circulating factors may influence the degree and duration of thrombus deposition at the time of disruption of the coronary plaque.[28]

THE INFLAMMATORY ROLE OF PLATELETS

Early evidence pointed to the involvement of inflammatory and immune-mediated mechanisms in the pathogenesis of atheroma.[36] In this context, the role of platelets goes beyond thrombosis. In fact, platelets became a critical actor linking atherosclerosis, thrombosis, and inflammation. Patients with ACS not only have increased interactions between platelets but also have increased interactions between platelets and leukocytes (heterotypic aggregates) detectable in blood. These aggregates form when activated platelets undergo degranulation, after which they adhere to circulating leukocytes. Early work suggested that these heterotypic aggregates form in inflammatory states.[51] Platelets bind via P-selectin (CD62P)

expressed on the surface of activated platelets to the leukocyte receptor, P-selectin glycoprotein ligand-1 (PSGL-1).[52] This initial association leads to increased expression of CD11b/CD18 (Mac-1) on leukocytes,[53] which itself supports interactions with platelets, possibly because bivalent fibrinogen links this integrin with its platelet surface counterpart GPIIb/IIIa.[54] The importance of platelet–leukocyte aggregates in vascular disease is supported by a recent study demonstrating that the infusion of recombinant human PSGL-1 in an animal model of vascular injury reduced myocardial reperfusion injury and preserved vascular endothelial function.[55]

Measurement of platelet–leukocyte aggregates might be a better reflection of plaque instability and ongoing vascular thrombosis and inflammation. Platelet–leukocyte aggregates may also be a more sensitive marker of platelet activation than surface P-selectin expression because degranulated platelets rapidly lose surface P-selectin in vivo but continue to be detected in circulation. This observation was recently reported by Michelson et al;[56] they demonstrated that after acute MI, circulating monocyte–platelet aggregates are a more sensitive marker of in-vivo platelet activation than platelet surface P-selectin. In addition, two recent publications[57,58] showed that the number of circulating monocyte–platelet aggregates in ACS patients was increased compared with subjects with non-cardiac chest pain.

The binding of platelets and monocytes in ACS highlights, once again, the interaction between inflammation and thrombosis in cardiovascular disease. Plaque rupture promotes activation of the inflammatory response, and increased expression of TF initiates extrinsic coagulation. The expression of TF on both ECs and monocytes is partially regulated by proinflammatory cytokines, including tumor necrosis factor (TNF) and interleukin-1 (IL-1).[59]

In addition to initiating coagulation, TF interacts with P-selectin, accelerating fibrin formation and deposition.[59] Platelet surface P-selectin also induces the expression of TF on monocytes, enhances monocyte cytokine expression, and promotes CD11b/CD18 expression.[53]

T lymphocytes in human plaque were known to stain positively for CD40L. The role of CD40L in lesion progression and thrombosis was established through gene-targeting studies utilizing murine knockout models. In an LDL-deficient knockout, treatment with an anti-CD40L monoclonal antibody significantly reduced atherosclerotic lesion size and macrophage, T lymphocyte, and lipid content.[60] Furthermore, Schonbeck et al, utilizing the same murine model in a temporally longer, randomized study, not only demonstrated that anti-CD40L monoclonal antibody limited atherosclerotic disease evolution but also conferred stable plaque characteristics.[61] Moreover, CD40L deficiency was shown to protect against microvascular thrombus formation, while recombinant soluble CD40L (sCD40L) restored normal thrombosis.[62] Recently, much attention has been focused on CD40L's cryptic existence in platelets and its potential role in mediating platelet-dependent inflammatory response associated with the atherothrombotic state. Pioneering work has shown platelet-associated CD40L to elicit an inflammatory response from ECs[63] and induce human monocytic,[64] endothelial,[65,66] and vascular smooth muscle[67] TF expression in a CD40/CD40L-dependent manner. Furthermore, Henn et al have demonstrated that upon platelet stimulation, CD40L is expressed on the surface and then subsequently cleaved to generate a soluble, trimeric fragment, sCD40L.[68] Although no definitive data identify platelets as the sole source of sCD40L found in the circulation[68,69] platelet counts[70] and platelet activation[71] have been shown to correlate with sCD40L. Additionally, sCD40L is able to ligate platelet GPIIb/IIIa complex, confering a thrombogenic proclivity, and through this mechanism may play a role in high-shear-dependent platelet aggregation.[62]

CD40L and sCD40L both consist of homologous, multifunctional structural domains. They both bind CD40 by way of their TNF homology domain[72–74] to induce cellular signaling. Moreover, they both bind the platelet GPIIb/IIIa receptor through their lysine–glycine aspartic acid (KGD) peptide sequence and may stabilize arterial thrombi in this manner.[62] GPIIb/IIIa receptor antagonists at clinically relevant doses inhibit platelet release of sCD40L in vitro.[75] On the other hand, subtherapeutic dosing of these potent antiplatelet agents increases the release of the sCD40L, explaining a potential mechanism by which suboptimal doses of GPIIb/IIIa antagonists may not only be non-protective and prothrombotic but may also be proinflammatory.[75] Interestingly, both GPIIb/IIIa-dependent platelet adhesion to endothelium and GPIIb/IIIa engagement up-regulate platelet-associated CD40L.[76] These data define a significant role for the GPIIb/IIIa receptor in modulating the platelet–CD40L system.

Platelet-derived CD40L is capable of initiating various inflammatory responses on ECs, including production of reactive oxygen species,[77] expression of adhesion molecules (e.g. VCAM-1, ICAM-1, and E-selectin), chemokines (e.g. monocyte chemoattractant protein-1 [MCP-1] and IL-8), cytokine IL-6,[63] and TF.[65] In contrast to CD40L constitutively stored in platelet cytoplasm, platelet IL-6 is synthesized upon platelet activation.[78] A portion of IL-6 is presented in its mature form on the platelet membrane and induces EC adhesiveness. Hence, these mediators are involved in the inflammatory process underlying atherosclerosis.

C-reactive protein (CRP) is a protein of the acute-phase response and a sensitive marker of low-grade inflammation. Increased levels of CRP have been reported to predict acute coronary events,[79,80] and it seems to be a useful marker in the prediction of thrombotic events. Whether CRP reflects the inflammatory component of atherosclerotic plaques or of the circulating blood, and whether it is a surrogate marker or a biologically active element in plaque development of thrombus formation at the site of the atherosclerotic vessel, are not known. However, recent studies support the hypothesis that CRP is an activator of blood monocyte and vessel-wall ECs.[81]

CLINICAL IMPLICATIONS

The clinical manifestations of atherosclerotic plaques depend on several factors, including the degree and speed of blood flow obstruction, the duration of decreased myocardial perfusion, and the myocardial oxygen demand at the time of obstruction. The thrombotic response at the time of disruption is also a major determinant. If the resulting thrombus is small (found in up to 8% of patients dying of non-cardiovascular causes), plaque rupture probably proceeds unnoticed. If however, the thrombus is large enough to compromise blood flow to the myocardium, the individual may experience an acute ischemic syndrome.

Following mild injury to the vessel wall, it is likely that the thrombogenic stimulus is relatively limited and the resulting thrombotic occlusion transient, as occurs in unstable angina. The relative lack of therapeutic response to fibrinolysis suggests that therapeutic agents do not access this fibrin within a platelet-rich mixture, although antiplatelet agents may be able to influence events on the thrombus surface. Deep vessel injury secondary to plaque rupture and ulceration results in exposure of collagen, lipids, and other elements of the vessel media, leading to relatively persistent thrombotic occlusion and MI (Figure 4.3).

In patients with stable coronary artery disease, angina commonly results from

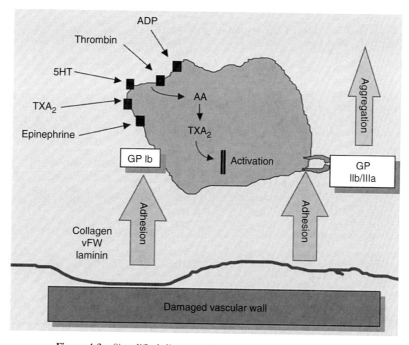

Figure 4.3 Simplified diagram of platelet receptors and ligands.

increases in myocardial oxygen demand beyond the ability of stenosed arteries to increase its delivery. By contrast, unstable angina, non-ST-elevation MI and ST-elevation MI represent a continuum and are usually characterized by an abrupt cessation in coronary blood flow. In unstable angina, plaque disruption may lead to acute changes in plaque morphology and reduction in coronary blood flow. In addition to plaque disruption, other mechanisms also contribute to reduce coronary blood flow. Platelets attach to the damaged endothelium and exposed media and release vasoactive substances, including thromboxane A_2 (TXA_2) and serotonin (5-hydroxytryptamine; 5HT), leading to further platelet aggregation and vasoconstriction. In non-ST-elevation infarction, the angiographic morphology of the culprit lesion is similar to that seen in unstable angina, suggesting that plaque disruption is similar in both syndromes. Approximately one-fourth of patients with non-ST-elevation infarction have a completely occluded infarct-related vessel at early angiography with the distal territory usually supplied by collaterals. In ST-elevation infarction, plaque rupture is frequently associated with deep arterial injury or ulceration, resulting in the formation of a fixed and persistent thrombus with abrupt cessation of myocardial perfusion and subsequent necrosis. The coronary lesion responsible for the infarction is usually only mildly stenotic, which suggests that plaque rupture with superimposed thrombosis is the primary determinant of acute occlusion rather than lesion severity.[11]

CONCLUSION

Direct evidence supports the conclusion that activated platelets play an important role in the development of atherosclerosis. Mechanisms for the participation of platelets in atherosclerosis have not been fully examined yet, but strongly emphasize the role of endothelial dysfunction, platelet reactivity, and TF activity in acute arterial thrombosis after atherosclerotic plaque disruption. Further investigation of these mechanisms may lead to new approaches for reducing the development and progression of atherosclerosis and for developing innovative and efficient therapies in the prevention of cardiac clinical manifestations.

REFERENCES

1. Broijersen A, Hamsten A, Eriksson M, Angelin B, Hjemdahl P. Platelet activity in vivo in hyperlipoproteinemia – importance of combined hyperlipidemia. Thromb Haemost 1998; 79(2):268–75.
2. Nityanand S, Pande I, Bajpai VK et al. Platelets in essential hypertension. Thromb Res 1993; 72(5):447–54.
3. Manduteanu I, Calb M, Lupu C, Simionescu N, Simionescu M. Increased adhesion of human diabetic platelets to cultured valvular endothelial cells. J Submicrosc Cytol Pathol 1992; 24(4):539–47.
4. Badimon L, Chesebro JH, Badimon JJ. Thrombus formation on ruptured atherosclerotic plaques and rethrombosis on evolving thrombi. Circulation 1992; 86(6 Suppl):III74–85.
5. Collaborative meta-analysis of randomised trials of antiplatelet therapy for prevention of death, myocardial infarction, and stroke in high risk patients. BMJ 2002; 324(7329):71–86.
6. Lusis AJ. Atherosclerosis. Nature 2000; 407(6801): 233–41.
7. Ruschitzka F, Moehrlen U, Quaschning T et al. Tissue endothelin-converting enzyme activity correlates with cardiovascular risk factors in coronary artery disease. Circulation 2000; 102(10):1086–92.
8. Kinlay S, Libby P, Ganz P. Endothelial function and coronary artery disease. Curr Opin Lipidol 2001; 12(4):383–9.
9. Barnes PJ, Karin M. Nuclear factor-kappaB: a pivotal transcription factor in chronic inflammatory diseases. N Engl J Med 1997; 336(15):1066–71.
10. Spieker LE, Sudano I, Hurlimann D et al. High-density lipoprotein restores endothelial function in hypercholesterolemic men. Circulation 2002; 105(12):1399–402.
11. Fuster V, Fayad ZA, Badimon JJ. Acute coronary syndromes: biology. Lancet 1999; 353 (Suppl 2):SII5–9.
12. Libby P. Current concepts of the pathogenesis of the acute coronary syndromes. Circulation 2001; 104(3):365–72.
13. Stary HC, Chandler AB, Glagov S et al. A definition of initial, fatty streak, and intermediate lesions of atherosclerosis. A report from the Committee on

Vascular Lesions of the Council on Arteriosclerosis, American Heart Association. Arterioscler Thromb 1994; 14(5):840–56.

14. Ambrose JA, Weinrauch M. Thrombosis in ischemic heart disease. Arch Intern Med 1996; 156(13): 1382–94.

15. Falk E, Shah PK, Fuster V. Coronary plaque disruption. Circulation 1995; 92(3):657–71.

16. Moreno PR, Bernardi VH, Lopez-Cuellar J et al. Macrophage infiltration predicts restenosis after coronary intervention in patients with unstable angina. Circulation 1996; 94(12):3098–102.

17. Libby P, Simon DI. Inflammation and thrombosis: the clot thickens. Circulation 2001; 103(13):1718–20.

18. Sata M, Saiura A, Kunisato A et al. Hematopoietic stem cells differentiate into vascular cells that participate in the pathogenesis of atherosclerosis. Nat Med 2002; 8(4):403–9.

19. Galis ZS, Johnson C, Godin D et al. Targeted disruption of the matrix metalloproteinase-9 gene impairs smooth muscle cell migration and geometrical arterial remodeling. Circ Res 2002; 91(9):852–9.

20. Scott J. ATVB In focus: lipoproteins, inflammation, and atherosclerosis. Arterioscler Thromb Vasc Biol 2003; 23(4):528.

21. Moreno PR, Falk E, Palacios IF et al. Macrophage infiltration in acute coronary syndromes. Implications for plaque rupture. Circulation 1994; 90(2):775–8.

22. Uzui H, Harpf A, Liu M et al. Increased expression of membrane type 3-matrix metalloproteinase in human atherosclerotic plaque: role of activated macrophages and inflammatory cytokines. Circulation 2002; 106(24):3024–30.

23. Toschi V, Gallo R, Lettino M et al. Tissue factor modulates the thrombogenicity of human atherosclerotic plaques. Circulation 1997; 95(3):594–9.

24. Badimon JJ, Lettino M, Toschi V et al. Local inhibition of tissue factor reduces the thrombogenicity of disrupted human atherosclerotic plaques: effects of tissue factor pathway inhibitor on plaque thrombogenicity under flow conditions. Circulation 1999; 99(14):1780–7.

25. Virmani R, Kolodgie FD, Burke AP, Farb A, Schwartz SM. Lessons from sudden coronary death: a comprehensive morphological classification scheme for atherosclerotic lesions. Arterioscler Thromb Vasc Biol 2000; 20(5):1262–75.

26. Mallat Z, Tedgui A. Current perspective on the role of apoptosis in atherothrombotic disease. Circ Res 2001; 88(10):998–1003.

27. Roque M, Reis ED, Fuster V et al. Inhibition of tissue factor reduces thrombus formation and intimal hyperplasia after porcine coronary angioplasty. J Am Coll Cardiol 2000; 36(7):2303–10.

28. Burke AP, Kolodgie FD, Farb A et al. Healed plaque ruptures and sudden coronary death: evidence that subclinical rupture has a role in plaque progression. Circulation 2001; 103(7):934–40.

29. Fuster V, Fallon JT, Nemerson Y. Coronary thrombosis. Lancet 1996; 348 (Suppl 1):S7–10.

30. Sambola A, Osende J, Hathcock J et al. Role of risk factors in the modulation of tissue factor activity and blood thrombogenicity. Circulation 2003; 107(7): 973–7.

31. Kabbani SS, Watkins MW, Holoch PA et al. Platelet reactivity in coronary ostial blood: a reflection of the thrombotic state accompanying plaque rupture and of the adequacy of anti-thrombotic therapy. J Thromb Thrombolysis 2001; 12(2):171–6.

32. Patrono C, Coller B, Dalen JE et al. Platelet-active drugs: the relationships among dose, effectiveness, and side effects. Chest 2001; 119(1 Suppl):39S-63S.

33. Osende JI, Badimon JJ, Fuster V et al. Blood thrombogenicity in type 2 diabetes mellitus patients is associated with glycemic control. J Am Coll Cardiol 2001; 38(5):1307–12.

34. Rauch U, Crandall J, Osende JI et al. Increased thrombus formation relates to ambient blood glucose and leukocyte count in diabetes mellitus type 2. Am J Cardiol 2000; 86(2):246–9.

35. Corti R, Badimon JJ. Value or desirability of hemorheological-hemostatic parameter changes as endpoints in blood lipid-regulating trials. Curr Opin Lipidol 2001; 12(6):629–37.

36. Ross R. Atherosclerosis is an inflammatory disease. Am Heart J 1999; 138(5 Pt 2):S419–20.

37. Sachais BS. Platelet–endothelial interactions in atherosclerosis. Curr Atheroscler Rep 2001; 3(5): 412–16.

38. Huo Y, Schober A, Forlow SB et al. Circulating activated platelets exacerbate atherosclerosis in mice deficient in apolipoprotein E. Nat Med 2003; 9(1):61–7.

39. Johnson RC, Chapman SM, Dong ZM et al. Absence of P-selectin delays fatty streak formation in mice. J Clin Invest 1997; 99(5):1037–43.

40. Dong ZM, Brown AA, Wagner DD. Prominent role of P-selectin in the development of advanced atherosclerosis in ApoE-deficient mice. Circulation 2000; 101(19):2290–5.

41. Burger PE, Coetzee S, McKeehan WL et al. Fibroblast growth factor receptor-1 is expressed by endothelial progenitor cells. Blood 2002; 100(10):3527–35.

42. Massberg S, Brand K, Gruner S et al. A critical role of platelet adhesion in the initiation of atherosclerotic lesion formation. J Exp Med 2002; 196(7):887–96.

43. Massberg S, Gawaz M, Gruner S et al. A crucial role of glycoprotein VI for platelet recruitment to the injured arterial wall in vivo. J Exp Med 2003; 197(1):41–9.

44. Theilmeier G, Michiels C, Spaepen E et al. Endothelial von Willebrand factor recruits platelets to atherosclerosis-prone sites in response to hypercholesterolemia. Blood 2002; 99(12):4486–93.

45. Tailor A, Granger DN. Hypercholesterolemia promotes p-selectin-dependent platelet–endothelial cell adhesion in postcapillary venules. Arterioscler Thromb Vasc Biol 2003; 23(4):675–80.

46. Methia N, Andre P, Denis CV, Economopoulos M, Wagner DD. Localized reduction of atherosclerosis in von Willebrand factor-deficient mice. Blood 2001; 98(5):1424–8.

47. Shpilberg O, Rabi I, Schiller K et al. Patients with Glanzmann thrombasthenia lacking platelet glycoprotein alpha(IIb)beta(3) (GPIIb/IIIa) and alpha(v)beta(3) receptors are not protected from atherosclerosis. Circulation 2002; 105(9):1044–8.

48. Ross R. The pathogenesis of atherosclerosis: a perspective for the 1990s. Nature 1993; 362(6423): 801–9.

49. Sachais BS, Kuo A, Nassar T et al. Platelet factor 4 binds to low-density lipoprotein receptors and disrupts the endocytic machinery, resulting in retention of low-density lipoprotein on the cell surface. Blood 2002; 99(10):3613–22.

50. De Meyer GR, De Cleen DM, Cooper S et al. Platelet phagocytosis and processing of beta-amyloid precursor protein as a mechanism of macrophage activation in atherosclerosis. Circ Res 2002; 90(11): 1197–204.

51. Arber N, Berliner S, Rotenberg Z et al. Detection of aggregated leukocytes in the circulating pool during stress-demargination is not necessarily a result of decreased leukocyte adhesiveness. Acta Haematol 1991; 86(1):20–4.

52. Rinder HM, Bonan JL, Rinder CS, Ault KA, Smith BR. Dynamics of leukocyte–platelet adhesion in whole blood. Blood 1991; 78(7):1730–7.

53. Neumann FJ, Zohlnhofer D, Fakhoury L et al. Effect of glycoprotein IIb/IIIa receptor blockade on platelet–leukocyte interaction and surface expression of the leukocyte integrin Mac-1 in acute myocardial infarction. J Am Coll Cardiol 1999; 34(5): 1420–6.

54. Simon DI, Ezratty AM, Francis SA, Rennke H, Loscalzo J. Fibrin(ogen) is internalized and degraded by activated human monocytoid cells via Mac-1 (CD11b/CD18): a nonplasmin fibrinolytic pathway. Blood 1993; 82(8):2414–22.

55. Hayward R, Campbell B, Shin YK, Scalia R, Lefer AM. Recombinant soluble P-selectin glycoprotein ligand-1 protects against myocardial ischemic reperfusion injury in cats. Cardiovasc Res 1999; 41(1):65–76.

56. Michelson AD, Barnard MR, Krueger LA, Valeri CR, Furman MI. Circulating monocyte–platelet aggregates are a more sensitive marker of in vivo platelet activation than platelet surface P-selectin: studies in baboons, human coronary intervention, and human acute myocardial infarction. Circulation 2001; 104(13):1533–7.

57. Sarma J, Laan CA, Alam S et al. Increased platelet binding to circulating monocytes in acute coronary syndromes. Circulation 2002; 105(18):2166–71.

58. Furman MI, Barnard MR, Krueger LA et al. Circulating monocyte–platelet aggregates are an early marker of acute myocardial infarction. J Am Coll Cardiol 2001; 38(4):1002–6.

59. Shebuski RJ, Kilgore KS. Role of inflammatory mediators in thrombogenesis. J Pharmacol Exp Ther 2002; 300(3):729–35.

60. Mach F, Schonbeck U, Sukhova GK, Atkinson E, Libby P. Reduction of atherosclerosis in mice by inhibition of CD40 signalling. Nature 1998; 394(6689): 200–3.

61. Schonbeck U, Sukhova GK, Shimizu K, Mach F, Libby P. Inhibition of CD40 signaling limits evolution of established atherosclerosis in mice. Proc Natl Acad Sci USA 2000; 97(13):7458–63.

62. Andre P, Prasad KS, Denis CV et al. CD40L stabilizes arterial thrombi by a beta3 integrin-dependent mechanism. Nat Med 2002; 8(3):247–52.

63. Henn V, Slupsky JR, Grafe M et al. CD40 ligand on activated platelets triggers an inflammatory reaction of endothelial cells. Nature 1998; 391(6667): 591–4.

64. Lindmark E, Tenno T, Siegbahn A. Role of platelet P-selectin and CD40 ligand in the induction of monocytic tissue factor expression. Arterioscler Thromb Vasc Biol 2000; 20(10):2322–8.

65. Slupsky JR, Kalbas M, Willuweit A et al. Activated platelets induce tissue factor expression on human umbilical vein endothelial cells by ligation of CD40. Thromb Haemost 1998; 80(6):1008–14.

66. Bavendiek U, Libby P, Kilbride M et al. Induction of tissue factor expression in human endothelial cells by CD40 ligand is mediated via activator protein 1, nuclear factor kappa B, and Egr-1. J Biol Chem 2002; 277(28):25032–9.

67. Schonbeck U, Mach F, Sukhova GK et al. CD40 ligation induces tissue factor expression in human vascular smooth muscle cells. Am J Pathol 2000; 156(1):7–14.

68. Henn V, Steinbach S, Buchner K, Presek P, Kroczek RA. The inflammatory action of CD40 ligand (CD154) expressed on activated human platelets is temporally limited by coexpressed CD40. Blood 2001; 98(4):1047–54.

69. Aukrust P, Muller F, Ueland T et al. Enhanced levels of soluble and membrane-bound CD40 ligand in patients with unstable angina. Possible reflection of T lymphocyte and platelet involvement in the pathogenesis of acute coronary syndromes. Circulation 1999; 100(6):614–20.

70. Viallard JF, Solanilla A, Gauthier B et al. Increased soluble and platelet-associated CD40 ligand in essential thrombocythemia and reactive thrombocytosis. Blood 2002; 99(7):2612–14.

71. Heeschen C, Dimmeler S, Hamm CW et al. Soluble CD40 ligand in acute coronary syndromes. N Engl J Med 2003; 348(12):1104–11.

72. Bajorath J, Aruffo A. Construction and analysis of a detailed three-dimensional model of the ligand binding domain of the human B cell receptor CD40. Proteins 1997; 27(1):59–70.

73. van Kooten C, Banchereau J. CD40-CD40 ligand. J Leukoc Biol 2000; 67(1):2–17.

74. Mazzei GJ, Edgerton MD, Losberger C et al. Recombinant soluble trimeric CD40 ligand is biologically active. J Biol Chem 1995; 270(13):7025–8.

75. Nannizzi-Alaimo L, Alves VL, Phillips DR. Inhibitory effects of glycoprotein IIb/IIIa antagonists and aspirin on the release of soluble CD40 ligand during platelet stimulation. Circulation 2003; 107(8):1123–8.

76. May AE, Kalsch T, Massberg S et al. Engagement of glycoprotein IIb/IIIa (alpha(IIb)beta3) on platelets upregulates CD40L and triggers CD40L-dependent matrix degradation by endothelial cells. Circulation 2002; 106(16):2111–17.

77. Urbich C, Dernbach E, Aicher A, Zeiher AM, Dimmeler S. CD40 ligand inhibits endothelial cell migration by increasing production of endothelial reactive oxygen species. Circulation 2002; 106(8): 981–6.

78. Hawrylowicz C, Santoro S, Platt F, Unanue E. Activated platelets express IL-1 activity. J Immunol 1989; 143(12):4015–18.

79. Ridker PM, Buring JE, Cook NR, Rifai N. C-reactive protein, the metabolic syndrome, and risk of incident cardiovascular events: an 8-year follow-up of 14719 initially healthy American women. Circulation 2003; 107(3):391–7.

80. Ridker PM, Rifai N, Rose L, Buring JE, Cook NR. Comparison of C-reactive protein and low-density lipoprotein cholesterol levels in the prediction of first cardiovascular events. N Engl J Med 2002; 347(20):1557–65.

81. Pasceri V, Cheng JS, Willerson JT, Yeh ET, Chang J. Modulation of C-reactive protein-mediated monocyte chemoattractant protein-1 induction in human endothelial cells by anti-atherosclerosis drugs. Circulation 2001; 103(21):2531–4.

82. Huo Y, Ley KF. Role of platelets in the development of atherosclerosis. Trends Cardiovasc Med 2004; 14(1):18–22.

Role of metalloproteinases in the vulnerable plaque

5

Jason L Johnson and Andrew C Newby

INTRODUCTION

Pioneering work by pathologists, including Erling Falk and the late Michael Davies, established that structural disruption of atherosclerotic plaques is the main mechanism underlying myocardial infarctions and strokes.[1] Key histologic features of disrupted plaques include thinning of the fibrous cap and depletion of structural collagens that provide most of the tensile strength.[1] These observations suggest that dysregulated protease activity is responsible for weakening the plaque cap. In this chapter, we consider the evidence that matrix metalloproteinases (MMPs) promote plaque vulnerability and are therefore an appropriate target for plaque-stabilizing therapy.

MMPs comprise at least 24 structurally related proteinases, each of which directly degrades several extracellular matrix (ECM) proteins (Table 5.1) as well as non-matrix proteins (Table 5.2).[2] Most MMPs are secreted, although they may be confined to the pericellular environment by binding to surface receptors (Figure 5.1). These membrane-bound proteinases known as membrane-type MMPs (MT-MMPs) are ecto-enzymes, i.e. integral membrane proteins with their catalytic domains on the cell surface (see Figure 5.1). The activity of MMPs is tightly controlled by regulating transcription and translation of genes, in a few cases by packaging and secretion from vesicles, by activation of pro-forms, and by binding to four tissue inhibitors of MMPs (TIMPs) (see Figure 5.1).[2]

In the context of atherosclerosis, MMPs could reduce plaque size and promote plaque instability simply by degrading major ECM structural proteins. For example, collagenases (MMP-1, MMP-2, MMP-8, MMP-13, and MMP-14) cleave structural type I and III collagens, whereas MMP-9 and MMP-12 actively degrade elastin (see Table 5.1). Several MMPs, including the stromelysins and matrilysins (e.g MMP-3 and MMP-7) have a broad specificity that includes the core proteins of proteoglycans, the third major structural component of the artery wall (see Table 5.1). On the other hand, some MMPs (particularly MMP-2, MMP-9, MMP-12, and MMP-14) promote migration of vascular smooth muscle cells (SMCs)[3] and infiltration of immune inflammatory cells.[4] These MMPs could therefore paradoxically promote plaque growth and even help to form a stable plaque fibrous cap. MMPs are also implicated in angiogenesis, an important feature associated with both growth and vulnerability of atherosclerotic plaques.[5] It is therefore important to consider critically the evidence implicating each individual MMP as well as MMPs in general in plaque vulnerability.

Table 5.1 Human matrix metalloproteinases (MMPs) and their extracellular matrix (ECM) substrates

Protein name	Alternative names	Collagenous substrates	Non-collagenous ECM substrates
MMP-1	Collagenase-1	Collagen types I, II, III, VII, VIII, X, and gelatin	Aggrecan, casein, serpins, versican, perlecan, proteoglycan link protein, and tenascin-C
MMP-2	Gelatinase-A	Collagen types I, IV, V, VII, X, XI, XIV, and gelatin	Aggrecan, elastin, fibronectin, laminin, proteoglycan link protein, and versican
MMP-3	Stromelysin-1	Collagen types II, IV, IX, X, and gelatin	Aggrecan, casein, decorin, elastin, fibronectin, laminin, perlecan, proteoglycan, and versican
MMP-7	Matrilysin-1	Collagen types I, II, III, V, VI, and X	Aggrecan, casein, elastin, entactin, laminin, and proteoglycan link protein
MMP-8	Collagenase-2 (neutrophil collagenase)	Collagen types I, II, III, V, VII, VIII, X, and gelatin	Aggrecan and laminin
MMP-9	Gelatinase-B	Collagen types V, VI, VII, X, and XIV	Fibronectin, laminin, proteoglycan link protein, and versican
MMP-10	Stromelysin-2	Collagen types II, IV, V, and gelatin	Fibronectin and laminin
MMP-11	Stromelysin-3	None known	Laminin
MMP-12	Macrophage metalloelastase	None known	Elastin
MMP-13	Collagenase-3	Collagen types I, II, III, IV, V, IX, X, XI, and gelatin	Aggrecan, fibronectin, laminin, perlecan, and tenascin
MMP-14	MT1-MMP	Collagen types I, II, III, and gelatin	Aggrecan, dermatan sulfate proteoglycan, fibrin, fibronectin, laminin, perlecan, tenascin, and vitronectin
MMP-15	MT2-MMP	Collagen types I, II, III, and gelatin	Aggrecan, fibronectin, laminin, perlecan, tenascin, and vitronectin
MMP-16	MT3-MMP	Collagen types I, III, and gelatin	Aggrecan, casein, fibronectin, laminin, perlecan, and vitronectin
MMP-17	MT4-MMP	Gelatin	Fibrin and fibronectin
MMP-19	RASI-1 (T-cell rheumatoid A)	Collagen types I, IV, and gelatine	Aggrecan, casein, fibronectin, laminin, and tenascin
MMP-20	Enamelysin		Aggrecan, amelogenin, and cartilage oligomeric protein
MMP-21			
MMP-23	CA-MMP (cysteine array)	Gelatin	Chondroitin sulfate, dermatan sulfate, and fibronectin
MMP-24	MT5-MMP	Gelatin	Fibrin and fibronectin
MMP-25	Leukolysin, MT6-MMP	Collagen type IV and gelatin	Casein, fibrinogen, and fibronectin
MMP-26	Matrilysin-2, endometase	Collagen type IV and gelatin	Casein
MMP-28	Epilysin		

Table 5.2 Non-traditional matrix metalloproteinase (MMP) substrates

Substrate	MMP	Biological effect
Pro-TGF-β (decorin)	MMP-2, -3, -7, and -9	Antiproliferative, antiapoptotic, and inhibits MMP expression
ProTNF-α	MMP-1, -2, -3, -7, -9, and -14	Proinflammatory cell chemotaxis, migration, and activation
FGF/perlecan complex	MMP-1, -3, and -13	Altered cellular growth and differentiation
IL-1β	MMP-1, -2, -3, and -9	Pro- and antiinflammatory
IL-2Rα	MMP-9	Anti-T-cell proliferation and migration
MCP-3	MMP-1, -2, -3, -13, and -14	Reduced chemotaxis (antiinflammatory)
Pro-vascular endothelial growth factor (VEGF)	MMP-9	Angiogenesis
β₄ integrin	MMP-7	Cell–cell and cell–matrix modulation
Pro-heparin-binding epidermal growth factor	MMP-3	Pro-SMC chemotaxis and proliferation
Tissue transglutaminase	MMP-14, -15, and -16	Reduced cell adhesion and spreading
Plasminogen	MMP-3, -7, -9, and -12	Generation of angiostatin (antiangiogenic)
Factor XII	MMP-12, -13, and -14	Suppress normal clotting mechanisms
Fibrinogen	MMP-1, -2, -3, -7, -8, -9, -10, -12, -13, -14, and -26	Suppress normal clotting mechanisms
Fibrin	MMP-1, -2, -3, -9, and -14	Proangiogenic and promigratory
Insulin-like growth factor binding proteins (IGFBPs)	MMP-1, -2, -3, and -11	Increased IGF (promigratory and proliferative)
CD44	MMP-14	Promigratory
Complement C1q	MMP-1, -2, -3, -8, -9, and -13	Enhanced inflammatory cell phagocytosis
E-cadherin	MMP-3 and MMP-7	Cell–cell modulation, promigratory
Fas-ligand	MMP-7	Fas receptor-mediated apoptosis
α₁-antichymotrypsin	MMP-1, -2, and -3	Proinflammatory
α₂-macroglobulin	MMP-1, -3, -8, -9, -11, -12, -13, and -14	Increased plasma proteinase activity
α₁-proteinase inhibitor	MMP-1, -2, -3, -7, -8, -9, -11, -12, -14, and -26	Proinflammatory (e.g. neutrophil chemotaxis)

INCREASED MMP EXPRESSION AND ACTIVITY IS FOUND IN HUMAN ATHEROSCLEROTIC PLAQUES, ESPECIALLY AT THE VULNERABLE SHOULDER REGIONS

Expression of MMP-1, MMP-3, and MMP-9 occurs in macrophage-derived foam cells, lymphocytes, SMCs, and endothelial cells (ECs), particularly at the rupture-prone shoulder regions of atherosclerotic plaques.[6-10] Normal arteries express only MMP-2, TIMP-1, and TIMP-2.[7,11,12] Moreover, in-situ zymography detects net MMP activity at the foam-cell rich, vulnerable shoulder regions of plaques

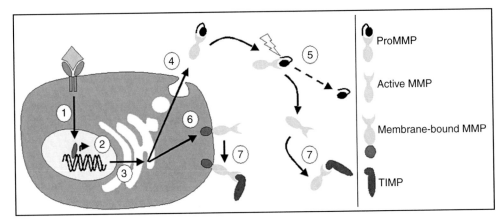

Figure 5.1 Schematic diagram illustrating the multiple levels of matrix metalliproteinase (MMP) regulation. These mechanisms include ligand-mediated signal transduction (1), transcriptional activation (2), post-transcriptional mRNA translation (3), vesicle packaging, constitutive and regulated secretion (4), proteolytic activation (5), cell surface expression (6), and active enzyme inhibition by tissue inhibitors of MMPs (TIMPs) (7).

but not in normal arteries. The collagenases MMP-1 and MMP-13 are overexpressed at sites of high circumferential tensile stress in the fibrous cap, where ruptures are most likely to occur, and co-localize with neo-epitopes of cleaved collagen.[13,14] Increased expression of MMP-2, MMP-8, MMP-11, MMP-14, and MMP-16 is also detected at rupture-prone regions of unstable plaques.[13,15-20] Increased MMP activity is often co-localized with macrophage accumulation,[13] which is another key histologic correlate of plaque instability.[21] Moreover, foam cell macrophages isolated from rabbit atherosclerotic plaques produce MMP-1 and MMP-3,[22] whereas alveolar and granuloma macrophages do not.[22,23] Furthermore, conditioned media from foam-cell macrophages, in contrast to SMC,[24] contain an excess of active MMPs over TIMPs.[23] In contrast to the MMPs discussed above, MMP-7 and MMP-12 localize to the borders between the lipid core and the macrophage-rich shoulder regions of human plaques[16] and could therefore have distinct roles.

MMP EXPRESSION AND ACTIVITY IS UP-REGULATED BY MEDIATORS PRESENT IN VULNERABLE PLAQUES

The cytokines, tumor necrosis factor-α (TNF-α) and interleukin-1 (IL-1), and the growth factors, transforming growth factor-β (TGF-β), fibroblast growth factor-2 (FGF-2), and platelet-derived growth factor (PDGF), all of which are present in plaques, have divergent effects on MMP and TIMP synthesis in SMCs, ECs, and macrophages.[8,25-28] For example, combinations of IL-1 and PDGF increase MMP-1, MMP-3, and MMP-9 synthesis and secretion from SMCs,[24,25,29] but do not alter TIMP-1 or TIMP-2 secretion.[8,24,25,29] Inflammatory mediators therefore shift the balance of MMPs and TIMPs so as to promote MMP activity.

Cell–cell contact between activated T lymphocytes and SMC or macrophages can also induce MMP expression. CD40 ligation, in particular, induces expression of MMP-1 and MMP-3,[30] MMP-9,[31] MMP-11,[17] and MMP-12,[32] in human monocytes/macrophages and SMCs.[33] CD40L and CD40 protein are co-localized in ECs, SMCs, and macrophages, and CD40L protein is found in T lymphocytes, in the shoulder regions of human atherosclerotic plaques.[30] This suggests that CD40 ligation orchestrates immune-modulated destabilization of human atherosclerotic plaques.[34–36]

GENETIC EPIDEMIOLOGY IMPLICATES MMPS IN PLAQUE VULNERABILITY

Since the pioneering study in 1995,[37] there have been a large number of independent studies on the 5A/6A promoter polymorphism in the MMP-3 gene. In summary, the 5A allele that drives greater transcription is associated with less advanced coronary[38,39] and carotid[40] atherosclerosis but with greater incidence of myocardial infarction (MI)[39,41,42] and strokes.[43] These data can be rationalized by the hypothesis that MMP-3 decreases ECM accumulation, leading to smaller but less-stable plaques. The MMP-1 gene has seven promoter polymorphisms. High levels of MMP-1 promoter activity appear to favor plaque instability and precipitate MI,[44] whereas lower promoter activity may worsen symptomatic coronary heart disease[45] and carotid artery stenosis.[40] Hence, MMP-1 activity may also cause less matrix protein accumulation and therefore smaller but less-stable plaques. Single-nucleotide polymorphisms have also been identified within the genes for MMP-7,[46] MMP-9,[47] and MMP-12,[48] and are related to the progression of coronary artery disease. In particular, the mutation in the MMP-9 gene resulting in greater promoter activity has been associated with increased disease severity,[47,49] contrary to the results with MMP-1 and MMP-3. These studies have been recently reviewed in depth.[50]

CIRCULATING MMP LEVELS ARE BIOMARKERS FOR UNSTABLE ATHEROSCLEROSIS

Increased levels of MMP-2,[51,52] MMP-3,[53] MMP-9,[49,51,54] and TIMP-1[54] have been detected in patients with acute coronary syndromes. However, these studies do not distinguish whether increased blood MMP levels are the consequence or cause of plaque rupture. For example, disruption of an atherosclerotic plaque triggers platelet aggregation and thrombus formation, both of which can induce MMP expression.[55,56] Additionally, the levels of plasma MMPs could be influenced by drugs commonly used to treat patients with coronary artery disease.[57,58] Perhaps the most persuasive evidence comes from a recent study utilizing a large cohort of patients with established coronary atherosclerosis, which reported a strong association between plasma levels of MMP-9 and subsequent 4-year risk for fatal coronary heart disease.[49]

CONTRARY EVIDENCE THAT SOME MMPS CONTRIBUTE TO FIBROUS CAP GROWTH AND STABILITY

Increased MMP-9 expression and MMP-2 activation accompany neointima formation in cultured human saphenous veins,[59] in the balloon injured rat[60] or porcine carotid artery,[61] and saphenous vein into carotid artery interposition grafts.[62] Adenovirus-mediated gene transfer of the human TIMP-1 and TIMP-2 genes into human saphenous vein segments[63,64] and the rat model of vascular balloon injury[65–67] reduces MMP activity and inhibits neointima formation, primarily by inhibiting medial SMC migration. Moreover, targeted disruption of the MMP-2 and MMP-9 genes retards SMC migration and inhibits neointima formation in the injured mouse carotid artery.[68–70] As recently reviewed[3] the permissive effects of MMP-2 and MMP-9 on SMC migration could result from removing ECM barriers to migration or by regulating signaling pathways that depend on MMP-mediated remodeling of cell–cell and cell–matrix contacts. Since MMP-2 and MMP-9 activity are both increased in atherosclerotic plaques,[7,9,15,71] their effect to promote SMC migration could contribute to fibrous cap formation and hence stabilize plaques.

INSIGHTS FROM GENETIC MANIPULATION IN MICE

Overexpression or deletion of individual MMP and TIMP genes in mice appears a potent strategy to elucidate their individual roles in plaque stability. Acute plaque rupture has been observed in the cholesterol-fed ApoE[−/−] mouse.[72] More often, however, surrogates for plaque instability have been used (see Figure 5.2). These include lower collagen and SMC content, increased macrophage content, and the presence of buried fibrous caps. Disruption of the medial elastic lamellae has also been observed, but whether this is a marker of plaque instability or aneurysm formation is not clear. Although each of these features is replicated in human atherosclerosis, there is obviously a huge difference in scale, and therefore biomechanics, between mouse and human lesions. There are also biochemical differences that could confound extrapolation from mouse to man. For example, up-regulation of MMP-3, MMP-11, MMP-12, and MMP-13 is readily detected in murine atherosclerotic plaques[17,73,74] but the MMP-1 gene seems not to be used in mice. Nevertheless, engineering macrophages to overexpress MMP-1 decreases atherosclerotic lesion size in apolipoprotein E[−/−] (ApoE[−/−]) mice,[75] perhaps due to increased collagen degradation or decreased deposition. Strangely, the anticipated destabilization of the lesions was not observed, presumably due to retarded plaque development. MMP-13 deletion in ApoE[−/−] mice caused more collagen to accumulate in aortic root lesions, implying greater stability, although no effects on lesion size or macrophage density were observed.[76] ApoE[−/−] mice engineered to express collagenase-resistant collagen I also demonstrated increased collagen accumulation in atherosclerotic plaques, implying greater stability.[77] These results demonstrate that collagenases modulate the collagen content in atherosclerotic plaques, but their effects

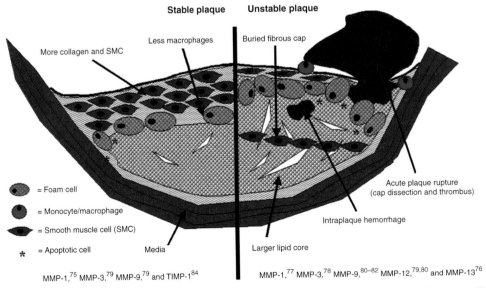

Figure 5.2 Divergent roles of matrix metalloproteinase (MMPs) in murine atherosclerotic plaque phenotype. The cardinal characteristics of atherosclerotic plaque phenotype and association of MMP and tissue inhibitor of MMP (TIMP) involvement generated by genetic studies in mice.

on plaque stability are perhaps less dramatic than expected.

Deficiency of MMP-3 in cholesterol-fed ApoE[-/-] mice[78] leads to larger atherosclerotic plaques throughout the thoracic aorta; the lesions exhibit a more stable phenotype, including increased collagen and decreased macrophage content. MMP-3/ApoE double knockout mice also demonstrate increased plaque burden in the brachiocephalic artery[79] but, in direct contrast, a less-stable plaque phenotype is observed.[79] Hence, while the studies concur that MMP-3 attenuates plaque progression, they imply opposite effects on plaque stability.

ApoE[-/-] mice deficient in MMP-9 show no difference in size or stability in early lesions from the descending aorta and aortic root, but lesion size in advanced plaques is reduced.[80] Fibrillar collagen is reduced, implying less stability, but macrophage content is also decreased, implying greater stability.[80] In another study,[79] MMP-9/ApoE double knockout mice had larger plaques in the brachiocephalic artery, with less collagen and

more macrophages, implying less stability (Figure 5.3). Two other studies have used gene transfer to overexpress MMP-9. Local overexpression of pro-MMP-9 in carotid atherosclerotic lesions of ApoE[-/-] mice had no effect on size of early or advanced lesions but promoted intraplaque hemorrhage in advanced lesions.[81] By contrast, macrophage-specific overexpression of wild-type pro-MMP-9 showed no effect on stability of advanced brachiocephalic artery plaques.[82] However, similar expression of an auto-activating form of pro-MMP-9 induced significant plaque disruption, without significantly affecting lesion size or macrophage content.[82] In summary, MMP-9 appears to promote, have no effect, or undermine plaque stability, depending on the anatomic location, the stage of plaque development, and the state of MMP activation.

Deletion of MMP-12 reduced elastin degradation but did not alter the size or cellular composition of early or advanced plaques in the aorta of ApoE[-/-] mice.[80] In contrast, MMP-12 deletion promoted smaller more stable lesions in the

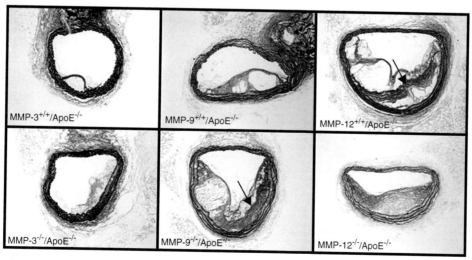

Figure 5.3 Representative atherosclerotic lesions from the brachiocephalic artery of matrix metalloproteinase/apolipoprotein E (MMP/ApoE) double knockout mice. Representative elastin van Gieson stained brachiocephalic arteries from ApoE knockout mice with a combined deficiency in either MMP-3, MMP-9, or MMP-12, and their respective wild-type controls. Arrows indicate the presence of buried fibrous layers, indicative of previous silent plaque ruptures.

brachiocephalic artery (see Figure 5.3).[79] In the only available study, deletion of MMP-7 had no effect on plaque growth or stability in the brachiocephalic artery.[79]

Two groups have studied the effect of TIMP-1 gene deletion in ApoE knockout mice, showing that local vessel wall MMP activity was increased and elastin degradation promoted.[83,84] However, the results on aortic plaque size were ambiguous; one study reported a decrease in plaque size in TIMP-1-deficient mice,[83] whereas no effect was observed in the other.[84] TIMP-1 has also been overexpressed in ApoE knockout mice by systemic delivery of an adenovirus, resulting in increased plasma levels of human TIMP-1;[74] aortic sinus lesion size and macrophage content were decreased. However, oral administration of synthetic MMP inhibitors had no effect on lesion size or stability in hypercholesterolemic mice.[85,86]

The results of these mouse experiments are summarized in Figure 5.2, which lists those MMPs that have been associated with features indicating increased plaque stability and those associated with plaque vulnerability. In many cases the conclusions are equivocal (see Figure 5.2). The experiments highlight the potential complexities of manipulating a system where MMPs may cause smaller, less-stable plaques by destroying the ECM or cause larger more or less stable plaques by promoting SMC and macrophage migration. Effects on endothelial cells might also be relevant. Hence, as we showed recently,[79] even within the same standardized model, deletion of one MMP (in this case MMP-12) was clearly deleterious for plaque stability, whereas deletion of others (MMP-3, MMP-9) was clearly protective (see Figure 5.3).

COULD INHIBITORS OF MMP ACTIVITY BE USED TO STABILIZE PLAQUES?

Some physiologic mediators present in the vessel wall can suppress MMP induction. Nitric oxide, for example, inhibits MMP-9 expression in SMCs by inhibiting superoxide generation and subsequent ERK activation.[87] Heparin and heparan sulfate proteoglycans also inhibit induction of MMP-1, MMP-3, and MMP-9 from SMCs.[88] TGF-β inhibits MMP-1, MMP-3, and MMP-7 induction in fibroblasts,[89] MMP-9[90] secretion in mast cells, and MMP-7[91] and MMP-9[92] in macrophages. Interferon-γ (IFN-γ) inhibits the CD40 ligation-induced secretion of MMP-1 and MMP-9 from SMCs,[33] and MMP-1, MMP-3, MMP-9, and MMP-12 from macrophages.[30,32] Apart from IFN-γ, these mediators have established atheroprotective roles that could be partly explained by effects on MMPs.

Statins are potent lipid-lowering drugs that prevent atherosclerosis progression and the onset of its acute thrombotic complications.[93,94] Statins may also have anti-inflammatory effects, including inhibition of MMP secretion, that are independent of their lipid-lowering action.[95] Statins reduce expression and secretion of MMP-1, MMP-2, MMP-3, and MMP-9 from macrophages and SMCs in vitro, and in rabbit and human atheroma,[96–100] but increase TIMP-1 expression,[98] in part by post-translational mechanisms.[100] Statin treatment may therefore tip the proteolytic balance from matrix degradation towards matrix accumulation, rendering plaques more stable.

Synthetic MMP inhibitors containing zinc-chelating groups such as thiol or hydroxamate groups have been developed, but clinical studies of broad-spectrum MMP inhibitors have demonstrated a narrow therapeutic window.[3] Experimental studies using such MMP inhibitors showed no effect on the development of atherosclerosis in hyperlipidemic mice[85] or atherosclerotic primates.[101]

Tetracyclines are a family of antibiotic drugs that have pluripotent effects, including efficient inhibition of MMP expression and activity.[102] The tetracycline derivative doxycycline is the most widely studied of this family and acts as a broad-spectrum MMP inhibitor. Recent studies have demonstrated inhibition of elastin degradation, and reduced MMP-2 and MMP-9 activity and expression, in the rat and human aortic wall after doxycycline treatment (as reviewed by Loftus et al[103]). Similarly, the presence of doxycycline attenuates MMP-2 and MMP-9 expression and retards intimal lesion development in vitro[104] and in vivo.[105] Similar results were observed when a non-antibiotic chemically modified tetracycline was utilized.[106] However, doxycycline treatment of hyperlipidemic mice had no effect on the extent of atherosclerosis.[86] Moreover, a small clinical trial[107] elegantly demonstrated that doxycycline penetrated human atherosclerotic carotid plaques and reduced MMP-1 tissue expression but found no beneficial effect on morphologic characteristics of the atherosclerotic lesions or patient outcome.

These disappointing initial results are perhaps because of the complexity of the MMP family and their diverse actions on ECM and non-ECM substrates. Studies with more selective MMP inhibitors are eagerly awaited.

SUMMARY

Histologic studies provide persuasive but largely correlative evidence that many MMPs play a role in plaque vulnerability in man. This is supported by genetic epidemiologic studies that imply, in particular, that MMP-1 and MMP-3 activity results in smaller but less-stable plaques. Contrary to expectation, however, knockout and transgenic studies fail to provide unequivocal evidence that MMPs promote plaque instability in the mouse. Indeed, some studies show clear protective effects. This could be due to limitations of the models or the complexities of manipulating the multiple effects of MMPs on different aspects of plaque biology. Possibly, for the same reason, broad-spectrum

MMP inhibitors appear to have little effect on plaque progression or vulnerability in animal models at clinically tolerable concentrations. In our view, more work is needed to elucidate the role of individual MMPs in plaque instability so as to tailor potential therapies using selective inhibitors.

ACKNOWLEDGMENT

The authors' work is supported by grants from the British Heart Foundation and the European Vascular Genomics Network.

REFERENCES

1. Davies MJ, Thomas A. Thrombosis and acute coronary-artery lesions in sudden cardiac ischemic death. N Engl J Med 1984; 310(18):1137–40.
2. Nagase H, Visse R, Murphy G. Structure and function of matrix metalloproteinases and TIMPs. Cardiovasc Res 2006; 69(3):562–73.
3. Newby AC. Matrix metalloproteinases regulate migration, proliferation, and death of vascular smooth muscle cells by degrading matrix and non-matrix substrates. Cardiovasc Res 2006; 69(3): 614–24.
4. Shipley JM, Wesselschmidt RL, Kobayashi DK, Ley TJ, Shapiro SD. Metalloelastase is required for macrophage-mediated proteolysis and matrix invasion in mice. Proc Natl Acad Sci USA 1996; 93:3942–6.
5. Virmani R, Kolodgie FD, Burke AP et al. Atherosclerotic plaque progression and vulnerability to rupture: angiogenesis as a source of intraplaque hemorrhage. Arterioscler Thromb Vasc Biol 2005; 25(10):2054–61.
6. Henney AM, Wakeley PR, Davies MJ et al. Localization of stromelysin gene expression in atherosclerotic plaques by in situ hybridization. Proc Natl Acad Sci 1991; 88:8154–8.
7. Galis ZS, Sukhova GK, Lark MW, Libby P. Increased expression of matrix metalloproteinases and matrix degrading activity in vulnerable regions of human atherosclerotic plaques. J Clin Invest 1994; 94:2493–503.
8. Galis ZS, Muszynski M, Sukhova GK et al. Cytokine-stimulated human vascular smooth muscle cells synthesize a complement of enzymes required for extracellular matrix digestion. Circ Res 1994; 75: 181–9.
9. Brown DL, Hibbs MS, Kearney M, Loushin C, Isner JM. Identification of 92-kD gelatinase in human coronary

atherosclerotic lesions. Association of active enzyme synthesis with unstable angina. Circulation 1995; 91: 2125–31.

10. Nikkari ST, Obrien KD, Ferguson M et al. Interstitial collagenase (MMP-1) expression in human carotid atherosclerosis. Circulation 1995; 92(6):1393–8.

11. Galis ZS, Sukhova GK, Libby P. Microscopic localisation of active proteases by in situ zymography: detection of matrix metalloproteinase activity in vascular tissue. FASEB J 1995; 9:974–80.

12. Johnson JL, Jackson CL, Angelini GD, George SJ. Activation of matrix-degrading metalloproteinases by mast cell proteases in atherosclerotic plaques. Arterioscler Thromb Vasc Biol 1998; 18:1707–15.

13. Sukhova GK, Schonbeck U, Rabkin E et al. Evidence for increased collagenolysis by interstitial collagenases-1 and -3 in vulnerable human atheromatous plaques. Circulation 1999; 99:2503–9.

14. Lee RT, Schoen FJ, Loree HM, Lark MW, Libby P. Circumferential stress and matrix metalloproteinase 1 in human coronary atherosclerosis – Implications for plaque rupture. Arterioscler Thromb Vasc Biol 1996; 16(8):1070–3.

15. Li Z, Li L, Zielke HR et al. Increased expression of 72-kd type IV collagenase (MMP-2) in human aortic atherosclerotic lesions. Am J Pathol 1996; 148:121–8.

16. Halpert I, Sires UI, Roby JD et al. Matrilysin is expressed by lipid-laden macrophages at sites of potential rupture in atherosclerotic lesions and localizes to areas of versican deposition, a proteoglycan substrate for the enzyme. Proc Natl Acad Sci USA 1996; 93(18):9748–53.

17. Schönbeck U, Mach F, Sukhova GK et al. Expression of stromelysin-3 in atherosclerotic lesions: regulation via CD40-CD40 ligand signaling in vitro and in vivo. J Exp Med 1999; 189:843–53.

18. Rajavashisth TB, Xu X-P, Jovinge S et al. Membrane type 1 matrix metalloproteinase expression in human atherosclerotic plaques: evidence for activation by proinflammatory mediators. Circulation 1999; 99:3103–9.

19. Uzui H, Harpf A, Liu M et al. Increased expression of membrane type 3-matrix metalloproteinase in human atherosclerotic plaque: role of activated macrophages and inflammatory cytokines. Circulation 2002; 106:3024–30.

20. Herman MP, Sukhova GK, Libby P et al. Expression of neutrophil collagenase (matrix metalloproteinase-8) in human atheroma: a novel collagenolytic pathway suggested by transcriptional profiling. Circulation 2001; 104:1899–904.

21. Davies MJ, Richardson PD, Woolf N, Katz DR, Mann J. Risk of thrombosis in human atherosclerotic plaques: role of extracellular lipid, macrophage, and smooth muscle cell content. Br Heart J 1993; 69(5):377–81.

22. Galis ZS, Sukhova GK, Kranzhöfer R, Clark S, Libby P. Macrophage foam cells from experimental atheroma constitutively produce matrix-degrading proteinases. Proc Natl Acad Sci USA 1995; 92:402–6.

23. Chase AJ, Bond M, Crook MF, Newby AC. Role of nuclear factor-κB activation in metalloproteinase-1,-3, and -9 secretion by human macrophages in vitro and rabbit foam cells produced in vivo. Arterioscler Thromb Vasc Biol 2002; 22:765–71.

24. Bond M, Chase AJ, Baker AH, Newby AC. Inhibition of transcription factor NF-kappaB reduces matrix metalloproteinase-1, -3 and -9 production by vascular smooth muscle cells. Cardiovasc Res 2001; 50(3): 556–65.

25. Yanagi H, Sasaguri Y, Sugama K, Morimatsu M, Nagase H. Production of tissue collagenase (matrix metalloproteinase 1) by human aortic smooth muscle cells in response to platelet-derived growth factor. Atherosclerosis 1992; 91:207–16.

26. Saren P, Welgus HG, Kovanen PT. TNF-α and IL-1β selectively induce expression of 92-kDa gelatinase by human macrophages. J Immunol 1996; 157:4159–65.

27. Fabunmi RP, Baker AH, Murray EJ, Booth RFG, Newby AC. Divergent regulation by growth factors and cytokines of 95 kDa and 72 kDa gelatinases and tissue inhibitors of metalloproteinases-1, -2 and -3 in rabbit aortic smooth muscle cells. Biochem J 1996; 315(Part 1):335–42.

28. Pickering JG, Ford CM, Tang B, Chow LH. Coordinated effects of fibroblast growth factor-2 on expression of fibrillar collagens, matrix metalloproteinases, and tissue inhibitors of matrix metalloproteinases by human vascular smooth muscle cells. Evidence for repressed collagen production and activated degradative capacity. Arterioscler Thromb Vasc Biol 1997; 17(3):475–82.

29. Bond M, Fabunmi RP, Baker AH, Newby AC. Synergistic upregulation of metalloproteinase-9 by growth factors and inflammatory cytokines: an absolute requirement for transcription factor NF-kappa B. FEBS Lett 1998; 11(1):29–34.

30. Mach F, Schönbeck U, Bonnefoy J-Y, Pober JS, Libby P. Activation of monocyte/macrophage functions related to acute atheroma complication by ligation of CD40. Induction of collagenase, stromelysin, and tissue factor. Circulation 1997; 96:396–9.

31. Malik N, Greenfield BW, Wahl AF, Kiener PA. Activation of human monocytes through CD40 induces matrix metalloproteinases. J Immunol 1996; 156:3952–60.

32. Wu L, Fan J, Matsumoto S-I, Watanabe T. Induction and regulation of matrix metalloproteinase-12 by cytokines and CD40 signaling in monocyte/macrophages. Biochem Bioph Res Commun 2000; 269:808–14.

33. Schönbeck U, Mach F, Sukhova GK et al. Regulation of matrix metalloproteinase expression in human vascular smooth muscle cells by T lymphocytes: a role for CD40 signaling in plaque rupture? Circ Res 1997; 81:448–54.

34. Mach F, Schönbeck U, Libby P. CD40 signaling in vascular cells: a key role in atherosclerosis? Atherosclerosis 1998; 137((Suppl)):S89–95.

35. Schönbeck U, Libby P. CD40 signaling and plaque instability. Circ Res 2001; 89:1092–103.

36. Lutgens E, Daemen MJAP. CD40–CD40L interactions in atherosclerosis. Trends Cardiovasc Med 2002; 12:27–32.

37. Ye S, Watts GF, Mandalia S, Humphries SE, Henney AM. Preliminary report: genetic variation in the human stromelysin promoter is associated with progression of coronary atherosclerosis. Br Heart J 1995; 73:209–15.

38. Hirashiki A, Yamada Y, Murase Y et al. Association of gene polymorphisms with coronary artery disease in low- or high-risk subjects defined by conventional risk factors. J Am Coll Cardiol 2003; 42(8): 1429–37.

39. Beyzade S, Zhang S, Wong Y et al. Influences of matrix metalloproteinase-3 gene variation on extent of coronary atherosclerosis and risk of myocardial infarction. J Am Coll Cardiol 2003; 41(12):2130–7.

40. Ghilardi G, Biondi ML, DeMonti M et al. Matrix metalloproteinase-1 and matrix metalloproteinase-3 gene promoter polymorphisms are associated with carotid artery stenosis. Stroke 2002; 33:2408–12.

41. Terashima M, Akita H, Kanazawa K et al. Stromelysin promoter 5A/6A polymorphism is associated with acute myocardial infarction. Circulation 1999; 99:2717–19.

42. Zhou X, Huang J, Chen J et al. Haplotype analysis of the matrix metalloproteinase 3 gene and myocardial infarction in a Chinese Han population. The Beijing atherosclerosis study. Thromb Haemost 2004; 92: 867–73.

43. Flex A, Gaetani E, Papaleo P et al. Proinflammatory genetic profiles in subjects with history of ischemic stroke. Stroke 2004; 35:2270–5.

44. Pearce E, Tregouet DA, Samnegard A et al. Haplotype effect of the matrix metalloproteinase-1 gene on risk of myocardial infarction. Circ Res 2005; 97(10):1070–6.

45. Ye S, Gale CR, Martyn CN. Variation in the matrix metalloproteinase-1 gene and risk of coronary heart disease. Eur Heart J 2003; 24(18):1668–71.

46. Jormsjo S, Wahtling C, Walter DH et al. Allele-specific regulation of matrix metalloproteinase-7 promoter activity is associated with coronary artery luminal dimensions among hypercholesterolemic patients. Arterioscler Thromb Vasc Biol 2001; 21:1834–9.

47. Zhang B, Ye S, Herrmann S-M et al. Functional polymorphism in the regulatory region of gelatinase B gene in relation to severity of coronary atherosclerosis. Circulation 1999; 99:1788–94.

48. Jormsjo S, Ye S, Moritz J et al. Allele-specific regulation of matrix metalloproteinase-12 gene activity is associated with coronary artery luminal dimensions in diabetic patients with manifest coronary artery disease. Circ Res 2000; 86:998–1003.

49. Blankenberg S, Rupprecht HJ, Poirier O et al. Plasma concentrations and genetic variation of matrix metalloproteinase 9 and prognosis of patients with cardiovascular disease. Circulation 2003; 107: 1579–85.

50. Ye S. Influence of matrix metalloproteinase genotype on cardiovascular disease susceptibility and outcome. Cardiovas Res 2006; 69(3):636–45.

51. Kai H, Ikeda H, Yasukawa H et al. Peripheral blood levels of matrix metalloproteinases-2 and -9 are elevated in patients with acute coronary syndromes. J Am Coll Cardiol 1998; 32(2):368–72.

52. Hojo Y, Ikeda U, Ueno S, Arakawa H, Shimada K. Expression of matrix metalloproteinases in patients with acute myocardial infarction. Jpn Circ J 2001; 65:71–5.

53. Wu TC, Leu HB, Lin WT et al. Plasma matrix metalloproteinase-3 level is an independent prognostic factor in stable coronary artery disease. Eur J Clin Invest 2005; 35:537–45.

54. Inokubo Y, Hanada H, Ishizaka H et al. Plasma levels of matrix metalloproteinase-9 and tissue inhibitor of metalloproteinase-1 are increased in the coronary circulation in patients with acute coronary syndrome. Am Heart J 2001; 141(2):211–17.

55. Duhamel-Clèrin E, Orvain C, Lanza F, Cazenave J-P, Klein-Soyer C. Thrombin receptor-mediated increase of two matrix metalloproteinases, MMP-1 and MMP-3, in human endothelial cells. Arterioscler Thromb Vasc Biol 1997; 17:1931–8.

56. Galt SW, Lindemann S, Medd D et al. Differential regulation of matrix metalloproteinase-9 by monocytes adherent to collagen and platelets. Circ Res 2001; 89(6):509–16.

57. Son JW, Koh KK, Ahn JY et al. Effects of statin on plaque stability and thrombogenicity in hypercholesterolemic patients with coronary artery disease. Int J Cardiol 2003; 88(1):77–82.

58. Death AK, Nakhla S, McGrath KCY et al. Nitroglycerin upregulates matrix metalloproteinase expression by human macrophages. J Am Coll Cardiol 2002; 39(12):1943–50.

59. George SJ, Zaltsman AB, Newby AC. Surgical preparative injury and neointima formation increase MMP-9 expression and MMP-2 activation in human saphenous vein. Cardiovasc Res 1997; 33:447–59.

60. Zempo N, Kenagy RD, Au T et al. Matrix metalloproteinases of vascular wall cells are increased in balloon-injured rat carotid. J Vasc Surg 1994; 20:209–17.

61. Southgate KM, Fisher M, Banning AP et al. Upregulation of basement membrane-degrading metalloproteinase secretion after balloon injury of pig carotid arteries. Circ Res 1996; 79(6):1177–87.

62. Southgate KM, Mehta D, Izzat MB, Newby AC, Angelini GD. Increased secretion of basement membrane-degrading metalloproteinases in pig saphenous vein into carotid artery interposition grafts. Arterioscler Thromb Vasc Biol 1999; 19:1640–9.

63. George SJ, Johnson JL, Angelini GD, Newby AC, Baker AH. Adenovirus-mediated gene transfer of the human TIMP-1 gene inhibits smooth muscle cell

migration and neointima formation in human saphenous vein. Hum Gene Ther 1998; 9:867–77.

64. George SJ, Baker AH, Angelini GD, Newby AC. Gene transfer of tissue inhibitor of metalloproteinase-2 inhibits metalloproteinase activity and neointima formation in human saphenous veins. Gene Therapy 1998; 5:1552–60.

65. Forough R, Koyama N, Hasenstab D et al. Overexpression of tissue inhibitor of matrix metalloprotienase-1 inhibits vascular smooth muscle cell functions in vitro and in vivo. Circ Res 1996; 79: 812–20.

66. Dollery CM, Humphries SE, McClelland A, Latchman DS, McEwan JR. Expression of tissue inhibitor of matrix metalloproteinases 1 by use of an adenoviral vector inhibits smooth muscle cell migration and reduces neointimal hyperplasia in the rat model of vascular balloon injury. Circulation 1999; 99(24):3199–205.

67. Cheng L, Mantile G, Pauly R et al. Adenovirus-mediated gene transfer of the human tissue inhibitor of metalloproteinase-2 blocks vascular smooth muscle cell invasiveness in vitro and modulates neointimal development in vivo. Circulation 1998; 98:2195–201.

68. Galis ZS, Johnson C, Godin D et al. Targeted disruption of the matrix metalloproteinase-9 gene impairs smooth muscle cell migration and geometrical arterial remodeling. Circ Res 2002; 91:852–9.

69. Cho A, Reidy MA. Matrix metalloproteinase-9 is necessary for the regulation of smooth muscle cell replication and migration after arterial injury. Circ Res 2002; 91:845–51.

70. Kuzuya M, Kanda S, Sasaki T et al. Deficiency of gelatinase a suppresses smooth muscle cell invasion and development of experimental intimal hyperplasia. Circulation 2003; 108(11):1375–81.

71. Zaltsman AB, Newby AC. Increased secretion of gelatinases A and B from the aortas of cholesterol fed rabbits: relationship to lesion severity. Atherosclerosis 1997; 130(1–2):61–70.

72. Johnson J, Carson K, Williams H et al. Plaque rupture after short periods of fat-feeding in the apolipoprotein E knockout mouse: model characterisation, and effects of pravastatin treatment. Circulation 2005; 111:1422–30.

73. Jeng AY, Chou M, Sawyer WK et al. Enhanced expression of matrix metalloproteinase-3, -12, and -13 mRNAs in the aortas of apolipoprotein E-deficient mice with advanced atherosclerosis. Ann NY Acad Sci 1999; 878:555–8.

74. Rouis M, Adamy C, Duverger N et al. Adenovirus-mediated overexpression of tissue inhibitor of metalloproteinase-1 reduces atherosclerotic lesions in apolipoprotein E-deficient mice. Circulation 1999; 100:533–40.

75. Lemaitre V, O'Byrne TK, Borczuk AC et al. ApoE knockout mice expressing human matrix metalloproteinase-1 in macrophages have less advanced atherosclerosis. J Clin Invest 2001; 107:1227–34.

76. Deguchi JO, Aikawa E, Libby P et al. Matrix metalloproteinase-13/collagenase-3 deletion promotes collagen accumulation and organization in mouse atherosclerotic plaques. Circulation 2005; 112(17): 2708–15.

77. Fukumoto Y, Deguchi J, Libby P et al. Genetically determined resistance to collagenase action augments interstitial collagen accumulation in atherosclerotic plaques. Circulation 2004; 110(14):1953–9.

78. Silence J, Lupu F, Collen D, Lijnen HR. Persistence of atherosclerotic plaque but reduced aneurysm formation in mice with stromelysin-1 (MMP-3) gene inactivation. Arterioscler Thromb Vasc Biol 2001; 21:1440–5.

79. Johnson JL, George SJ, Newby AC, Jackson CL. Divergent effects of matrix metalloproteinases -3, -7,-9 and -12 on atherosclerotic plaque stability in mouse brachiocephalic arteries. Proc Natl Acad Sci USA 2005; 102(43):15575–80.

80. Luttun A, Lutgens E, Manderveld A et al. Loss of matrix metalloproteinase-9 or matrix metalloproteinase-12 protects apolipoprotein E-deficient mice against atherosclerotic media destruction but differentially affects plaque growth. Circulation 2004; 109(11):1408–14.

81. de Nooijer R, Verkleij CJ, von der Thuesen JH et al. Lesional overexpression of matrix metalloproteinase-9 promotes intraplaque hemorrhage in advanced lesions, but not at earlier stages of atherogenesis. Arterioscler Thromb Vasc Biol 2006; 26:340–6.

82. Gough PJ, Gomez IG, Wille PT, Raines EW. Macrophage expression of active MMP-9 induces acute plaque disruption in apoE-deficient mice. J Clin Invest 2006; 116(1):59–69.

83. Silence J, Collen D, Lijnen HR. Reduced atherosclerotic plaque but enhanced aneurysm formation in mice with inactivation of the tissue inhibitor of metalloproteinase-1 (TIMP-1) gene. Circ Res 2002; 90: 897–903.

84. Lemaître V, Soloway PD, D'Armiento J. Increased medial degradation with pseudo-aneurysm formation in apolipoprotein E-knockout mice deficient in tissue inhibitor of metalloproteinases-1. Circulation 2003; 107:333–8.

85. Prescott MF, Sawyer WK, Von Linden-Reed J et al. Effect of matrix metalloproteinase inhibition on progression of atherosclerosis and aneurysm in LDL receptor-deficient mice overexpressing MMP3, MMP-12, and MMP-13 and on restenosis in rats after balloon injury. Ann NY Acad Sci 1999; 878: 179–90.

86. Manning MW, Cassis LA, Daugherty A. Differential effects of doxycycline, a broad-spectrum matrix metalloproteinase inhibitor, on angiotensin II-induced atherosclerosis and abdominal aortic aneurysms. Arterioscler Thromb Vasc Biol 2003; 23:483–8.

87. Gurjar MV, DeLeon J, Sharma RV, Bhalla RC. Mechanism of inhibition of matrix metalloproteinase-9

induction by NO in vascular smooth muscle cells. J Appl Physiol 2001; 91(3):1380–6.

88. Kenagy RD, Nikkari ST, Welgus HG, Clowes AW. Heparin inhibits the induction of three matrix metalloproteinases (stomelysin, 92-kD gelatinase, and collagenase) in primate arterial smooth muscle cells. J Clin Invest 1994; 93:1987–93.

89. Uria JA, Jimenez MG, Balbin M, Freije JMP, Lopez-Otin C. Differential effects of transforming growth factor-β on the expression of collagenase-1 and collagenase-3 in human fibroblasts. J Biol Chem 1998; 273(16):9769–77.

90. Fang KC, Wolters PJ, Steinhoff M et al. Mast cell expression of gelatinases A and B is regulated by kit ligand and TGF-β. J Immunol 1999; 162:5528–35.

91. Busiek DF, Baragi VM, Nehring LC, Parks WC, Welgus HG. Matrilysin expression by human mononuclear phagocytes and its regulation by cytokines and hormones. J Immunol 1995; 154: 6484–91.

92. Feinberg MW, Jain MK, Werner F et al. Transforming growth factor-β1 inhibits cytokine-mediated induction of human metalloelastase in macrophages. J Biol Chem 2000; 275(33):25766–73.

93. Libby P. Current concepts of the pathogenesis of the acute coronary syndromes. Circulation 2001; 104: 365–72.

94. Libby P, Aikawa M. Stabilization of atherosclerotic plaques: new mechanisms and clinical targets. Nat Med 2002; 8(11):1257–62.

95. Palinski W, Napoli. Unraveling pleiotropic effects of statins on plaque rupture. Arterioscler Thromb Vasc Biol 2002; 22:1745–50.

96. Bellosta S, Via D, Canavesi M et al. HMG-CoA reductase inhibitors reduce MMP-9 secretion by macrophages. Arterioscler Thromb Vasc Biol 1998; 18:1671–8.

97. Aikawa M, Rabkin E, Sugiyama S et al. An HMG-CoA reductase inhibitor, cerivastatin, suppresses growth of macrophages expressing matrix metalloproteinases and tissue factor in vivo and in vitro. Circulation 2001; 103:276–83.

98. Crisby M, Nordin-Fredriksson G, Shah PK et al. Pravastatin treatment increases collagen content and decreases lipid content, inflammation, metalloproteinases, and cell death in human carotid plaques. Circulation 2001; 103:926–33.

99. Fukumoto Y, Libby P, Rabkin E et al. Statins alter smooth muscle cell accumulation and collagen content in established atheroma of Watanabe heritable hyperlipidemic rabbits. Circulation 2001; 103: 993–9.

100. Luan Z, Chase AJ, Newby AC. Statins inhibit secretion of metalloproteinases-1, -2, -3 and -9 from vascular smooth muscle cells and macrophages. Arterioscler Thromb Vasc Biol 2003; 23(5):769–75.

101. Cherr GS, Motew SJ, Travis JA et al. Metalloproteinase inhibition and the response to angioplasty and stenting in atherosclerotic primates. Arterioscler Thromb Vasc Biol 2002; 22:161–6.

102. Golub LM, Lee HM, Ryan ME et al. Tetracyclines inhibit connective tissue breakdown by multiple non-antimicrobial mechanisms. Adv Dent Res 1998; 12(2):12–26.

103. Loftus IM, Naylor AR, Bell PR, Thompson MM. Matrix metalloproteinases and atherosclerotic plaque instability. Br J Surg 2002; 89:680–94.

104. Porter KE, Thompson MM, Loftus IM et al. Production and inhibition of the gelatinolytic matrix metalloproteinases in a human model of vein graft stenosis. Eur J Vasc Endovasc Surg 1999; 14:404–12.

105. Bendeck MP, Conte M, Zhang M et al. Doxycycline modulates smooth muscle cell growth, migration, and matrix remodeling after arterial injury. Am J Pathol 2002; 160:1089–95.

106. Islam MM, Franco CD, Courtman DW, Bendeck MP. A nonantibiotic chemically modified tetracycline (CMT-3) inhibits intimal thickening. Am J Pathol 2003; 163(4):1557–66.

107. Axisa B, Loftus IM, Naylor AR et al. Prospective, randomized, double-blind trial investigating the effect of doxycycline on matrix metalloproteinase expression within atherosclerotic carotid plaques. Stroke 2002; 33:2858–64.

Oxidative stress and the vulnerable plaque

6

Donald D Heistad and Yi Chu

INTRODUCTION

An extremely hot topic in vascular biology is the role of superoxide and other reactive oxygen species (ROS) in cell signaling and in pathophysiology of vascular disease. The role of ROS in the vulnerable plaque has received remarkably little attention, but may be central to understanding development and rupture of the vulnerable plaque.[1]

Two recent clinical studies are particularly important in implication of ROS in the vulnerable plaque. First, in coronary atherectomy samples from patients with unstable and stable angina, generation of ROS was greater in patients with unstable angina (Figure 6.1).[2] Secondly, impairment of an endogenous antioxidant enzyme which protects against ROS is associated with increased incidence of ischemic heart disease.[3]

In this chapter, we briefly summarize:

- the role of ROS, especially superoxide, in the pathophysiology of atherosclerosis
- sources of ROS in atherosclerotic plaques
- antioxidant mechanisms
- some targets of ROS
- the potential role of ROS in the vulnerable plaque
- superoxide after catheter-induced vascular injury.

We speculate that superoxide may destabilize the vulnerable plaque, and impairment of the endothelial thrombomodulin/protein C anticoagulant system may predispose to propagation of arterial thrombosis downstream from a vulnerable plaque.

REACTIVE OXYGEN SPECIES IN ATHEROSCLEROSIS

Atherosclerosis and a variety of risk factors for cardiovascular disease are associated with oxidative stress, with increased levels of superoxide in the arterial wall.[4,5] An important aspect of oxidative stress is that superoxide (O_2^{-}) inactivates nitric oxide ($NO^{.}$) and thus produces endothelial dysfunction.[6,7] Endothelial dysfunction is associated with, and probably contributes to, increased risk of cardiovascular events.[8] Thus, at least in part through its role in endothelial dysfunction, superoxide may contribute to increased risk of cardiovascular events.

High levels of superoxide in atherosclerotic arteries[9,10] may have several consequences. Oxidation of low-density lipoprotein (LDL) plays an important role in atherosclerosis.[11] At normal levels, ROS play a key role in cell signaling.[12] At excess levels, however, ROS damage lipids in the cell membrane, proteins, and DNA.[13]

Endothelium not only modulates vasomotor tone but also plays a key role in endogenous anticoagulant mechanisms. For example, thrombin is not only a

Figure 6.1 Reactive oxygen species in coronary atherectomy sample from a patient with unstable angina. Dihydroethidium fluoresces (red) in the presence of superoxide. (Reproduced from Azumi et al,[2] with permission.)

procoagulant but it also binds to thrombomodulin in endothelium and thereby activates protein C, which is an extremely potent anticoagulant. In atherosclerosis, however, the endothelial thrombomodulin/protein C anticoagulant system is impaired,[14] which may contribute to the risk of thrombosis in atherosclerotic arteries.

Treatment of hypercholesterolemia produces relatively rapid improvement in endothelial function in atherosclerotic

monkeys[15–17] and humans.[18,19] Levels of superoxide in arteries decrease greatly during regression of atherosclerosis (Figure 6.2).[10] Reduction of superoxide during regression of atherosclerosis presumably accounts for improvement in endothelial function. Regression of atherosclerosis in monkeys is also accompanied by improvement in the endothelial thrombomodulin/protein C anticoagulant system.[20] The finding may provide insight into an important mechanism by which treatment of hypercholesterolemia reduces risk of cardiovascular events.

SOURCES OF REACTIVE OXYGEN SPECIES IN ATHEROSCLEROTIC PLAQUES

In light of the inflammatory response in atherosclerosis,[21] it is not surprising that leukocytes are an important source of superoxide in atherosclerotic arteries. A surprising finding, however, was that smooth muscle cells in the media become an important source of superoxide in atherosclerotic arteries (Figure 6.3).[9] Angiotensin II activates NAD(P)H oxidase,[22] and it is likely that activation of

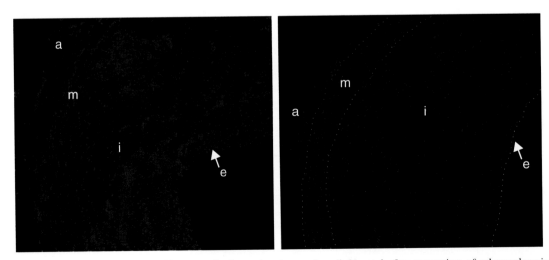

Figure 6.2 Superoxide in carotid artery of atherosclerotic monkey (left), and after regression of atherosclerosis (right), as indicated by fluorescence of dihydroethidium: a = adventitia, m = media, i = intima, and e = endothelium. (Reproduced from Hathaway et al,[10] with permission.)

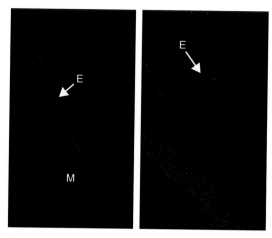

Figure 6.3 Superoxide in aorta of normal rabbit (left) and Watanabe hypercholesterolemic rabbit (right). Elevated levels of superoxide in atherosclerotic arteries occur throughout the vascular wall, including smooth muscle cells. (Reproduced from Miller et al,[9] with permission.)

NAD(P)H oxidase in smooth muscle cells is an important mechanism for generation of superoxide in atherosclerotic monkeys.

Other enzymatic sources also may contribute to generation of superoxide in atherosclerotic arteries. Xanthine oxidase and lipoxygenases also may generate superoxide in atherosclerotic arteries.[13] 'Uncoupling' of nitric oxide synthase (NOS), with generation of superoxide as well as NO, occurs when a cofactor of NOS (tetrahydrobiopterin) is deficient.[23,24] Uncoupling of NOS may occur in atherosclerotic arteries, and contribute to generation of superoxide. Mitochondria also are an important potential source for generation of superoxide in atherosclerotic arteries.

ANTIOXIDANT MECHANISMS

Superoxide dismutases (SODs) catalyze the reaction which dismutes superoxide ($O_2{}^{\cdot-}$) to H_2O_2. The three isoforms of SOD are copper–zinc SOD (CuZnSOD), which is localized in cytosol (and the nucleus), manganese SOD (MnSOD) in mitochondria, and extracellular SOD (ecSOD) in the extracellular space.[25] CuZnSOD and ecSOD are the predominant isoforms in arteries.

CuZnSOD plays a critical role in regulation of basal levels of superoxide in blood vessels, and of NO bioavailability.[25] When MnSOD is deficient, there is enhanced mitochondrial DNA damage and amelioration of atherosclerosis.[13]

Despite its high concentrations and activity in blood vessels, ecSOD has received far less attention than the other SODs. ecSOD is localized preferentially in the extracellular space between smooth muscle and endothelium, and a major function of ecSOD may be to protect NO as it diffuses from endothelium to vascular muscle.[26]

A recent study[3] has brought new attention to the importance of ecSOD. The study reported that a common gene variant of ecSOD (ecSOD$_{R213G}$) is associated with increased risk of ischemic heart disease.[3] The R213G gene variant occurs in the heparin-binding domain (HBD) of ecSOD, which accounts for binding of ecSOD to the external membrane of cells. Because ecSOD fails to bind to the outer surface of endothelium and other cells, serum levels of ecSOD are increased in humans with the R213G gene variant.

We have reported that the HBD is essential for normal vascular function of ecSOD.[27] Recently we found that ecSOD$_{R213G}$ fails to protect endothelial function.[28] Thus, it appears that each of the isoforms of SOD plays an important role in protection of blood vessels against oxidative stress.[5]

Catalase and glutathione peroxidase are important enzymes that also protect against damage from ROS. Finally, nonenzymatic antioxidants, including glutathione, ascorbic acid, and α-tocopherol, also protect against oxidant injury.

SOME TARGETS OF REACTIVE OXYGEN SPECIES

Low levels of superoxide and other ROS play an important physiologic role in signaling.[12] During a variety of pathophysiologic states, however, high levels of superoxide are generated, and may become destructive. Oxidation of LDL is important in the pathophysiology of atherosclerosis.[11] Activation of matrix metalloproteinases (MMPs) by ROS may lead to degradation of matrix.[29] High levels of superoxide and other ROS also produce necrosis, and perhaps apoptosis.[30]

Superoxide reacts with NO to produce peroxynitrite, which is very toxic to cells. It is of interest that peroxynitrite can inactivate tetrahydrobiopterin (BH_4) a cofactor for each of the nitric oxide synthases.[12] Deficiency of BH_4 leads to 'uncoupling' of NOS,[23,24] which leads to generation of superoxide by NOS. Thus, generation of peroxynitrite by the reaction of $O_2{}^{.-}$ and $NO^{.}$, inactivation of BH_4, and uncoupling of NOS have the potential to feed forward, and generate more superoxide and peroxynitrite.

REACTIVE OXYGEN SPECIES IN THE VULNERABLE PLAQUE

A very important study reported that coronary arteries of patients with acute coronary syndrome have high levels of superoxide.[2] The authors used two independent methods to demonstrate, in atherectomy samples, that superoxide levels were much higher in coronary arteries of patients with unstable angina than in patients with stable angina. Sources of ROS in the coronary arteries of patients with unstable angina were inflammatory cells, smooth muscle cells, and fibroblasts.

The authors[2] also demonstrated increased expression of p22[phox], a component of NAD(P)H oxidase. The finding implicates the oxidase as a source of superoxide in atherosclerotic coronary arteries. They also demonstrated spatial colocalization of p22[phox] and oxidized LDL, which thereby implicates NAD(P)H oxidase as a mediator of oxidation of LDL.

What are the implications of these findings for the vulnerable plaque? The study provides direct evidence that coronary arteries of patients with acute coronary syndrome have high levels of superoxide. Because MMPs are activated by superoxide,[31] the study[2] provides evidence for a mechanism to activate MMPs, and presumably destabilize plaques, in patients with acute coronary syndrome (Figure 6.4).

As discussed above, atherosclerosis impairs the endothelial thrombomodulin/protein C pathway,[14] and regression of atherosclerosis restores this potent anticoagulant pathway towards normal.[20] We speculate that these changes may be especially relevant to the vulnerable plaque. When thrombin initiates formation of a thrombus in an artery with normal endothelium (e.g. at the site of a puncture), activation of the thrombomodulin/protein C pathway prevents propagation of the thrombus. In contrast, when thrombin initiates formation of a thrombus at the site of a vulnerable plaque, endothelium of the atherosclerotic artery is abnormal, activation of the thrombomodulin/protein C pathway is impaired, and the thrombus may propagate downstream from the initial thrombus.

As demonstrated in many clinical trials, 'statins' (or HMG-CoA reductase inhibitors) greatly reduce the risk of cardiovascular events. It seems likely that the protective effect of statins is mediated at least in part by beneficial effects on the vulnerable plaque. In this context, it is of interest that statins inhibit the assembly of components of NAD(P)H oxidase.[32] Thus, perhaps, statins attenuate the risk of vulnerable plaques in part by inhibition of NAD(P)H oxidase.

Human monocytes contain angiotensin II,[33] which is a strong stimulus for activation of NAD(P)H oxidase.[22] Macrophages in atherosclerotic lesions of monkeys (especially in the vulnerable 'shoulder' region of plaques) contain angiotensin II, and angiotensin II-containing cells decrease during regression of atherosclerosis.[34]

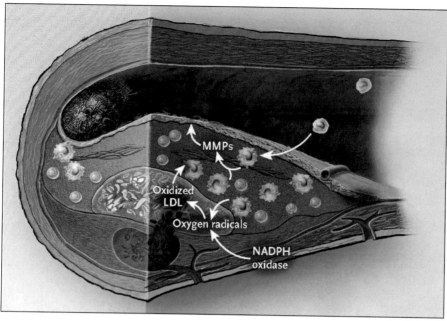

Figure 6.4   In a vulnerable plaque, superoxide and other oxygen radicals may be generated from NAD(P)H oxidase, inflammatory cells, and by other enzymatic mechanisms. Superoxide oxidizes low-density lipoprotein (LDL), and also activates matrix metalloproteinases (MMPs), thus contributing to destabilization of the plaque. (Modified from Heistad,[1] with permission.)

We speculate that reduction of angiotensin II-containing cells during regression of atherosclerosis results in decreased activation of NAD(P)H oxidase, and a reduction in generation of superoxide in the vulnerable plaque during regression of atherosclerosis.

SUPEROXIDE AFTER VASCULAR INJURY

Catheter-induced injury of arteries produces an acute burst of superoxide,[30,35] which is sustained for at least 2 weeks (Figure 6.5).[36] The findings are especially important because ROS modulate proliferation and migration of smooth muscle cells,[37] and may thereby contribute to restenosis. Several antioxidants have been reported to reduce neointimal proliferation and perhaps restenosis.

An NAD(P)H oxidase appears to be involved in generation of superoxide after balloon injury.[35] It is of particular interest that two homologs of gp91phox, nox 1 and nox 4, both of which generate superoxide, appear to serve different functions. Nox 1 is expressed early in arterial injury, and may contribute to formation of neointima, and nox 4 is expressed 2 weeks after arterial injury, and may serve to terminate the response.[38] Thus, generation of superoxide by different noxes, in different locations within the cell and artery, may contribute to both initiation and termination of the vascular responses to injury.

SUMMARY

The role of superoxide and other ROS in blood vessels has been studied in atherosclerosis and a variety of other vascular diseases. There is strong evidence that oxidative injury plays a central role in the pathophysiology of vascular disease.

There is a paucity of studies of the role of superoxide and other ROS in the

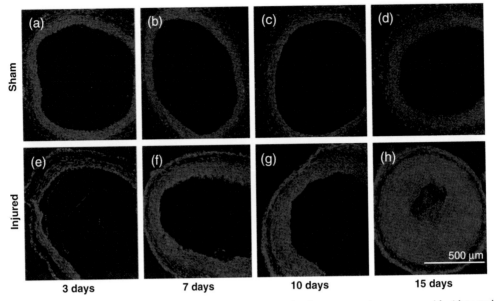

Figure 6.5 After balloon injury of the carotid artery in rats, but not in sham-operated rats, superoxide (detected with dihydroethidium) is increased at 3, 7, 10, and 15 days after injury. (Reproduced from Szocs et al,[38] with permission.)

vulnerable plaque. There is strong rationale for suggesting that superoxide may destabilize the vulnerable plaque, and an important study suggests that superoxide is increased in coronary arteries of patients with acute coronary syndrome. It is likely that studies of the role of ROS in the vulnerable plaque will be a fruitful area of research.

ACKNOWLEDGMENTS

Original studies described in this chapter were supported by NIH grants HL 62984, HL 16066, NS 24621, HL 14388, HL 38901, DK 54759, DK 15843, DK 52617, funds provided by the VA Medical Service, and a Carver Trust Research Program of Excellence.

REFERENCES

1. Heistad DD. Unstable coronary-artery plaques. N Engl J Med 2003; 349:2285–87.
2. Azumi H, Inoue N, Ohasha Y et al. Superoxide generation in directional coronary atherectomy specimens of patients with angina pectorism; important role of NAD(P)H oxidase. Arterioscler Thromb Vasc Biol 2002; 22:1838–44.
3. Juul K, Tybjaerg-Hansen A, Marklund S et al. Genetically reduced antioxidative protection and increased ischemic heart disease risk: The Copenhagen City Heart Study. Circulation 2004; 109:59–65.
4. Ohara Y, Peterson TE, Harrison DG. Hypercholesterolemia increases endothelial superoxide anion production. J Clin Invest 1993; 91:2546–51.
5. Heistad D. Oxidative stress and vascular disease: 2005 Duff lecture. Arterioscler Thromb Vasc Biol 2006; 26: 689–95.
6. Wei EP, Kontos HA, Christman CW, DeWitt DS, Povlishock JT. Superoxide generation and reversal of acetylcholine-induced cerebral arteriolar dilation after acute hypertension. Circ Res 1985; 57:781–7.
7. Rubanyi GM, Vanhoutte PM. Superoxide anions and hyperoxia inactivate endothelium-derived relaxing factor. Am J Physiol 1986; 250:H822–7.
8. Bonetti PO, Lerman LO, Lerman A. Endothelial dysfunction: A marker for atherosclerotic risk. Arterioscler Thromb Vasc Biol 2003; 23:168–75.
9. Miller FJ, Gutterman DD, Rios CD, Heistad DD, Davidson BL. Superoxide production in vascular smooth muscle contributes to oxidative stress and impaired relaxation in atherosclerosis. Circ Res 1998; 82:1298–305.
10. Hathaway C, Heistad DD, Piegors DJ, Miller FM. Regression of atherosclerosis in monkeys reduces vascular superoxide levels. Circ Res 2002; 90: 277–83.

11. Steinberg D. Low density lipoprotein oxidation and its pathobiological significance. J Biol Chem 1997; 272:20963–6.

12. Mueller CFH, Laude K, McNally JS, Harrison DG. Redox mechanisms in blood vessels. Arterioscler Thromb Vasc Biol 2005; 25:274–8.

13. Madamanchi NR, Vendrov A, Runge MS. Oxidative stress and vascular disease. Arterioscler Thromb Vasc Biol 2005; 25:29–38.

14. Lentz SR, Fernandez, JA, Griffin JH et al. Impaired anticoagulant response to infusion of thrombin in atherosclerotic monkeys associated with acquired defects in the protein C system. Arterioscler Thromb Vasc Biol 1999; 19:1744–50.

15. Harrison DG, Armstrong ML, Freiman PC, Heistad DD. Restoration of endothelium-dependent relaxation by dietary treatment of atherosclerosis. J Clin Invest 1987; 80:1808–11.

16. Heistad DD, Mark AL, Marcus ML, Piegors DJ, Armstrong ML. Dietary treatment of atherosclerosis abolishes hyperresponsiveness to serotonin: implications for vasospasm. Circ Res 1987; 61:346–51.

17. Benzuly KH, Padgett RC, Kaul S et al. Functional improvement precedes structural regression of atherosclerosis. Circulation 1994; 89:1810–18.

18. Leung WH, Lau CP, Wong CK. Beneficial effect of cholesterol–lowering therapy on coronary endothelium-dependent relaxation in hypercholesterolemic patients. Lancet 1993; 341:1496–500.

19. Treasure CB, Klein JL, Weintraub JD et al. Beneficial effects of cholesterol-lowering therapy on the coronary endothelium in patients with coronary artery disease. N Engl J Med 1995; 332:481–7.

20. Lentz SR, Miller FM Jr, Piegors DJ et al. Anticoagulant responses to thrombin are enhanced during regression of atherosclerosis in monkeys. Circulation 2002; 106:842–6.

21. Hansson G. Inflammation, atherosclerosis, and coronary artery disease. N Engl J Med 2005; 352:1685–95.

22. Griendling K, Ollerenshaw JD, Minieri CA, Alexander RW. Angiotensin II stimulates NADH and NADPH activity in cultured vascular smooth muscle cells. Circ Res 1994; 74:1141–8.

23. Alp NJ, Channon KM. Regulation of endothelial nitric oxide synthase by tetrahydrobiopterin in vascular disease. Arterioscler Thromb Vasc Biol 2004; 24:413–20.

24. Vasquez-Vivar J, Kalyanaraman B, Martasek P et al. Superoxide generation by endothelial nitric oxide synthase: the influence of cofactors. Proc Natl Acad Sci USA 1998; 95:9220–5.

25. Faraci FM, Didion SP. Vascular protection: superoxide dismutase isoforms in the vessel wall. Arterioscler Thromb Vasc Biol 2004; 24:1367–73.

26. Oury TD, Day BJ, Crapo JD. Extracellular superoxide dismutase: a regulator of nitric oxide bioavailability. Lab Invest 1996; 75:617–36.

27. Chu Y, Iida S, Lund DD et al. Gene transfer of extracellular superoxide dismutase reduces arterial pressure in spontaneously hypertensive rats: role of heparin binding domain. Circ Res 2003; 92:461–8.

28. Chu Y, Alwahdani A, Iida S et al. Vascular effects of human extracellular SOD_{R213G} variant. Circulation 2005; 112:1047–53.

29. Lee RT, Libby P. The unstable atheroma. Arterioscler Thromb Vasc Biol 1997; 17:1859–67.

30. Pollman MJ, Hall JL, Gibbons GH. Determinants of vascular smooth muscle cell apoptosis after balloon angioplasty injury: influence of redox state and cell phenotype. Circ Res 1999; 84:113–21.

31. Libby P. Molecular bases of the acute coronary syndromes. Circulation 1995; 91:2844–50.

32. Wagner AH, Kohler T, Ruckschloss U et al. Improvement of nitric oxide-dependent vasodilation by HMG-CoA reductase inhibitors through attenuation of endothelial superoxide anion formation. Arterioscler Thromb Vasc Biol 2000; 20:61–9.

33. Kitazono T, Padgett RC, Armstrong ML, Tompkins PK, Heistad DD. Evidence that angiotensin II is present in human monocytes. Circulation 1995; 91: 1129–34.

34. Potter DD, Sobey CG, Tompkins PK, Rossen JD, Heistad DD. Evidence that macrophages in atherosclerotic lesions contain angiotensin II. Circulation 1998; 98:800–7.

35. Souza HP, Souza LC, Anastacio VM et al. Vascular oxidant stress early after balloon injury: evidence for increased NAD(P)H oxidoreductase activity. Free Radic Biol Med 2000; 28:1232–42.

36. Nunes GL, Robinson K, Kalynch A et al. Vitamins C and E inhibit O_2^- production in the pig coronary artery. Circulation 1997; 96:3593–601.

37. Sundaresan M, Zu-Xi Y, Ferrans VJ et al. Requirement for generation of H_2O_2 for platelet-derived growth factor signal transduction. Science 1995; 270:296–9.

38. Szocs K, Lassegue B, Sorescu D et al. Upregulation of Nox-based NAD(P)H oxidases in restenosis after carotid injury. Arterioscler Thromb Vasc Biol 2002; 22:21–7.

Carotid vulnerable plaque 7

Erica CS Camargo and Karen L Furie

BACKGROUND

Carotid artery disease is one of the major causes of ischemic stroke.[1,2] The predominant mechanisms by which it causes stroke are:

- arterial embolism from atherosclerotic plaques
- hemodynamic changes, leading to 'watershed' infarcts
- distal propagation of thrombus originating from acute carotid occlusion.[3]

Clinical studies favor atherosclerotic artery-to-artery embolism as the principal mechanism related to carotid stroke.[4,5] Multiple studies have shown a direct relationship between degree of carotid stenosis and risk of subsequent ipsilateral stroke.[6,7] However, it has been demonstrated that even severe carotid stenosis may not necessarily lead to a high rate of arterial embolization.[8,9] Hence, lumenal narrowing may not be the core determinant of ischemic cerebrovascular events. Similarly, in the coronary arterial bed, the majority of atherosclerotic lesions have <50% stenosis on the initial vascular imaging prior to an acute coronary event.[10,11] In the coronaries, compensatory enlargement of the arteries occurs in response to plaque formation, such that functionally important lumenal stenosis may be delayed until the lesion occupies 40% of the internal elastic lamina area.[12]

Hence, plaque stability, or plaque vulnerability to (1) embolization of atherosclerotic debris, (2) formation and embolization of thrombus from the lumenal surface, or (3) progression of lumenal compromise could be the added factor accounting for the variability in the behavior of atherosclerotic vessels.[13] We will consider 'vulnerable plaque' to be an atherosclerotic lesion prone to cause symptoms by one of these mechanisms. It is important to consider that other factors, such as hypercoagulable states ('vulnerable blood') and local tissue predisposition may also play a role in the pathogenesis of thrombotic occlusion. A broader term that encompasses all these factors has been proposed, the 'vulnerable patient', in whom systemic vulnerability to thrombosis plays a major role in the pathogenesis of cardiovascular and cerebrovascular events.[14,15]

In this chapter, we focus on the definition and pathophysiology of carotid 'vulnerable' plaque, the diagnostic tools used to assess this disease, and the therapeutic strategies for the prevention of strokes secondary to carotid vulnerable plaques.

DEFINITION

The concept of vulnerable plaque was introduced into the literature in 1994 by Muller et al, and defined functionally as a plaque that had a high likelihood of becoming disrupted and initiating thrombosis in a coronary artery.[16] The plaques that corresponded to this functional definition had large lipid content, a thin atheromatous cap, and macrophage-dense inflammation on or below its surface. Subsequent histologic studies by Virmani et al revealed that there are several histologic subtypes of vulnerable coronary plaque: plaque erosion (de-endothelialized surface upon which thrombus forms); thin fibrous cap atheroma (the most common type); ruptured plaque; and calcified nodule. Other histologic plaque variants, such as intimal thickening, intimal xanthoma, and fibrocalcific plaque, are not commonly associated with thrombosis.[17]

In 2003, additional criteria for the determination of plaque vulnerability were proposed to further standardize its classification. The statement by Naghavi et al proposed the following diagnostic criteria: [14]

Major criteria:

- active inflammation, with infiltration of monocytes/macrophages and T cells
- thin cap with a large lipid core (>40% of the plaque volume)
- endothelial denudation with superficial platelet aggregation
- fissured plaque
- severe stenosis.

Minor criteria:

- superficial calcified nodule within or close to the cap
- glistening yellow color (suggestive of thin cap with large lipid core)
- intraplaque hemorrhage (suggestive of plaque instability)
- endothelial dysfunction (predictor of coronary heart disease and stroke)
- outward or positive remodeling (compensatory enlargement of non-stenotic lesions, preceding significant occlusion of the vascular lumen).

While the most frequent final mechanism producing clinical events differs for ischemic stroke and myocardial infarction (embolism for the former, in-situ thrombosis for the latter), the initial steps of plaque disruption leading to localized thrombosis are similar, as are the histologic features of plaques causing the diseases.

Patients with carotid atherosclerosis are very likely to have coronary artery disease as well. In the Asymptomatic Carotid Atherosclerosis Study (ACAS), 69% of patients with >60% asymptomatic carotid stenosis had concomitant coronary artery disease.[9] In the Atherosclerosis Risk in Communities (ARIC) Study cohort, mean carotid far wall intimal–medial thickness was significantly larger in subjects with cardiovascular disease than in healthy participants.[18] Additionally, the risk factors for carotid and coronary disease appear to be similar. Hence, it seems reasonable to utilize the term 'vulnerable plaque' in the same manner for both carotid and coronary arteries.

PATHOLOGY AND PATHOPHYSIOLOGY

Atherosclerosis is a systemic disease that begins early in life. Inflammation may be the critical factor in the evolution of a stable atheroma to an unstable, vulnerable plaque. In this process, platelet-derived growth factor (PDGF) stimulates proliferation of smooth muscle cells, which subsequently deposit collagen in the extracellular matrix. Macrophage-derived cytokines also promote collagen synthesis by vascular smooth muscle cells. Collagen is involved in the formation of the atheromatous fibrous cap. Macrophages and T lymphocytes may, however, also decrease plaque stability by secretion of cytokines and proteases that degrade the extracellular matrix and promote plaque rupture, such as serine proteases, cysteine proteases, and matrix metalloproteinases (MMPs).[19] MMPs have been shown in high levels at the site of carotid plaque inflammatory infiltrates, and are associated with symptomatic carotid disease and spontaneous carotid embolization.[20] Thus, MMPs may override the action of tissue inhibitors of metalloproteinases (TIMPs) in atheromatous plaques. MMPs are overexpressed in regions of increased mechanical stress to the plaque, which contributes to plaque instability.[21] Significantly higher concentrations of active MMP-8, and of MMP-1 and MMP-12 transcripts, have been encountered in carotid plaques of symptomatic patients than in non-symptomatic cases. MMP-8 also correlated with higher rates of thrombus embolization, as seen by transcranial Doppler (TCD), MMP-1 transcripts with thin caps, and MMP-12 transcripts with ruptured plaques.[22,23] In an experimental model, MMP-9 has been shown to be significantly associated with intraplaque hemorrhage and decreased mean cap thickness in advanced carotid lesions.[24] Additionally, other cytokines produced by the inflammatory cells – interferon-γ (IFN-γ), interleukin-1 (IL-1), and tumor necrosis factor-α (TNF-α) – stimulate smooth muscle cell production of MMPs.[19] IFN-γ also suppresses collagen gene expression on smooth muscle cells and promotes their apoptosis, compromising repair of ruptured plaques.[19,25,26]

Tissue factor expression in the necrotic core and in the fibrous cap resulting from inflammation contributes to the thrombogenicity of the plaque.[27,28] CD40+, a cell surface protein expressed on the surface of monocytes and B-lymphocytes, can activate intraplaque macrophages and trigger tissue factor expression. Neovascularization and inflammation detected by monoclonal antibodies to von Willebrand factor, CD31+, and CD34+, and proliferation of inflammatory cells, particularly at the shoulder of carotid plaques, may contribute to plaque destabilization.[29–31] Imbalances between pro- and antioxidant systems in the plaques also contribute to plaque vulnerability, as seen by significantly higher levels of oxidized low-density lipoprotein (LDL) and lower levels of superoxide dismutase in vulnerable carotid plaques as compared to stable ones.[32]

Inflammation is more commonly found in plaques associated with symptoms of cerebral ischemia.[33–35] Macrophages appear to be more commonly found in carotid plaques with a high lipid content and hemorrhage, than in calcified and fibrous plaques.[36] There are conflicting results about the endothelial expression of adhesion molecules. Levels of intercellular adhesion molecule-1 (ICAM-1), vascular cell adhesion molecule-1 (VCAM-1), P-selectin, and E-selectin have not consistently been found to be increased in the symptomatic carotid plaques, as compared to asymptomatic plaques.[37]

Plaque rupture, fibrous cap thinning, and macrophage infiltration of the fibrous cap are more common in symptomatic carotid plaques.[38] Lumen thrombus and intraplaque hemorrhage were equally frequent in symptomatic and asymptomatic patients.[4,20,39,40] Thrombotic occlusion of a vessel is not necessarily causally associated with plaque rupture, as has been shown in the cardiac literature, where erosive plaques have been shown to be responsible for 25–30% of coronary thrombi.[17,41]

High rates of microemboli have been associated with ischemic symptoms and echolucent plaques. In patients with ischemic symptoms and the presence of microemboli on TCD, histologic studies of carotid endarterectomy (CEA) specimens demonstrated tissue factor expression (>40% by semiquantitative assessment) in 44% of patients vs 11% of patients without embolic features. Plaque infiltration by CD68+ macrophages and T cells was also increased.[42]

BIOMARKERS

As inflammation is believed to play an important role in the development of atherosclerosis, multiple inflammatory biomarkers have been identified that may help diagnose this disease in the early stages of plaque vulnerability.

Fibrinogen has been associated with an increased risk of stroke and of cardiovascular events in asymptomatic patients.[43–47]

In patients with symptomatic carotid disease, the highest tertile of fibrinogen concentrations was associated with a greater number of CD68+ macrophages and CD3+ lymphocytes, mainly in the fibrous cap, and with thinning of the fibrous cap (< 210 μm cap in 83% of highest tertile of fibrinogen cases).[48] In a study of ischemic stroke, patients who had a fibrinogen level in the highest vs lowest tertile had a relative risk (RR) of 4.18 (95% CI 1.46–11.97).[43] Another study, pooling data from 5113 patients with recent minor ischemic stroke or transient ischemic attack (TIA) showed a hazard ratio (HR) for subsequent ischemic stroke of 1.34 in patients with fibrinogen level above the median (95% CI 1.13–1.60, $P = 0.001$).[49]

C-reactive protein (CRP) has been associated with increased cardiac risk in both symptomatic and asymptomatic individuals.[50–57] It has been associated specifically with ischemic stroke.[43,47,58] Fibrinogen and CRP have been shown to be highly correlated in patients with coronary artery disease and ischemic stroke.[47,59] The RR for highest (>33 mg/L) vs lowest (<5 mg/L) tertile of CRP was 8.5 (95% CI 2.62–27.58) for the endpoints of death, TIA/stroke, and angina/myocardial infarction (MI) within 1 year of the ischemic stroke.[43] In multiple logistic regression, only CRP was predictive of a new ischemic event or death (odds ratio [OR] = 2.39, 95% CI 1.28–4.49).[43] A Japanese study found that over approximately 3 years, high-sensitivity CRP (hsCRP) was associated with progression of very early carotid plaques (focal intima–media thickness [IMT] ≥ 1.1 mm) but not with the sum of all the plaques or the number of discrete plaques.[60] This holds true for hypertensive patients as well.[61]

Antibodies to heat-shock protein 65 (Hsp65) have been associated with coronary artery disease and carotid atherosclerosis.[62,63] Elevated levels are associated with progressive atherosclerosis in the carotids and predictive of 5-year mortality.[63,64] The anti-Hsp65 antibody titer was 360 ± 373 in patients without progression of the carotid atherosclerosis and 501 ± 711 in patients with progression.[62]

Other systemic markers of inflammation have been shown to be associated with carotid atherosclerosis. A recent imaging study correlating carotid artery magnetic resonance imaging (MRI) findings with levels of inflammation found that study participants with evidence of increased wall thickening, increased T2-signal, or gadolinium enhancement had higher levels of interleukin-6 (IL-6), CRP, VCAM-1, and ICAM-1.[65] Soluble CD-40 ligand levels are higher in ischemic stroke patients than in controls.[66] In a cross-sectional study by Elkind et al, the highest quartile of white blood cell counts was associated with maximal internal carotid artery plaque thickness in African-Americans and Hispanics, but not in non-Hispanic Whites.[67] Leukocyte and blood myeloperoxidase levels were associated with an OR of 11.9 and 20.4, respectively, for the highest vs lowest quartiles.[68]

The activation of inflammatory cells may have secondary effects on plaque constituents and the genetic regulation of the expression of endothelial factors.[69] Many genetic polymorphisms associated with the development of coronary and carotid atherosclerosis are being discovered, and the importance of gene–gene interactions and effect modification of clinical outcomes are under study.[70] Some of the genes and polymorphisms implicated with atherosclerosis are phosphodiesterase 4D gene; allele 2 for the IL-1 receptor antagonist; toll-like receptor-4 Asp299Gly, IL-6 GG and GC, among others.[70–72]

In a large multiethnic cohort, total homocysteine level >15 μmol/L was an independent risk factor for ischemic stroke (HR = 2.01, 95% CI 1.00–4.05), particularly in Whites and Hispanics.[73]

Cronin et al have shown, in a meta-analysis, a graded increase in ischemic stroke risk with increasing 5,10-methylene tetrahydrofolate reductase 677T allele dose, suggesting an influence of this polymorphism as a genetic stroke risk factor and supporting evidence indicating a causal relationship between elevated homocysteine and stroke.[74]

NEUROIMAGING

Plaques with similar morphology with respect to their lipid core content and to their fibrous cap may look alike when only structural neuroimaging is used. However, with diagnostic methods that permit the detection of plaque activity and physiology, major differences can be seen that highlight the vulnerability of plaques. The combination of structural and functional neuroimaging can significantly improve the diagnosis of plaque vulnerability.[14]

Magnetic resonance imaging

High-resolution MRI using a phased-array coil enables determination of plaque composition using sequences that produce bright-blood and dark-blood images.[75] Tissue quantification of carotid plaques has been shown to be reproducible and accurate.[76,77] In order to better differentiate between the multiple constituents of vulnerable plaques, paramagnetic contrast agents are used. These help to demonstrate increased neovascularization of the carotid plaque, and highlight the differences between the plaque's necrotic core and its fibrous cap.[78,79] With high-resolution MRI, one can determine the age of the intraluminal thrombus and establish the location of a hemorrhage (intraluminal vs intraplaque).[80]

MRI techniques have further advanced toward molecular imaging, which applies intravenously injected nanoparticles that interfere with metabolic pathways to produce detectable imaging signs, similar to the tracers used in nuclear medicine studies.[79] These techniques have been used not only to analyze specific biomarkers of atherosclerosis but also to better identify the thrombus itself and neovascularization.

High-resolution MRI with flow suppression has also been used to evaluate the efficacy of lipid-reducing medications and other potential anti-inflammatory therapies, and promises to be an important tool for future therapeutic trials of vulnerable carotid plaque.[79]

Positron emission tomography

While PET (positron-emission tomography) scanning provides data on inflammation, it is costly, time-consuming, and requires radiation. The tracers used for PET imaging are very sensitive, as they can be detected at low concentrations.[79] However, PET provides very poor localization and therefore may not be ideal for targeting specific regions of a plaque for analysis. Anatomic resolution can be optimized with the use of PET/CT (computed tomography) scanners.[13] ^{18}F-fluorodeoxyglucose (FDG) is taken up by macrophages, and can be used as a measure of inflammation within the plaque.[81–83] Rudd et al demonstrated FDG uptake in human carotid atherosclerotic lesions using PET/CT.[84]

Ultrasound

Carotid duplex ultrasound (CDUS) can be used to determine plaque morphology. However, CDUS interpretation is highly dependent on reader expertise, leading to low inter-rater reliability. Hence, the ability of ultrasound to detect plaque ulceration varies widely between studies (sensitivity 29–93%, specificity 32–100%).[85] Compound B-mode ultrasound has better signal-to-noise ratio and better agreement on plaque surface characteristics when compared with conventional B-mode ultrasound; four-dimensional ultrasound permits analysis of plaque motion.

Echolucent, heterogeneous plaques appear to more likely be symptomatic than those echodense and homogeneous.[86–92] CDUS provides limited information about plaque vulnerability. Integrated backscatter correlates with vascular risk factors and plaque thickness. Yamagami et al studied 246 patients with carotid atherosclerosis and used the backscatter pattern to determine echogenicity and to correlate it with levels of IL-6 and hsCRP. IL-6 was inversely associated with echogenicity.[93] In addition, a recent study investigated whether the mean gray scale on ultrasound correlated with inflammation on histopathology. Studying 26 CEA patients, they found that mean gray levels correlated positively with smooth muscle cells and inversely with macrophages. There was no correlation with lymphocytes.[94]

Carotid plaque area, as measured by CDUS, has been correlated with 5-year risk of stroke, MI, and vascular death.[95] Carotid plaque progression is a significant predictor of vascular events.

THE NEUROLOGIST'S APPROACH TO MANAGEMENT OF CAROTID VULNERABLE PLAQUE

Medical procedures

Carotid endarterectomy

The degree of carotid stenosis is a major predictor of subsequent stroke. In the North American Symptomatic Carotid Endarterectomy Trial (NASCET) and in the European Carotid Surgery Trial (ECST), patients with >69% stenosis of a symptomatic carotid had a significant reduction in stroke risk with CEA, provided the surgical risk was inferior than 3%.[6,7] However, in patients with moderate carotid stenosis, the benefit of surgical treatment is less clear. The NASCET investigators subsequently demonstrated a significant

reduction in the 5-year rate of ipsilateral stroke in symptomatic patients with 50–69% carotid stenosis when treated with endarterectomy, as compared to patients treated medically; and a non-significant reduction in symptomatic patients with <50% carotid stenosis when treated surgically, again compared to patients that received medical therapy.[96]

In patients who have not had a large infarction, or who have suffered a TIA, CEA should be undertaken preferably early (within 3–30 days post stroke/TIA) rather than only 6–8 weeks after the ictus.[97,98] Patients with non-significant carotid stenosis are not stroke-risk free. Although the risk of having a stroke with <50% stenosis is small, the attributable risk of stroke is high, since the prevalence of low-grade carotid stenosis is elevated in the general population.[99]

The Medical Research Council (MRC) Asymptomatic Carotid Surgery Trial (ACST) Collaborative Group randomized 3120 asymptomatic patients with significant carotid stenosis to 'immediate CEA' (1 month to 1 year) and to 'indefinite deferral of CEA' (4% per year in this group received CEA). Comparing all patients allocated immediate CEA vs all allocated deferral, but excluding perioperative events, the 5-year stroke risks were 3.8% vs 11% (gain 7.2% [95% CI 5.0–9.4], $P < 0.0001$). This benefit was not seen for patients over 75 years old.[100]

Endovascular therapy

Endovascular therapy may provide an alternative to CEA for treatment of severe carotid stenosis. The Carotid and Vertebral Artery Transluminal Angioplasty Study (CAVATAS) trial randomized 504 symptomatic and asymptomatic patients with >70% stenosis of the common or internal carotid artery, and requiring intervention, to CEA or endovascular therapy (angioplasty or stenting). At 30 days, the rates of stroke or death, or of disabling stroke/ death were similar in the two arms, and no difference in stroke rates was detected at 3 years. More patients had ≥70% stenosis of the ipsilateral carotid artery 1 year after endovascular treatment than after endarterectomy (18.5% vs 5.2%, P = 0.0001). However, angioplasty had a much lower rate of cranial neuropathy and hematoma formation. All seven deaths in the endovascular group were caused by stroke, whereas only one death in the CEA group was stroke-related, suggesting that endovascular therapy may have directly contributed to fatal outcomes.[101,102] In a non-inferiority trial, stenting with an emboli-protection device proved to be non-inferior to CEA in patients with symptomatic carotid artery stenosis ≥50% or asymptomatic stenosis ≥80%, in preventing major cardiovascular events at 1 year, or death/ipsilateral stroke at 1–12 months.[103]

Two ongoing clinical trials will further address CEA vs endovascular therapy for carotid disease. The Carotid Revascularization Using Endarterectomy or Stenting Systems (CaRESS) phase I clinical trial recently released its 1-year results, suggesting that the 30-day and 1-year risk of death, stroke, or MI for stenting with cerebral protection is equivalent to that of CEA in symptomatic and asymptomatic patients with carotid stenosis.[104] The Carotid Revascularization Endarterectomy versus Stent Trial (CREST) investigators released interim results from the lead-in phase of the study, showing that the periprocedural risk of stroke and death after stenting increases with age, particularly in octogenarians.[105]

Medical therapies

Clearly, to address the mechanisms by with atherosclerotic plaques become vulnerable, optimal medical treatments would target plaque inflammation. Several studies have documented decreases in clinical events that are presumably due to stabilization of plaques, in both the coronary and carotid arteries.

Antiplatelet agents have been the mainstay of medical management for secondary prevention of strokes in patients with symptomatic carotid disease. Antiplatelets can reduce the risk of stroke by 11–15%.[79] The combination of antiplatelets, however, will increase the risk of major bleeding in patients under dual antiplatelet therapy. In a recent study (Clopidogrel and Aspirin for Reduction of Emboli in Symptomatic Carotid Stenosis [CARESS] trial), patients with symptomatic carotid disease, and that had microembolic signals (MES) seen on TCD, were randomized to clopidogrel + aspirin or aspirin monotherapy. Intention-to-treat analysis revealed a significant reduction in MES: 43.8% of dual-therapy patients had MES at day 7, as compared with 72.7% of monotherapy patients (RR reduction = 39.8%; 95% CI 13.8–58.0; P = 0.0046). The risk of ischemic stroke or TIA within the first week post randomization was also higher in the monotherapy group.[106]

The Study to Evaluate Carotid Ultrasound Changes in Patients Treated with Ramipril and Vitamin E (SECURE) trial – a substudy of the Heart Outcomes Prevention Evaluation (HOPE) trial – was a prospective double-blind trial that evaluated an angiotensin-converting enzyme (ACE) inhibitor (ramipril) and vitamin E (400 IU/day) on the progression of carotid atherosclerosis over an average of 4.5 years in high-risk patients (≥55 years old, vascular disease, or diabetes mellitus and at least one other risk factor). Progression of atherosclerosis was determined through serial measurements of IMT using CDUS. Ramipril use slowed the progression of IMT and reduced risk of cardiovascular death, MI, or stroke, whereas the addition of vitamin E had no effect on progression of IMT or the development of a clinical endpoint.[107]

The potential anti-inflammatory role of statins has also been studied. Statins have been shown to reduce stroke risk, owing to their effect on multiple predisposing factors.[3] Patients with symptomatic carotid stenosis treated with pravastatin for 3 months prior to carotid endarterectomy had fewer macrophages (15 ± 10% vs 25.3 ± 12.5%), less lipid (8.2 ± 8.4% vs 23.9 ± 21.1%), less oxidized LDL immunoreactivity, greater TIMP-1 immunoreactivity, and higher collagen content than those treated with placebo. ICAM-1, VCAM-1, MMP-1, MMP-9, TIMP-2 immunoreactivity, and nuclear factor kappa B (NF-κB) immunoreactivity were not significantly different in the two groups.[108] Similarly, 18 patients with asymptomatic aortic and/or carotid plaques and hypercholesterolemia were treated with simvastatin with demonstrable reduction in wall thickness and wall area, but not lumen area, on in-vivo black-blood MRI scans after 12 months of therapy. There were no changes observable after 6 months of therapy.[109]

Doxycycline has been studied with respect to its effect on MMP expression in human carotid plaques. One hundred patients requiring CEA were randomized either to 200 mg/day of doxycycline or placebo for 2–8 weeks prior to the procedure. The CEA specimens from patients that were treated with doxycycline had significantly reduced concentrations of MMP-1, but not of other MMPs.[110] Other trials are warranted that address these potential new medical therapies for vulnerable plaque stabilization.

REFERENCES

1. Fisher CM. Occlusion of the internal carotid artery. Arch Neurol Psychiatry 1951; 65:346–77.
2. Madden KP, Karanjia PN, Adams HP Jr, Clarke WR. Accuracy of initial stroke subtype diagnosis in the TOAST study. Trial of ORG 10172 in Acute Stroke Treatment. Neurology 1995; 45(11):1975–9.
3. Golledge J, Greenhalgh RM, Davies AH. The symptomatic carotid plaque. Stroke 2000; 31(3):774–81.
4. Sitzer M, Muller W, Siebler M et al. Plaque ulceration and lumen thrombus are the main sources of cerebral microemboli in high-grade internal carotid artery stenosis. Stroke 1995; 26(7):1231–3.
5. Markus HS, Thomson ND, Brown MM. Asymptomatic cerebral embolic signals in symptomatic and asymptomatic carotid artery disease. Brain 1995; 118(Pt 4):1005–11.
6. Beneficial effect of carotid endarterectomy in symptomatic patients with high-grade carotid stenosis. North American Symptomatic Carotid Endarterectomy Trial Collaborators. N Engl J Med 1991; 325(7):445–53.
7. Randomised trial of endarterectomy for recently symptomatic carotid stenosis: final results of the MRC European Carotid Surgery Trial (ECST). Lancet 1998; 351(9113):1379–87.
8. Hobson RW 2nd, Weiss DG, Fields WS et al. Efficacy of carotid endarterectomy for asymptomatic carotid stenosis. The Veterans Affairs Cooperative Study Group. N Engl J Med 1993; 328(4):221–7.
9. Endarterectomy for asymptomatic carotid artery stenosis. Executive Committee for the Asymptomatic Carotid Atherosclerosis Study. JAMA 1995; 273(18):1421–8.
10. Little WC, Constantinescu M, Applegate RJ et al. Can coronary angiography predict the site of a subsequent myocardial infarction in patients with mild-to-moderate coronary artery disease? Circulation 1988; 78(5 Pt 1):1157–66.
11. Mulcahy D, Husain S, Zalos G et al. Ischemia during ambulatory monitoring as a prognostic indicator in patients with stable coronary artery disease. JAMA 1997; 277(4):318–24.
12. Glagov S, Weisenberg E, Zarins CK, Stankunavicius R, Kolettis GJ. Compensatory enlargement of human atherosclerotic coronary arteries. N Engl J Med 1987; 316(22):1371–5.
13. Chen JW, Wasserman BA. Vulnerable plaque imaging. Neuroimaging Clin N Am 2005; 15(3):609–21.
14. Naghavi M, Libby P, Falk E et al. From vulnerable plaque to vulnerable patient: a call for new definitions and risk assessment strategies: Part I. Circulation 2003; 108(14):1664–72.
15. Naghavi M, Libby P, Falk E et al. From vulnerable plaque to vulnerable patient: a call for new definitions and risk assessment strategies: Part II. Circulation 2003; 108(15):1772–8.
16. Muller JE, Abela GS, Nesto RW, Tofler GH. Triggers, acute risk factors and vulnerable plaques: the lexicon of a new frontier. J Am Coll Cardiol 1994; 23(3):809–13.
17. Virmani R, Kolodgie FD, Burke AP, Farb A, Schwartz SM. Lessons from sudden coronary death: a comprehensive morphological classification scheme for atherosclerotic lesions. Arterioscler Thromb Vasc Biol 2000; 20(5):1262–75.
18. Burke GL, Evans GW, Riley WA et al. Arterial wall thickness is associated with prevalent cardiovascular disease in middle-aged adults. The Atherosclerosis Risk in Communities (ARIC) Study. Stroke 1995; 26(3):386–91.
19. Arroyo LH, Lee RT. Mechanisms of plaque rupture: mechanical and biologic interactions. Cardiovasc Res 1999; 41(2):369–75.

20. Loftus IM, Naylor AR, Goodall S et al. Increased matrix metalloproteinase-9 activity in unstable carotid plaques. A potential role in acute plaque disruption. Stroke 2000; 31(1):40–7.

21. Lee RT, Schoen FJ, Loree HM, Lark MW, Libby P. Circumferential stress and matrix metalloproteinase 1 in human coronary atherosclerosis. Implications for plaque rupture. Arterioscler Thromb Vasc Biol 1996; 16(8):1070–3.

22. Molloy KJ, Thompson MM, Jones JL et al. Unstable carotid plaques exhibit raised matrix metalloproteinase-8 activity. Circulation 2004; 110(3):337–43.

23. Morgan AR, Rerkasem K, Gallagher PJ et al. Differences in matrix metalloproteinase-1 and matrix metalloproteinase-12 transcript levels among carotid atherosclerotic plaques with different histopathological characteristics. Stroke 2004; 35(6):1310–15.

24. de Nooijer R, Verkleij CJ, von der Thusen JH et al. Lesional overexpression of matrix metalloproteinase-9 promotes intraplaque hemorrhage in advanced lesions but not at earlier stages of atherogenesis. Arterioscler Thromb Vasc Biol 2006; 26(2): 340–6.

25. Amento EP, Ehsani N, Palmer H, Libby P. Cytokines and growth factors positively and negatively regulate interstitial collagen gene expression in human vascular smooth muscle cells. Arterioscler Thromb 1991; 11(5):1223–30.

26. Bennett MR, Evan GI, Schwartz SM. Apoptosis of human vascular smooth muscle cells derived from normal vessels and coronary atherosclerotic plaques. J Clin Invest 1995; 95(5):2266–74.

27. Moreno PR, Bernardi VH, Lopez-Cuellar J et al. Macrophages, smooth muscle cells, and tissue factor in unstable angina. Implications for cell-mediated thrombogenicity in acute coronary syndromes. Circulation 1996; 94(12):3090–7.

28. Toschi V, Gallo R, Lettino M et al. Tissue factor modulates the thrombogenicity of human atherosclerotic plaques. Circulation 1997; 95(3):594–9.

29. Mach F, Schonbeck U, Bonnefoy JY, Pober JS, Libby P. Activation of monocyte/macrophage functions related to acute atheroma complication by ligation of CD40: induction of collagenase, stromelysin, and tissue factor. Circulation 1997; 96(2):396–9.

30. McCarthy MJ, Loftus IM, Thompson MM et al. Angiogenesis and the atherosclerotic carotid plaque: an association between symptomatology and plaque morphology. J Vasc Surg 1999; 30(2):261–8.

31. Moreno PR, Purushothaman KR, Fuster V et al. Plaque neovascularization is increased in ruptured atherosclerotic lesions of human aorta: implications for plaque vulnerability. Circulation 2004; 110(14):2032–8.

32. Uno M, Kitazato KT, Suzue A et al. Contribution of an imbalance between oxidant–antioxidant systems to plaque vulnerability in patients with carotid artery stenosis. J Neurosurg 2005; 103(3):518–25.

33. Jander S, Sitzer M, Schumann R et al. Inflammation in high-grade carotid stenosis: a possible role for macrophages and T cells in plaque destabilization. Stroke 1998; 29(8):1625–30.

34. DeGraba TJ, Siren AL, Penix L et al. Increased endothelial expression of intercellular adhesion molecule-1 in symptomatic versus asymptomatic human carotid atherosclerotic plaque. Stroke 1998; 29(7):1405–10.

35. Bassiouny HS, Sakaguchi Y, Mikucki SA et al. Juxtalumenal location of plaque necrosis and neoformation in symptomatic carotid stenosis. J Vasc Surg 1997; 26(4):585–94.

36. Gronholdt ML, Nordestgaard BG, Bentzon J et al. Macrophages are associated with lipid-rich carotid artery plaques, echolucency on B-mode imaging, and elevated plasma lipid levels. J Vasc Surg 2002; 35(1):137–45.

37. Nuotio K, Lindsberg PJ, Carpen O et al. Adhesion molecule expression in symptomatic and asymptomatic carotid stenosis. Neurology 2003; 60(12):1890–9.

38. Carr S, Farb A, Pearce WH, Virmani R, Yao JS. Atherosclerotic plaque rupture in symptomatic carotid artery stenosis. J Vasc Surg 1996; 23(5): 755–65; discussion 765–6.

39. Bassiouny HS, Davis H, Massawa N et al. Critical carotid stenoses: morphologic and chemical similarity between symptomatic and asymptomatic plaques. J Vasc Surg 1989; 9(2):202–12.

40. Seeger JM, Barratt E, Lawson GA, Klingman N. The relationship between carotid plaque composition, plaque morphology, and neurologic symptoms. J Surg Res 1995; 58(3):330–6.

41. Arbustini E, Grasso M, Diegoli M et al. Coronary atherosclerotic plaques with and without thrombus in ischemic heart syndromes: a morphologic, immunohistochemical, and biochemical study. Am J Cardiol 1991; 68(7):36–50B.

42. Jander S, Sitzer M, Wendt A et al. Expression of tissue factor in high-grade carotid artery stenosis: association with plaque destabilization. Stroke 2001; 32(4):850–4.

43. Di Napoli M, Papa F, Bocola V. Prognostic influence of increased C-reactive protein and fibrinogen levels in ischemic stroke. Stroke 2001; 32(1):133–8.

44. Heinrich J, Balleisen L, Schulte H, Assmann G, van de Loo J. Fibrinogen and factor VII in the prediction of coronary risk. Results from the PROCAM study in healthy men. Arterioscler Thromb 1994; 14(1): 54–9.

45. Kannel WB, Wolf PA, Castelli WP, D'Agostino RB. Fibrinogen and risk of cardiovascular disease. The Framingham Study. JAMA 1987; 258(9):1183–6.

46. Meade TW, North WR, Chakrabarti R et al. Haemostatic function and cardiovascular death: early results of a prospective study. Lancet 1980; 1(8177):1050–4.

47. Woodward M, Lowe GD, Campbell DJ et al. Associations of inflammatory and hemostatic variables with the risk of recurrent stroke. Stroke 2005; 36(10):2143–7.

48. Mauriello A, Sangiorgi G, Palmieri G et al. Hyperfibrinogenemia is associated with specific histocytological composition and complications of atherosclerotic carotid plaques in patients affected by transient ischemic attacks. Circulation 2000; 101(7):744–50.

49. Rothwell PM, Howard SC, Power DA et al. Fibrinogen concentration and risk of ischemic stroke and acute coronary events in 5113 patients with transient ischemic attack and minor ischemic stroke. Stroke 2004; 35(10):2300–5.

50. Ridker PM, Cushman M, Stampfer MJ, Tracy RP, Hennekens CH. Inflammation, aspirin, and the risk of cardiovascular disease in apparently healthy men. N Engl J Med 1997; 336(14):973–9.

51. Ridker PM, Glynn RJ, Hennekens CH. C-reactive protein adds to the predictive value of total and HDL cholesterol in determining risk of first myocardial infarction. Circulation 1998; 97(20):2007–11.

52. Ridker PM, Hennekens CH, Buring JE, Rifai N. C-reactive protein and other markers of inflammation in the prediction of cardiovascular disease in women. N Engl J Med 2000; 342(12):836–43.

53. Kuller LH, Tracy RP, Shaten J, Meilahn EN. Relation of C-reactive protein and coronary heart disease in the MRFIT nested case-control study. Multiple Risk Factor Intervention Trial. Am J Epidemiol 1996; 144(6):537–47.

54. Haverkate F, Thompson SG, Pyke SD, Gallimore JR, Pepys MB. Production of C-reactive protein and risk of coronary events in stable and unstable angina. European Concerted Action on Thrombosis and Disabilities Angina Pectoris Study Group. Lancet 1997; 349(9050):462–6.

55. Morrow DA, Rifai N, Antman EM et al. C-reactive protein is a potent predictor of mortality independently of and in combination with troponin T in acute coronary syndromes: a TIMI 11A substudy. Thrombolysis in Myocardial Infarction. J Am Coll Cardiol 1998; 31(7):1460–5.

56. Biasucci LM, Liuzzo G, Grillo RL et al. Elevated levels of C-reactive protein at discharge in patients with unstable angina predict recurrent instability. Circulation 1999; 99(7):855–60.

57. Chew DP, Bhatt DL, Robbins MA et al. Incremental prognostic value of elevated baseline C-reactive protein among established markers of risk in percutaneous coronary intervention. Circulation 2001; 104(9):992–7.

58. Beamer NB, Coull BM, Clark WM, Hazel JS, Silberger JR. Interleukin-6 and interleukin-1 receptor antagonist in acute stroke. Ann Neurol 1995; 37(6):800–5.

59. Banerjee AK, Pearson J, Gilliland EL et al. A six year prospective study of fibrinogen and other risk factors associated with mortality in stable claudicants. Thromb Haemost 1992; 68(3):261–3.

60. Hashimoto H, Kitagawa K, Hougaku H et al. C-reactive protein is an independent predictor of the rate of increase in early carotid atherosclerosis. Circulation 2001; 104(1):63–7.

61. Hashimoto H, Kitagawa K, Hougaku H, Etani H, Hori M. Relationship between C-reactive protein and progression of early carotid atherosclerosis in hypertensive subjects. Stroke 2004; 35(7):1625–30.

62. Xu Q, Kiechl S, Mayr M et al. Association of serum antibodies to heat-shock protein 65 with carotid atherosclerosis: clinical significance determined in a follow-up study. Circulation 1999; 100(11):1169–74.

63. Hoppichler F, Koch T, Dzien A, Gschwandtner G, Lechleitner M. Prognostic value of antibody titre to heat-shock protein 65 on cardiovascular events. Cardiology 2000; 94(4):220–3.

64. Xu Q, Willeit J, Marosi M et al. Association of serum antibodies to heat-shock protein 65 with carotid atherosclerosis. Lancet 1993; 341(8840):255–9.

65. Weiss CR, Arai AE, Bui MN et al. Arterial wall MRI characteristics are associated with elevated serum markers of inflammation in humans. J Magn Reson Imaging 2001; 14(6):698–704.

66. Garlichs CD, Kozina S, Fateh-Moghadam S et al. Upregulation of CD40-CD40 ligand (CD154) in patients with acute cerebral ischemia. Stroke 2003; 34(6):1412–18.

67. Elkind MS, Cheng J, Boden-Albala B, Paik MC, Sacco RL. Elevated white blood cell count and carotid plaque thickness: Northern Manhattan Stroke Study. Stroke 2001; 32(4):842–9.

68. Zhang R, Brennan ML, Fu X et al. Association between myeloperoxidase levels and risk of coronary artery disease. JAMA 2001; 286(17):2136–42.

69. Haley KJ, Lilly CM, Yang JH et al. Overexpression of eotaxin and the CCR3 receptor in human atherosclerosis: using genomic technology to identify a potential novel pathway of vascular inflammation. Circulation 2000; 102(18):2185–9.

70. DeGraba TJ. Immunogenetic susceptibility of atherosclerotic stroke: implications on current and future treatment of vascular inflammation. Stroke 2004; 35(11 Suppl 1):2712–19.

71. Worrall BB, Azhar S, Nyquist PA et al. Interleukin-1 receptor antagonist gene polymorphisms in carotid atherosclerosis. Stroke 2003; 34(3):790–3.

72. Flex A, Gaetani E, Papaleo P et al. Proinflammatory genetic profiles in subjects with history of ischemic stroke. Stroke 2004; 35(10):2270–5.

73. Sacco RL, Anand K, Lee HS et al. Homocysteine and the risk of ischemic stroke in a triethnic cohort: the NOrthern MAnhattan Study. Stroke 2004; 35(10):2263–9.

74. Cronin S, Furie KL, Kelly PJ. Dose-related association of MTHFR 677T allele with risk of ischemic stroke: evidence from a cumulative meta-analysis. Stroke 2005; 36(7):1581–7.

75. Cai JM, Hatsukami TS, Ferguson MS et al. Classification of human carotid atherosclerotic lesions with in vivo multicontrast magnetic resonance imaging. Circulation 2002; 106(11):1368–73.

76. Saam T, Ferguson MS, Yarnykh VL et al. Quantitative evaluation of carotid plaque composition by in vivo MRI. Arterioscler Thromb Vasc Biol 2005; 25(1):234–9.

77. Cai J, Hatsukami TS, Ferguson MS et al. In vivo quantitative measurement of intact fibrous cap and lipid-rich necrotic core size in atherosclerotic carotid plaque: comparison of high-resolution, contrast-enhanced magnetic resonance imaging and histology. Circulation 2005; 112(22):3437–44.

78. Kerwin W, Hooker A, Spilker M et al. Quantitative magnetic resonance imaging analysis of neovasculature volume in carotid atherosclerotic plaque. Circulation 2003; 107(6):851–6.

79. Nighoghossian N, Derex L, Douek P. The vulnerable carotid artery plaque: current imaging methods and new perspectives. Stroke 2005; 36(12):2764–72.

80. Kampschulte A, Ferguson MS, Kerwin WS et al. Differentiation of intraplaque versus juxtaluminal hemorrhage/thrombus in advanced human carotid atherosclerotic lesions by in vivo magnetic resonance imaging. Circulation 2004; 110(20):3239–44.

81. Libby P. Inflammation in atherosclerosis. Nature 2002; 420(6917):868–74.

82. Kubota R, Yamada S, Kubota K et al. Intratumoral distribution of fluorine-18-fluorodeoxyglucose in vivo: high accumulation in macrophages and granulation tissues studied by microautoradiography. J Nucl Med 1992; 33(11):1972–80.

83. Ogawa M, Ishino S, Mukai T et al. (18)F-FDG accumulation in atherosclerotic plaques: immunohistochemical and PET imaging study. J Nucl Med 2004; 45(7):1245–50.

84. Rudd JH, Warburton EA, Fryer TD et al. Imaging atherosclerotic plaque inflammation with [18F]-fluorodeoxyglucose positron emission tomography. Circulation 2002; 105(23):2708–11.

85. Widder B, Paulat K, Hackspacher J et al. Morphological characterization of carotid artery stenoses by ultrasound duplex scanning. Ultrasound Med Biol 1990; 16(4):349–54.

86. Gronholdt ML. Ultrasound and lipoproteins as predictors of lipid-rich, rupture-prone plaques in the carotid artery. Arterioscler Thromb Vasc Biol 1999; 19(1):2–13.

87. Langsfeld M, Gray-Weale AC, Lusby RJ. The role of plaque morphology and diameter reduction in the development of new symptoms in asymptomatic carotid arteries. J Vasc Surg 1989; 9(4):548–57.

88. O'Holleran LW, Kennelly MM, McClurken M, Johnson JM. Natural history of asymptomatic carotid plaque. Five year follow-up study. Am J Surg 1987; 154(6):659–62.

89. Bock RW, Gray-Weale AC, Mock PA et al. The natural history of asymptomatic carotid artery disease. J Vasc Surg 1993; 17(1):160–9; discussion 170–1.

90. Gronholdt ML, Nordestgaard BG, Schroeder TV, Vorstrup S, Sillesen H. Ultrasonic echolucent carotid plaques predict future strokes. Circulation 2001; 104(1):68–73.

91. Gronholdt ML, Wiebe BM, Laursen H et al. Lipid-rich carotid artery plaques appear echolucent on ultrasound B-mode images and may be associated with intraplaque haemorrhage. Eur J Vasc Endovasc Surg 1997; 14(6):439–45.

92. Mathiesen EB, Bonaa KH, Joakimsen O. Echolucent plaques are associated with high risk of ischemic cerebrovascular events in carotid stenosis: the tromso study. Circulation 2001; 103(17):2171–5.

93. Yamagami H, Kitagawa K, Nagai Y et al. Higher levels of interleukin-6 are associated with lower echogenicity of carotid artery plaques. Stroke 2004; 35(3): 677–81.

94. Puato M, Faggin E, Rattazzi M et al. In vivo noninvasive identification of cell composition of intimal lesions: a combined approach with ultrasonography and immunocytochemistry. J Vasc Surg 2003; 38(6):1390–5.

95. Spence JD, Eliasziw M, DiCicco M et al. Carotid plaque area: a tool for targeting and evaluating vascular preventive therapy. Stroke 2002; 33(12): 2916–22.

96. Barnett HJ, Taylor DW, Eliasziw M et al. Benefit of carotid endarterectomy in patients with symptomatic moderate or severe stenosis. North American Symptomatic Carotid Endarterectomy Trial Collaborators. N Engl J Med 1998; 339(20):1415–25.

97. Gasecki AP, Ferguson GG, Eliasziw M et al. Early endarterectomy for severe carotid artery stenosis after a nondisabling stroke: results from the North American Symptomatic Carotid Endarterectomy Trial. J Vasc Surg 1994; 20(2):288–95.

98. Ballotta E, Da Giau G, Baracchini C et al. Early versus delayed carotid endarterectomy after a nondisabling ischemic stroke: a prospective randomized study. Surgery 2002; 131(3):287–93.

99. Wasserman BA, Wityk RJ, Trout HH 3rd, Virmani R. Low-grade carotid stenosis: looking beyond the lumen with MRI. Stroke 2005; 36(11):2504–13.

100. Halliday A, Mansfield A, Marro J et al. Prevention of disabling and fatal strokes by successful carotid endarterectomy in patients without recent neurological symptoms: randomised controlled trial. Lancet 2004; 363(9420):1491–502.

101. Endovascular versus surgical treatment in patients with carotid stenosis in the Carotid and Vertebral Artery Transluminal Angioplasty Study (CAVATAS): a randomised trial. Lancet 2001; 357(9270):1729–37.

102. McCabe DJ, Pereira AC, Clifton A, Bland JM, Brown MM. Restenosis after carotid angioplasty, stenting, or endarterectomy in the Carotid and Vertebral Artery Transluminal Angioplasty Study (CAVATAS). Stroke 2005; 36(2):281–6.

103. Yadav JS, Wholey MH, Kuntz RE et al. Protected carotid-artery stenting versus endarterectomy in high-risk patients. N Engl J Med 2004; 351(15): 1493–501.

104. Carotid Revascularization Using Endarterectomy or Stenting Systems (CaRESS) phase I clinical trial: 1-year results. J Vasc Surg 2005; 42(2):213–19.

105. Hobson RW 2nd, Howard VJ, Roubin GS et al. Carotid artery stenting is associated with increased complications in octogenarians: 30-day stroke and death rates in the CREST lead-in phase. J Vasc Surg 2004; 40(6):1106–11.

106. Markus HS, Droste DW, Kaps M et al. Dual antiplatelet therapy with clopidogrel and aspirin in symptomatic carotid stenosis evaluated using doppler embolic signal detection: the Clopidogrel and Aspirin for Reduction of Emboli in Symptomatic Carotid Stenosis (CARESS) trial. Circulation 2005; 111(17):2233–40.

107. Lonn E, Yusuf S, Dzavik V et al. SECURE Investigators. Effects of ramipril and vitamin E on atherosclerosis: the study to evaluate carotid ultrasound changes in patients treated with ramipril and vitamin E (SECURE). Circulation 2001; 103(7): 919–25.

108. Crisby M, Nordin-Fredriksson G, Shah PK, Yano J, Zhu J, Nilsson J. Pravastatin treatment increases collagen content and decreases lipid content, inflammation, metalloproteinases, and cell death in human carotid plaques: implications for plaque stabilization. Circulation 2001; 103(7):926–33.

109. Corti R, Fayad ZA, Fuster V et al. Effects of lipid-lowering by simvastatin on human atherosclerotic lesions: a longitudinal study by high-resolution, noninvasive magnetic resonance imaging. Circulation 2001; 104(3):249–52.

110. Axisa B, Loftus IM, Naylor AR et al. Prospective, randomized, double-blind trial investigating the effect of doxycycline on matrix metalloproteinase expression within atherosclerotic carotid plaques. Stroke 2002; 33(12):2858–64.

Psychological triggers for plaque rupture

8

Geoffrey H Tofler and Thomas Buckley

INTRODUCTION

Emotional stress has long been associated with myocardial infarction (MI) and sudden cardiac death; however, the evidence for a causal link has been uncertain. Advances over the last two decades in understanding the mechanism of onset and treatment of acute cardiovascular disease (CVD) have coincided with increased acceptance of the role of psychological factors, both acute and chronic, in the onset of MI, sudden cardiac death, and stroke. The purpose of this chapter is to review the evidence for triggering of plaque rupture and acute CVD by psychological triggers.

EVIDENCE FOR PSYCHOLOGICAL TRIGGERS OF CARDIOVASCULAR DISEASE

Evidence for psychological factors as triggers includes the following points:

1. MI results from plaque rupture or erosion and thrombosis.[1]
2. Thrombotic occlusion frequently occurs at coronary artery sites that did not have severe stenosis prior to the acute plaque rupture.[2]
3. There is a morning peak in frequency of MI, sudden cardiac death, and stroke[3–7] that coincides with heightened blood pressure, heart rate, vasoconstriction, and prothrombotic changes.[8]
4. Emotional stressors cause similar acute physiologic changes to those seen in the morning period, and can transiently increase the risk of plaque rupture and thrombosis.[9]
5. Epidemiologic studies, stimulated by the development of the case-crossover study design, have confirmed and characterized several acute triggers of MI and sudden cardiac death.[10–14]
6. Cardioprotective agents such as aspirin and β-blockers modify the physiologic responses to acute stressors and have been shown to reduce the likelihood of morning and trigger-induced MI.[15–18]

It is useful to define several of the trigger-related concepts:

- *Trigger*: an activity that produces acute physiologic changes that may lead directly to onset of acute cardiovascular disease.[9]
- *Acute risk factor*: a transient physiologic change, such as a surge in arterial pressure or heart rate, an increase in coagulability, or vasoconstriction, that follows a trigger and may result in disease onset.[9]
- *Hazard period*: the time interval after trigger initiation associated with an increased risk of disease onset due to the trigger. The onset and offset times of the hazard period, which could also be designated a '*vulnerable period*', may be sharply defined, as in heavy exertion, or less well-defined as with respiratory infection. The duration of the hazard period may also vary, from less than 1 hour during heavy physical exertion, to weeks, to months with bereavement.[18]

- *Triggered acute risk prevention*: a conceptual framework to consider risk reduction that focuses on the transient increase in CVD risk associated with a trigger. Triggered acute risk prevention (TARP) can be considered analogous to the way a tarpaulin (often abbreviated as tarp) can be placed when rain is imminent.[18]

PSYCHOLOGICAL TRIGGERS OF ACUTE CADIOVASCULAR DISEASE

In the Multicenter Investigation of Limitation of Infarct Size (MILIS) study, almost half (48%) of the patients reported a possible trigger, of whom 13% reported a combination of two or more possible triggers[19] (Figure 8.1). Emotional upset was the most commonly reported potential precipitant (18%), together with moderate physical activity (14%), heavy physical activity (9%), and lack of sleep (8%). This analysis is limited by a lack of control data, since exposure to potential triggers such as emotional upset is common, yet MI occurs rarely. The case-crossover study design has helped to address this and other limitations in the study of triggering.[10,20] A feature of the case-crossover design is that each person is self-matched, with a hazard and control period, to determine the relative risk (RR) of a potential trigger leading to MI.

Anger

In the Determinants of Onset of Myocardial Infarction Study (ONSET), 2.4% of patients reported anger ≥ 5 on a 7-point scale in the 2-hour period before MI. This level of anger, which corresponded with 'very angry, body tense, clenching fists or teeth' up to 'furious or enraged', was associated with an RR of 2.3 (95% CI 1.2–3.2) compared with a control period of usual annual frequency.[11] The RR was 4.0 (95% CI 1.9–9.4) when the control period was the same 2-hour period the day before MI. The most frequently reported contributors to anger were arguments with family members (25%), conflicts at work (22%), and legal problems (8%). In the Stockholm Heart Epidemiology Program (SHEEP), the RR was 9-fold for anger as a trigger.[21] Koton et al showed an odds ratio (OR) of 14 (95% CI 3–253) for anger triggering stroke in the subsequent 2 hours.[22]

While the RRs during anger are significantly increased compared with baseline periods, the most important information for clinical significance is not the RR of a potential trigger, but the absolute difference in risk the activity produces. To estimate absolute risk, data on RR can be combined with baseline risk from populations similar to that from which the study patients originated. For instance, Framingham Heart Study data indicate that

Figure 8.1 Possible triggers of acute myocardial infarction. A possible trigger was reported by 412 of 849 patients (48.5%) from the Multicenter Investigation of Limitation of Infarct Size (MILIS); 109 patients (13%) reported two or more possible triggers. (Adapted from Tofler et al.[19])

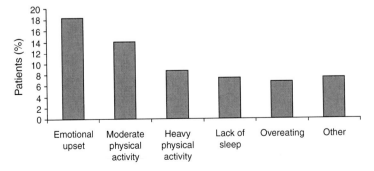

the risk that a 50-year-old, non-smoking, non-diabetic man will experience an MI is approximately 1% per year, or 1 chance in a million per hour. If the RR of MI was increased 4-fold by a single episode of severe anger, this activity would only increase his hourly risk to 4 in a million, and only for a 2-hour period. Even for a person at increased overall absolute risk, such as post-MI, the incremental increase in risk from a specific episode would probably be very small.

Anxiety

A significantly elevated RR of 1.6 (95% CI 1.1–2.2) was associated with episodes of anxiety above the 75th percentile on an anxiety scale within the 2 hours prior to MI.[11]

Bereavement

Increased cardiac mortality in bereaved individuals is well described, and has been described as 'the broken heart'.[23–28] In a cohort of middle-aged widowers, a 40% increase in the mortality rate was observed in the first 6 months following bereavement.[25] In an analysis of psychosocial factors in the INTERHEART study, stressful life events had occurred more frequently within the prior year among patients than among controls (16.1 vs 13.0%; OR = 1.48; 95% CI 1.33–1.64).[29] Stressful life events specified included marital separation or divorce, loss of job or retirement, loss of crop or business failure, violence, major family conflict, major personal injury or illness, death or major illness of a close family member, death of a spouse, or other major stress.

Work-related stress

A high-pressure work deadline in the prior 24 hours was associated with a 6-fold increase in RR of MI in the SHEEP study,[30] whereas in ONSET, the RR for a high-pressure deadline over a 7-day hazard period was 2.3 (95% CI 1.4–4.0), and

2.2 (95% CI 1.0–5.0) for firing somebody.[11] The emotional significance of a job stress influenced its contribution to RR of MI. Thus, when increased work responsibilities affected men in a very or fairly negative way in the SHEEP study, the RR, adjusted for other risk factors, was 6.3 (95% CI 2.7–14.7), whereas the RR was only 1.5 (95% CI 0.9–2.3) when the increased work responsibilities did not mean very much, and 0.7 (95% CI 0.5–0.9) when it had a positive effect. Corresponding RRs among women were 3.8 (1.3–11.0), 0.8 (0.3–2.5), and 1.0 (0.6–1.8).[30]

Population stressors

Earthquakes[31,32] and wartime missile attack[33] have been linked with acute increases in CVD. In the week after the Los Angeles earthquake of 1994, which occurred at 4:31 a.m. there was a 35% increase in non-fatal MI compared with the week before, and a 4-fold increase in sudden cardiac death on the day of the earthquake[32,34] (Figure 8.2). For the 6 days after this spike, however, the number of sudden deaths fell below the baseline, suggesting that some of the initial deaths may have been moved forward by several days in individuals who were predisposed, rather than being excess deaths.[34] The 1989 Loma Prieta, San Francisco Bay earthquake, which occurred at 5:04 p.m. was not associated with increased MI, leading Brown to suggest that the added stress of abrupt awakening in the 4:31 a.m. Los Angeles earthquake contributed to the triggered events.[35]

During the first week of Iraqi missile attacks on Israel in 1991, Meisel and colleagues found a doubling of non-fatal MI compared with a control period 1 year previously.[33] This was mirrored by a near doubling of sudden out-of-hospital deaths for the corresponding 1-month period.[33] In the 60 days following the World Trade Center bombing of September 11, 2001, Allegra et al reported a 49% increase in

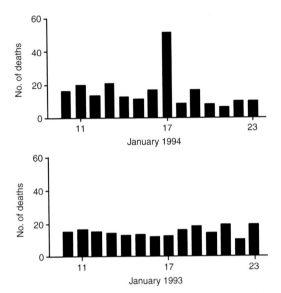

Figure 8.2 Daily numbers of cardiovascular deaths in Los Angeles County in January 1993 and 1994. On the day of the Northridge earthquake (January 17, 1994), there was a sharp rise in the number of deaths related to atherosclerotic cardiovascular disease (relative risk = 2.6; 95% CI 1.8–3.7). The daily number of CVD deaths declined in the 6 days after the earthquake (P = 0.002). (From Leor J et al.[34])

patients admitted with MI through 16 Emergency Departments within a 50-mile radius of the World Trade Center, compared with the 60 days beforehand (118 after vs 79 before, P = 0.01).[36]

Sporting events provide another example of population stress. On the day of the 1996 European football championship that Holland were eliminated after narrowly losing to France on penalties, Dutch men had an increased relative risk of MI or stroke of 1.5 (95% CI 1.1–2.1), whereas there was no increased risk for Dutch women or French men and women.[37,38]

Environmental stress

Exposure to traffic, related to both pollution and emotional stress, has been associated with an increased RR of MI of 2.7 (95% CI 2.1–3.6).[39]

Seasonal and other variations

A seasonal variation in the incidence of MI, cardiac death, and stroke is consistently described, with a winter peak up to 60% greater than the summer nadir.[40,41] The mechanisms underlying this variation, which holds true in both cold and warmer climates, are not fully understood.[42,43] Besides cold ambient temperature, hypotheses advanced include respiratory infections, hypercoagulable state, and increases in blood pressure, serum lipids, and glucose.[44,45] The seasonal variation may also reflect a decreased risk during summer months, which may include vacation and reduced emotional stress. A daily variation in CVD and stroke has also been described with a peak incidence on Mondays.[41,46–48] Holidays such as Christmas and New Year's Day have also been associated with increased cardiac mortality.[49]

Takotsubo cardiomyopathy

The transient left ventricular apical ballooning syndrome, also known as takotsubo cardiomyopathy, is frequently preceded by acute emotional stress.[50] The syndrome typically affects postmenopausal women, and presents as chest pain with ST-segment elevation in the precordial leads, relatively minor cardiac enzyme elevation, and transient apical systolic left ventricular dysfunction, despite the absence of obstructive coronary disease. Although the cause is uncertain, proposed mechanisms include epicardial or microvascular spasm, neurogenically or catecholamine-associated myocardial stunning.[51] Abnormalities of cardiac sympathetic innervation have been described, with sympathetic hyperactivity at the apex.[52]

CHRONIC STRESS AND PROGRESSION OF ATHEROSCLEROSIS

There is increasing evidence for long-term psychological stress contributing to progression of vascular disease. The link may be both direct, via damage to the endothelium, and indirect, via aggravation of traditional risk factors such as smoking, hypertension, and lipid metabolism.[53,54] Takano et al reported an average of 1.67 ruptured plaques per person in non-culprit vessels of patients with acute coronary syndromes.[55]

Insights into the role of psychological stress in progression of atherosclerosis come from animal and human studies. Cynomolgus monkeys display complex patterns of social interactions characterized by hierarchies of dominant (aggressive) and subordinate (submissive) animals. Several observations were made. Animals exposed to a socially stressful situation had more extensive atherosclerosis than animals within a stable environment. Those who responded with aggressive behavior to stressful environments had the most atherosclerosis. In addition, those with a high heart rate reaction to stress had intimal lesions that were twice as extensive as those seen in low reactors.[56] Moreover, the administration of propranolol, associated with a 20% reduction in heart rate, resulted in significantly less atherosclerosis.[57]

In the INTERHEART study, sources of chronic stress were divided into work stress, home stress, and financial stress.[29] Patients with a first MI reported significantly more stress in each of these categories than controls. The proportion of MI patients experiencing moderate or severe work or home stress varied widely among regions, from 43.8% in North America to 15.6% in China and Hong Kong.

During a 2-year follow-up of 33 999 subjects who were aged 42–77 years and initially free of diagnosed disease, the age-adjusted RR of fatal cardiovascular disease was 3-fold greater for those with the highest levels of phobic anxiety compared with those with the lowest levels. There was also a significant trend of increasing risk with increasing symptoms of phobic anxiety.[58]

There is mounting evidence that depressive symptoms are associated with increased cardiovascular risk.[59–61] In the Women's Health Initiative Observational Study, those with current or previous depression had significantly higher rates of cardiovascular death (0.79 vs 0.52%) and all-cause mortality (2.87 vs 2.18%) than those without depression. In the INTERHEART study, depression was significantly more common among patients with a first MI than among controls (24.0 vs 17.6%).[29] In the Cardiovascular Health Study, each 5-unit increase in depression score was associated with an adjusted hazard ratio (HR) of 1.15 and 1.16 for the development of coronary heart disease and all-cause mortality, respectively.[62] In one study, new-onset depression among men was of higher risk than long-term depressed mood.[61]

Whereas studies of the role of personality in the etiology of coronary artery disease have yielded inconsistent results, there is evidence that hostility, cynicism, and anger form a critical 'toxic' component of type A behavior that is associated with enhanced cardiovascular risk.[63] In the Atherosclerosis Risk in Communities (ARIC) study,[64] normotensive subjects with high trait anger were at higher risk for acute MI or cardiac mortality than normotensive subjects with low trait anger (HR = 2.69). In a 36-year follow-up of 1055 medical students, in whom anger reaction to stress was self-reported on a questionnaire, those with the highest level of anger, compared to those with lower levels, had an increased risk of premature cardiovascular disease developing before the age of 55 (adjusted RR = 3.1), coronary heart disease (adjusted RR = 3.5), and MI (RR = 6.4).[65]

PATHOPHYSIOLOGY

There are several mechanisms by which emotional stress might trigger an acute MI (Figure 8.3).[8] Mental stress produces significant increases in heart rate and blood pressure that may lead to rheologic changes at the site of a plaque and precipitate plaque rupture.[9,66] Mental stress may also lead to vasoconstriction and aggravate

Figure 8.3 Potential mechanisms by which a trigger may increase the risk of myocardial infarction or sudden cardiac death. The relative contribution of each physiologic change may vary depending on the specific trigger, and differences in pathophysiology between infarction and sudden cardiac death. VT/VF, ventricular tachycardia/ventricular fibrillation.

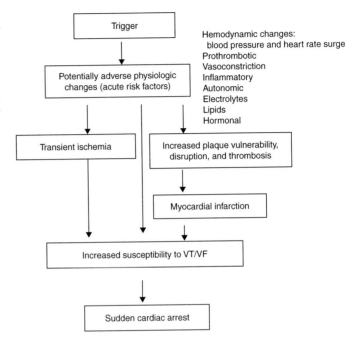

endothelial dysfunction.[67] Whereas coronary arteries of normal patients dilate during mental stress, impaired dilation and even constriction have been demonstrated in atherosclerotic arteries.[68] The vasoconstriction induced by stress may not be immediate. In a dog model, profound coronary vasoconstriction could be demonstrated 2–3 minutes following elicitation of anger.[69] The vasoconstriction persisted well after heart rate and arterial blood pressure recovered.

Studies have also shown that mental stress may increase platelet activation.[70–73] Although this may be balanced by a compensatory increase in fibrinolytic activity following acute stress, the fibrinolytic response may be diminished in the presence of endothelial dysfunction, leading to a prothrombotic imbalance. Although the effects of chronic stress on cardiovascular risk factors are less clear, a systemic stress response can include activation of neuroendocrinological pathways such as the sympathetic nervous system, hypothalamic–pituitary axis, and the renin–angiotensin system, with the release of stress hormones

(catecholamines, corticosteroids, growth hormone, and renin), with macrophage activation and cytokine release.[74,75]

STRATEGY FOR TRIGGERED ACUTE RISK PREVENTION

Five broad approaches can be considered for acute risk protection (Box 8.1) Because of the limited evidence to date, these approaches provide more a framework for future research than a guide for clinical management.

First, one can adopt a long-term behavioral and pharmaceutical approach that focuses on absolute risk reduction. This corresponds to traditional risk factor modification, emphasizing optimal blood pressure and lipids, not smoking, being physically active, and maintaining optimal weight. By reducing the atherosclerotic burden and the number of vulnerable plaques, such a long-term strategy would probably reduce the risk that a trigger would produce an acute CVD event.

Secondly, a long-term preventive approach can be directed against a specific

Box 8.1   Potential strategies for triggered acute risk prevention

1. Long-term general preventive therapy
2. Long-term trigger-specific preventive therapy
3. Ignore added risk of the trigger, since the absolute risk is so low
4. Modify or avoid the trigger
5. Therapy to sever the link between the trigger and its potential pathophysiologic consequences

trigger. At a public health level, provision of defibrillators and rapid cardiac resuscitation capability in sporting arenas, aircraft terminals, and as part of response preparedness for natural and man-made disasters may reduce cardiac death where large numbers of people congregate and are exposed to increased stress levels.[76–79]

Anger management or stress reduction training could be used to limit the responses of anger and anxiety. Psychosocial interventions appear to improve depressive symptoms and reduce social isolation in patients post-MI, but it is not clear whether these benefits translate into improved cardiovascular outcome. Several non-randomized studies suggested that targeted stress reduction post-MI may have cardiovascular benefits. However, a mortality benefit was not seen in the much larger and controlled ENRICHD trial, which evaluated 2481 patients post-MI who had either depression or a low level of perceived social support or both.[80] All patients were randomly assigned to 6 months of usual medical care with or without psychosocial intervention with individual and group cognitive therapy and social support counseling; antidepressant drugs were added for up to 12 months if there was severe depression or no response to cognitive therapy. After a mean follow-up of 29 months, patients receiving psychosocial intervention had less depression and better levels of perceived social support, but there was no reduction in mortality.

Thirdly, one can determine that the absolute risk of the trigger is very low and does not require intervention. In an individual considered to be at low risk for having atherosclerotic disease or vulnerable plaques, a maximal emotional stress should pose little absolute risk. Nonetheless, even in individuals without significant atherosclerosis, repeated surges in catecholamines due to severe emotional stress may be a mechanism for progression of atherosclerosis and subclinical plaque disruption.[53,54,81]

Fourthly, individuals could avoid or modify the specific triggering activity. Although data are limited, a person at increased absolute risk could avoid a direct angry confrontation with a neighbor or perform relaxation exercises at the time of severe emotional stress. Providing social support and sensitivity at the time of bereavement could be beneficial.

Finally, protective therapy can be taken in an effort to sever the link between the stressor and the potential pathophysiologic consequences. Many individuals known to be at high absolute risk are already taking daily β-blocker, aspirin, statin, and angiotensin-converting enzyme (ACE) inhibitor. It is useful to consider how these agents may modify stress-induced triggering.

β-blockers

β-Blockers provide the most compelling evidence for protection against the emotional triggers of acute coronary syndromes. Their protective effect against transient myocardial ischemia, MI, and sudden cardiac death is pronounced during the morning peak in frequency of these events, a time associated with emotional stress.[3,16,18,82–84] Although statistical power is limited for subgroup analyses of triggering studies, trends suggest that β-blockers reduce the likelihood of MI being triggered by emotional stress.[7,11,19] β-blockers reduce perioperative MI[85] and attenuate morning and stress-related surges in heart rate, blood pressure, and ischemia.[18]

Deedwania and Nelson noted that most transient ischemic episodes were preceded by increases in heart rate and blood pressure.[86] Andrews et al found that 81% of ischemic episodes were preceded by an increase in heart rate ≥5 beats/min, and that propranolol reduced these episodes more than diltiazem or nifedipine.[87] Compared with placebo, propranolol reduced ischemic episodes associated with an increased heart rate by 65%, and reduced episodes not associated with a heart rate increase by 45%. Of note, McLenachan et al found that propranolol was effective in reducing episodes occurring at a heart rate ≥80 beats/min but increased the number of events occurring at rates <80 beats/min,[88] possibly due to vasoconstriction, which can occur in response to stressors in the presence of atherosclerosis.[89–91] An animal model of takotsubo cardiomypathy suggested that combined α-β blockade was more effective than β-blockade alone.[92] The importance of heart rate in CVD onset is supported by an analysis of patients who underwent two coronary angiograms within 6 months, in whom higher heart rate was associated with coronary plaque disruption, and β-blocker use was protective.[81] By reducing flow velocity, turbulence, and vortex formation at regions of high circumferential tensile stress,[66] β-blockers could reduce endothelial damage and plaque rupture. This would be analogous to the protective role of β-blockers in acute dissection.[93] Some studies suggest beneficial effects of β-blockers on coagulability, although these findings have not been consistent.[94–96] The demonstration that β-blockers reduce the somatic symptoms associated with anxiety has led to an informal use for performance anxiety.[97,98]

Aspirin

In the Physicians Health study, aspirin preferentially reduced the morning peak of MI that corresponds with a morning peak of platelet reactivity.[17] Catecholamine excess associated with physical and emotional stress has been shown to increase platelet activation.[70,99] Aspirin inhibits epinephrine-induced platelet aggregation, and reduces platelet aggregates in the Folts model of stenosis, although the inhibitory effect was attenuated in a high catecholamine state.[100]

Lipid-lowering therapy

Statins protect against CVD in part through reduced inflammation, plaque stabilization, and inhibition of thrombus deposition.[101] While statins are used long term, evidence suggests an early benefit, both in lipid lowering, whereby a 20% cholesterol lowering was achieved after five daily doses of 80 mg atorvastatin in one study,[102] and by modifying other processes such as endothelial function, bioavailability of nitric oxide, and ischemia-reperfusion injury.[103,104] These rapid effects suggest that statins could play a protective role in triggering situations whose hazard period extends over days and weeks. Emotional stress is associated with higher lipid levels, only in part due to hemoconcentration.[105–107]

Angiotensin-converting enzyme inhibitors

ACE inhibitors have been shown to improve stress-induced endothelial dysfunction.[108–110] Endothelium-dependent vasodilator responsiveness to stressors is impaired in patients with atherosclerosis and risk factors.[89,103]

Calcium channel blockers

Heart rate lowering agents, such as verapamil and diltiazem, may inhibit stress-related surges in heart rate and reduce platelet reactivity.[73,111]

Nitrates

Nitroglycerin counters the stressor-induced vasoconstriction that can occur at the site of dysfunctional endothelium.[68,89,90] Nitroglycerin has an antiplatelet effect,[112] and may be helpful in prophylaxis against stress-induced angina.

Other potential therapy

Selective serotonin reuptake inhibitors (SSRIs) have been studied post-MI in the SADHART study (Sertraline Antidepressant Heart Attack Randomized Trial). In this study, 369 patients with depression who had been hospitalized for an MI or unstable angina were randomly assigned to 24 weeks of treatment with the SSRI sertraline or placebo.[113] Sertraline was no different from placebo in its effect on any measure of cardiovascular safety, including the left ventricular ejection fraction (the primary endpoint), blood pressure, heart rate, arrhythmias, or QTc prolongation. The incidence of severe cardiovascular adverse events tended to be lower in the sertraline group (14.5% vs 22.4%), although this difference was not statistically significant. Depression scale ratings did not improve significantly in the total study population with sertraline therapy compared with placebo. However, the subset of patients who had a history of major depression prior to their MI did have significant improvements in depressive symptoms with sertraline. The findings from SADHART were encouraging, although sample sizes were too small to formally evaluate CVD endpoints and treatment was not initiated until an average of 34 days following an MI; thus, the safety in the immediate post-MI period is not clear.

AREAS FOR FUTURE RESEARCH

Characterization of triggers

Although there has been much progress in defining the psychological triggers of acute CVD, there remains a need to better characterize the frequency of specific triggers; their relative, absolute, and attributable risk and hazard duration; and to better understand the modifiers of risk, including individual differences in response to the same trigger.[114] Incorporating triggering questions into prospective trials of therapy, including among individuals with implantable defibrillators, would be useful. Further study is needed to differentiate excess CVD events from earlier cases that would have occurred several hours or days later if the patient had not been exposed to the earlier trigger. The mechanisms by which emotional stress triggers MI, sudden cardiac death, and stroke, and the potential protective role of therapies, need to be better characterized, in human and animal models. For instance, a better understanding of the role of tachycardia and acute inflammation in acute plaque rupture may lead to evaluation of heart rate-lowering drugs or agents such as matrix metalloproteinase (MMP) inhibitors against triggered events.

Multiple triggers

One-quarter of the individuals reporting a possible trigger in the MILIS study identified two or more possible triggers. Further study is required of the effect on risk of multiple concurrent triggers, such as heavy exertion at the time of emotional stress, e.g. hurrying to catch a plane while carrying a suitcase.

Progression of atherosclerosis

The contribution of triggers such as severe emotional stress to the progression of vascular disease, mediated by catecholamine-mediated uptake of low-density lipoprotein (LDL) into vessel walls, endothelial dysfunction,[57,115] and asymptomatic plaque rupture requires further study. It may be difficult to separate patients for whom MI is the first clinical event from those with premonitory symptoms that may have been triggered by a stressor, or those in whom culprit plaque rupture occurred unrecognized 1–2 weeks prior to the MI.

Relationship between triggering and plaque vulnerability

An inverse relation probably exists between the degree of plaque vulnerability and the intensity of the trigger required to produce rupture and thrombosis. Thus, an individual with an extremely vulnerable plaque or severe stenosis may develop occlusion without a demonstrable trigger, whereas someone with no vulnerable lesions or stenosis may require a major identifiable stressor to trigger plaque rupture and thrombosis. Since plaque disruption is often present at more than one location, in these individuals, there may be a general increase in inflammatory activity and transient increase in plaque vulnerability.

Therapeutic approach

Many individuals at moderate to high risk of CVD are already taking daily therapy that – as part of their mechanism of action – may be protective against triggered events. Indeed, protection against triggers, some of which cannot be anticipated, provides a further rationale for daily evidence-based therapy. Although unproven, the presence of the circadian morning peak of events supports the use of daily medication of sufficient duration that, when taken on one day, it is active the following morning.

For those on daily evidence-based therapy or for whom regular therapy is not considered indicated, it remains unknown whether incremental therapy during a hazard period of increased risk is useful. Large numbers of randomized individuals would be required to test whether strategies directed at specific emotional triggers would be feasible or would lower CVD events beyond current preventive approaches. However, the recognition that bereavement and other prolonged periods of severe stress are associated with increased CVD risk should provide an impetus for physicians to review such individuals more closely for symptoms, or changes in blood pressure, lipids, and other risk factors. Although the physician is best placed to initiate and monitor therapy, actively involving patients in their care is consistent with moves towards greater patient awareness and may improve compliance and stimulate individuals to lower their overall cardiac risk.[116] Underutilization of evidence-based therapies, such as β-blockers, is well recognized among patients prior to MI, despite known CVD or risk factors,[117] and long-term adherence in secondary prevention remains suboptimal. Whereas focus has been on prevention, a benefit of medications such as an aspirin in the wallet or handbag is that it is immediately available if symptoms of MI develop.

CONCLUSION

Triggering findings, such as the observation that MIs may be triggered by episodes of anger, provide insight into the mechanism of onset of CVD and the interaction with plaque vulnerability. However, from a clinical perspective, the data on triggering must be balanced against the recognition that the absolute risk for any potential triggering activity to cause MI is the most important clinical measure. If the absolute risk is extremely small, then even a substantial increase in that risk may not be clinically meaningful or warrant a specific therapy. It would be cause for significant concern if a focus on small risks associated with stressors of daily living, which are frequently unavoidable, led to excessive caution and reduced enjoyment of life, since many pleasures of life are associated with adrenergic activation. Nonetheless, depression, anxiety, and issues regarding anger management, which are common, important, and worthy of greater attention, may also contribute to progression of atherosclerosis.

Although the proportion of individuals with plaques that are vulnerable to rupture at any given moment is likely to be very low, the recognition that stressors trigger cardiovascular events also supports the need for wider availability of cardiac care, including defibrillators at large gatherings of individuals who may experience mental stress, and as part of an optimal acute response to disasters.

The means of prevention would not be to eliminate all potential triggering activities – an undesirable and unattainable goal – but to design strategies that can be evaluated in randomized studies for their ability to sever the linkage between a trigger and its potentially adverse consequence.

A preventive approach to acute risk could have made a significant difference to John Hunter (1728–93), Surgeon and Medical Educator at St George's Hospital, London who presciently stated, 'My life is at the mercy of any rogue who chooses to provoke me,' and indeed died shortly after an acrimonious meeting with hospital administrators.

REFERENCES

1. Davies MJ, Thomas AC. Plaque fissuring – the cause of acute myocardial infarction, sudden ischemic death, and crescendo angina. Br Heart J 1985; 53:363–73.
2. Ambrose JA, Tannenbaum MA, Alexopoulos D et al. Angiographic progression of coronary artery disease and the development of myocardial infarction. J Am Coll Cardiol 1988; 12:56–62.
3. Muller JE, Stone PH, Turi ZG et al. Circadian variation in the frequency of onset of acute myocardial infarction. N Engl J Med 1985; 313:1315–22.
4. Willich SN, Levy D, Rocco MB et al. Circadian variation in the incidence of sudden cardiac death in the Framingham Heart Study population. Am J Cardiol 1987; 60:801–6.
5. Marler JR, Price TR, Clark GL et al. Morning increase in onset of ischemic stroke. Stroke 1989; 20:473–6.
6. Behar S, Halabi M, Reicher-Reiss H et al. Circadian variation and possible external triggers of onset of myocardial infarction. SPRINT Study Group. Am J Med 1993; 94:395–400.
7. Tofler GH, Muller JE, Stone PH et al. Modifiers of timing and possible triggers of acute myocardial infarction in the Thrombolysis in Myocardial Infarction Phase II (TIMI II) Study Group. J Am Coll Cardiol 1992; 20:1049–55.
8. Muller JE, Tofler GH, Stone PH. Circadian variation and triggers of onset of acute cardiovascular disease. Circulation 1989; 79:733–43.
9. Muller JE, Abela GS, Nesto RW, Tofler GH. Triggers, acute risk factors and vulnerable plaques: the lexicon of a new frontier. J Am Coll Cardiol 1994; 23: 809–13.
10. Mittleman MA, Maclure M, Tofler GH et al. Triggering of acute myocardial infarction by heavy physical exertion. Protection against triggering by regular exertion. Determinants of Myocardial Infarction Onset Study Investigators. N Engl J Med 1993; 329:1677–83.
11. Mittleman MA, Maclure M, Sherwood JB et al. Triggering of acute myocardial infarction onset by episodes of anger. Circulation 1995; 92:1720–5.
12. Giri S, Thompson PD, Kiernan FJ et al. Clinical and angiographic characteristics of exertion-related acute myocardial infarction. JAMA 1999; 282:1731–6.
13. Willich SN, Lewis M, Lowel H et al. For the Triggers and Mechanisms of Myocardial Infarction Study Group. Physical exertion as a trigger of acute myocardial infarction. N Engl J Med 1993; 329:1684–90.
14. Smeeth L, Thomas SH, Hall AJ, Hubbard R, Farrington P, Vallance P. Risk of myocardial infarction and stroke after acute infection or vaccination. N Engl J Med 2004; 351:2611–18.
15. Peters RW, Muller JE, Goldstein S, Byington R, Friedman LM. Propranolol and the morning increase in the frequency of sudden cardiac death (BHAT Study). Am J Cardiol 1989; 63:1518–20.
16. Ridker PM, Manson JE, Buring JE, Muller JE, Hennekens CH. Circadian variation of acute myocardial infarction and the effect of low-dose aspirin in a randomized trial of physicians. Circulation 1990; 82:897–902.
17. Parker JD, Testa MA, Jimenez AH et al. Morning increase in ambulatory ischemia in patients with stable coronary artery disease. Importance of physical activity and increased cardiac demand. Circulation 1994; 89:604–14.
18. Tofler GH, Muller JE. Triggering of acute cardiovascular disease and potential preventive strategies. Circulation 2006; 114:1863–72.
19. Tofler GH, Stone PH, Maclure M et al. Analysis of possible triggers of acute myocardial infarction (the MILIS study). Am J Cardiol 1990; 66:22–7.
20. Maclure M. The case-crossover design: a method for studying transient effects on the risk of acute events. Am J Epidemiol 1991; 133:144–53.
21. Moller J, Hallqvist J, Diderichsen F et al. Do episodes of anger trigger myocardial infarction? A case-crossover analysis in the Stockholm Heart Epidemiology Program (SHEEP). Psychosom Med 1999; 61:842–9.

22. Koton S, Tanne D, Bornstein NM, Green MS. Triggering risk factors for ischaemic stroke: a case-crossover study. Neurology 2004; 63:2006–10.

23. Jacobs S. An epidemiological review of the mortality of bereavement. Psychosom Med 1977; 39:344–57.

24. Stroebe MS. The broken heart phenomenon: an examination of the mortality of bereavement. J Commun and Appl Soc Psychol 1994; 4:47–61.

25. Young M, Benjamin B, Wallis C. The mortality of widowers. Lancet 1963; 2:454–6.

26. O'Connor M, Allen J, Kasniak A. Autonomic and emotion regulation in bereavement and depression. J Psychosom Res 2002; 52:183–5.

27. Tennant C. Life stress, social support and coronary heart disease. Aust NZ J Psychiatry 1999; 33:636–41.

28. Rees WD, Lutkins SG. Mortality of bereavement. Br Med J 1967; 4:13–16.

29. Rosengren A, Hawken S, Ounpuu S et al; for the INTERHEART Investigators. Association of psychosocial risk factors with risk of acute myocardial infarction in 11 119 cases and 13 648 controls from 52 countries (the INTERHEART study): case-control study. Lancet 2004; 364:953–62.

30. Moller J, Theorell T, de Faire U, Ahlbom A, Hallqvist J. Work related stressful life events and the risk of myocardial infarction. Case-control and case-crossover analyses within the Stockholm heart epidemiology programme (SHEEP). J Epidemiol Community Health 2005; 59:23–30.

31. Trichopoulos D, Zavitsanos X, Katsouyanni K, Tzonou A, Dalla-Vorgia P. Psychological stress and fatal heart attack: the Athens earthquake natural experiment. Lancet 1983; 1:441–3.

32. Leor J, Kloner RA. The Northridge earthquake as a trigger for acute myocardial infarction. Am J Cardiol 1996; 77:1230–2.

33. Meisel SR, Kutz I, Dayan KI et al. Effect of Iraqi missile war on incidence of acute myocardial infarction and sudden death in Israeli civilians. Lancet 1991; 338:660–1.

34. Leor J, Poole WK, Kloner RA. Sudden cardiac death triggered by an earthquake. N Engl J Med 1996; 334: 413–9.

35. Brown DL. Disparate effects of the 1989 Loma Prieta and 1994 Northbridge earthquakes on hospital admissions for acute myocardial infarction: importance of superimposition of triggers. Am Heart J 1999; 137:830–6.

36. Allegra JR, Mostashari F, Rothman J, Milano P, Cochrane DG. Cardiac events in New Jersey after the September 11, 2001, terrorist attack. J Urban Health 2005; 82:358–63.

37. Witte DR, Bois MI, Hoes AW, Grobbee DE. Cardiovascular mortality in Dutch men during 1996 European football championship: longitudinal population study. BMJ 2000; 321:1552–4.

38. Toubiana L, Hanslik T, Letrilliart L. French cardiovascular mortality did not increase during football championship. BMJ 2001; 322:1306.

39. Peters A, von Klot S, Heier M, Trentiaglia I et al. Cooperative Health Research in the Region of Augsburg Study Group. Exposure to traffic and the onset of myocardial infarction. N Engl J Med 2004; 351:1721–30.

40. Ornato JP, Siegel L, Craren EJ, Nelson N. Increased incidence of cardiac death attributed to acute myocardial infarction during winter. Coronary Artery Disease 1990; 1:199–203.

41. Kelly-Hayes M, Wolf PA, Kase CS et al. Temporal patterns of stroke onset: the Framingham study. Stroke 1995; 26:1343–7.

42. Spencer FA, Goldberg RJ, Bucker RC, Gore JM. Seasonal distribution of acute myocardial infarction in the National Registry of Myocardial Infarction. J Am Coll Cardiol 1998; 31:1226–33.

43. Seto TB, Mittleman MA, Davis RB, Taira DA, Kawachi I. Seasonal variation in coronary artery disease mortality in Hawaii: observational study. BMJ 1998; 316:1946–7.

44. Woodhouse PR, Khaw KT, Plummer M, Foley A, Meade TW. Seasonal variation of plasma fibrinogen and factor VII activity in the elderly: winter infections and death from cardiovascular disease. Lancet 1994; 343:435–9.

45. Mavri A, Guzic-Salobir B, Salobir-Pajnic B et al. Seasonal variation of some metabolic and hemostatic risk factors in subjects with and without coronary artery disease. Blood Coag Fibrinol 2001; 12:359–65.

46. Gnecchi-Ruscone T, Piccaluga E, Guzzetti S et al. Morning and Monday: critical periods for the onset of acute myocardial infarction – the GISSI 2 study experience. Eur Heart J 1994; 15:882–7.

47. Peters RW, McQuillan S, Kaye SA, Gold MR. Increased Monday incidence of life-threatening ventricular arrhythmias. Experience with a third-generation implantable defibrillator. Circulation 1995; 94:1346–9.

48. Barnett AG, Dobson AJ. Excess in cardiovascular events on Mondays: a meta-analysis and prospective study. J Epidemiol Community Health 2005; 59:109–14.

49. Phillips DP, Jarvinen JR, Abramson IS, Phillips RR. Cardiac mortality is higher around Christmas and New Year's that at any other time. Circulation 2004; 110:3781–8.

50. Wittstein IS, Thiemann DR, Lima JAC et al. Neurohormonal features of myocardial stunning due to sudden emotional stress. N Engl J Med 2005; 352:539–48.

51. Bybee KA, Kara T, Prasad A et al. Systematic review: transient left ventricular apical ballooning: a syndrome that mimics ST-segment elevation myocardial infarction. Ann Intern Med 2004; 141:858–65.

52. Owa M, Aizawa K, Urasawa N et al. Emotional stress-induced "ampulla cardiomyopathy": discrepancy between the metabolic and sympathetic innervation imaging performed during the recovery course. Jpn Circ J 2001; 65:349–52.

53. Cardona-Sanclemente LE, Born GV. Adrenaline increases the uptake of low-density lipoproteins in carotid arteries of rabbits. Atherosclerosis 1992; 96:215–18.

54. Burke AP, Kolodgie FD, Farb A et al. Healed plaque ruptures and sudden coronary death: evidence that subclinical rupture has a role in plaque progression. Circulation 2001; 103:934–40.

55. Takano M, Inami S, Ishibashi F et al. Angioscopic follow-up study of coronary ruptured plaques in non culprit lesions. J Am Coll Cardiol 2005; 45:652–8.

56. Manuck SB, Kaplan JR, Clarkson TB. Behaviorally induced heart rate reactivity and atherosclerosis in cynomolgus monkeys. Psychosom Med 1983; 45:95–108.

57. Kaplan JR, Manuck SB, Adams MR, Weingand KW, Clarkson TB. Inhibition of coronary atherosclerosis by propranolol in behaviorally predisposed monkeys fed an atherogenic diet. Circulation 1987; 76: 1364–72.

58. Kawachi I, Colditz GA, Ascherio A et al. Prospective study of phobic anxiety and risk of coronary heart disease in men. Circulation 1994; 89:1992–7.

59. Wassertheil-Smoller S, Shumaker S, Ockene JT et al. Depression and cardiovascular sequelae in postmenopausal women. The Women's Health Initiative (WHI). Arch Intern Med 2004; 164:289–98.

60. Wulsin LR, Evans JC, Vasan RS et al. Depressive symptoms, coronary heart disease, and overall mortality in the Framingham Heart Study. Psychosom Med 2005; 67:697–702.

61. Penninx BW, Guralnik JM, Mendes de Leon CF et al. Cardiovascular events and mortality in newly and chronically depressed persons >70 years of age. Am J Cardiol 1998; 81:988–94.

62. Ariyo AA, Haan M, Tangen CM et al. Depressive symptoms and risks of coronary heart disease and mortality in elderly Americans. Cardiovascular Health Study Collaborative Research Group. Circulation 2000; 102:1773–9.

63. Shekelle RB, Gale M, Ostfeld AM, Paul O. Hostility, risk of coronary heart disease and mortality. Psychosom Med 1983; 45:109–14.

64. Williams JE, Paton CC, Siegler IC et al. Anger proneness predicts coronary heart disease risk: prospective analysis from the Atherosclerosis Risk in Communities (ARIC) Study. Circulation 2000; 101:2034–9.

65. Chang PP, Ford DE, Meoni IC et al. Anger in young men and subsequent cardiovascular disease: The Precursors Study. Arch Intern Med 2002; 162:901.

66. Richardson PD, Davies MJ, Born GV. Influence of plaque configuration and stress distribution on fissuring of coronary atherosclerotic plaques. Lancet 1989; 2:941–4.

67. Ghiadoni L, Donald AE, Cropley M et al. Mental stress induces transient endothelial dysfunction in humans. Circulation 2000; 102:2473–8.

68. Yeung AC, Vekshtein VI, Krantz DS et al. The effect of atherosclerosis on the vasomotor response of coronary arteries to mental stress. N Engl J Med 1991; 325:1551–6.

69. Verrier RL, Hagestad EL, Lown B. Delayed myocardial ischemia induced by anger. Circulation 1987; 75:249–54.

70. Levine SP, Towell BL, Saurez AM et al. Platelet activation and secretion associated with emotional stress. Circulation 1985; 71:1129–34.

71. Musumeci V, Baroni S, Cardillo C et al. Cardiovascular reactivity, plasma markers of endothelial and platelet activity and plasma renin activity after mental stress in normals and hypertensives. J Hypertens 1987; 5 (Suppl 5):S1–S4.

72. Wagner CT, Kroll MH, Chow TW, Hellums JD, Schafer AI. Epinephrine and shear stress synergistically induce platelet aggregation via a mechanism that partially bypasses vWF–GPIB interactions. Biorheology 1996; 33:209–29.

73. Gebara OCE, Jimenez AH, McKenna C et al. Stress-induced hemodynamic and hemostatic changes in subjects with systemic hypertension: Effect of Verapamil. Clin Cardiol 1996; 19:205–11.

74. Adams DO. Molecular biology of macrophage activation: a pathway whereby psychosocial factors can potentially affect health. Psychosom Med 1994; 56:316–27.

75. Black PH. Stress and the inflammatory response: a review of neurogenic inflammation. Brain Behav Immun 2002; 16:622–53.

76. O'Rourke MF, Donaldson E, Geddes JS. An airline cardiac arrest program. Circulation 1997; 96:2849–53.

77. Galea S. Disasters and the health of urban populations. J Urban Health 2006; 82:347–49.

78. Hallsrom AP, Ornato JP, Weisfeldt M et al. Public Access Defibrillation Trial Investigators. Public-access defibrillation and survival after out-of-hospital cardiac arrest. N Engl J Med 2004; 351:637–46.

79. Hazinski MF, Idris AH, Kerber RE et al. Rescuer automated axternal defibrillator ("public access defibrillation") programs: lessons learned from an international multicenter trial: advisory statement from the American Heart Association Emergency Cardiovascular Committee; the Council on Cardiopulmonary, Perioperative, and Critical Care; and the Council on Clinical Cardiology. Circulation 2005; 111:3336–40.

80. Berkman LF, Blumenthal J, Burg M et al. Enhancing Recovery in Coronary Heart Disease Patients Investigators (ENRICHD). Effects of treating depression and low perceived social support on clinical events after myocardial infarction: the Enhancing Recovery in Coronary Heart Disease Patients (ENRICHD) Randomized Trial. JAMA 2003; 289:3106–16.

81. Heidland UE, Strauer BE. Left ventricular muscle mass and elevated heart rate are associated with coronary plaque disruption. Circulation 2001; 104:1477–82.

82. Deedwania PC, Carbajal EV. Role of beta blockade in the treatment of myocardial ischemia. Am J Cardiol 1997; 80(9B):23J–28J.

83. Frishman WH, Furberg DC, Friedewald WT. Beta-adrenergic blockade for survivors of acute myocardial infarction. N Engl J Med 1984; 310:830–6.

84. Frishman WH. Multifactorial actions of beta-adrenergic blocking drugs in ischemic heart disease: current concepts. Circulation 1983; 67:11–18.

85. Mangano DT, Layug EL, Wallace A, Tateo I; for the Multicenter Study of Perioperative Ischaemia Research Group. Effect of atenolol on mortality and cardiovascular morbidity after noncardiac surgery. N Engl J Med 1996; 335:1713–20.

86. Deedwania PC, Nelson JR. Pathophysiology of silent myocardial ischemia during daily life: hemodynamic evaluation by simultaneous electorcardiographic and blood pressure monitoring. Circulation 1990; 82:1296–304.

87. Andrews TC, Fenton T, Toyosaki N et al. Subsets of ambulatory myocardial ischemia based on heart rate activity. Circadian distribution and response to anti-ischemia medication. The Angina and Silent Ischemia Study Group (ASIS). Circulation 1993; 88:92–100.

88. McLenachan JM, Weidinger FF, Barry J et al. Relations between heart rate, ischemia, and drug therapy during daily life in patients with coronary artery disease. Circulation 1991; 83:1263–70.

89. Gordon JB, Ganz P, Nabel EG et al. Atherosclerosis influences the vasomotor response of epicardial coronary arteries to exercise. J Clin Invest 1989; 83:1946–52.

90. Nabel EG, Selwyn AP, Ganz P. Paradoxical narrowing of atherosclerotic coronary arteries induced by increases in heart rate. Circulation 1990; 81:1147–50.

91. Nabel EG, Ganz P, Gordon JB, Alexander RW, Selwyn AP. Dilatation of normal and constriction of atherosclerotic coronary arteries caused by the cold pressor test. Circulation 1988; 77:43–52.

92. Ueyama T. Emotional stress-induced Tako-tsubo cardiomyopathy: animal model and molecular mechanism. Ann NY Acad Sci 2004; 1018:437–44.

93. Nienaber CA, Eagle KA. Aortic dissection: new frontiers in diagnosis and management. Part II: therapeutic management and follow-up. Circulation 2003; 108:772–8.

94. Frishman WH, Weksler B, Christodoulou JP, Smithen C, Killip T. Reversal of abnormal platelet aggregability and change in exercise tolerance in patients with angina pectoris following oral propranolol. Circulation 1974; 50:887–96.

95. Horn EH, Jalihal S, Bruce M, Dean A, Rubin PC. The effect on platelet behaviour of treatment with atenolol and the combination of atenolol and nifedipine in healthy volunteers. Platelets 1992; 3:15–21.

96. Willich SN, Pohjola-Sintonen S, Bhatia SJ et al. Suppression of silent ischemia by metoprolol without alteration of morning increase of platelet aggregability in patients with stable coronary artery disease. Circulation 1989; 79:557–65.

97. Sherman DG, Easton JD. Beta-adrenergic blockade and anxiety. Lancet 1976; 2:911–12.

98. Fishbein M, Middlestadt SE. The ICSOM medical questionnaire. Senza Sordino 1987; 25:1–8.

99. Kestin AS, Ellis PA, Barnard MR et al. Effect of strenuous exercise on platelet activation state and reactivity. Circulation 1983; 88:1502–11.

100. Folts JD, Rowe GG. Epinephrine potentiation of in vivo stimuli reverses aspirin inhibition of platelet thrombus formation in stenosed canine coronary arteries. Thromb Res 1988; 50:507–16.

101. Sukhova GK, Williams JK, Libby P. Statins reduce inflammation in atheroma of nonhuman primates independent of effects on serum cholesterol. Arterioscl Thromb Vasc Biol 2002; 22:1452–8.

102. Correia LCL, Sposito AC, Lima JC et al. Anti-inflammatory effect of atorvastatin (80 mg) in unstable angina pectoris and non-Q-wave acute myocardial infarction. Am J Cardiol 2003; 92:298–301.

103. John S, Schneider MP, Delles C, Jacobi J, Schmieder RE. Lipid-independent effects of statins on endothelial function and bioavailability of nitric oxide in hypercholesterolemic patients. Am Heart J 2005; 149(3):473.

104. Mensah K, Mocanu MM, Yellon DM. Failure to protect the myocardium against ischemia/reperfusion injury after chronic atorvastatin treatment is recaptured by acute atorvastatin treatment. J Am Coll Cardiol 2005; 45:1287–91.

105. Friedman M, Rosenman RH, Carroll V, Tat RJ. Changes in the serum cholesterol and blood clotting time in men subjected to cyclic variation of occupational stress. Circulation 1958; 17:852–61.

106. Bachen EA, Muldoon MF, Matthews KA, Manuck SB. Effect of hemoconcentration and sympathetic activation on serum lipid responses to brief mental stress. Psychosom Med 2002; 64:587–94.

107. Siegrist J, Peter R, Cremer P, Siedel D. Chronic work stress is associated with atherogenic lipids and elevated fibrinogen in middle-aged men. J Intern Med 1997; 242:149–56.

108. Watanabe S, Tagawa T, Yamakawa K, Shimabukuro M, Ueda S. Inhibition of the renin-angiotensin system prevents free fatty acid-induced acute endothelial dysfunction in humans. Arterioscl Thromb Vasc Biol 2005; 25:2376–80.

109. Koh KK, Bui MN, Hathaway L et al. Mechanism by which quinapril improves vascular function in coronary artery disease. Am J Cardiol 1999; 83:327–31.

110. Wiel W, Pu Q, Leclerc J et al. Effects of the angiotensin-converting enzyme inhibitor perindopril on endothelial injury and hemostasis in rabbit endotoxic shock. Intensive Care Med 2004; 8:1652–9.

111. Gibson RS, Hansen JF, Messerli F, Schechtman KB, Boden WE. Long-term effects of diltiazem and verapamil on mortality and cardiac events in non-Q-wave acute myocardial infarction without pulmonary congestion: Post hoc subset analysis of the Multicenter Postinfarction Trial and the second Danish Verapamil Infarction Trial Studies. Am J Cardiol 2000; 86:275–9.

112. Folts JD, Stamler J, Loscalzo J. Intravenous nitroglycerin infusion inhibits cyclic blood flow responses caused by periodic platelet thrombus formation in stenosed canine coronary arteries. Circulation 1991; 83:2122–7.

113. Glassman AH, O'Connor CM, Califf RM et al. Sertraline Antidepressant Heart Attack Randomised Trial (SADHEART) Group. Sertraline treatment of major depression in patients with acute MI or unstable angina. JAMA 2002; 288:701–9.

114. Rothman KJ. Modern Epidemiology. Boston, MA: Little Brown; 1986.

115. Strawn WB, Bondjers G, Kaplan JR et al. Endothelial dysfunction in response to psychosocial stress in monkeys. Circ Res 1991; 68:1270–9.

116. Rosner F. Patient noncompliance: causes and solutions. Mt Sinai J Med 2006; 773:553–9.

117. Miller RR, Li Y-F, Sun H et al. Underuse of cardioprotective medications in patients prior to acute myocardial infarction. Am J Cardiol 2003; 92:209–11.

Animal models of vulnerable plaque　9

Juan F Granada and Robert S Schwartz

INTRODUCTION

Acute thrombus formation on the surface of a complex atherosclerotic lesion appears responsible for the majority of acute coronary events.[1–4] Autopsy studies show that most of these thrombotic events are associated with disruption of an atherosclerotic plaque that contains specific structural and biologic features.[5–7] Although extensive literature describes the morphology and biology of these lesions, little data exist regarding their long-term course in living humans.[8,9] The search for an accurate animal model of plaque vulnerability should thus be a priority in vascular biology research.

Animal models facilitate our understanding of human disease by providing a controlled environment that allows testing mechanistic and pathophysiologic hypotheses followed by assessing therapeutic interventions. An accurate vulnerable plaque model has proven difficult to create, in part due to imprecision of what a 'vulnerable plaque' truly is.[10] This is complicated by a poorly defined natural course of the disease.[8,10] and uncertainty about the impact of plaque rupture on coronary artery thrombosis.[11,12] This chapter reviews current animal models of complex atherosclerosis that display histopathologic features of arterial and plaque vulnerability, regardless of plaque rupture.

DESIRABLE FEATURES OF AN ANIMAL MODEL OF VULNERABLE PLAQUE

The ideal animal model of vulnerable plaque does not yet exist. Several principles must be fulfilled for an accurate animal model of complex atherosclerosis (Table 9.1). The animal model should exhibit vascular lesions structurally and biologically similar to human atherosclerotic tissue. These lesions must occur in regions accessible to diagnostic and/or interventional manipulation to satisfy the objectives of the proposed therapies. For basic research, small animals such as mice are cost-effective to test mechanistic hypotheses related to molecular aspects of vascular disease.[13] In this setting, morphologic appearance or anatomic location of the lesions is not as important as when imaging must be validated. For validating invasive or non-invasive diagnostic technology, the morphology, location, and presence of specific structural plaque components such as calcium are of pivotal importance for developing tissue characterization algorithms.[14–17] If molecular imaging is involved, specific biologic components such as macrophages and thrombotic components including fibrin and platelets must be involved.[18,19] A more complex environment is needed to validate potential therapeutic strategies, such as demonstrating the effects of therapies

Table 9.1   Desirable features of an animal model of vulnerable plaque

Feature	Mice	Rabbit	Pig
Nature of atherosclerotic lesions similar to humans	+	++	+++
Known genetic background	+++	++[a]	++[b]
Simple development method	++	++	+
Metabolic profile similar to humans	+	+	++
Short development time (<6 months)	++	++	+
Ability to perform non-invasive imaging	+	++	++
Ability to perform invasive imaging	−	++	+++
Ability to perform systemic therapeutic interventions	++	++	++
Ability to perform invasive therapeutic procedures	−	++	+++
Low development cost	+	++	+++

[a]The Watanabe heritable hyperlipidemic rabbit.
[b]The inherited hyper-LDL (low-density lipoprotein) cholesterolemia-bearing mutant alleles for apolipoprotein B (ApoB).

directed toward limiting vascular inflammation, necrosis, remodeling, and healing. Regardless of the animal model used, researchers, industry, and regulatory agencies must reach a consensus for standardizing definitions that allow comparison among validation studies for emerging cardiovascular therapies.

VULNERABILITY ENDPOINTS IN ANIMAL MODELS OF VULNERABLE PLAQUE

One major initial consideration in developing a vulnerable plaque model is to define the vascular lesion components that will predominate. Autopsy studies suggest that acute coronary thrombosis arises from several different pathologic substrates. Disruption of a thin-cap fibroatheroma (TCFA) is probably responsible for many acute coronary events.[7,20–23] An animal model of vulnerable plaque should thus include vascular lesions comparable to the human TCFA (Table 9.2). These lesions should demonstrate non-stenotic, eccentric plaques preferentially located in positively remodeled vessel segments.[24–26] Such lesions should display

Table 9.2   Vulnerability endpoints in animal models of vulnerable plaque for basic research and technology validation studies

Feature	Basic research	Imaging validation	Therapy validation
Cellular markers	+++	++	++
Immunologic markers	+++	++	++
Proteolytic enzymes	+++	+	+
Cellular apoptosis	+++	++	+
Vascular remodeling	+	++	+
Prominent necrotic core	+	+++	++
Thinned fibrous cap	+	+++	+++
Macrophage infiltration	+++	+++	+++
Neovascularization	++	++	+
Calcification	++	++	+
Stem cell kinetics	+++	++	++

a high lipid content (with or without a lipidic pool), inflammatory cells (macrophages), and a thinned fibrous cap.[20,27,28] Variants of these plaques may contain confluent cellular lesions with extracellular lipid intermixed with normal intima, which may predominate as an outer layer or cap, or possess an extracellular lipid core covered by an acquired fibrous cap. The fibrous cap must be thinner than 65 μm and contain collagen types I and VIII, proteoglycans,[20] and inflammatory cells at the shoulders of the plaque.[29] Sophisticated lesion characterization may be needed for basic science research and validation of molecular imaging or therapies including the detailed characterization of cholesterol ester types, monocyte-derived macrophages, T lymphocytes, and smooth muscle cells (SMCs).[20,30–34] Secondary features such as medial thinning,[35] hemorrhage, calcification, apoptosis, and growth of vasa vasorum are also desirable.[36–39] Finally, while the morphologic appearance of the atherosclerotic lesion is one the most important variables in animal model development, it is the ability to reproduce these lesions in anatomic location, obstruction, and composition, that will eventually make possible comparison with human studies.

PLAQUE RUPTURE AND ANIMAL MODELS OF VULNERABLE PLAQUE

The mainstream hypothesis of coronary thrombosis suggests that plaque disruption is responsible for most coronary events.[5,20,21,40] This observation is based on autopsy and angiographic studies, and is compelling though imperfect. Plaque rupture and subsequent ulceration accounts for at least two-thirds of acute coronary events, but most rupture cases are multiple, silent, and may be responsible only for plaque progression.[41] Also, many thrombotic lesions occur on non-ruptured lesions containing minimal macrophage infiltration and abundant SMCs.[40,42] Conversely, plaque rupture may follow a benign course toward stabilization and healing and not necessarily lead to acute vessel occlusion.[43–46] Besides the mechanical failure associated with plaque disruption, several interrelated cellular immunologic and hematologic variables may play central roles in the acute phase of vascular thrombosis.[47–49] Therefore, while plaque rupture may be a good indicator of plaque vulnerability and is a desirable feature in animal models of vulnerable plaque, the lack of this phenomenon should not preclude the inclusion of any given animal model in technology validation studies.

ANIMAL MODELS OF COMPLEX ATHEROSCLEROSIS

Several animal atherosclerotic models have emerged in the past 50 years.[50] Since multiple unanswered questions exist regarding the definition and natural history of the disease, one very practical approach is to use current animal atherosclerosis models that display histopathologic features of plaque vulnerability. Some of these models have been used to test mechanistic hypotheses in basic research and for validating diagnostic modalities and emerging therapeutic technologies in interventional cardiology.[50–54] In general, rats and dogs are poor animal models because they do not develop spontaneous lesions despite dietary modification. Primates are not widely used because of ethical issues, risk to experimenters, and maintenance costs. In this chapter, we discuss atherosclerotic models developed in mice, rabbits, and pigs, regardless of the presence of rupture or vascular thrombosis.

Mouse models

The mouse is the most cost-effective animal species used for studying complex atherosclerosis, mainly because of easy handling and the large amount of genetic information available. Although mice are naturally resistant to atherosclerosis due to naturally occurring high HDL (high-density lipoprotein) and low LDL (low-density lipoprotein), significant atherosclerotic lesions nevertheless occur when genetic manipulation is performed.[55–61] A common feature of the genetically manipulated mice is the accumulation of very low-density lipoprotein (VLDL) and/or LDL in the plasma. The most important models achieved by genetic manipulations are apoprotein E (ApoE)-deficient mice (ApoE$^{-/-}$) and LDL receptor-deficient mice (LDLR$^{-/-}$).[55,56,59–61] Mice carrying a mutant ApoE gene were described in 1992.[61] When this strain of animals is placed on a Western-type diet, their cholesterol levels exceed 2000 mg/dl and they develop advanced fibrotic atherosclerotic plaques located in the aortic root and composed of thin luminal elastin and collagen fibers capping small lipoid-rich globular aggregates[60,61] (Figure 9.1). Preliminary studies using this model reported that the aortic lesions developed by the animals could be

mechanically disrupted by the use of forceps.[62] Subsequent reports localized these complex atherosclerotic lesions to the innominate artery of 60-week-old ApoE knockout mice.[63] Such lesions are collagen-rich, fibrofatty nodules and xanthomas containing necrotic areas and intramural bleeding.[59] Recently, Johnson and co-workers described ApoE knockout mice with a different genetic background (C57BL6/129SvJ) that develop atherosclerotic plaques that rupture at a mean age of 14 months.[13,64] In this model, atherosclerotic lesions are covered by thin fibrous caps composed of elastin and SMCs that rupture preferentially at the innominate artery bifurcation. They are associated with intraluminal thrombus (Figure 9.2). Interestingly, though most mice died suddenly, the incidence of sudden death did not differ between the ruptured and unruptured groups.[13,64] The LDL receptor-deficient mouse (LDL receptor-knockout), described in 1994 by Ishibashi et al,[65] develops modest atherosclerotic lesions when placed on a regular chow diet (cholesterol levels 200–300 mg/dl).[56] However, when these mice

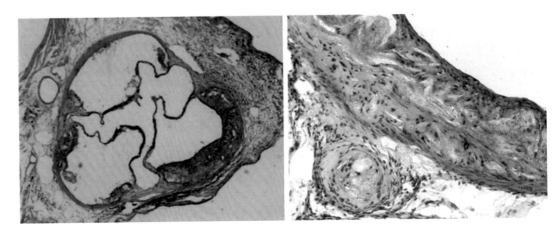

Figure 9.1   ApoE1 knockout mice model of atherosclerosis. Histologic section obtained above the level of the aortic leaflets (Sudan IV and H&E stains). Left panel (4×), section of the aortic root at the aortic valve level. Right panel (20×), eccentric lesion with multiple layers of SMCs, mature fibrous cap, necrosis, and cholesterol clefts. At the bottom, there is a coronary vessel occluded by a concentric atheroma. (Original picture courtesy of Dr Nobuyo Maeda, Department of Pathology, University of North Carolina, Chapel Hill, NC, USA.)

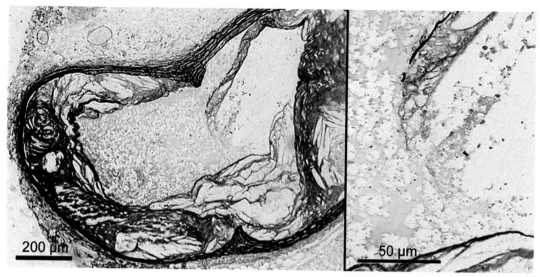

Figure 9.2 ApoE1 knockout mice model of atherosclerosis. Histologic section obtained from a female ApoE knockout mouse that died suddenly after receiving a high-cholesterol diet for 1 year (elastin–van Gieson stain). Left panel (4×), origin of the brachiocephalic artery at the level of the aortic origin with rupture of a thinned fibrous cap and a thrombus filling the lumen of the vessel. Right panel, magnified view of the plaque showing that the thrombus has penetrated a highly lipidic region below the fibrous cap. (Original picture courtesy of Drs Chris Jackson and Helen Williams, Bristol Heart Institute, Bristol, UK.)

are placed on a Western-type diet (21% fat, 0.15% cholesterol), they reach cholesterol levels greater than 1500 mg/dl and develop widely distributed complex atherosclerotic lesions similar to those seen in the ApoE knockout model.[60,65] Other models less well-characterized are the LDLR⁻/ApoB⁻ mice,[66] the ApoB100/LDLR⁻ transgenic mice[67] and the Dahl salt-sensitive hypertensive rats transgenic for human cholesteryl ester transfer protein.[68]

The ApoE knockout model of atherosclerosis has contributed to the understanding of critical pathophysiologic mechanisms associated with plaque vulnerability and rupture. Using this model, several investigators described the cellular and molecular events occurring during the process of vascular remodeling[69,70] and the contribution of transforming growth factor-β (TGF-β),[71] vascular endothelial growth factor (VEGF),[72] P-selectin,[72,73] and interleukin-6 (IL-6)[72,74] on atherosclerosis plaque progression and destabilization. ApoE(−/−)/LDL(−/−)

double knockout mice develop significant vasa vasorum during the process of atherosclerosis plaque progression, permitting the study of this phenomenon and its contribution to plaque progression.[75,76] Important lessons have been learned from mice models in regards to plaque rupture. The role of plaque overexpression of interleukins IL-8, and IL-18 and matrix metalloproteinase-9 (MMP-9) on collagen loss, intraplaque hemorrhage, and plaque rupture has been widely described[77–79] and advanced the field of vulnerable plaque detection through the use of molecular imaging.[18,80,81]

A principal limitation of murine models results from significant differences in lipid metabolism. Mice do not develop atherosclerosis without genetic manipulation,[82,83] therefore making difficult the extrapolation of data from a genetically manipulated model that aims to study a complex genetically acquired disease.[84] Another challenge relates to differences in anatomic size and composition of the mouse vascular system. The vessel wall of the mouse consists of endothelial cells lying directly on the internal elastic lamina and a thin layer of SMCs. Therefore, the pathologic results seen in genetically manipulated mice may not reflect either the pathologic vascular changes seen during complex atherosclerotic lesion progression or the biologic events leading to thrombosis-triggering in humans. In addition, the size of the animals complicates this model for validating endovascular imaging devices and therapies. In summary, murine models of complex atherosclerosis are particularly cost-effective in the study of specific molecular mechanisms of atherosclerotic vascular disease and in the early stage of development of non-invasive imaging techniques.

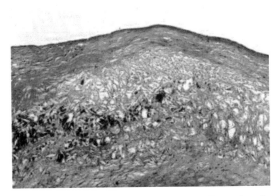

Figure 9.3 New Zealand rabbit model of atherosclerosis. Histologic section (4×) of a typical atherosclerotic lesion seen in the aorta of a 4-year-old New Zealand hypercholesterolemic rabbit. The lesions induced at 4 years show similar features to human TCFA, with an eccentric lumen, fibrous cap, necrotic core, and calcification. (Original picture courtesy of Dr Pedro R Moreno, Mount Sinai School of Medicine, New York, USA.)

Rabbit models

While the rabbit differs considerably from humans in its metabolism, nourishment, and arterial wall responses to an atherogenic diet, the New Zealand rabbit is the most commonly used animal species in interventional cardiology research today. This is because complex atherosclerotic lesions can be induced if the animals are maintained for at least 8 months on a high-cholesterol diet (>0.15%).[85–88] The lesions occur mostly on the dorsal aspect of the aorta and are composed of lipid-rich necrotic cores filled with cellular debris and cholesterol clefts covered by a well-developed fibrous cap consisting of SMCs, extracellular matrix, and focal foam-cell infiltrates.[87] Moreno and co-workers showed that in 4-year-old New Zealand rabbits these atherosclerotic lesions display complex features of atherosclerosis such as necrosis, intraplaque hemorrhage, calcification, and cholesterol crystallization[4] (Figure 9.3). A major drawback of the New Zealand rabbit is the location of the disease, selective in the aorta and not the coronary arteries. In the cases where the epicardial vessels are involved, these lesions are more fibrotic and less complex than the plaques seen in the aorta.[87] Rekhter et al created a rabbit model to study characteristics of atherosclerotic plaque mechanics. In this model, plaque rupture was created by introducing a balloon catheter system into the vessel wall of a previously injured aorta and progressively inflating the balloon to induce plaque rupture. This model, though suitable for measuring the mechanical properties of different atherosclerotic lesions, provides no insight into biologic aspects of plaque vulnerability.[89] A recent study by Pakala et al proposed ionizing radiation to accelerate and induce complex atherosclerotic lesions in hypercholesterolemic rabbits.[90] In this study, New Zealand White rabbits were placed on a 1% hypercholesterolemic diet for 7 days, followed by balloon denudation (7 days) and radiation (4 weeks with 192-Ir, 15 Gy) of both iliac arteries. At 8 weeks, the radiated lesions were significantly larger and contained more macrophages, MMP-1 expression, and fewer SMCs than non-radiated arteries.[90] Other variations of the rabbit model have been used to study the pathogenesis of vascular thrombosis by injecting several pharmacologic agents in hypercholesterolemic rabbits.[91–93]

The Watanabe heritable hyperlipidemic rabbit (WHHL rabbit) is a strain with an inherited hyperlipidemic trait discovered in 1980.[94] These rabbits show abnormally increased serum levels of cholesterol and triglycerides (>600 mg/dl) and develop complex atherosclerotic lesions over 6 months of age[95–97] (Figure 9.4). Shiomi et al developed a rabbit strain exhibiting spontaneous myocardial infarction by selectively breeding coronary atherosclerosis-prone WHHL rabbits.[98] Almost all such rabbits developed significant coronary atherosclerotic lesions and started to die suddenly by the 11th month of follow-up. The typical plaques were frequently found in large vascular branches and were associated with calcification, intraplaque hemorrhage, a thinned fibrous cap, macrophages, lipid cores, and calcium deposits (Figure 9.5). Despite the widespread presence of these atherosclerotic lesions, the authors could not detect plaque rupture or thrombus formation to explain the premature rabbit's death.[98]

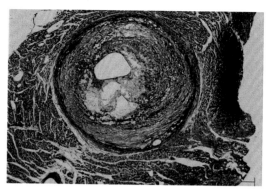

Figure 9.5 Watanabe heritable hypercholesterolemic rabbit (WHHL rabbit) model of atherosclerosis with plaque rupture. Photomicrograph of a plaque observed in the left circumflex artery of a 24-month WHHLMI rabbit (WHHL rabbit with myocardial infarction) that died suddenly. The area of ischemic myocardial lesion was 30% in the left ventricular wall. The cellular components of the plaque are decreased, but collagen fibers, extracellular lipid accumulation, and cholesterol cleft are increased. (Original picture courtesy of Dr Masashi Shiomi, Kobe University School of Medicine, Kobe, Japan.)

Rabbit models of complex atherosclerosis are used most commonly today in interventional vascular research because they are relatively inexpensive, yet easy to maintain and reproduce. One major advantage of these rabbits is the easy access to major vascular territories affected by disease such as the abdominal aorta and iliacs. These vascular segments are specifically attractive for imaging and catheter-based therapy validation studies.[99,100] Also, because of the widespread distribution of disease and adequate size of the animal, this model has been widely utilized for imaging validation studies such as computed tomography (CT) or magnetic resonance imaging (MRI) technologies.[101] A major limitation of the rabbit model is that it develops atherosclerotic lesions (xanthomatous macrophage-rich plaques) that are histopathologically different from complex human atherosclerotic disease. Also, because of the preferential peripheral location of the lesions and vascular size, this model may be of limited use to validate technologies

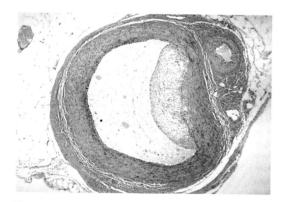

Figure 9.4 Watanabe heritable hypercholesterolemic rabbit (WHHL rabbit) model of atherosclerosis. H&E section (4×) of a typical atherosclerotic lesion seen in the aorta of a WHHL rabbit. These lesions are described as eccentric, xanthomatous, and macrophage-rich atherosclerotic plaques. (Original picture courtesy of Dr Deborah Vela, Texas Heart Institute, Houston, TX, USA.)

designed to target the coronary vasculature. However, rabbit models of atherosclerosis remain the most cost-effective for preliminary evaluation of imaging and therapeutic technologies in interventional cardiology.

Porcine models

The pig is one of the most useful animal atherosclerosis models because of its close anatomic and biologic resemblance to the human coronary vasculature. If maintained on a regular chow diet for a prolonged time, pigs develop generalized atherosclerosis resembling early-stage human disease.[102–104] Marked intraplaque cellular proliferation, cellular necrosis, cholesterol crystal deposition, and calcification have been reported among pigs maintained on a high-cholesterol diet for more than 1 year.[102–104] The Yucatan pig is quite sensitive to these dietary manipulations and may be especially useful in long-term experiments, since the animal maintains a relatively constant size over time.[102–104] A different strain of pigs bearing three immunogenetically defined lipoprotein-associated allotypes develop hypercholesterolemia (>240 mg/dl) even if maintained on a low-fat, cholesterol-free diet.[105–107] Unlike genetically manipulated animal models or the WHHL rabbit, the affected pigs have a normal LDL receptor activity. By 2 years, these animals develop eccentric lesions that consist predominantly of macrophage-derived foam cells with admixed SMCs. By the third year, large areas of necrosis, fibrous cap formation, mononuclear cell infiltration and intraplaque hemorrhage are commonly seen in these lesions (Figure 9.6).[105–107] A more elaborate model of porcine atherosclerosis has been developed by the induction of chemical diabetes in normal pigs by intravenously injecting streptozocin, resulting in a >80% reduction in pancreatic β cells.[108–110] In this model, accelerated

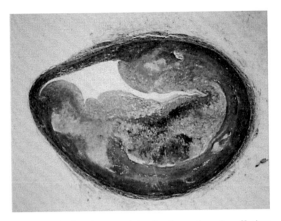

Figure 9.6 Porcine model of atherosclerosis-suffering inherited LDL (low-density lipoprotein) hypercholesterolemia. Histologic section (Masson trichrome-elastin stain) of a coronary artery of a 29-month-old female pig with inherited LDL hypercholesterolemia. This lesion shows a mature fibrous cap, central necrosis, intraplaque hemorrhage, and calcification. (Original picture courtesy of Dr Erlin Falk, Skejby University Hospital, Aarhus, Denmark.)

atherosclerotic lesions develop in the first 2–3 cm of the proximal arteries as early as 20 weeks after the induction of diabetes. When fed a high-cholesterol diet, the diabetic hypercholesterolemic pigs develop lesions with acellular necrotic cores covered by fibrous caps with medial thinning, hemorrhage, and calcification (Figure 9.7).[108–110]

The principal limitations of porcine atherosclerosis models are related to development and maintenance costs. Multiple attempts have been made to accelerate the atherosclerotic process by inducing vascular injury [111] using external radiation,[112] wire-induced endothelial denudation,[113] or barotrauma.[102] Using this combined approach, complex vascular lesions composed of SMCs and extracellular matrix are seen as early as 8 weeks.[102] In 2001, Keelan and Schwartz introduced the concept of 'accelerating' the process of atherosclerosis formation by combining balloon injury (Infiltrator catheter, Boston Scientific, Minneapolis, MN, USA) and

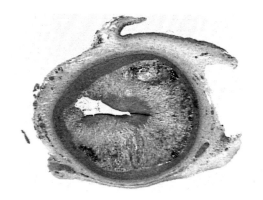

Figure 9.7 Porcine model of diabetes and hypercholesterolemia. Characteristic appearance of a lesion developed by a diabetic pig with induced hypercholesterolemia at 20 weeks of age (H&E stain). The lesion was harvested from the proximal segment of the left anterior coronary artery. The plaque shows humanoid features of eccentric lumen, fibrous cap, necrotic core, and calcification. (Original picture courtesy of Dr Ross Gerrity, Department of Pathology, Medical College of Georgia, Augusta, GA, USA.)

the triggering of inflammation by directly injecting large amount of lipids into the vessel wall of hypercholesterolemic pigs.[114] The lesions produced with this model are significant in size and contain a large amount of lipids, inflammation, and SMCs. However, due to the barotrauma associated with the delivery device, the potential to produce a disproportionate component of neointimal hyperplasia remains significant.[115–117] Granada et al have recently published the preliminary experience with the local delivery of human oxidized LDL (oxLDL) and cholesterol esters into the adventitia of hypercholesterolemic pigs using an endovascular needle injection catheter.[118] Longitudinal follow-up using intravascular ultrasound (IVUS) has shown that lesions are identifiable within 4 weeks of lipid delivery. The histopathologic progression of these lesions has been documented in a prospective fashion. At 4 weeks, microscopic sections of these plaques are similar to human fatty streaks, with a high lipidic content and few intraplaque macrophages

(type 2). By 7 weeks, these plaques are more prominent in size and contain scattered extracellular lipid droplets and particles that disrupt the coherence of SMC (type 3). By 10 weeks, these plaques are seen as eccentric and constitute less than half the vessel circumference. Oil Red O staining shows lipid clefts mainly in the neointima of the vessel. Also, these plaques are significant in size (percent, mean plaque area = $58.9 \pm 14\%$), lipidic (percent mean lipidic area = $12.9 \pm 5.5\%$), and contain abundant neovessels (mean number per plaque = 33 ± 12) and macrophages (mean number per plaque = 322 ± 134).[119] At 10 weeks, these lesions are still immature with no evidence of necrotic core formation, intraplaque hemorrhage, or calcium deposits (Figure 9.8). A very important feature seen in the lesions induced in this model is the ability to consistently reproduce these lesions. In general, all the lesions had a similar morphologic appearance, size, and length, regardless of anatomic location (Figure 9.9). Recently, a novel model has been developed by attaching a segment of a cadaveric human coronary artery from the aorta to the right atrium in normal pigs.[120] Using this model, in-vivo imaging of human plaques using IVUS has been performed, demonstrating expansion of arterial and luminal dimensions during the cardiac cycle (Figure 9.10).

Porcine models have the great advantage of providing anatomic and histopathologic vascular lesions similar to human tissue in both size and composition. The limitations in porcine model development are logistics involved in developing the models, the infrastructure for animal maintenance, the long follow-up period needed to induce the lesions, and development costs. Further development involving innovative ways to accelerate the process of atherosclerosis in already-diseased pigs will probably emerge as the most important animal models for the preclinical validation of technologies in vulnerable plaque research.

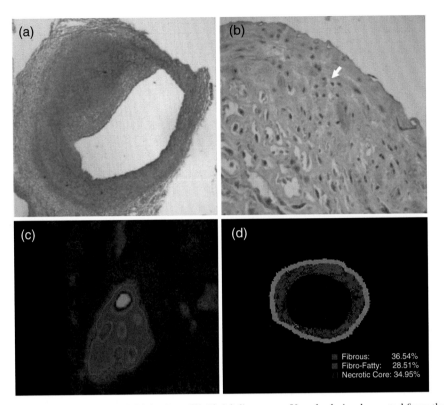

Figure 9.8   Porcine model of adventitial injection of lipid-rich liposomes. Vascular lesion harvested from the proximal left anterior descending artery 10 weeks following adventitial liposome delivery. (a) H&E stain of the lesion at 4×; (b) 40× magnification showing macrophage infiltration (arrow); (c) In vivo imaging of 3 separate lesions (left anterior descending artery and right coronary artery) using PET imaging; (d) In vivo plaque characterization using IVUS-based on gray level median of echogenicity. (Original picture courtesy of Dr Juan F Granada, The Methodist DeBakey Heart Center and The Methodist Research Institute, Houston, TX, USA.)

CONCLUSIONS

Predicting future cardiovascular events by accurately detecting and characterizing complex atherosclerotic lesions has become a dynamic research niche in interventional cardiology. Innovative imaging detection and therapeutic technologies will ultimately depend on successful animal models that permit preclinical validation of the technology in a controlled environment. Small animal models, particularly genetically manipulated mice, are important for the testing of mechanistic hypotheses that permit advancing our understanding of plaque vulnerability. Larger animals, such as rabbits, are cost-effective for validating non-invasive imaging modalities and preliminary experiences with endovascular therapies. Porcine models, while more expensive and difficult to produce, are already available for the validation of imaging technologies. Because of uncertainty regarding the definition and natural history of the disease, the use of these models for validation of therapeutic interventions is unknown. Regardless, animal models of complex atherosclerosis will become perhaps the most critical part of the preclinical validation phases of diagnostic and therapeutic emerging technology in the vulnerable plaque field.

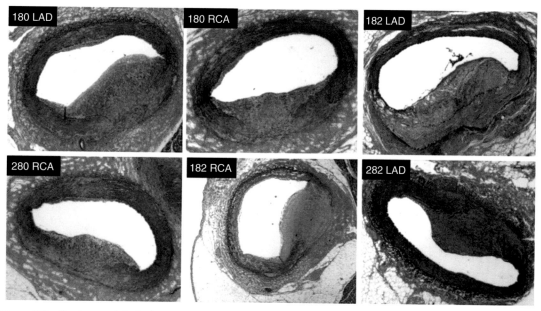

Figure 9.9 Porcine model of adventitial injection of lipid-rich liposomes. Six representative examples of lesions harvested from pigs 10 weeks after the adventitial injection of cholesterol esters and human oxidized LDL (Movat Pentachrome stain, magnification 2×). Lesions are described as eccentric, and contain lipids, macrophages, and neovessels. RCA, right coronary artery; LAD, left anterior descending coronary artery. (Original picture courtesy of Dr Juan F Granada, The Methodist DeBakey Heart Center and The Methodist Research Institute, Houston, TX, USA.)

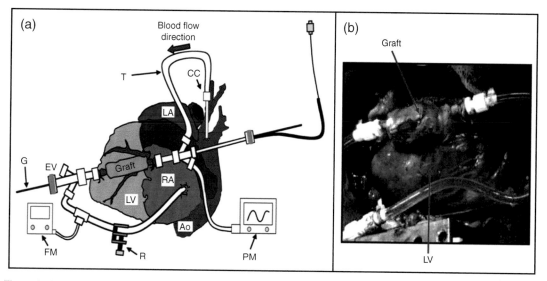

Figure 9.10 Schematic representation of the xenograft model (a) and photograph of implanted graft in the pig (b). The aorta and right atrium are cannulated and connected end-to-end with the human coronary xenograft, forming an aorto–atrial conduit. The graft is sutured to the anterior wall of the heart. A 'Y' connector with a valve and sideport are attached proximal to the graft to measure pressure, inject contrast and saline, and introduce an imaging catheter. A flow meter (FM) is connected distal to the graft. The direction of flow is indicated by the red arrow. Ao, aorta, CC, cardioplegia cannula; EV, endoscope valve; G, guidewire; LA, left atrium; LV, left ventricle; PM, pressure monitor; R, rotating valve; RA, right atrium; T, tubing. (Original picture courtesy of Dr Sergio Waxman, Lahey Clinic, Boston, MA, USA.)

REFERENCES

1. Davies MJ, Fulton WF, Robertson WB. The relation of coronary thrombosis to ischaemic myocardial necrosis. J Pathol 1979; 127:99–110.

2. Davies MJ, Thomas A. Thrombosis and acute coronary-artery lesions in sudden cardiac ischemic death. N Engl J Med 1984; 310:1137–40.

3. Davies MJ. The contribution of thrombosis to the clinical expression of coronary atherosclerosis. Thromb Res 1996; 82:1–32.

4. Fuster V, Moreno PR, Fayad ZA, Corti R, Badimon JJ. Atherothrombosis and high-risk plaque: part I: evolving concepts. J Am Coll Cardiol 2005; 46:937–54.

5. Davies MJ, Thomas AC. Plaque fissuring – the cause of acute myocardial infarction, sudden ischaemic death, and crescendo angina. Br Heart J 1985; 53: 363–73.

6. Falk E. Plaque rupture with severe pre-existing stenosis precipitating coronary thrombosis. Characteristics of coronary atherosclerotic plaques underlying fatal occlusive thrombi. Br Heart J 1983; 50:127–34.

7. Virmani R, Kolodgie FD, Burke AP, Farb A, Schwartz SM. Lessons from sudden coronary death: a comprehensive morphological classification scheme for atherosclerotic lesions. Arterioscler Thromb Vasc Biol 2000; 20:1262–75.

8. Granada JF, Kaluza GL, Raizner AE, Moreno PR. Vulnerable plaque paradigm: prediction of future clinical events based on a morphological definition. Catheter Cardiovasc Interv 2004; 62:364–74.

9. Maseri A, Fuster V. Is there a vulnerable plaque? Circulation 2003; 107:2068–71.

10. Schaar JA, Muller JE, Falk E et al. Terminology for high-risk and vulnerable coronary artery plaques. Report of a meeting on the vulnerable plaque, June 17 and 18, 2003, Santorini, Greece. Eur Heart J 2004; 25:1077–82.

11. Goldstein JA. Multifocal coronary plaque instability. Prog Cardiovasc Dis 2002; 44:449–54.

12. Rioufol G, Finet G, Ginon I et al. Multiple atherosclerotic plaque rupture in acute coronary syndrome: a three-vessel intravascular ultrasound study. Circulation 2002; 106:804–8.

13. Williams H, Johnson JL, Carson KG, Jackson CL. Characteristics of intact and ruptured atherosclerotic plaques in brachiocephalic arteries of apolipoprotein E knockout mice. Arterioscler Thromb Vasc Biol 2002; 22:788–92.

14. Fayad ZA. Noncoronary and coronary atherothrombotic plaque imaging and monitoring of therapy by MRI. Neuroimaging Clin N Am 2002; 12:461–71.

15. Fayad ZA, Fuster V, Nikolaou K, Becker C. Computed tomography and magnetic resonance imaging for noninvasive coronary angiography and plaque imaging: current and potential future concepts. Circulation 2002; 106:2026–34.

16. Nair A, Kuban BD, Obuchowski N, Vince DG. Assessing spectral algorithms to predict atherosclerotic plaque composition with normalized and raw intravascular ultrasound data. Ultrasound Med Biol 2001; 27:1319–31.

17. Nair A, Kuban BD, Tuzcu EM et al. Coronary plaque classification with intravascular ultrasound radiofrequency data analysis. Circulation 2002; 106:2200–6.

18. Jaffer FA, Libby P, Weissleder R. Molecular and cellular imaging of atherosclerosis: emerging applications. J Am Coll Cardiol 2006; 47:1328–38.

19. Sirol M, Fuster V, Toussaint JF, Fayad ZA. Molecular imaging for the diagnosis of high-risk plaque. Arch Mal Coeur Vaiss 2003; 96:1219–24.

20. Burke AP, Farb A, Malcom GT et al. Coronary risk factors and plaque morphology in men with coronary disease who died suddenly. N Engl J Med 1997; 336:1276–82.

21. Virmani R, Burke AP, Farb A. Plaque morphology in sudden coronary death. Cardiologia 1998; 43:267–71.

22. Virmani R, Burke AP, Farb A. Plaque rupture and plaque erosion. Thromb Haemost 1999; 82 (Suppl 1):1–3.

23. Virmani R, Burke AP, Kolodgie FD, Farb A. Vulnerable plaque: the pathology of unstable coronary lesions. J Interv Cardiol 2002; 15:439–46.

24. Glagov S, Weisenberg E, Zarins CK, Stankunavicius R, Kolettis GJ. Compensatory enlargement of human atherosclerotic coronary arteries. N Engl J Med 1987; 316:1371–5.

25. Ward MR, Pasterkamp G, Yeung AC, Borst C. Arterial remodeling. Mechanisms and clinical implications. Circulation 2000; 102:1186–91.

26. Tronc F, Mallat Z, Lehoux S et al. Role of matrix metalloproteinases in blood flow-induced arterial enlargement: interaction with NO. Arterioscler Thromb Vasc Biol 2000; 20:E120–6.

27. Moreno PR, Falk E, Palacios IF et al. Macrophage infiltration in acute coronary syndromes. Implications for plaque rupture. Circulation 1994; 90:775–8.

28. Davies MJ. Stability and instability: two faces of coronary atherosclerosis. The Paul Dudley White Lecture 1995. Circulation 1996; 94:2013–20.

29. Libby P. Atherosclerosis: the new view. Sci Am 2002; 286:46–55.

30. Daugherty A, Rateri DL. T lymphocytes in atherosclerosis: the yin-yang of Th1 and Th2 influence on lesion formation. Circ Res 2002; 90:1039–40.

31. Libby P, Ridker PM, Maseri A. Inflammation and atherosclerosis. Circulation 2002; 105:1135–43.

32. Stary HC. Composition and classification of human atherosclerotic lesions. Virchows Arch A Pathol Anat Histopathol 1992; 421:277–90.

33. Stary HC, Chandler AB, Glagov S et al. A definition of initial, fatty streak, and intermediate lesions of atherosclerosis. A report from the Committee on Vascular Lesions of the Council on Arteriosclerosis, American Heart Association. Arterioscler Thromb 1994; 14:840–56.

34. Stary HC, Chandler AB, Dinsmore RE et al. A definition of advanced types of atherosclerotic lesions and

a histological classification of atherosclerosis. A report from the Committee on Vascular Lesions of the Council on Arteriosclerosis, American Heart Association. Arterioscler Thromb Vasc Biol 1995; 15:1512–31.

35. Moreno PR, Purushothaman KR, Fuster V, O'Connor WN. Intimomedial interface damage and adventitial inflammation is increased beneath disrupted atherosclerosis in the aorta: implications for plaque vulnerability. Circulation 2002; 105:2504–11.

36. Kolodgie FD, Gold HK, Burke AP et al. Intraplaque hemorrhage and progression of coronary atheroma. N Engl J Med 2003; 349:2316–25.

37. Moreno PR, Purushothaman KR, Fuster V et al. Plaque neovascularization is increased in ruptured atherosclerotic lesions of human aorta: implications for plaque vulnerability. Circulation 2004; 110:2032–8.

38. Ware JA. Too many vessels? Not enough? The wrong kind? The VEGF debate continues. Nat Med 2001; 7:403–4.

39. Williams JK, Heistad DD. [The vasa vasorum of the arteries]. J Mal Vasc 1996; 21 (Suppl C):266–9.

40. Burke AP, Farb A, Malcom GT et al. Plaque rupture and sudden death related to exertion in men with coronary artery disease. JAMA 1999; 281:921–6.

41. Mailhac A, Badimon JJ, Fallon JT et al. Effect of an eccentric severe stenosis on fibrin(ogen) deposition on severely damaged vessel wall in arterial thrombosis. Relative contribution of fibrin(ogen) and platelets. Circulation 1994; 90:988–96.

42. Burke AP, Kolodgie FD, Farb A et al. Healed plaque ruptures and sudden coronary death: evidence that subclinical rupture has a role in plaque progression. Circulation 2001; 103:934–40.

43. Farb A, Tang AL, Burke AP et al. Sudden coronary death. Frequency of active coronary lesions, inactive coronary lesions, and myocardial infarction. Circulation 1995; 92:1701–9.

44. Farb A, Burke AP, Tang AL et al. Coronary plaque erosion without rupture into a lipid core. A frequent cause of coronary thrombosis in sudden coronary death. Circulation 1996; 93:1354–63.

45. van der Wal AC, Becker AE, van der Loos CM, Das PK. Site of intimal rupture or erosion of thrombosed coronary atherosclerotic plaques is characterized by an inflammatory process irrespective of the dominant plaque morphology. Circulation 1994; 89:36–44.

46. van der Wal AC, Becker AE, Koch KT et al. Clinically stable angina pectoris is not necessarily associated with histologically stable atherosclerotic plaques. Heart 1996; 76:312–16.

47. Badimon JJ, Lettino M, Toschi V et al. Local inhibition of tissue factor reduces the thrombogenicity of disrupted human atherosclerotic plaques: effects of tissue factor pathway inhibitor on plaque thrombogenicity under flow conditions. Circulation 1999; 99:1780–7.

48. Badimon L, Badimon JJ, Turitto VT, Vallabhajosula S, Fuster V. Platelet thrombus formation on collagen type I. A model of deep vessel injury. Influence of blood rheology, von Willebrand factor, and blood coagulation. Circulation 1988; 78:1431–42.

49. Toschi V, Gallo R, Lettino M et al. Tissue factor modulates the thrombogenicity of human atherosclerotic plaques. Circulation 1997; 95:594–9.

50. Rekhter MD. How to evaluate plaque vulnerability in animal models of atherosclerosis? Cardiovasc Res 2002; 54:36–41.

51. Lowe HC, Jang IK, Khachigian LM. Animal models of vulnerable plaque. Clinical context and current status. Thromb Haemost 2003; 90:774–80.

52. Fuster V, Ip JH, Badimon L et al. Importance of experimental models for the development of clinical trials on thromboatherosclerosis. Circulation 1991; 83:IV15–25.

53. Badimon L. Atherosclerosis and thrombosis: lessons from animal models. Thromb Haemost 2001; 86:356–65.

54. Cullen P, Baetta R, Bellosta S et al. Rupture of the atherosclerotic plaque: does a good animal model exist? Arterioscler Thromb Vasc Biol 2003; 23:535–42.

55. Lichtman AH, Clinton SK, Iiyama K et al. Hyperlipidemia and atherosclerotic lesion development in LDL receptor-deficient mice fed defined semipurified diets with and without cholate. Arterioscler Thromb Vasc Biol 1999; 19:1938–44.

56. Moore RE, Kawashiri MA, Kitajima K et al. Apolipoprotein A-I deficiency results in markedly increased atherosclerosis in mice lacking the LDL receptor. Arterioscler Thromb Vasc Biol 2003; 23:1914–20.

57. Nakashima Y, Plump AS, Raines EW, Breslow JL, Ross R. ApoE-deficient mice develop lesions of all phases of atherosclerosis throughout the arterial tree. Arterioscler Thromb 1994; 14:133–40.

58. Piedrahita JA, Zhang SH, Hagaman JR, Oliver PM, Maeda N. Generation of mice carrying a mutant apolipoprotein E gene inactivated by gene targeting in embryonic stem cells. Proc Natl Acad Sci USA 1992; 89:4471–5.

59. Plump AS, Smith JD, Hayek T et al. Severe hypercholesterolemia and atherosclerosis in apolipoprotein E-deficient mice created by homologous recombination in ES cells. Cell 1992; 71:343–53.

60. Reardon CA, Blachowicz L, Lukens J, Nissenbaum M, Getz GS. Genetic background selectively influences innominate artery atherosclerosis: immune system deficiency as a probe. Arterioscler Thromb Vasc Biol 2003; 23:1449–54.

61. Zhang SH, Reddick RL, Piedrahita JA, Maeda N. Spontaneous hypercholesterolemia and arterial lesions in mice lacking apolipoprotein E. Science 1992; 258:468–71.

62. Reddick RL, Zhang SH, Maeda N. Aortic atherosclerotic plaque injury in apolipoprotein E deficient mice. Atherosclerosis 1998; 140:297–305.

63. Rosenfeld ME, Polinsky P, Virmani R et al. Advanced atherosclerotic lesions in the innominate artery of

the ApoE knockout mouse. Arterioscler Thromb Vasc Biol 2000; 20:2587–92.

64. Johnson JL, Jackson CL. Atherosclerotic plaque rupture in the apolipoprotein E knockout mouse. Atherosclerosis 2001; 154:399–406.

65. Ishibashi S, Goldstein JL, Brown MS, Herz J, Burns DK. Massive xanthomatosis and atherosclerosis in cholesterol-fed low density lipoprotein receptor-negative mice. J Clin Invest 1994; 93:1885–93.

66. Powell-Braxton L, Veniant M, Latvala RD et al. A mouse model of human familial hypercholesterolemia: markedly elevated low density lipoprotein cholesterol levels and severe atherosclerosis on a low-fat chow diet. Nat Med 1998; 4:934–8.

67. Sanan DA, Newland DL, Tao R et al. Low density lipoprotein receptor-negative mice expressing human apolipoprotein B-100 develop complex atherosclerotic lesions on a chow diet: no accentuation by apolipoprotein(a). Proc Natl Acad Sci USA 1998; 95:4544–9.

68. Herrera VL, Makrides SC, Xie HX et al. Spontaneous combined hyperlipidemia, coronary heart disease and decreased survival in Dahl salt-sensitive hypertensive rats transgenic for human cholesteryl ester transfer protein. Nat Med 1999; 5:1383–9.

69. Hollestelle SC, De Vries MR, Van Keulen JK et al. Toll-like receptor 4 is involved in outward arterial remodeling. Circulation 2004; 109:393–8.

70. Ivan E, Khatri JJ, Johnson C et al. Expansive arterial remodeling is associated with increased neointimal macrophage foam cell content: the murine model of macrophage-rich carotid artery lesions. Circulation 2002; 105:2686–91.

71. Lutgens E, Gijbels M, Smook M et al. Transforming growth factor-beta mediates balance between inflammation and fibrosis during plaque progression. Arterioscler Thromb Vasc Biol 2002; 22:975–82.

72. Celletti FL, Waugh JM, Amabile PG et al. Vascular endothelial growth factor enhances atherosclerotic plaque progression. Nat Med 2001; 7:425–9.

73. Dong ZM, Brown AA, Wagner DD. Prominent role of P-selectin in the development of advanced atherosclerosis in ApoE-deficient mice. Circulation 2000; 101:2290–5.

74. Schieffer B, Selle T, Hilfiker A et al. Impact of interleukin-6 on plaque development and morphology in experimental atherosclerosis. Circulation 2004; 110:3493–500.

75. Langheinrich AC, Michniewicz A, Sedding DG et al. Correlation of vasa vasorum neovascularization and plaque progression in aortas of apolipoprotein E(–/–)/low-density lipoprotein(–/–) double knockout mice. Arterioscler Thromb Vasc Biol 2006; 26:347–52.

76. Moulton KS, Vakili K, Zurakowski D et al. Inhibition of plaque neovascularization reduces macrophage accumulation and progression of advanced atherosclerosis. Proc Natl Acad Sci USA 2003; 100:4736–41.

77. de Nooijer R, von der Thusen JH, Verkleij CJ et al. Overexpression of IL-18 decreases intimal collagen content and promotes a vulnerable plaque phenotype in apolipoprotein-E-deficient mice. Arterioscler Thromb Vasc Biol 2004; 24:2313–19.

78. de Nooijer R, Verkleij CJ, von der Thusen JH et al. Lesional overexpression of matrix metalloproteinase-9 promotes intraplaque hemorrhage in advanced lesions but not at earlier stages of atherogenesis. Arterioscler Thromb Vasc Biol 2006; 26:340–6.

79. Gough PJ, Gomez IG, Wille PT, Raines EW. Macrophage expression of active MMP-9 induces acute plaque disruption in apoE-deficient mice. J Clin Invest 2006; 116:59–69.

80. Schneider JE, McAteer MA, Tyler DJ et al. High-resolution, multicontrast three-dimensional-MRI characterizes atherosclerotic plaque composition in ApoE–/– mice ex vivo. J Magn Reson Imaging 2004; 20:981–9.

81. Trogan E, Fayad ZA, Itskovich VV et al. Serial studies of mouse atherosclerosis by in vivo magnetic resonance imaging detect lesion regression after correction of dyslipidemia. Arterioscler Thromb Vasc Biol 2004; 24:1714–19.

82. Ishida BY, Blanche PJ, Nichols AV, Yashar M, Paigen B. Effects of atherogenic diet consumption on lipoproteins in mouse strains C57BL/6 and C3H. J Lipid Res 1991; 32:559–68.

83. Nishina PM, Verstuyft J, Paigen B. Synthetic low and high fat diets for the study of atherosclerosis in the mouse. J Lipid Res 1990; 31:859–69.

84. Sigmund CD. Viewpoint: are studies in genetically altered mice out of control? Arterioscler Thromb Vasc Biol 2000; 20:1425–9.

85. Clarkson TB. Atherosclerosis – Spontaneous and induced. Adv Lipid Res 1963; 64:211–52.

86. Hunt CE, Duncan LA. Hyperlipoproteinaemia and atherosclerosis in rabbits fed low-level cholesterol and lecithin. Br J Exp Pathol 1985; 66:35–46.

87. Kolodgie FD, Katocs AS Jr, Largis EE et al. Hypercholesterolemia in the rabbit induced by feeding graded amounts of low-level cholesterol. Methodological considerations regarding individual variability in response to dietary cholesterol and development of lesion type. Arterioscler Thromb Vasc Biol 1996; 16:1454–64.

88. Wissler RW, Eilert ML, Schroeder MA, Cohen L. Production of lipomatous and atheromatous arterial lesions in the albino rat. AMA Arch Pathol 1954; 57:333–51.

89. Rekhter MD, Hicks GW, Brammer DW et al. Animal model that mimics atherosclerotic plaque rupture. Circ Res 1998; 83:705–13.

90. Pakala R, Leborgne L, Cheneau E et al. Radiation-induced atherosclerotic plaque progression in a hypercholesterolemic rabbit: a prospective vulnerable plaque model? Cardiovasc Radiat Med 2003; 4:146–51.

91. Abela GS, Picon PD, Friedl SE et al. Triggering of plaque disruption and arterial thrombosis in an atherosclerotic rabbit model. Circulation 1995; 91:776–84.

92. Constantinides P, Booth J, Carlson G. Production of advanced cholesterol atherosclerosis in the rabbit. Arch Pathol 1960; 70:712–24.

93. Constantinides P, Chakravarti RN. Rabbit arterial thrombosis production by systemic procedures. Arch Pathol 1961; 72:197–208.

94. Watanabe Y. Serial inbreeding of rabbits with hereditary hyperlipidemia (WHHL-rabbit). Atherosclerosis 1980; 36:261–8.

95. Buja LM, Kita T, Goldstein JL, Watanabe Y, Brown MS. Cellular pathology of progressive atherosclerosis in the WHHL rabbit. An animal model of familial hypercholesterolemia. Arteriosclerosis 1983; 3:87–101.

96. Shiomi M, Ito T, Watanabe Y. Hypercholesterolemia and atherosclerosis in the WHHL rabbit, an animal model of familial hypercholesterolemia. Prog Clin Biol Res 1987; 229:35–40.

97. Watanabe Y, Ito T, Shiomi M. The effect of selective breeding on the development of coronary atherosclerosis in WHHL rabbits. An animal model for familial hypercholesterolemia. Atherosclerosis 1985; 56:71–9.

98. Shiomi M, Ito T, Yamada S, Kawashima S, Fan J. Development of an animal model for spontaneous myocardial infarction (WHHLMI rabbit). Arterioscler Thromb Vasc Biol 2003; 23:1239–44.

99. Verheye S, De Meyer GR, Van Langenhove G, Knaapen MW, Kockx MM. In vivo temperature heterogeneity of atherosclerotic plaques is determined by plaque composition. Circulation 2002; 105: 1596–601.

100. Zimmermann-Paul GG, Quick HH, Vogt P et al. High-resolution intravascular magnetic resonance imaging: monitoring of plaque formation in heritable hyperlipidemic rabbits. Circulation 1999; 99:1054–61.

101. Viles-Gonzalez JF, Poon M, Sanz J et al. In vivo 16-slice, multidetector-row computed tomography for the assessment of experimental atherosclerosis: comparison with magnetic resonance imaging and histopathology. Circulation 2004; 110:1467–72.

102. Gal D, Rongione AJ, Slovenkai GA et al. Atherosclerotic Yucatan microswine: an animal model with high-grade, fibrocalcific, nonfatty lesions suitable for testing catheter-based interventions. Am Heart J 1990; 119:291–300.

103. Reitman JS, Mahley RW, Fry DL. Yucatan miniature swine as a model for diet-induced atherosclerosis. Atherosclerosis 1982; 43:119–32.

104. Thorpe PE, Hunter WJ III, Zhan XX, Dovgan PS, Agrawal DK. A noninjury, diet-induced swine model of atherosclerosis for cardiovascular-interventional research. Angiology 1996; 47:849–57.

105. Prescott MF, McBride CH, Hasler-Rapacz J, Von LJ, Rapacz J. Development of complex atherosclerotic lesions in pigs with inherited hyper-LDL cholesterolemia bearing mutant alleles for apolipoprotein B. Am J Pathol 1991; 139:139–47.

106. Prescott MF, Hasler-Rapacz J, Von Linden-Reed J, Rapacz J. Familial hypercholesterolemia associated with coronary atherosclerosis in swine bearing different alleles for apolipoprotein B. Ann NY Acad Sci 1995; 748:283–92.

107. Rapacz J, Hasler-Rapacz J, Taylor KM, Checovich WJ, Attie AD. Lipoprotein mutations in pigs are associated with elevated plasma cholesterol and atherosclerosis. Science 1986; 234:1573–7.

108. Feldman DL, Hoff HF, Gerrity RG. Immunohistochemical localization of apoprotein B in aortas from hyperlipemic swine. Preferential accumulation in lesion-prone areas. Arch Pathol Lab Med 1984; 108:817–22.

109. Gerrity RG, Naito HK, Richardson M, Schwartz CJ. Dietary induced atherogenesis in swine. Morphology of the intima in prelesion stages. Am J Pathol 1979; 95:775–92.

110. Gerrity RG, Natarajan R, Nadler JL, Kimsey T. Diabetes-induced accelerated atherosclerosis in swine. Diabetes 2001; 50:1654–65.

111. Steele PM, Chesebro JH, Stanson AW et al. Balloon angioplasty. Natural history of the pathophysiological response to injury in a pig model. Circ Res 1985; 57:105–12.

112. Lee KT, Jarmolych J, Kim DN et al. Production of advanced coronary atherosclerosis, myocardial infarction and "sudden death" in swine. Exp Mol Pathol 1971; 15:170–90.

113. Mihaylov D, van Luyn MJ, Rakhorst G. Development of an animal model of selective coronary atherosclerosis. Coron Artery Dis 2000; 11:145–9.

114. Keelan P. A novel porcine model for in vivo detection of vulnerable plaque: deposition and localization of lipid-rich lesions in the coronary arterial wall. Circulation 2001; 104:67.

115. Schwartz RS, Murphy JG, Edwards WD et al. Restenosis after balloon angioplasty. A practical proliferative model in porcine coronary arteries. Circulation 1990; 82:2190–200.

116. Schwartz RS, Holmes DR Jr, Topol EJ. The restenosis paradigm revisited: an alternative proposal for cellular mechanisms. J Am Coll Cardiol 1992; 20:1284–93.

117. Schwartz RS, Huber KC, Murphy JG et al. Restenosis and the proportional neointimal response to coronary artery injury: results in a porcine model. J Am Coll Cardiol 1992; 19:267–74.

118. Granada JF, Moreno PR, Burke AP et al. Endovascular needle injection of cholesteryl linoleate into the arterial wall produces complex vascular lesions identifiable by intravascular ultrasound: early development in a porcine model of vulnerable plaque. Coron Artery Dis 2005; 16:217–24.

119. Granada JF, Wallace-Bradley D, Alviar CL et al. In vivo plaque characterization using intravascular ultrasound–virtual histology in a porcine model of complex coronary lesions. Arterioscler Thromb Vasc Biol 2007; in press.

120. Waxman S, Khabbaz KR, Connolly RJ et al. An animal model for in vivo imaging of human coronaries: a new tool to evaluate emerging technologies to detect vulnerable plaques. J Am Coll Cardiol 2004; 43:73A.

SECTION II

Biomarkers

Endothelial biomarkers of vulnerable plaque progression

10

Victoria LM Herrera

INTRODUCTION

The real-time monitoring of vulnerable plaque progression and detection of vulnerable plaque destabilization prior to an acute coronary syndrome (ACS) event (myocardial infarction, unstable angina, coronary death) are major goals for cardiovascular research. Endothelial biomarkers of endothelial dysfunctions, along with other biomarkers of key interacting players in ACS, could allow real-time monitoring of vulnerable plaque progression and/or destabilization. While current analytical designs detect significant predictive values supporting the concept of biomarkers of endothelial dysfunction, the potential for real-time monitoring has not been realized. This shortfall is not surprising given the complex pathogenic interactions in ACS, thus elucidating the necessity for a systematic, mechanism-based context analysis of biomarkers.

As an emerging field, clarification of terminology usage is important:

- *Biomarker*: a measurable quantitative or qualitative parameter reflecting a physiologic or pathologic state or change.
- *Endothelial biomarker*: biomarker giving insight into the status of the endothelium specific to one or more of its multiple functions as barrier, crosstalk mediator, regulator of inflammation, hemostasis, vascular tone, and angiogenesis.
- *Endothelial biomarkers of acute coronary syndromes*: biomarkers of endothelial dysfunction; determinants of

vulnerable plaque progression and/or destabilization.
- *Endothelial dysfunction*: represents a pathophysiologic state in which collective homeostatic properties of normal endothelial cells are impaired or lost, thereby promoting a pathologic (atherogenic) milieu.[1]

RATIONALE AND CONCEPTS

The rationale for the development of endothelial biomarkers of ACS is based on:

1. The clinical need for biomarkers that could detect and monitor – in real-time – coronary vulnerable plaque progression and/or imminent vulnerable plaque destabilization in ACS.
2. The likelihood of informativeness of endothelial biomarkers deriving from endothelial turnkey roles in the progression of the vulnerable plaque and vulnerable patient.[1]
3. The inherent potential for real-time monitoring derived from the accessibility of endothelial biomarkers for detection with current and emerging technologies.

Aside from clinical relevance, analysis of endothelial biomarkers will also allow the assessment of the scope and severity of endothelial dysfunctions, thus giving new insight into endothelial dysfunction determinants of vulnerable plaque progression and/or destabilization in ACS.

It should be noted that since ACS is complex and typified by vulnerable/culprit plaque heterogeneity, biomarkers for ACS should comprehensively monitor said complex of multiple cellular and molecular events in vulnerable plaque progression – and, as such, are not limited to endothelial biomarkers. Endothelial biomarkers, representing endothelial dysfunctions in ACS pathogenesis, constitute but one important piece of the puzzle, and while a likely 'master switch' player in ACS, the endothelium should really be evaluated in the context of other key players in ACS (Figure 10.1).

Biomarker design concepts should integrate multiple key issues addressing the complexity of endothelial functions and dysfunctions, as well as the complexity and heterogeneity of ACS.

Knowing normal endothelial functions is critical to deciphering endothelial biomarkers

Because of the multiple functions of the endothelium, no single test provides a comprehensive physiologic assessment of endothelial function.[1] Although difficult, development of biomarkers of endothelial dysfunctions can and should be done, guided by a framework addressing the complexities and dynamic interactions of endothelial functions. Comparative analysis of normal endothelial functions and endothelial dysfunctions associated with ACS reveals a multiparadigm framework with which to develop endothelial biomarkers for vulnerable plaque progression and/or destabilization.

As summarized in Table 10.1, normal endothelial functions require an orchestrated balance and regulation of multiple endothelial products with diametrical functions (pro- and anti-inflammatory, pro- and anticoagulant, etc.). Endothelial dysfunctions therefore, represent the pathophysiologic, disordered loss of said homeostatic equilibrium with dysregulation and imbalance of multiple endothelial products. This multiplayer paradigm of dysregulation and imbalance would be expected to require a panel of biomarkers and context analysis of biomarkers for accurate representation, since analysis of a single endothelial product or pathway

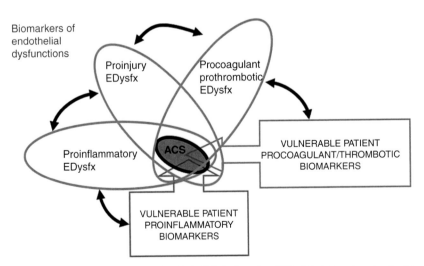

Figure 10.1 Interactions among biomarkers of endothelial dysfunction (EDysfx) determinants of vulnerable plaques and vulnerable patient biomarkers in acute coronary syndromes (ACS).

Table 10.1 Comparative profiles of normal endothelial functions vs endothelial dysfunctions

			Paradigms of normal endothelial functions: Multiplayer paradigms of balance and regulation		
1 Crosstalk for homeostatic equilibrium	*2* Vascular tone regulation	*3* Barrier function	*4* Regulation of inflammation	*5* Regulation of hemostasis	*6* Regulation of angiogenesis and vascular cell growth
• normal panel and levels of receptors, channels, pumps, signal transduction mechanisms • no pathology-associated receptors, e.g. LOX-1	• homeostatic balance of vasodilators and vasoconstrictors • antioxidant capacity >oxidative stress • normal NO production	• surface integrity and continuity • repair ability greater than turnover • tight junctions intact	• non-adhesive endothelium • quiescent but 'on-the-ready' cytokine and chemokine release • homeostatic balance of constitutive anti- and proinflammatory endothelial products	• quiescent but 'on-the-ready' procoagulant, prothrombotic response mechanism • homeostatic balance of platelet inhibitors and activators	• quiescent angiogenesis system • maintenance of circulatory networks • homeostatic balance of cell growth inhibitors and promoters

Continued

Table 10.1 Comparative profiles of normal endothelial functions vs dysendothelial functions—cont'd

	Endothelial dysfunctions in acute coronary syndromes: multiplayer paradigms of imbalance and dysregulation				
_1_	_2_	_3_	_4_	_5_	_6_
Setpoint changes that: enhance proinjury, proinflammatory, and procoagulant dysfunctions	Proconstriction dysfunction: results in loss of NO-dependent vasodilation	Proinjury dysfunction: results in loss of endothelial integrity	Proinflammatory dysfunction: results in plaque inflammation, pro injury, prothrombosis	Procoagulant/prothrombotic dysfunction: facilitates atherothrombotic event	Pathologic angiogenesis: results in leaky PLQ neovessels (vulnerable PLQ) deficient myocardial collateral formation (vulnerable PT)
e.g.	e.g.	e.g.	e.g.	e.g.	e.g.
• increased EC MMP/decreased EC TIMP expression • increased oxidative stress/decreased antioxidant capacity • oxLDL-mediated positive feedback loop upregulation of LOX-1	• vasoconstrictor-to-vasodilator imbalance • antioxidant-to-oxidant imbalance • decreased NO; and NO-mediated vasodilation (first referred to as 'endothelial dysfunction')	• imbalance of turnover & repair resulting in erosion or disruption _increased turnover:_ increased apoptosis, EMPs _decreased repair:_ decreased EC proliferation, altered EC–EPC crosstalk • endothelial leakiness	• endothelial activation: increased adhesion molecules, increased cytokines and chemokines	• imbalance of pro- and anticoagulants • dysregulated pro- and antifibrinolysis • increased platelet adhesion molecules	• altered VEGF/Ang1/Ang2 ratios, resulting in leaky neovessels • intraplaque neovessels • deficient myocardial angiogenesis and collateral formation
Vulnerable PLQ _Vulnerable PT_	– _Vulnerable PT_	_Vulnerable PLQ_ –	_Vulnerable PLQ_ –	_Vulnerable PLQ_ _Vulnerable PT_	_Vulnerable PLQ_ _Vulnerable PT_

_e.g._, representative examples given, not all inclusive; Ang1, angiopoietin-1; Ang2, angiopoietin-2; EC, endothelial cell; EMP, endothelial microparticles; EPC, endothelial progenitor cell; LOX-1, lectin-like oxidized LDL endothelial receptor; MMP, matrix metalloproteinase; NO, nitric oxide; oxLDL, oxidized LDL; PLQ, plaque; PT, patient; TIMP, tissue inhibitor of metalloproteinase; TF, tissue factor; VEGF, vascular endothelial growth factor.

will undoubtedly be incomplete. Context analysis of endothelial biomarkers refers to analysis of biomarker trend and/or threshold as a function of a dynamic, multifunctional, and interactive endothelium factoring in pertinent variables, such as status of diametrical functions, interactive partners, and spectrum of endothelial dysfunctions.

Multifaceted endothelial involvement in vulnerable plaque progression requires biomarker panel

The singleton 'best-marker' concept would most likely not apply to ACS since molecular players and mechanisms underlying endothelial dysfunctions associated with ACS are multifaceted, redundant, and overlapping, as well as interactive and synergistic. Instead, a 'best marker panel' concept would better represent the complex and dynamic endothelial involvement in vulnerable plaque destabilization. Furthermore, since physiologic disturbances associated with endothelial dysfunctions are detected from early atherosclerosis,[1] endothelial biomarkers that distinguish vulnerable plaque destabilization are necessary. The concept of coronary artery disease (CAD) stage-specific endothelial biomarkers is supported by experimental evidence, since transcription profiles distinguish overt CAD (animal model equivalent of ACS) from quiescent and/or attenuated CAD in a transgenic rat model of CAD.[2] This concept of transcription profile changes along progression of CAD and in response to risk factor interaction (e.g. diabetes) is also demonstrated in human CAD,[3] thus confirming differential transcription profile changes as a molecular basis for biomarker differences in different severities of CAD plaque grades. Whereas the number of altered endothelial functions as marked by respective elevated biomarkers could be expected to be proportional to increased risk for vulnerable

plaque progression or imminence of adverse cardiac events, mechanism-based strategies would better facilitate identification of the informative biomarker panel of endothelial dysfunction determinants of acute coronary syndromes.

Factoring in biomarker functional significance facilitates analysis

In order to optimize the value of biomarker-derived information, functional significance should be addressed within the relevant pathogenic framework of the disease in question, in this case vulnerable plaque progression and/or destabilization. For example, if interleukin-18 (IL-18) elevation is detected, greater functional significance could be deduced if biomarkers for its downstream effects are also evaluated. Determination of IL-18 elevation and its downstream effects relevant to ACS pathogenesis should provide greater insight into vulnerable plaque progression status. More specifically, since IL-18 receptors are detected in plaque endothelium[4] and are constitutively expressed in neutrophils,[5] IL-18-mediated changes in endothelial cells and neutrophils present a logical, accessible downstream-effect paradigm for biomarker evaluation of IL-18 functional significance. Among IL-18-mediated effects is the induction of cell death in endothelial cells.[6] Biomarkers for endothelial cell death, such as endothelial microparticles (EMPs) with apoptotic phenotype, could therefore be informative when partnered with IL-18 biomarker analysis. Additionally, since IL-18 is known to prime neutrophil oxidative burst upon activation and induce neutrophil myeloperoxidase release,[7] myeloperoxidase could also be partnered with IL-18 biomarker evaluation. Altogether, detecting increased IL-18, increased neutrophil priming/activation, and increased myeloperoxidase, along with biomarkers of endothelial injury, would constitute a logical panel for evaluation in predicting/ monitoring vulnerable plaque progression and, more critically, risk for plaque destabilization.

Biomarker selection should be based on mechanisms with emphasis on positive feedback loops

While deciphering the complexity of vulnerable plaque progression is a daunting challenge, with multiple cell players involved in a spectrum of diverse and interacting pathways such as oxidative stress, inflammation, apoptosis, matrix degradation, procoagulant/prothrombotic changes, etc., biomarkers based on pathogenic mechanisms constitute a logical strategy of candidate biomarkers to be tested. This selection strategy can be further honed by focusing on positive-feedback loop mechanisms that underlie self-sustaining set-point changes which contribute to vulnerable plaque progression and/or destabilization. Increased expression of endothelial genes with positive-feedback loop regulation has been observed in transcription profiles associated with overt CAD in a transgenic rat model of CAD,[2] thus providing experimental basis for this strategy of endothelial biomarker selection. This strategy is demonstrated in the case of LOX-1, the lectin-like oxidized LDL (low-density lipoprotein) endothelial receptor, which is markedly increased in overt CAD transcription profile compared with age-, gender-, diet-matched quiescent CAD,[2] and has been demonstrated to be induced by its ligand, oxidized LDL, which then allows greater oxLDL (oxidized LDL) uptake, hence oxidative stress, and still greater LOX-1 expression.[8] Increased endothelial LOX-1 expression can be expected to contribute to vulnerable plaque progression/destabilization as LOX-1 induces ACS-associated events such as CD40/ CD40L signaling,[9] endothelial apoptosis,[10] and platelet–endothelium interactions.[11]

Concordantly, soluble LOX-1 is elevated in association with ACS.[12]

Context analysis of multiple biomarkers is ideal, if not necessary

When multiple players are involved, or when key players can play dual and even diametrical roles (proapoptosis vs antiapoptosis in different microenvironments), or when net outcome depends also on the state of interacting partners, it becomes clear that context analysis of biomarkers becomes imperative. Several paradigms of context analysis can be applied to the identification of biomarkers of endothelial dysfunction determinants of ACS.

- Paradigm 1. Cause-and-effect: evaluating biomarker A (e.g. IL-18) and its downstream effects as biomarker B (endothelial cell death),[4] biomarker C (neutrophil activation)[5,7] etc.
- Paradigm 2. Cognate partners or 'reciprocal activation': evaluating biomarkers that coactivate the other (e.g. increased sICAM-1 (soluble intercellular adhesion molecule-1) and CD11b+ activated-monocytes).[13]
- Paradigm 3. Imbalanced ratios: evaluating biomarker A/B ratio with alteration of normal/adaptive relative ratios (e.g. increased VEGF (vascular endothelial growth factor) levels[14] with low EPC (endothelial progenitor cell) counts[15]).
- Paradigm 4. Set-point change: evaluating biomarkers that result in resetting endothelial set points such that subsequent endothelial response and/or interactions are altered, as demonstrated in sepsis.[16]

These paradigms of context analysis could hone the determination of the clinical significance of specific endothelial biomarkers, and may be better able to represent the complex, dynamic pathogenesis of vulnerable plaque progression/ destabilization.

Prioritization strategies should focus on combinatorial interactions and 'master switches'

Although there are multiple mechanisms involved in vulnerable plaque progression, focusing on proinjury, proinflammatory, and prothrombotic mechanisms of endothelial dysfunctions constitutes a logical first-pass prioritization scheme based on their respective key roles in plaque instability, and, more importantly, their synergistic interactions. The interactions among proinflammatory, prothrombotic, and proinjury mechanisms are well characterized,[17–19] such that detection of biomarkers for all three paradigms of endothelial dysfunction could be expected to correlate with risk for plaque instability. Along with detection of other (non-endothelial) vulnerable plaque/patient proinflammatory and prothrombotic biomarkers, detection of this triad of synergistic endothelial dysfunctions could be expected to indicate highest risk for ACS. Support for this biomarker design concept is emerging with the report of ACS-associated significant elevations of endothelial biomarkers of damage/dysfunction, circulating endothelial cells (CECs), and von Willebrand factor (vWF), with circulating procoagulant (tissue factor) and proinflammatory (IL-6) biomarkers.[20]

Furthermore, while knowledge of complex and interactive roles of the endothelium in vulnerable plaque progression is critical, we note that detecting changes in endothelial cells is not enough. Value-added prioritization is necessary and should focus on the detection of endothelial changes that (1) trigger or facilitate overcoming a threshold, or that (2) result in self-sustaining positive-feedback loop phenomena, or that (3) reset endothelial set points such that endothelial responses are altered in a manner that facilitates vulnerable plaque progression, akin to observations in sepsis.[16]

Endothelial biomarkers are not 'stand-alone' tests

Since the endothelium is involved in multiple disease entities that are distinct from and easily distinguished from CAD such as autoimmune diseases, sepsis, and vasculitides, endothelial biomarkers of endothelial dysfunction can also be expected to be elevated in different disease entities other than vulnerable plaque progression. As with all medical diagnoses, even 'perfect' endothelial biomarkers, when identified, are not stand-alone tests. Disease-specific context should be evaluated in combination with biomarkers of endothelial dysfunction. Ideally, high-resolution and/or molecular imaging of coronary plaques can provide specific disease context to real-time evaluation of biomarkers.

CURRENT LIST OF ENDOTHELIAL BIOMARKERS – PROOF OF CONCEPT

Recent clinical studies show that plasma levels of direct and indirect (functional impact) markers of dysfunctional endothelium can have predictive values in patients with acute coronary syndromes (see Table 10.1) – establishing proof of concept that endothelial biomarkers may play a contributory role in risk stratification, and, one day, real-time monitoring of CAD progression and treatment response.

INSIGHTS AND LESSONS FROM CURRENT LIST OF ENDOTHELIAL BIOMARKERS

Feasibility of detectable levels demonstrated

The predictive serum/plasma values reported in Table 10.2 indicate the feasibility of accessible monitoring in the systemic circulation. Whereas current endothelial biomarkers are not indicative of the site of

Table 10.2   Current biomarkers of endothelial dysfunctions in acute coronary syndromes

Marker studies	Mechanism	Observations	Threshold levels
I. Biomarkers of proinflammatory endothelial dysfunction			
sVCAM-1[28] • 91 pts UA or non-Q-wave MI who were sorted for major adverse events	• soluble CAMs reflect surface expression of CAMS • sCAMs might function as competitive inhibitors for membrane-bound CAMs • VCAM fx: rolling and firm adhesion of lymphocytes and monocytes • distribution not specific to ECs	• CRP, sVCAM, sICAM, E-selectin and P-selectin are elevated in UA and NQMI patients • CRP and sVCAM-1 correlated with recurrent UA, non-fatal MI, and cardiovascular death 6 months later, but not E-selectin, P-selectin, or sICAM-1 levels • sVCAM exhibited greater specificity than CRP	90% sensitivity for predicting future events: • CRP >3 mg/L • sVCAM-1 >780 ng/ml
sICAM-1[29] • 241 males <65 years: AMI, UA, non-ischemic chest pain	• ICAM-1 fx: firm adhesion monocytes and pmn • distribution not specific to ECs	• sICAM-1, IL-6, and CRP were elevated at baseline but no correlation with events at 3 months	Not specified
sE-selectin, sP-selectin, sL-selectin[30] • 23 pts UA, 26 pts SA, 15 control	• E-selectin: mediates slow leukocyte rolling and initial pmn adhesion note: EC specific • P-selectin: mediates platelet and fast leukocyte rolling • L-selectin: mediates neutrophil recruitment	• E-, P-, and L-selectins were significantly higher in UA patients compared with SA and controls (P<0.001–0.005)	Not specified
sICAM-1, sVCAM-1, E-selectin[31] • subgroup of 1246 pts with angiographically proven CAD (ACS + elective cath)	See above	• higher levels of sVCAM-1, sICAM-1 and sE-selectin were observed in pts with cardiac deaths (mean 2.7 years follow-up)	Not specified
PECAM-1 (CD31)[32] 20 pts AMI, 16 pts UA, 20 pts SA, 28 controls	• PECAM-1: mediates migration of leukocytes and platelet–endothelium interactions; plays significant role in thrombus formation	• PECAM-1 was higher in AMI and UA than in SA and controls (decreases after 1 week) • sICAM-1 higher in AMI, UA and SA compared with controls but not among the three coronary syndromes • P-selectin not informative in this study	Not specified

PECAM-1[33] • 144 CAD, 150 age- and gender-matched controls		• PECAM-1 is elevated in CAD patients (P = 0.005) and correlated with platelet activation marked by increased sP-selectin	Not specified
sP-selectin, D-dimer[34] • 391 pts with acute chest pain but normal cTNI: 1-year incidence of death/MI	• P-selectin: see above • D-dimer as a marker for ongoing thrombosis formation-resolution on prothrombotic activated endothelium (indirect marker)	• forward stepwise logistic regression model including sICAM-1, sVCAM-1, sP-selectin, d-dimer, fibrinogen, and ECG parameters • d-dimer detected as predictor of death/MI (P = 0.005) • weak trend for sP-selectin (P = 0.06)	d-dimer >580 ng/ml sP-selectin >152 ng/ml
sP-selectin[35] • 23 UA, 20 SA, 13 healthy controls		• higher in UA (87.6 ± 30 ng/ml) than SA (36.2 ± 13.8 ng/ml) and controls (16.7 ± 8.6 ng/ml)	Not specified
IL-6[24] • From 10000 men prospective PRIME study: 158 with MI, 142 with angina, 563 controls	• cytokine released by activated ECs	• only risk factor that remained significantly associated with MI when 3 inflammatory markers (IL-6, CRP, fibrinogen) were included in the same model	Not specified
IL-18[25] • 11 pts UA, 21 pts non-Q-MI; 21 pts Q-wave MI, 9 pts SA, 11 controls	• activation of IL-18 receptor-bearing cells: neutrophils, monocytes, plaque endothelial cells, SMCs, and macrophages • IL-18 induces cell death	• increased in UA and MI compared with SA and controls (P <0.01); correlates with severity of myocardial dysfunction	Not specified
IL-18[36]		• significantly higher in AMI than in UA	Not specified
IL18[37] • 27 ACS with 15 MI, nl CK, 10 controls		• on admission, increased IL-18 in ACS and preceded creatine kinase MB elevation in MI patients	Not specified
MCP-1[38]	• involved in the recruitment of monocytes into vessel wall	• elevated in patients with CAD compared with controls, along with sICAM-1 and sE-selectin	Not specified
PAPP-A[39] • 20 pts UA; 17 pts AMI	• member of metzincin superfamily of metalloproteinases • produced by activated ECs and SMCs in unstable plqs (eroded and ruptured plqs), minimally in stable plqs	• increased in 85% UA pts (ROC P = 0.01) • increased in 94% AMI pts (ROC P = 0.03) CRP increased in 50%; TnI increased in 15% • no correlation with CK-MB • valuable for unstable coronary disease when Tn and CRP are not elevated	>10 mIU/L

Continued

Table 10.2   Current biomarkers of endothelial dysfunctions in acute coronary syndromes—cont'd

Marker studies	Mechanism	Observations	Threshold levels
PAPP-A[40] • 136 ACS patients TnI(–) 6 months follow-up for events		• independent predictor • 4.6-fold higher adjusted risk (P = 0.002) for adverse outcome • CRP >2 mg/L (RR 2.6; P = 0.03)	>2.9 mIU/L
PAPP-A[41] • 547 pts with angiographically validated ACS; 644 pts with acute chest pain in ER		• predictive value almost entirely restricted to low anti-inflammatory IL-10 levels • did not interfere with predictive power of sCD40L • PAPP-1, sCD40L and TnT are all independent predictors of death or MI in ACS	>12.6 mIU/L
II. Biomarkers of prothrombotic endothelial dysfunction			
vWF[24] • 10 000 men prospective PRIME study: 158 with MI, 142 with angina pectoris, 563 controls	• mediates platelet adhesion and plays a role in thrombus formation • levels increase with EC damage	• independent risk factor for 'hard CHD events', i.e. fatal or non-fatal MI, but not angina pectoris (UA, SA) • vWF in highest quartile and f-TFPI in lowest 10th percentile predicted 6.9-fold increased risk for hard CHD events	Not specified
f-TFPI[24] • 10 000 men prospective PRIME study: 158 with MI, 142 with angina pectoris, 563 controls	• main physiologic inhibitor of tissue factor-induced coagulation	• independent risk factor for 'hard CHD events', i.e. fatal or non-fatal MI, but not angina pectoris (UA, SA) • vWF in highest quartile and f-TFPI in lowest 10th percentile predicted 6.9-fold increased risk for hard CHD events	Not specified
Thrombomodulin[24] • 10 000 men prospective PRIME study: 158 with MI, 142 with angina pectoris, 563 controls	• EC surface receptor for thrombin that functions as an anticoagulant by accelerating thrombin-induced activation of protein C; soluble truncated form in plasma with no known function	• not associated with UA, SA, or MI	Not specified

III. Biomarkers of proinjury endothelial dysfunction – loss of integrity

Biomarker / patients	Mechanism	Findings	
EMPs, annexin + EMPs[42] • 27 ACS, 12 SA, 12 controls	• microparticles released from activated or apoptotic endothelial cells released by vesiculation • activates ECs and leukocytes	• EMPs increased in ACS compared with CAD or non-coronary patients • procoagulant EMPs (prothrombinase assay)	Not specified
EMPs[43] • 43 pts undergoing coronary angiography (15 MI, 20 UA, 5 SA, 3 CHF)		• 2.5-fold increase in EMP counts in eccentric type II or multiple irregular lesions than low-risk type I (concentric lesion) ($P<0.05$) • 3-fold higher EMP in lesions with thrombi than lesions without ($P = 0.05$) • mild stenosis (>20% to < 45%) had 5-fold higher EMP than those without stenosis ($P<0.01$)	>2.5-fold increase
CD51+ EMPs[44] • 66 ST-elevation AMI; 10 controls		• Higher in AMI compared with control $P < 0.042$	Not specified
EPCs[45] • 519 pts with angiography-proven CAD	• circulating EPCs provide an endogenous repair mechanism to counteract endothelial injury and/or to replace dysfunctional endothelium • believed to support the integrity of the vascular endothelium	• baseline cd34+/KDR+ EPC levels predict the occurrence of cardiovascular events and cardiac death prior to and by 12 months • EPC counts were not predictive of MI infarction	Not specified
EPCs[15] 120 pts: 43 controls, 44 stable CAD, 33 ACS		• reduced number of CD34+/KDR+ EPCs were associated with higher incidence of cardiovascular events (death, UA, MI, PTCA, CABG, ischemic stroke) in 10 month follow-up • reduced EPCs are an independent predictor of poor prognosis (hazard ratio 3.9, $P<0.05$)	Not specified

Continued

Table 10.2 Current biomarkers of endothelial dysfunctions in acute coronary syndromes—cont'd

Marker studies	Mechanism	Observations	Threshold levels
CECs[46] 60 non-ST-elevation ACS, 40 controls	• shedding of endothelial cells from damaged endothelium occurs in several vascular disorders • could represent endothelial erosion or disruption	• 32/60 had high CEC counts (median 25.5 cells/ml) • CEC count is an early, specific, independent diagnostic marker for non-ST-elevation ACS at H4 and H8 post admission for chest pain, combined use of CEC and troponin was significantly better as a marker of ACS than CEC alone or TNI alone • CEC count did not correlate with sICAM-1, sVCAM-1, sP-selectin, sE-selectin	>>3 cells/ml
MMP-3 or stromelysin[26] 150 significant CAD, 15 cardiac syndrome X, 17 normal	• expressed in endothelial cells, as well as in plaque SMCs and macrophages[47]	• only MMP-3 level was an independent predictor of adverse events in CAD, rather than hsCRP, MMP-2, MMP-9 • hsCRP, MMP-2, -3 and -9 were all elevated in CAD compared to controls and cardiac syndrome X	Not specified
IV. Biomarkers of crosstalk set-point changes facilitating proinflammatory, procoagulation/thrombosis, proinjury dysfunctions			
sLOX-1[12] 521 pts: 80 ACS, 173 symptomatic CAD, 122 significant CAD without ischemia	• endothelial receptor for oxLDL • Also detected on activated platelets	• elevated in ACS from its early stage – early diagnostic marker of ACS • higher in ACS (median 2.91 ng/ml, range 0.5–170 ng/ml) compared with 6 groups: nl coronary (0.5–1.3 ng/ml), controlled CHD (0.5–3.4 ng/ml), ischemic CHD (0.5–14 ng/ml) and chronic illness (0.5–3.3 ng/ml)	>1 ng/ml sLOX-1 can discriminate ACS from non-ACS CAD ($P<0.001$) with 81% and 75% sensitivity and specificity, respectively

V. Biomarkers of dysregulated angiogenesis and/or hypoxia-responsive angiogenesis

PlGF[48]
- 547 pts with angiographically validated ACS; 626 pts with acute chest pain in ER

- ligand for VEGFR1; implicated in pathophysiologic angiogenesis

- increased sPlGF levels indicated increased risk for events at 30 days ($P = 0.001$)
- multivariate analysis: TnT, sCD40L, and PlGF were independent predictors, while elevated hsCRP was not
- patients negative for all 3 were at very low risk

>27 ng/L

VEGF, Ang-1, Ang-2; Tie-2[14]
- 126 pts ACS (82 MI, 44 UA), 40 healthy controls, 40 pts SA

- VEGF, Ang-1, Ang-2, and Tie-2 regulate angiogenesis and may therefore contribute to myocardial collateral formation[14]
- VEGF contributes to intraplaque and vaso vasorum angiogenesis

- plasma Ang-2, Tie-2 and VEGF were increased in ACS, but not Ang-1

Not specified

VI. Biomarkers of dysregulated vascular tone

- assessed by degree of endothelium-dependent dilation
- detected in all stages of CAD in coronary arteries with and without plaques, and in peripheral vasculature[49,50]

ACS, acute coronary syndromes; AMI, acute myocardial infarction; Ang1, angiopoietin-1; Ang2, angiopoietin-2; CAD, coronary artery disease; CAMs, cellular adhesion molecules; CEC, circulating endothelial cells; CHD, coronary heart disease; CHF, congestive heart failure; CRP, C-reactive protein; EC, endothelial cell; CABG, coronary artery bypass graft; EMPs, endothelial microparticles; EPCs, endothelial progenitor cells; ER, emergency room; f-TFPI, free tissue factor pathway inhibitor; H4, hour 4 after presentation; H8, hour 8 after presentation; hsCRP, high-sensitivity CRP; ICAM-1, intercellular adhesion molecule-1; IL, interleukin; KDR, kinase domain receptor or VEGF-receptor 2; MCP-1, monocyte chemoattractant protein-1; MI, myocardial infarction; MMP, matrix metalloproteinase; nl, normal; NQMI, non-Q-wave MI; OXLDL, oxidized low-density lipoprotein PTCA, percutaneous transluminal coronary angiography; PCAM-1, platelet-endothelial cell adhesion molecule-1; pts, patients; PAPP-A, pregnancy-associated plasma protein-A; PlGF, placental growth factor; plq, plaque; pmn, polymorphonuclear cells; s, soluble; SA, stable angina; SMCs, smooth muscle cells; Tie-2, angiopoietin receptor; Tn, troponin; UA, unstable angina; VCAM-1, vascular cell adhesion molecule-1; VEGF, vascular endothelial growth factor; VEGFR1, vascular endothelial growth factor receptor-1 or flt-1; vWF, von Willebrand factor.

endothelial activation (whether plaque surface, plaque neovessels, plaque subjacent adventitial vaso vasorum, or other-site vascular endothelium) or the stimulus or stimuli of endothelial dysfunction, the fact that serum/plasma levels are indeed informative suggests the robust potential of endothelial biomarkers as a monitoring paradigm for ACS. Alternatively, systemic circulation detection could also be indicative of generalized dysfunctional endothelium, or more generalized plaque burden, rather than coronary plaque-specific changes.

Making the case for biomarkers of proinjury endothelial dysfunctions

As summarized in Table 10.2, a preponderance of endothelial biomarkers studied to date assess endothelial activation. Although prominent, endothelial activation biomarkers will not be enough, as observed in conflicting results – association as well as non-association with ACS (see Table 10.2). Since the loss of the endothelial cell barrier is the main trigger for the formation of a thrombus[19] and represents a likely plaque event rather than a generalized endothelial event, assessment of proinjury pathways could represent a central point in biomarker context analysis. Detection of proinjury endothelial dysfunctions could also indicate surpassing a threshold towards destabilization, since proinflammatory pathways can further injure endothelial cells, and procoagulant pathways can further proinflammatory pathways. Intuitively, the detection of informative biomarker elevation in all three would probably reflect significant endothelial dysfunctions contributing to ACS.

Multiple interacting pathways require combinatorial mechanism-based treatments

The detection of biomarkers representing proinflammatory, prothrombotic, and proinjury endothelial dysfunctions with predictive value for ACS (see Table 10.2) indicates the involvement of all three in vulnerable plaque progression and destabilization. Based on known interactions among this triad, it follows that treatment strategies should address this interacting triad in order to effectively address endothelial determinants of ACS. Biomarkers of these endothelial dysfunction determinants can also serve as 'surrogate endpoints' for successful treatment strategies.

A normal endothelial biomarker for one parameter or pathway does not imply normal endothelium – other pathways may be abnormal and/or other biomarkers more informative

Verheggen et al[21] reported that inflammatory status is a main determinant of outcome in patients with unstable angina, independent of coagulation activation and endothelial cell function. We note, however, that parameters used for coagulation and endothelial function (prothrombin fragments 1 + 2, thrombin–antithrombin complex levels, tissue type plasminogen activator, von Willebrand factor, and plasminogen activator inhibitor levels) do not represent the full assessment of procoagulant changes or endothelial dysfunctions. This would imply that a panel of biomarkers will be needed to comprehensively analyze coagulation and multiple endothelial dysfunctions.

Current limitations

Although endothelial biomarkers of ACS are still a developing clinical paradigm for monitoring, recognition of limitations is necessary. Foremost of current limitations revolve around the source of biomarker elevation and the interpretation of elevated levels (extent of CAD vs instability). Additionally, plasma/serum biomarkers of dysfunctional endothelium will not be able to discern the anatomic site of the dysfunctional endothelium – coronary artery disease vs peripheral vascular disease, since the latter also exhibits procoagulant, proinflammatory endothelial dysfunctions.[22] Testing of transcoronary levels could narrow the site to the coronary vasculature. Distinction of plaque surface endothelium from plaque neovessels is currently not available, but may be possible through emerging molecular imaging technologies.

Distinguishing the extent of CAD vs instability is also a key limitation at present. A study by Yildirir et al[23] reveals correlation of vascular cell adhesion molecule-1 (VCAM-1) and soluble E-selectin (sE-selectin) levels with extent of coronary atherosclerosis rather than stability, whereas C-reactive protein (CRP), troponin 1, and leukocyte count were predictors of clinical stability. These observations raise a critical issue of discerning instability and extent of coronary atherosclerosis.

FURTHER CONCEPT DEVELOPMENT – BEYOND PREDICTING RISK, REAL-TIME DISEASE MONITORING

With the above proof of concept, advancing translation to the clinics would require further investigation. Some key points for systematic evaluation span the following.

Investigation of balance of endothelial products with diametrical roles

Context analysis of endothelial biomarkers needs to address the diametrical homeostatic roles of the endothelium. For example, in its hemostatic regulatory role, the endothelium synthesizes both procoagulant von Willebrand factor (vWF) and anticoagulant free tissue factor pathway inhibitor (f-TFPI) and soluble thrombomodulin (sTM) factors; in its vascular tone regulatory role, the endothelium synthesizes and releases both vasodilatory (nitric oxide) and vasoconstrictive (endothelin-1) regulators of vascular tone.

These opposite diametrical roles can be discerned by testing biomarkers that reflect the balance of opposing endothelial functions, as done for pro/anticoagulant functions: vWF, f-TFPI, and sTM.[24] Detecting the balance or changes in the equilibrium of opposing diametrical endothelial functions will be critical, and could be more informative in deciphering the dynamic processes involved in vulnerable plaque progression and destabilization. Invariably, informative endothelial biomarkers would also facilitate assessment of treatment responses.

Investigation in the context of CAD pathophysiology

Robustness of clinical relevance of endothelial biomarkers would require assessment within the CAD pathologic context determining:

- endothelial cell (EC) status (plaque EC apoptosis, injury, decreased EC repair, extraplaque EC activation)
- plaque vulnerability parameters (inflammation, neovascularization, large core: cap ratio, matrix degradation, smooth muscle cell paucity, etc.
- vulnerable patient parameters (risk factors, genetic susceptibility, prothrombotic, procoagulant, and proinflammatory changes).

Investigation of the site of endothelial activation

Since it could be expected that endothelial activation from any site can result in an inflammatory cascade which can then interact with the plaque, thereby resulting in plaque destabilization, it is therefore relevant to monitor endothelial activation regardless of source and the inflammatory response in the presence of CAD. However, localizing the plaque as a source of endothelial activation biomarkers, or for any other endothelial dysfunction, would more likely carry greater indication of impending plaque destabilization.

Investigation of plaque type-specific biomarkers

Since inflammation is implicated in all stages of CAD (initiation, progression, destabilization) and since there is lesion heterogeneity, determination as to whether there are plaque type-specific (early, stable, vulnerable plaque, destabilized plaque) characteristics of endothelial activation should be done. The fact that overt CAD (animal model equivalent of ACS) stage-specific transcription profiles can be distinguished from quiescent, advanced CAD and attenuated CAD in the transgenic rat model of CAD[2] suggests that differential transcriptional regulation represents a molecular mechanism for CAD stage-specific set-point changes and, hence, biomarkers. More specifically, transcription profiling and/or immuno-histochemical analysis elucidated the marked up-regulation of matrix metalloproteinase (MMP-3), IL-18, and LOX-1 in overt CAD in the transgenic rat model of CAD[2] prior to, and concordant with; their respective reports as biomarkers for acute coronary syndromes in humans: IL-18,[25] LOX-1,[12] and MMP-3.[26] These concordant observations provide key experimental and molecular mandates, as well as key insights for continued biomarker development in human ACS.

A stepwise framework of analysis could facilitate biomarker development

This framework could conceivably include the following paradigms.

1. Using a quantitative threshold paradigm, determine thresholds of biomarker levels above which risk for ACS increases significantly.
2. Using a multipathway paradigm, determine the panel of biomarkers which represent multiple interactive endothelial dysfunctions (e.g. proinflammatory + prothrombotic + proinjury). This could be expected to carry more weight than a single endothelial dysfunction parameter.
3. Using a combinatorial paradigm, enhance biomarker-panel specificity and sensitivity through functionally significant context analysis which uses a combination of parameters that mechanistically lead to a self-sustaining vicious circle and/or set-point changes which subsequently forward vulnerable plaque progression, as illustrated in Table 10.3.

Assessment of projected functional impact of endothelial activation

At the outset, to discern an impending cardiac event, endothelial biomarkers must be taken in the context of their interacting partners, which are also implicated in ACS. The detection of primed and/or activated leukocytes and/or platelets in addition to biomarkers of endothelial dysfunctions would be a harbinger of plaque instability. This mechanism-based projection needs to be tested systematically.

Establishment of uniformity of parameters used or comparative analysis designs

In order to correlate different studies, and make headway collectively, common methodologies and language of analysis are necessary. While ideal methodologies and analytical schemes are still being investigated along with the biomarker in question, uniformity in parameters and panels of biomarkers would allow the retrospective analysis of multiple studies.

Investigation of mechanisms of release and half-lives of biomarkers

Big unknowns are the half-lives and mechanisms of biomarker elevation. Although clinical studies are trying to address these issues, there are too many complexities

Table 10.3 Examples of combinatorial paradigms for endothelial biomarker development

Endothelial biomarker	Other (non-endothelial) biomarker	Mechanism	Reference
• Cause-and-effect paradigm			
e.g.			
IL-18	CRP	• Human recombinant CRP induced IL-18 release in human endothelial cells	36
IL-18 and endothelial cell death		• IL-18 induced apoptosis in human cardiac microvascular endothelial cells	6
IL-18	MPO, CD11b+ neutrophils	• IL-18 primes neutrophils and induces myeloperoxidase release	7
IL-18, ICAM-1	IL-6, ICAM-1, MMP-1, MMP-9, MMP-13	• IL-18 induces IL-6, IL-8, MMP-1, MMP-9, MMP-13	4
IL-6 and EMP31		• IL-6 levels correlate with EMPs with an apoptotic phenotype, CD31+/CD42 – EMPs	51
• Cognate partners paradigm			
e.g.			
sICAM-1	CD11B + monocytes	• Coordinated up-regulation of endothelial and monocyte activation	13
sICAM-1, SVCAM-1	PF4/heparin complex	• PF4/heparin was detected as predictor of 30-day MI (OR = 9.0) and was associated with higher sICAM-1 and sVCAM-1	52
PECAM-1	sP-selectin, platelet count	• PECAM-1 levels were associated with CAD, along with sP-selectin and platelet count	33
• Imbalance/mismatch paradigm			
e.g.			
IL-6 and MCP-1 Increase injury: CECs apoptotic EMPs	PMN-mps Decreased repair: EPCs as a biomarker for endothelial repair capacity	• PMN microparticles stimulate endothelial release of IL-6 and MCP-1 • EPCs may contribute to ongoing endothelial repair by homing to denuded areas or replacing dysfunctional ECs	53 15
IL-18	IL-10	• Serum IL-18/IL-10 ratio is an independent predictor of in-hospital adverse events in patients with ACS; significantly higher ORs compared with individual IL-18 and IL-10 levels	54

e.g., representative examples given, not all inclusive; ACS, acute coronary syndromes; CAD, coronary artery disease; CRP, C-reactive protein; CD11b, MAC-1; CD31, platelet-endothelial cell adhesion molecule or PECAM-1; CD42, platelet-specific marker; CEC, circulating endothelial cells; ECs, endothelial cells; EMPs, endothelial microparticles; EMP31, CD31+EMPss; EPCs, endothelial progenitor cells; ICAM-1, intercellular adhesion molecule-1; IL, interleukin; MCP-1, monocyte chemoattractant protein-1; MI, myocardial infarction; MMP, matrix metalloproteinase; MPO, myeloperoxidase; OR, odds ratio; PF4/heparin, platelet factor 4/heparin complex; PMN, polymorphonuclear cells S, soluble.

in clinical studies such that complementary studies of animal models of CAD are required. To eliminate confounders from biomarker half-lives, biomarker two-point trends will need to be assessed and compared wtih known half-lives. Increased or unchanged levels beyond half-life expectations indicate increase in the endothelial dysfunction determinant and increased ACS risk. Decreased levels upon repeat biomarker analysis beyond half-lives indicate reversal of the endothelial dysfunction pathway represented by the biomarker.

Beyond statistics – combinatorial assessment modalities for individualized treatment

Modeled after oncologic treatment paradigms in breast cancer biology,[27] future goals should aim for the identification of a panel of biomarkers and molecular imaging markers (assessing plaque and EC status; i.e. activation, injury, erosion) that will constitute strategic tests to reflect CAD plaque biology, and guide individualized treatment beyond predicting statistical relative risk. Such a panel of biomarkers could be assessed in an *endothelial dysfunction score*, with information for both the vulnerable plaque and vulnerable patient. This endothelial dysfunction score, in conjunction with assessment of platelet and leukocyte (monocyte, neutrophil, and T-cell) priming and/or activation, and ideally plaque imaging, could collectively elucidate clinical mandates for intervention and prevention strategies.

REFERENCES

1. Gokce N, Loscalzo J. Endothelial dysfunction and atherothrombosis. In: Wilson PWF, ed. Atlas of Atherosclerosis: Risk Factors and Treatment, Singapore: Current Medicine Inc; 2000: 21–40.
2. Herrera VM, Didishvili T, Lopez LV, Ruiz-Opazo N. Differential regulation of functional gene clusters in overt coronary artery disease in a transgenic atherosclerosis-hypertensive rat model. Mol Med 2002; 8:367–75.
3. King JY, Ferrara R, Tabibiazar R et al. Pathway analysis of coronary atherosclerosis. Physiol Genomics 2005; 23:103–18.
4. Gerdes N, Sukhova GK, Libby P et al. Expression of IL-18 and functional IL-18 receptor on human vascular endothelial cells, smooth muscle cells, and macrophages: implications for atherogenesis. J Exp Med 2002; 195:245–57.
5. Leung BP, Culshaw A, Gracie JA et al. A role for IL-18 in neutrophil activation. J Immunol 2001; 167: 2879–86.
6. Chandrasekar B, Valente AJ, Freeman GL, Mahimainathan L, Mummidi S. Interleukin-18 induces human cardiac endothelial cell death via a novel signaling pathway involving NF-kappaB-dependent PTEN activation. Biochem Biophys Res Commun 2006; 339:956–63.
7. Elbim C, Guichard C, Dang PM et al. Interleukin-18 primes the oxidative burst of neutrophils in response to formyl-peptides: role of cytochrome b558 translocation and N-formyl peptide receptor endocytosis. Clin Diagn Lab Immunol 2005; 12:436–46.
8. Aoyama T, Fujiwara H, Masak T, Sawamura T. Induction of lectin-like oxidized LDL receptor by oxidized LDL and lysophosphatidylcholine in cultured endothelial cells, J Mol Cell Cardiol 1999; 31: 2101–14.
9. Li D, Liu L, Chen H, Swamura T, Mehta JL. LOX-1, an oxidized LDL endothelial receptor, induces CD40/CD40L signaling in human coronary artery endothelial cells. Arterioscler Thromb Vasc Biol 2003; 23:816–21.
10. Shin HK, Kim YK, Kim KY, Lee JH, Hong KW. Remnant lipoprotein particles induce apoptosis in endothelial cells by NAD(P)H oxidase-mediated production of superoxide and cytokines via lectin-like oxidized low-density lipoprotein receptor-1 activation: prevention by cilostazol. Circulation 2004; 109:1022–8.
11. Kakutani M, Masaki T, Kawamura T. A platelet–endothelium interaction mediated by lectin-like oxidized low-density lipoprotein receptor-1. Proc Natl Acad Sci USA 2000; 97:360–4.
12. Hayashida K, Kume N, Murase T et al. Serum soluble lectin-like oxidized low-density lipoprotein receptor-1 levels are elevated in acute coronary syndrome: a novel marker for early diagnosis. Circulation 2004; 112:812–18.
13. Murphy RT, Foley JB, Crean P, Walsh MJ. Reciprocal activation of leukocyte–endothelial adhesion molecules in acute coronary syndromes. Int J Cardiol 2003; 90:247–52.
14. Lee KW, Lip GY, Blann AD. Plasma angiopoietin-1, angiopoietin-2, angiopoietin receptor tie-2, and vascular endothelial growth factor levels in acute coronary syndromes. Circulation 2004; 110:2355–60.
15. Schmidt-Lucke C, Rossig L, Fichtlscherer S et al. Reduced number of circulating endothelial progenitor cells predicts future cardiovascular events: proof

of concept for the clinical importance of endogenous vascular repair. Circulation 2005; 111:2981–7.

16. Wada Y, Out H, Wu S et al. Preconditioning of primary human endothelial cells with inflammatory mediators alters the 'set point' of the cell. FASEB J 2005; 19:1914–16.

17. Binder CJ, Chang MK, Shaw PX et al. Innate and acquired immunity in atherogenesis. Nat Med 2002; 8:1218–26.

18. Libby P, Aikawa M. Stabilization of atherosclerotic plaques: new mechanisms and clinical targets. Nat Med 2002; 8:1257–62.

19. Ruggeri ZM. Platelets in atherothrombosis. Nat Med 2002; 8:1227–34.

20. Lee KW, Blann AD, Lip GY. Inter-relationships of indices of endothelial damage/dysfunction [circulating endothelial cells, von Willebrand factor and flow-mediated dilatation] to tissue factor and interleukin-6 in acute coronary syndromes. Int J Cardiol 2006; 111:302–8.

21. Verheggen PW, de Maat MP, Cats VVM et al. Inflammatory status as a main determinant of outcome in patients with unstable angina, independent of coagulation activation and endothelial cell function. Eur Heart J 1999; 20:567–74.

22. Cassar K, Bachoo P, Ford I, Greaves M, Brittenden J. Markers of coagulation activation, endothelial stimulation and inflammation in patients with peripheral arterial disease. Eur J Vasc Endovasc Surg 2005; 29: 171–6.

23. Yildirir A, Tokgozoglu SL, Haznedaraglu I et al. Extent of coronary atherosclerosis and homocysteine affect endothelial markers. Angiology 2001; 52:589–96.

24. Morange PE, Simon C, Alessi MC et al.; PRIME Study Group. Endothelial cell markers and the risk of coronary heart disease. Circulation 2004; 109:1343–8.

25. Mallat Z, Henry P, Fressonnet R et al. Increased plasma concentrations of interleukin-18 in acute coronary syndromes. Heart 2002; 88:467–9.

26. Wu TC, Leu HB, Lin WT et al. Plasma matrix metalloproteinase-3 level is an independent prognostic factor in stable coronary artery disease. Eur J Clin Invest 2005; 35:537–45.

27. Yarden Y, Baselga J, Miles D. Molecular approach to breast cancer treatment. Semin Oncol 2004; 31 (5 Suppl 10):6–13.

28. Mulvihill NT, Foley JB, Murphy RT et al. Risk stratification in unstable angina and non-Q wave myocardial infarction using soluble cell adhesion molecules. Heart 2001; 85:623–7.

29. O'Malley T, Ludlam CA, Riemersma RA et al. Early increase in level of soluble inter-cellular adhesion molecule-1 (sICAM-1): potential risk factor for the acute coronary syndromes. Eur Heart J 2001; 22: 1226–34.

30. Atalar E, Aytemir K, Haznedaroglu I et al. Increased plasma levels of soluble selectins in patients with unstable angina. Int J Cardiol 2001; 78:69–73.

31. Blankenberg S, Rupprecht HJ, Bickel C et al; for the AtheroGene Investigators. Circulating cell adhesion molecules and death in patients with coronary artery disease. Circulation 2001; 104:1336–42.

32. Soeki T, Tamura Y, Shinohara H et al. Increased soluble platelet/endothelial cell adhesion molecule-1 in the early stages of acute coronary syndromes. Int J Cardiol 2003; 90:261–8.

33. Wei H, Fang L, Chowdhury SH et al. Platelet–endothelial cell adhesion molecule-1 gene polymorphism and its soluble level are associated with severe coronary artery stenosis in Chinese Singaporean. Clin Biochem 2004; 37:1091–7.

34. Menown IBA, Mathew TP, Gracey HM et al. Prediction of recurrent events by D-dimer and inflammatory markers in patients with normal cardiac troponin I (PREDICT) study. Am Heart J 2003; 145:986–92.

35. Draz N, Hamdy MS, Gomaa Y, Ramzy AA. Soluble P-selectin is a marker of plaque destabilization in unstable angina. Egypt J Immunol 2003; 10:83–7.

36. Yamaoka-Tojo M, Tojo T, Masuda T et al. C-reactive protein-induced production of interleukin-18 in human endothelial cells: a mechanism of orchestrating cytokine cascade in acute coronary syndrome. Heart Vessels 2003; 18:183–7.

37. Kawasaki D, Tsijino T, Morimoto S et al. Plasma interleukin-18 concentration: a novel marker of myocardial ischemia rather than necrosis in humans. Coron Artery Dis 2005; 16:437–41.

38. Martinovic I, Abegunewardene N, Seul M et al. Elevated monocyte chemoattractant protein-1 serum levels in patients at risk for coronary artery disease. Circ J 2005; 69:1484–9.

39. Bayes-Genis A, Conover CA, Overgaard MT et al. Pregnancy-associated plasma protein A as a marker of acute coronary syndromes. N Engl J Med 2001; 345:1022–9.

40. Lund J, Qin QP, Ilva T et al. Circulating pregnancy-associated plasma protein A predicts outcome in patients with acute coronary syndrome but no troponin I elevation. Circulation 2003; 108:1924–6.

41. Heeschen C, Dimmeler S, Hamm CW et al. Pregnancy-associated plasma protein-A levels in patients with acute coronary syndromes. J Am Coll Cardiol 2005; 45:229–37.

42. Mallat Z, Benamer H, Hugel B et al. Elevated levels of shed membrane microparticles with procoagulant potential in the peripheral circulating blood of patients with acute coronary syndromes. Circulation 2000; 101:841–3.

43. Bernal-Mizrachi L, Jy W, Fierro C et al. Endothelial microparticles with high-risk angiographic lesions in acute coronary syndromes. Int J Cardiol 2004; 97:439–46.

44. Zielinska M, Koniarek W, Goch JH et al. Circulating endothelial microparticles in patients with acute myocardial infarction. Kardiol Pol 2005; 62: 531–42.

45. Werner N, Kosiol S, Schiegl T et al. Circulating endothelial progenitor cells and cardiovascular outcomes. N Engl J Med 2005; 353:999–1007.

46. Quilici J, Banzet N, Paule P et al. Circulating endothelial cell count as a diagnostic marker for non-ST-elevation acute coronary syndromes. Circulation 2004; 110:1586–91.

47. Kanaki T, Bujo H, Mori S et al. Functional analysis of aortic endothelial cells expressing mutant PDGF receptors with respect to expression of matrix metalloproteinase-3. Biochem Biophys Res Commun 2002; 294:231–7.

48. Heeschen C, Dimmeler S, Fichtlscherer S et al. Prognostic value of placental growth factor in patients with acute chest pain. JAMA 2004; 291:435–41.

49. Elbaz M, Carrie D, Baudeux JL et al. High frequency of endothelial vasomotor dysfunction after acute coronary syndromes in non-culprit and angiographically normal coronary arteries: a reversible phenomenon. Atherosclerosis 2005; 181:311–19.

50. Thanyasiri P, Celermajer DS, Adams MR. Endothelial dysfunction occurs in peripheral circulation patients with acute and stable coronary artery disease. Am J Physiol Heart Circ Physiol 2005; 289:H513–17.

51. Chirinos JA, Zambrano JP, Virani SS et al. Correlation between apoptotic endothelial microparticles and serum interleukin-6 and C-reactive protein in healthy men. Am J Cardiol 2005; 95:1258–60.

52. Mascelli MA, Deliargyris EN, Damaraju LV et al. Antibodies to platelet factor 4/heparin are associated with elevated endothelial cell activation markers in patients with acute coronary ischemic syndromes. J Thromb Thrombolysis 2004; 18:171–5.

53. Mesri M, Altieri D. Leukocyte microparticles stimulate endothelial cell cytokine release and tissue factor induction in a JNK1 signaling pathway. J Biol Chem 1999; 274:23111–18.

54. Chalikias GK, Tziakas DN, Kaski JC et al. Interleukin-18:interleukin-10 ratio and in-hospital adverse events in patients with acute coronary syndrome. Atherosclerosis 2005; 182:135–43.

Biomarkers

11

Michael Weber and Christian W Hamm

BACKGROUND

In recent years the pathophysiology of coronary artery disease (CAD) has been unraveled, yielding a much deeper understanding of the mechanisms leading to acute coronary syndromes (ACS). Atherosclerosis is currently regarded as a dynamic process originating from endothelial dysfunction to plaque initiation, plaque progression, and finally to the development of either stable or unstable vulnerable plaques. Whereas stable plaques might cause myocardial ischemia and angina pectoris at exertion because of relevant lumen narrowing, rupture or erosion of high-risk vulnerable plaques with subsequent thrombus formation is responsible for the development of acute ischemic events. In this atherothrombotic process the interaction of endothelial dysfunction, inflammation, and enhanced blood thrombogenicity plays the key role.

The identification of high-risk patients with vulnerable plaques, the 'vulnerable patient', before an acute event, remains a major challenge. Development and further improvement of diagnostic techniques aim to accurately detect high-risk atherosclerotic plaques. Several invasive and non-invasive imaging techniques such as magnetic resonance imaging (MRI), intravascular ultrasound (IVUS), optical coherence tomography (OCT), virtual histology, intravascular elastography/palpography, and thermography are under investigation. In addition to these imaging techniques, biomarkers have gained great interest. Traditional biomarkers of myocardial damage, e.g. cardiac troponins, are established in clinical routine and play a pivotal role for the diagnostic work-up and management of patients with ACS.

The determination of a variety of enzymes, adhesion molecules, cytokines, and chemokines has provided important insights into the pathophysiology of atherosclerosis and has substantially contributed to the advanced understanding of mechanisms leading to ACS. Promising results of recently published studies suggest that these new markers of inflammation, cell activation, and plaque destabilization might also be of diagnostic use for identifying patients at high risk for acute ischemic events (Figure 11.1, Box 11.1).

It is the aim of this overview to summarize current knowledge on new biomarkers and their diagnostic potential to detect the vulnerable patient. Since it is not possible to cover all possible biomarkers linked to vulnerable plaques in this chapter, the focus will be put on a selection of biomarkers that (in the opinion of the authors) may enter clinical routine in the future.

ENDOTHELIAL DYSFUNCTION – INFLAMMATION – PLAQUE PROGRESSION

The endothelium separates the blood from the vessel wall. It is an autocrine and paracrine organ that is involved in the regulation of vascular homeostasis. The main signaling molecule released from the endothelium is nitric oxide (NO), which mediates a number of physiologic functions.

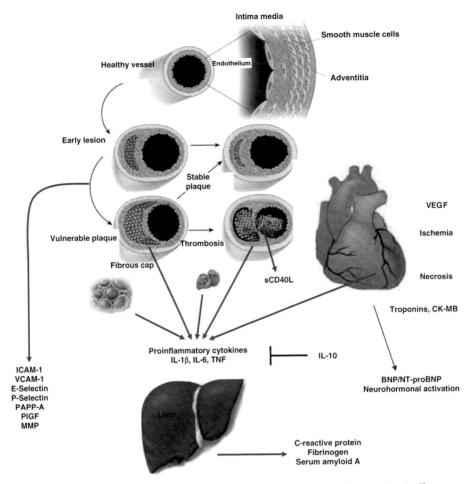

Figure 11.1 Pathophysiology of acute coronary syndromes. (Modified from Rader.[65])

Disturbances of physiologic blood flow and increased shear stress lead to endothelial cell activation and endothelial dysfunction. Moreover, traditional risk factors such as hypertension, smoking, and hypercholesterolemia are also associated with the development of endothelial dysfunction. Endothelial dysfunction is considered to be the earliest manifestation of atherosclerosis and is characterized by decreased NO synthesis, which facilitates vasoconstriction, oxidation of lipoproteins, internalization of lipoproteins, and inflammatory cells. Furthermore, endothelial cell activation leads to the expression of the chemokine monocyte chemoattractant protein 1 (MCP-1), inflammatory cytokines, and adhesion molecules (ICAM and VCAM), which causes adherence and internalization of monocytes and further perpetuates inflammation. In return, the systemic inflammatory response then amplifies endothelial dysfunction. Internalization of macrophages and oxidized low-density lipoprotein (oxLDL), smooth muscle cell proliferation, and extracellular matrix formation yields plaque initiation and plaque progression. Thus, atherosclerosis is a complex process that involves interaction of endothelial cells, inflammatory cells, and cells of the vessel wall itself. The ongoing

Box 11.1 Selection of candidate biomarkers that might become applicable for clinical use in the future for diagnosis and risk stratification of patients with acute coronary syndromes

Marker of inflammation

CRP[a]	C-reactive protein
IL-6[a]	Interleukin-6
IL-18	Interleukin-18
IL-10[a]	Interleukin-10
TNF-α	Tumor necrosis factor-α
SAA	Serum amyloid A

Marker of plaque destabilization

MPO[a]	Myeloperoxidase
sCD40L[a]	Soluble CD40 ligand
Lp-PLA$_2$[a]	Lipoprotein-associated phospholipase A$_2$
MMP-9	Matrix metalloproteinases-9
PlGF[a]	Placental growth factor
VGEF	Vascular endothelial growth factor
PAPP-A	Pregnancy-associated plasma protein-A
ICAM	Intercellular adhesion molecule
VCAM	Vascular adhesion molecule

Marker of ischemia and necrosis

IMA	Ischemia-mediated albumin
h-FABP	Heart-type fatty acid binding protein
Choline	Choline
cTnT	Cardiac troponin T
cTnI	Cardiac troponin I

Marker of myocardial stress

BNP	B-type natriuretic peptide
NT-proBNP	N-terminal B-type natriuretic peptide

[a]Biomarkers covered in this chapter.

inflammation augments the development of unstable, so-called vulnerable plaques, which are characterized by a thin, fibrous cap, a lipid-rich core, inflammatory cell infiltration, and a diminished number of smooth muscle cells. These plaques are prone for rupture or erosion, causing intravascular thrombosis, which is the anatomic correlate for acute ischemic coronary events.

MARKERS OF INFLAMMATION

Inflammation is one of the key players in the process that ends in destabilization and rupture of vulnerable plaques. Several inflammatory and anti-inflammatory markers have been investigated in recent years. The major objective of all studies is the question of whether increased levels of inflammatory biomarkers are able to identify vulnerable patients and to predict future coronary events.

C-reactive protein

The most widely studied inflammatory marker is C-reactive protein (CRP), which has been investigated extensively in large-scale studies. CRP is an acute phase reactant that plays a major role in human innate immune response. The main source of CRP is the liver, where it is produced from hepatocytes in response to interleukin-6 (IL-6) stimulation. However, CRP is also synthesized in smooth muscle cells within human coronary arteries and is expressed in atherosclerotic lesions.[1,2] Initially, CRP was thought to be only a downstream marker of inflammation. However, recently it has been suggested that CRP plays an active role in coronary artery disease, promoting atherosclerotic progress and inflammation.[3] CRP inhibits endothelial nitric oxide synthase (eNOS), leading to diminished NO release and thus to disturbances of vascular homeostasis.[4] Furthermore, it stimulates endothelin-1 (ET-1), IL-6, and MCP-1 release and expression of adhesion molecules, facilitating the internalization of inflammatory cells (Figure 11.2).[5]

In several epidemiologic studies it has been consistently found that CRP is a strong independent predictor for future cardiovascular events among apparently healthy men and women.[6] Likewise, CRP has been found to be elevated in patients with an adverse outcome, providing additional independent prognostic information

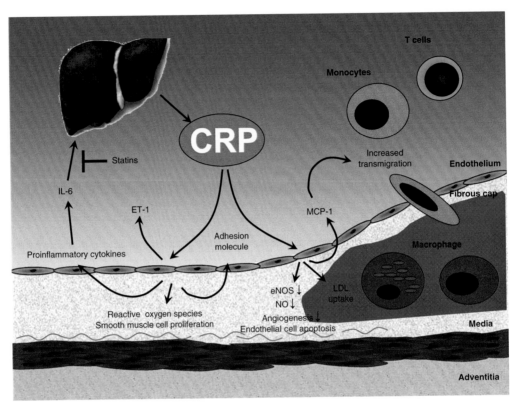

Figure 11.2 Pathophysiologic effects of CRP on the endothelium of atherosclerotic plaques. (Modified from Szmitko et al.[3])

in the setting of ACS.[7–9] Comparable results have been obtained in patients who have been treated by very early revascularization therapy.[10]

Statins were originally introduced as cholesterol-lowering drugs. However, beyond this effect, statin therapy has been shown to lower CRP levels.[11,12] The Air Force/Texas Coronary Atherosclerosis Prevention Study (AFCAPS/TexCAPS) aimed to test statin therapy vs placebo in primary prevention for acute coronary events. In this study, CRP was a predictor for an adverse outcome, and statin therapy was highly effective in reducing cardiac events in individuals with high CRP values and low LDL cholesterol.[13] Furthermore, in the Pravastatin or Atorvastatin Evaluation and Infection Therapy (PROVE IT-TIMI 22) trial, it has been demonstrated that

patients with an ACS in whom CRP levels could be lowered under statin therapy had a better clinical outcome, independent of the LDL cholesterol levels.[14]

Overall, these data suggest that CRP is not only a risk marker but also an active player in atherosclerosis, which can be attenuated by anti-inflammatory treatment with statins, resulting in an improved clinical outcome.

Interleukin-6

IL-6 is produced and released from activated monocytes and macrophages within the atheroma and from activated endothelial cells. IL-6 is thought to be the major determinant for the production of CRP and other acute phase reactants by hepatocytes in the liver.[15,16]

The IL-6-induced CRP synthesis can be attenuated by statin therapy, which is a newly identified mechanism for the anti-inflammatory properties of statins.[17] IL-6 is also directly involved in a number of proinflammatory and procoagulant processes that play a role in the patho-physiology of plaque progression and destabilization.[18,19] In a population-based study, it has been demonstrated that IL-6 levels were able to identify a subgroup of patients with high risk for subsequent death among older women with pre-existing cardiovascular disease, and in another study elevated levels of IL-6 were associated with an increased risk for future myocardial infarction in apparently healthy men.[20,21] In patients with unstable angina, raised levels of IL-6 have been commonly detected with a correlation to CRP and an association to the prognosis of the patients.[22] In a substudy of the Fast Revascularization during InStability in Coronary disease (FRISC II) trial, which included 3269 patients with unstable CAD, elevated values of IL-6 were independently associated with increased mortality at 6 and 12 months. Moreover, it could be demonstrated that elevated IL-6 was predictive for a benefit from an early invasive therapy and from a treatment with low-molecular-weight heparin.[23]

Interleukin-10

Interleukin-10 (IL-10) is secreted by activated monocytes/macrophages and lymphocytes. It inhibits the transcription factor nuclear factor-κB (NF-κB), leading to suppression of cytokine production, inhibition of matrix metalloproteinases, and reduction of tissue factor expression.[24,25] Therefore, IL-10 is a potent anti-inflammatory cytokine that induces plaque stabilization. Subsequently, in experimental studies in animals, increased susceptibility to atherosclerosis in IL-10-deficient mice has been demonstrated,[26] and in another study atherosclerotic lesion formation was

significantly less in transgenic mice over-expressing IL-10 compared with wild-type or IL-10-deficient mice.[27] It was also found that IL-10 serum levels were associated with improved systemic endothelial vasore-activity in patients with elevated CRP and documented CAD. These findings underscore the importance of the balance between pro- and anti-inflammatory mediators as a determinant for endothelial dysfunction and for plaque progression.[28]

In clinical studies it has been shown that low IL-10 levels are associated with unstable atherosclerotic disease.[29] In ACS, elevated serum levels of IL-10 were associated with an improved outcome, and the predictive value of IL-10 was independent of troponin T and CRP.[30] Thus, reduced IL-10 serum levels are not only a marker of plaque instability, favoring the development of ACS, but also, more importantly, they indicate adverse prognosis.

MARKER OF CELLULAR ACTIVATION AND PLAQUE DESTABILIZATION

In addition to markers of inflammation, markers that are thought to reflect cellular activation and are active contributors in the process leading to plaque destabilization have been identified and investigated. These markers are of special interest, since they display the final pathway of the mechanisms leading to acute coronary events.

Soluble CD40 ligand

The CD40–CD40 ligand system is expressed on a variety of cell types, including activated platelets, vascular endothelial cells, vascular smooth muscle cells, monocytes, and macrophages. Following expression on the cell surface, CD40L is partly cleaved by proteases and subsequently released into the circulation as soluble CD40 ligand (sCD40L), which can be detected in serum and plasma. The main sources

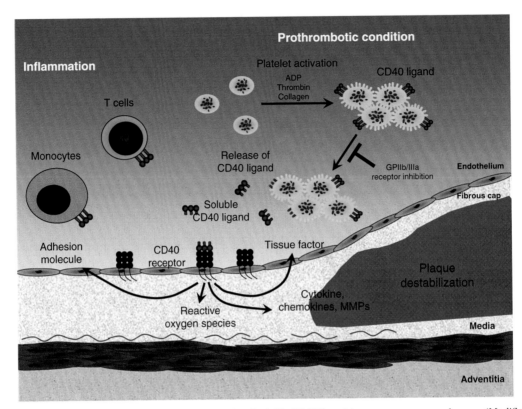

Figure 11.3   Pathophysiologic effects of CD40 ligand and soluble CD40 ligand in acute coronary syndromes. (Modified from Heeschen et al.[40])

of circulating sCD40L are platelets.[31] Membrane-bound CD40L executes a variety of biologic effects on the vasculature and is involved in the pathophysiology of ACS (Figure 11.3).[31–34] Binding of CD40L to the CD40 receptor mediates an inflammatory and prothrombotic response via the release of inflammatory cytokines, expression of adhesion molecules, activation of matrix metalloproteinases, and expression of tissue factor.[32] Furthermore, the interaction of CD40L with its receptor inhibits endothelial cell migration by increasing reactive oxygen species.[34] CD40L also binds to the major platelet integrin αIIbβ3 (GP IIb/IIIa receptor), promoting further platelet activation and thrombus stabilization.[35] Thus, CD40L binding enhances inflammation, has a prothrombotic action, leads to plaque destabilization, and inhibits endothelial

regeneration. To what extent released sCD40L displays comparable inflammatory and prothrombotic effects has not yet been fully elucidated and is controversial.[36]

In clinical studies it has been shown that sCD40L is of predictive value for an adverse outcome in apparently healthy women[37] and for the development of restenosis after percutaneous coronary intervention (PCI).[38] Circulating sCD40L is elevated in patients with ACS and provides prognostic information with therapeutical implications. According to the data derived from the Chimeric 7E3 AntiPlatelet Therapy in Unstable angina Refractory to standard treatment (CAPTURE) trial, patients with high sCD40L values had a clinical benefit from the treatment with the GP IIb/IIIa inhibitor abciximab even if they were troponin-negative. In contrast, patients with low sCD40L values had no advantage from abciximab treatment.[39–41] Thus, there is optimism that sCD40L may serve as a clinically useful biomarker for risk stratification and for therapeutical decision making in the setting of ACS.[42]

Myeloperoxidase

Myeloperoxidase (MPO) is a member of the heme peroxidase superfamily, and is traditionally regarded as a microbicidal enzyme. It is released at sites of inflammation from activated polymorphonuclear neutrophils (PMNs) and monocytes, where it is stored in azurophilic granules.[43] In ACS, increased numbers of MPO-expressing macrophages have been described in eroded or ruptured plaques, whereas macrophages in fatty streaks contained no or only small amounts of MPO (Figure 11.4). The accumulation of MPO-containing macrophages

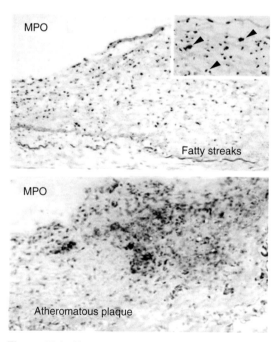

Figure 11.4 Expression of myeloperoxidase (MPO) immunoreactivity localized in advanced human atherosclerosis (lower image). Arteries with fatty streaks exhibited little MPO (upper image), but some samples contained MPO in the intima (arrowheads; inset).[44]

in vulnerable plaques is in part regulated by granulocyte–macrophage colony-stimulating factor (GM-CSF) and probably also by inflammatory cytokines.[44] MPO produces reactive oxygen species (ROS), consumes endothelium-derived NO, oxidizes LDL cholesterol, and activates metalloproteinases.[45] Thus, MPO actively promotes endothelial dysfunction and plaque destabilization. In a case-control study, Zhang et al [46] found elevated levels of circulating MPO and leukocyte inherent MPO in patients with stable CAD compared with controls. In a substudy of the population from the CAPTURE trial, elevated levels of MPO provided independent predictive information for an adverse outcome of patients with ACS.[47] Similarly, Brennan et al[48] reported that MPO was an independent predictor for an unfavorable course of patients presenting with chest pain to the emergency department. In both studies, the predictive value of MPO was independent of other biomarkers, especially of troponins.

Lipoprotein-associated phospholipase A$_2$

Lipoprotein-associated phospholipase A$_2$ (Lp-PLA$_2$) is produced mainly by monocytes and macrophages, T lymphocytes, and mast cells. Its synthesis is regulated by inflammatory cytokines. In the systemic circulation, 70–80% of Lp-PLA$_2$ is bound to LDL cholesterol. Lp-PLA$_2$ is an enzyme that hydrolyzes oxidized phospholipids to generate lysophosphatidylcholine and oxidized fatty acids, which both display proinflammatory properties and promote atherogenesis. Conversely, Lp-PLA$_2$ hydrolyzes platelet-activating factor. Thus, it is not entirely clear whether the atheroprotective properties outweigh the proinflammatory properties of Lp-PLA$_2$.[49] In a case-control study, the West of Scotland Coronary Prevention (WOSCOP) study, a primary prevention study including men with elevated LDL cholesterol and no history of myocardial infarction, Lp-PLA$_2$ levels were strongly associated with the risk of coronary heart disease. This suggests that Lp-PLA$_2$ is a potential risk factor playing a direct role in atherogenesis.[50] Similar results, indicating a predictive value of Lp-PLA$_2$ for future cardiovascular events, have been reported from the population-based MONItoring trends and determinants in CArdiovascular disease (MONICA) Augsburg survey and from the Atherosclerosis Risk in Communities (ARIC) study.[51,52] In contrast, in the Women's Health Study (WHS), Lp-PLA$_2$ was not a predictor of future cardiac events in apparently healthy middle-aged women.[53] In patients with stable coronary artery disease, Lp-PLA$_2$ was associated with traditional cardiovascular risk factors, with the extent of angiographically detected coronary lesions, and with major adverse events.[54] To date, no published data of Lp-PLA$_2$ in acute coronary syndromes are available. However, preliminary data presented at the American Heart meeting 2005 raised doubts on how strongly Lp-PLA$_2$ is associated with an unfavorable outcome, and thus is of predictive value in patients with ACS.[55]

Placental growth factor

PlGF is a member of the vascular endothelial growth factor (VGEF) family, originally identified in the placenta. However, it has been shown that PlGF is also up-regulated in early and advanced atherosclerotic lesions (Figure 11.5).[56] PlGF, by interacting with its receptor, Fms-like tyrosine kinase (Flt-1), stimulates vascular smooth muscle cell proliferation, enhances recruitment of macrophages, augments release of tumor necrosis factor-α (TNF-α), and MCP-1, and also stimulates pathologic angiogenesis.[57] Inhibition of the PlGF receptor in an animal model suppressed atherosclerotic plaque growth and vulnerability via inhibition of inflammatory cell infiltration (see Figure 11.5).[56] Thus, these preclinical studies demonstrate that PlGF may be used as a marker for plaque instability. The translation of these findings in clinical practice has been evaluated in a substudy of the CAPTURE trial.

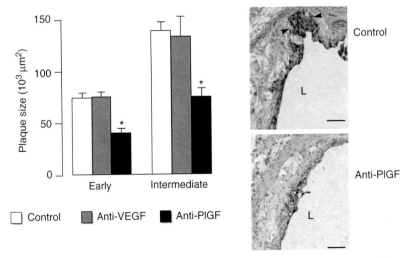

Figure 11.5 Anti-Flt1, an inhibitor of the PlGF receptor (black bars, lower figure), but not anti-Flk1, an inhibitor of the VEGF receptor (gray bars, upper figure) suppresses atherosclerotic plaque growth.[56]

Here it was found that PlGF levels at presentation are of prognostic value for the clinical outcome in patients with suspected ACS. The predictive value of PlGF was independent of myocardial necrosis, evidenced by troponin, or platelet activation, evidenced by sCD40L, and was superior to CRP.[58] Thus, PlGF represents a clinically valuable biomarker for vascular inflammation and plaque instability and, consequently, for an adverse outcome in patients presenting with ACS.

Pregnancy-associated plasma protein A

Pregnancy-associated plasma protein-A (PAPP-A) is a zinc-binding metalloproteinase that was originally identified in plasma of pregnant women and is used for screening of fetal trisomy. Recently, PAPP-A has been found to be elevated in patients with CAD related to the extent of disease[59] and to the angiographically determined plaque complexity;[60] it was also elevated in patients with ACS.[61,62] PAPP-A is thought to be produced by activated cells within the atherosclerotic plaque, either from macrophages, endothelial cells, or smooth muscle cells.[63] Its role in the pathophysiologic process of plaque progression and destabilization is not yet fully elucidated. PAPP-A specifically degrades insulin-like growth factor binding proteins (IGFBPs) and thus leads to release of insulin-like growth factor 1 (IGF-1), which exhibits proatherogenic properties. Free IGF-1 promotes smooth muscle cell proliferation, extracellular matrix synthesis, macrophage activation, chemotaxis, LDL cholesterol uptake by macrophages, and cytokine release.[64] However, this might not be the only pathway for PAPP-A involvement in the evolution of atherosclerosis. PAPP-A is a member of the metalloproteinase family, a group of proteases known to degrade extracellular matrix and thus promote plaque destabilization,

rupture, and erosion. Whether PAPP-A itself is able to degrade extracellular matrix remains unclear. The association of PAPP-A with atherosclerosis and vulnerable plaques has been demonstrated in a landmark study of Bayes–Genis et al.[63] They found PAPP-A abundantly expressed in ruptured or eroded plaques but not in stable plaques in tissue samples obtained at autopsy from eight patients who died of sudden cardiac death (Figure 11.6). Furthermore, they reported on higher circulating PAPP-A values in patients with ACS than in patients with stable CAD or in controls. The clinical relevance of these findings has been conclusively demonstrated by two independent studies. Heeschen et al found that PAPP-A is a strong and independent predictor of cardiovascular events in patients with ACS.[61] Similar results were reported by Lund et al.[62] In both studies PAPP-A consistently identified patients at risk who were troponin-negative, which renders expectations that PAPP-A might be able to recognize vulnerable patients ahead of an acute atherothrombotic event.

SUMMARY

The transition of stable atherosclerotic plaques to vulnerable plaques finally resulting in the clinical manifestation of an acute coronary syndrome is the consequence of an inflammatory reaction. This process involves complex cellular interactions engaging a great number of mediators, chemokines, and cytokines which can be measured in serum and plasma and thus serve as biomarkers that reflect different pathophysiologic phases of disease progression. In clinical investigations, several new biomarkers have been identified which provide incremental diagnostic and prognostic information. However, more confirmatory studies are required until these new markers are qualified for clinical routine. Furthermore, assays for automized

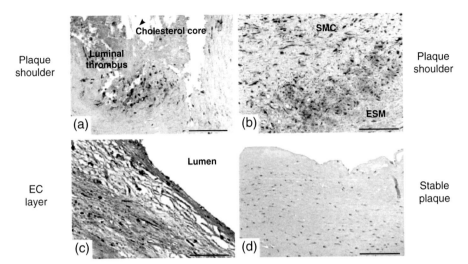

Figure 11.6 Expression of pregnancy-associated plasma protein-A (PAPP-A) in unstable and stable coronary athero-sclerotic plaques. (a) PAPP-A in an inflammatory shoulder area densely infiltrated by macrophages. The inflammatory infiltrate is present between the cholesterol core (arrowhead) and the luminal thrombus (asterisk). (b) There is intense staining for PAPP-A within spindle-shaped smooth muscle cells (SMC) and in the extracellular matrix (ECM) of an eroded plaque. (c) PAPP-A is present in non-eroded endothelial cells (EC) of an eroded plaque. (d) PAPP-A is absent in a stable plaque.[63]

use have to be developed, decision limits need to be defined, and preanalytic conditions for samples need to be standardized.[42]

REFERENCES

1. Calabro P, Willerson JT, Yeh ET. Inflammatory cytokines stimulated C-reactive protein production by human coronary artery smooth muscle cells. Circulation 2003; 108:1930–2.

2. Jabs WJ, Theissing E, Nitschke M et al. Local generation of C-reactive protein in diseased coronary artery venous bypass grafts and normal vascular tissue. Circulation 2003; 108:1428–31.

3. Szmitko PE, Wang CH, Weisel RD et al. New markers of inflammation and endothelial cell activation: Part I. Circulation 2003; 108:1917–23.

4. Verma S, Wang CH, Li SH et al. A self-fulfilling prophecy: C-reactive protein attenuates nitric oxide production and inhibits angiogenesis. Circulation 2002; 106:913–19.

5. Verma S, Li SH, Badiwala MV et al. Endothelin antagonism and interleukin-6 inhibition attenuate the proatherogenic effects of C-reactive protein. Circulation 2002; 105:1890–6.

6. Blake GJ, Ridker PM. C-reactive protein and other inflammatory risk markers in acute coronary syndromes. J Am Coll Cardiol 2003; 41:37–42S.

7. Heeschen C, Hamm CW, Bruemmer J, Simoons ML. Predictive value of C-reactive protein and troponin T in patients with unstable angina: a comparative analysis. CAPTURE Investigators. Chimeric c7E3 AntiPlatelet Therapy in Unstable angina REfractory to standard treatment trial. J Am Coll Cardiol 2000; 35:1535–42.

8. Liuzzo G, Biasucci LM, Gallimore JR et al. The prognostic value of C-reactive protein and serum amyloid a protein in severe unstable angina. N Engl J Med 1994; 331:417–24.

9. Lindahl B, Toss H, Siegbahn A, Venge P, Wallentin L. Markers of myocardial damage and inflammation in relation to long-term mortality in unstable coronary artery disease. FRISC Study Group. Fragmin during Instability in Coronary Artery Disease. N Engl J Med 2000; 343:1139–47.

10. Mueller C, Buettner HJ, Hodgson JM et al. Inflammation and long-term mortality after non-ST elevation acute coronary syndrome treated with a very early invasive strategy in 1042 consecutive patients. Circulation 2002; 105:1412–15.

11. Macin SM, Perna ER, Farias EF et al. Atorvastatin has an important acute anti-inflammatory effect in patients with acute coronary syndrome: results of a randomized, double-blind, placebo-controlled study. Am Heart J 2005; 149:451–7.

12. Kinlay S, Schwartz GG, Olsson AG et al. High-dose atorvastatin enhances the decline in inflammatory markers in patients with acute coronary syndromes in the MIRACL study. Circulation 2003; 108:1560–6.

13. Ridker PM, Rifai N, Clearfield M et al. Measurement of C-reactive protein for the targeting of statin therapy

in the primary prevention of acute coronary events. N Engl J Med 2001; 344:1959–65.

14. Ridker PM, Cannon CP, Morrow D et al. C-reactive protein levels and outcomes after statin therapy. N Engl J Med 2005; 352:20–8.

15. Moshage HJ, Roelofs HM, van Pelt JF et al. The effect of interleukin-1, interleukin-6 and its interrelationship on the synthesis of serum amyloid A and C-reactive protein in primary cultures of adult human hepatocytes. Biochem Biophys Res Commun 1988; 155:112–17.

16. Morrone G, Ciliberto G, Oliviero S et al. Recombinant interleukin 6 regulates the transcriptional activation of a set of human acute phase genes. J Biol Chem 1988; 263:12554–8.

17. Arnaud C, Burger F, Steffens S et al. Statins reduce interleukin-6-induced C-reactive protein in human hepatocytes: new evidence for direct antiinflammatory effects of statins. Arterioscler Thromb Vasc Biol 2005; 25:1231–6.

18. Xing Z, Gauldie J, Cox G et al. IL-6 is an antiinflammatory cytokine required for controlling local or systemic acute inflammatory responses. J Clin Invest 1998; 101:311–20.

19. van der Poll T, Levi M, Hack CE et al. Elimination of interleukin 6 attenuates coagulation activation in experimental endotoxemia in chimpanzees. J Exp Med 1994; 179:1253–9.

20. Volpato S, Guralnik JM, Ferrucci L et al. Cardiovascular disease, interleukin-6, and risk of mortality in older women: the women's health and aging study. Circulation 2001; 103:947–53.

21. Ridker PM, Rifai N, Stampfer MJ, Hennekens CH. Plasma concentration of interleukin-6 and the risk of future myocardial infarction among apparently healthy men. Circulation 2000; 101:1767–72.

22. Biasucci LM, Vitelli A, Liuzzo G et al. Elevated levels of interleukin-6 in unstable angina. Circulation 1996; 94:874–7.

23. Lindmark E, Diderholm E, Wallentin L, Siegbahn A. Relationship between interleukin 6 and mortality in patients with unstable coronary artery disease: effects of an early invasive or noninvasive strategy. JAMA 2001; 286:2107–13.

24. de Vries JE. Immunosuppressive and anti-inflammatory properties of interleukin 10. Ann Med 1995; 27: 537–41.

25. de Waal Malefyt R, Abrams J, Bennett B, Figdor CG, de Vries JE. Interleukin 10 (IL-10) inhibits cytokine synthesis by human monocytes: an autoregulatory role of IL-10 produced by monocytes. J Exp Med 1991; 174:1209–20.

26. Mallat Z, Besnard S, Duriez M et al Protective role of interleukin-10 in atherosclerosis. Circ Res 1999; 85:e17–24.

27. Pinderski Oslund LJ, Hedrick CC, Olvera T et al. Interleukin-10 blocks atherosclerotic events in vitro and in vivo. Arterioscler Thromb Vasc Biol 1999; 19:2847–53.

28. Fichtlscherer S, Breuer S, Heeschen C, Dimmeler S, Zeiher AM. Interleukin-10 serum levels and systemic endothelial vasoreactivity in patients with coronary artery disease. J Am Coll Cardiol 2004; 44:44–9.

29. Smith DA, Irving SD, Sheldon J, Cole D, Kaski JC. Serum levels of the antiinflammatory cytokine interleukin-10 are decreased in patients with unstable angina. Circulation 2001; 104:746–9.

30. Heeschen C, Dimmeler S, Hamm CW et al. Serum level of the antiinflammatory cytokine interleukin-10 is an important prognostic determinant in patients with acute coronary syndromes. Circulation 2003; 107:2109–14.

31. Henn V, Steinbach S, Buchner K, Presek P, Kroczek RA. The inflammatory action of CD40 ligand (CD154) expressed on activated human platelets is temporally limited by coexpressed CD40. Blood 2001; 98: 1047–54.

32. Schonbeck U, Libby P. The CD40/CD154 receptor/ligand dyad. Cell Mol Life Sci 2001; 58:4–43.

33. Henn V, Slupsky JR, Grafe M et al. CD40 ligand on activated platelets triggers an inflammatory reaction of endothelial cells. Nature 1998; 391:591–4.

34. Urbich C, Dernbach E, Aicher A, Zeiher AM, Dimmeler S. CD40 ligand inhibits endothelial cell migration by increasing production of endothelial reactive oxygen species. Circulation 2002; 106:981–6.

35. Andre P, Prasad KS, Denis CV et al. CD40L stabilizes arterial thrombi by a beta3 integrin—dependent mechanism. Nat Med 2002; 8:247–52.

36. Andre P, Nannizzi-Alaimo L, Prasad SK, Phillips DR. Platelet-derived CD40L: the switch-hitting player of cardiovascular disease. Circulation 2002; 106:896–9.

37. Schonbeck U, Varo N, Libby P, Buring J, Ridker PM. Soluble CD40L and cardiovascular risk in women. Circulation 2001; 104:2266–8.

38. Cipollone F, Ferri C, Desideri G et al. Preprocedural level of soluble CD40L is predictive of enhanced inflammatory response and restenosis after coronary angioplasty. Circulation 2003; 108:2776–82.

39. Aukrust P, Muller F, Ueland T et al. Enhanced levels of soluble and membrane-bound CD40 ligand in patients with unstable angina. Possible reflection of T lymphocyte and platelet involvement in the pathogenesis of acute coronary syndromes. Circulation 1999; 100:614–20.

40. Heeschen C, Dimmeler S, Hamm CW et al. Soluble CD40 ligand in acute coronary syndromes. N Engl J Med 2003; 348:1104–11.

41. Varo N, de Lemos JA, Libby P et al. Soluble CD40L: risk prediction after acute coronary syndromes. Circulation 2003; 108:1049–52.

42. Apple FS, Wu AH, Mair J et al. Future biomarkers for detection of ischemia and risk stratification in acute coronary syndrome. Clin Chem 2005; 51:810–24.

43. Arnhold J. Properties, functions, and secretion of human myeloperoxidase. Biochemistry (Mosc) 2004; 69:4–9.

44. Sugiyama S, Okada Y, Sukhova GK et al. Macrophage myeloperoxidase regulation by granulocyte macrophage colony-stimulating factor in human atherosclerosis and implications in acute coronary syndromes. Am J Pathol 2001; 158:879–91.

45. Podrez EA, Schmitt D, Hoff HF, Hazen SL. Myeloperoxidase-generated reactive nitrogen species convert LDL into an atherogenic form in vitro. J Clin Invest 1999; 103:1547–60.

46. Zhang R, Brennan ML, Fu X et al. Association between myeloperoxidase levels and risk of coronary artery disease. JAMA 2001; 286:2136-42.

47. Baldus S, Heeschen C, Meinertz T et al. Myeloperoxidase serum levels predict risk in patients with acute coronary syndromes. Circulation 2003; 108:1440–5.

48. Brennan ML, Penn MS, Van Lente F et al. Prognostic value of myeloperoxidase in patients with chest pain. N Engl J Med 2003; 349:1595–604.

49. Zalewski A, Macphee C. Role of lipoprotein-associated phospholipase A2 in atherosclerosis: biology, epidemiology, and possible therapeutic target. Arterioscler Thromb Vasc Biol 2005; 25:923–31.

50. Packard CJ, O'Reilly DS, Caslake MJ et al. Lipoprotein-associated phospholipase A2 as an independent predictor of coronary heart disease. West of Scotland Coronary Prevention Study Group. N Engl J Med 2000; 343:1148–55.

51. Koenig W, Khuseyinova N, Lowel H, Trischler G, Meisinger C. Lipoprotein-associated phospholipase A2 adds to risk prediction of incident coronary events by C-reactive protein in apparently healthy middle-aged men from the general population: results from the 14-year follow-up of a large cohort from southern Germany. Circulation 2004; 110:1903–8.

52. Ballantyne CM, Hoogeveen RC, Bang H et al. Lipoprotein-associated phospholipase A2, high-sensitivity C-reactive protein, and risk for incident coronary heart disease in middle-aged men and women in the Atherosclerosis Risk in Communities (ARIC) study. Circulation 2004; 109:837–42.

53. Blake GJ, Dada N, Fox JC, Manson JE, Ridker PM. A prospective evaluation of lipoprotein-associated phospholipase A(2) levels and the risk of future cardiovascular events in women. J Am Coll Cardiol 2001; 38:1302–6.

54. Brilakis ES, McConnell JP, Lennon RJ et al. Association of lipoprotein-associated phospholipase A2 levels with coronary artery disease risk factors, angiographic coronary artery disease, and major adverse events at follow-up. Eur Heart J 2005; 26:137–44.

55. Oldgren J, James S, Siegbahn A, Wallentin L. Lp-PLA$_2$ does not predict mortality or new ischemic events in acute coronary syndrome patients. Circulation 2005; 112:II387.

56. Luttun A, Tjwa M, Moons L et al. Revascularization of ischemic tissues by PlGF treatment, and inhibition of tumor angiogenesis, arthritis and atherosclerosis by anti-Flt1. Nat Med 2002; 8:831–40.

57. Autiero M, Luttun A, Tjwa M, Carmeliet P. Placental growth factor and its receptor, vascular endothelial growth factor receptor-1: novel targets for stimulation of ischemic tissue revascularization and inhibition of angiogenic and inflammatory disorders. J Thromb Haemost 2003; 1:1356–70.

58. Heeschen C, Dimmeler S, Fichtlscherer S et al. Prognostic value of placental growth factor in patients with acute chest pain. JAMA 2004; 291:435–41.

59. Cosin-Sales J, Kaski JC, Christiansen M et al. Relationship among pregnancy associated plasma protein-A levels, clinical characteristics, and coronary artery disease extent in patients with chronic stable angina pectoris. Eur Heart J 2005; 26:2093–8.

60. Cosin-Sales J, Christiansen M, Kaminski P et al. Pregnancy-associated plasma protein A and its endogenous inhibitor, the proform of eosinophil major basic protein (proMBP), are related to complex stenosis morphology in patients with stable angina pectoris. Circulation 2004; 109:1724–8.

61. Heeschen C, Dimmeler S, Hamm CW et al. Pregnancy-associated plasma protein-A levels in patients with acute coronary syndromes: comparison with markers of systemic inflammation, platelet activation, and myocardial necrosis. J Am Coll Cardiol 2005; 45:229–37.

62. Lund J, Qin QP, Ilva T et al. Circulating pregnancy-associated plasma protein A predicts outcome in patients with acute coronary syndrome but no troponin I elevation. Circulation 2003; 108:1924–6.

63. Bayes-Genis A, Conover CA, Overgaard MT et al. Pregnancy-associated plasma protein A as a marker of acute coronary syndromes. N Engl J Med 2001; 345:1022–9.

64. Laursen LS, Overgaard MT, Soe R et al. Pregnancy-associated plasma protein-A (PAPP-A) cleaves insulin-like growth factor binding protein (IGFBP)-5 independent of IGF: implications for the mechanism of IGFBP-4 proteolysis by PAPP-A. FEBS Lett 2001; 504:36–40.

65. Rader DJ. Inflammatory markers of coronary risk. N Engl J Med 2000; 343:1179–82.

Epidemiology of lipoprotein-associated phospholipase A₂

Isabella Kardys and Jacqueline CM Witteman

12

INTRODUCTION

Inflammation has been shown to play a central role in all phases of the atherosclerotic process.[1] Inflammatory pathways are implicated in early atherogenesis, in the progression of lesions, and in thrombotic complications. Clinical studies have shown associations of circulating markers of inflammation, such as C-reactive protein (CRP) and fibrinogen, with cardiovascular events.[2,3] Circulating inflammatory mediators may not only mark increased risk for cardiovascular events but also, in some cases, contribute to their pathogenesis. An inflammatory marker that has come under study recently with regard to cardiovascular disease is lipoprotein-associated phospholipase A₂ (Lp-PLA₂).

Lp-PLA₂ belongs to the superfamily of phospholipase A₂ enzymes.[4] It is a 45 kDa, Ca^{2+} independent protein, up-regulated in atherosclerotic plaques and strongly expressed in macrophages within the fibrous cap of rupture-prone lesions.[5] It is called lipoprotein-associated PLA₂ because of its tight association with lipoproteins: 80% of the enzyme in human plasma is located on low-density lipoprotein (LDL) and around 10% resides on high-density lipoprotein (HDL); in minor amounts, it associates with very low-density lipoprotein (VLDL) and lipoprotein(a).[6]

Lp-PLA₂ has been suggested to have both proatherogenic and antiatherogenic properties. When first identified, it was named platelet-activating factor acetylhydrolase (PAF-AH) owing to its ability to hydrolyze platelet-activating factor (PAF), a potent proinflammatory phospholipid. This ability suggests an antiatherogenic role of Lp-PLA₂, supported by research using mouse models.[7] However, in mice, Lp-PLA₂ is predominantly associated with HDL, and therefore the proposed antiatherogenic role of Lp-PLA₂ is, at least in part, based on its association with the antiatherogenic HDL. In addition to PAF hydrolysis, Lp-PLA₂ can hydrolyze a broad spectrum of substrates, including oxidized and polar phosphatidylcholines.[8] In humans, Lp-PLA₂ is bound predominantly to LDL cholesterol particles, and remains latent until the LDL-cholesterol particles undergo oxidative damage. Hereafter, Lp-PLA₂ cleaves the oxidized phosphatidylcholine into lysophosphatidylcholine and free fatty acid metabolites.[9] These mediators have been suggested to elicit proatherogenic effects.[10] These proatherogenic effects may outweigh the antiatherogenic effects in humans.

A substantial epidemiologic body of research is emerging on Lp-PLA₂ and risk of cardiovascular disease in humans. First, several, mostly small, case-control studies have suggested that Lp-PLA₂ may play a part in cardiovascular disease.[11–18] Hereafter, large cohort studies have examined Lp-PLA₂ in relation to incident cardiovascular events. Furthermore, studies were performed on Lp-PLA₂ and measures of atherosclerosis. Finally, Lp-PLA₂ genotypes have been used to shed more light on the relation between Lp-PLA$_2$ and cardiovascular disease. What follows is an overview of epidemiologic studies on Lp-PLA$_2$ and cardiovascular outcomes.

LP-PLA$_2$ AND INCIDENT CARDIOVASCULAR EVENTS

West of Scotland Coronary Prevention Study (WOSCOPS)

Studies on the association between Lp-PLA$_2$ and incident cardiovascular events are summarized in Table 12.1. The first study was performed within WOSCOPS, a trial in which 6595 men who had cholesterol levels between 4.5 and 6.0 mmol/L, but who had no history of a myocardial infarction, were randomly assigned to receive 40 mg of pravastatin or placebo daily. The present study was a case-control study, including 580 men who had an incident coronary event (non-fatal myocardial infarction, death from coronary heart disease, or revascularization), and 1160 controls matched on age and smoking status.[19] The study showed a relative risk (RR) of 1.18 (95% CI 1.05–1.33) per standard deviation (SD) of Lp-PLA$_2$ level for having a coronary event after adjustment for age, systolic blood pressure, plasma triglycerides, LDL and HDL cholesterol, fibrinogen, white cell count, and CRP. The multivariable adjusted RR for having a coronary event for the highest vs the lowest quintile of Lp-PLA$_2$ was significant and nearly doubled. There was no significant interaction with pravastatin use.

Women's Health Study (WHS)

The Women's Health Study is an ongoing randomized, double-blind, placebo-controlled trial of aspirin and vitamin E being conducted among 28 263 women aged ≥45 years with no history of cardiovascular disease or cancer. For the present study, 123 cases and 123 controls, matched for age and smoking status, were selected.[20]

Cases were defined as study participants who provided a baseline blood sample and who subsequently had a cardiovascular event as defined by death due to coronary heart disease, non-fatal myocardial infarction, or stroke. The mean follow-up period was 3 years. In univariate analyses, baseline levels of Lp-PLA$_2$ were higher among cases than controls (mean 1.20 vs 1.05 mg/L, $P = 0.016$). However, after adjustment for random assignment to aspirin or vitamin E, LDL and HDL cholesterol, body mass index (BMI), history of hypertension, history of diabetes, parental history of myocardial infarction, frequency of exercise, and current use of hormone replacement therapy, the effect was minimal and no longer statistically significant.

Atherosclerosis Risk in Communities (ARIC)

The ARIC study is a biracial cohort study of 15 792 men and women 45–64 years old, followed up for the subsequent development of a coronary heart disease event, including coronary heart disease-related death. A case-cohort design was constructed, the final sample size for the analysis being 608 cases and 740 non-cases.[21] The age-, race-, and sex-adjusted mean level of Lp-PLA$_2$ was higher in cases than in non-cases (404 vs 372 µg/L, $P < 0.001$). Lp-PLA$_2$ levels in the highest tertile were associated with increased coronary heart disease risk in a model adjusted for age, sex, and race (HR = 1.78, 95% CI 1.33–2.38); however, after additional adjustment for LDL and HDL cholesterol, smoking status, systolic blood pressure, diabetes, and CRP, the RR was attenuated and no longer significant. Further analyses revealed that in individuals with low LDL cholesterol, elevated Lp-PLA$_2$ was associated with a significantly higher risk for incident coronary heart disease, even after multivariable adjustment (HR = 2.08, 95% CI 1.20–3.62). No significant associations

Table 12.1 Lipoprotein-associated phospholipase A$_2$ (Lp-PLA$_2$) and cardiovascular events

Study	Authors, year	Subjects	Design	Cases	Non-cases	Determinant	Outcome	Association (multivariable adjusted)
WOSCOPS[19]	Packard et al, 2000	Hyperlipidemic men, mean age 56.8 years	Nested case control	580	1160	Lp-PLA$_2$ level (mg/L)	Non-fatal myocardial infarction, death from coronary heart disease, revascularization	RR = 1.18 (95% CI 1.05–1.33) per SD Lp-PLA$_2$ level
WHS[20]	Blake et al, 2001	Apparently healthy women aged ≥45 years	Nested case control	123	123	Lp-PLA$_2$ level (mg/L)	Non-fatal myocardial infarction, death from coronary heart disease, stroke	RR = 1.17 (95% CI 0.45–3.05) for highest vs lowest quartile of Lp-PLA$_2$ level
ARIC[21]	Ballantyne et al, 2004	Apparently healthy men and women aged 45–64 years	Case-cohort	608	740	Lp-PLA$_2$ level (µg/L)	Incident coronary heart disease, including coronary heart disease-related death	HR = 1.15 (95% CI 0.81–1.63) for highest vs lowest tertile of Lp-PLA$_2$ level. LDL cholesterol <130 mg/dl: HR = 2.08 (95% CI 1.20–3.62) for highest vs lowest tertile of Lp-PLA$_2$ level
ARIC[22]	Ballantyne et al, 2005	Apparently healthy men and women aged 45–64 years	Case-cohort	194	766	Lp-PLA$_2$ level (µg/L)	Ischemic stroke	HR = 1.93 (95% CI 1.14–3.27) for highest vs lowest tertile of Lp-PLA$_2$ level
MONICA[23]	Koenig et al, 2004	Apparently healthy men aged 45–64 years	Cohort	97	837	Lp-PLA$_2$ level (ng/ml)	Incident fatal or non-fatal acute myocardial infarction and sudden cardiac death	HR = 1.21 (95% CI 1.01–1.45) per SD Lp-PLA$_2$ level
Rotterdam Study[24]	Oei et al, 2005	Men and women aged ≥55 years	Case-cohort	308	1820	Lp-PLA$_2$ activity (nmol min^{-1} ml^{-1})	Coronary heart disease	HR = 1.20 (95% CI 1.04–1.39) per SD Lp-PLA$_2$ activity

Continued

Table 12.1 Lipoprotein-associated phospholipase A$_2$ (Lp-PLA$_2$) and cardiovascular events—cont'd

Study	Authors, year	Subjects	Design	Cases	Non-cases	Determinant	Outcome	Association (multivariable adjusted)
Rotterdam Study[24]	Oei et al, 2005	Men and women aged ≥55 years	Case-cohort	110	1820	Lp-PLA$_2$ activity (nmol min^{-1} ml^{-1})	Ischemic stroke	HR = 1.24 (95% CI 1.02–1.52) per SD Lp-PLA$_2$ activity
	Brilakis et al, 2005[25]	Men and women aged 26–76 years, undergoing clinically indicated coronary angiography	Cohort	61	405	Lp-PLA$_2$ level (ng/ml)	Death, myocardial infarction, coronary revascularization, stroke	HR = 1.30 (95% CI 1.06–1.59) per SD Lp-PLA$_2$ level

CI, confidence interval; HR, hazard ratio; SD, standard deviation; RR, relative risk.

were seen for individuals with higher LDL cholesterol.

The association between Lp-PLA$_2$ and ischemic stroke was also evaluated in the ARIC study using a case-cohort design.[22] Mean Lp-PLA$_2$ levels adjusted for sex, race, and age were higher in the 194 cases than the 766 non-cases (443 vs 374 μg/L). In a model adjusted for age, sex, race, smoking status, systolic blood pressure, LDL and HDL cholesterol levels, diabetes, hs-CRP level, antihypertensive medication and body mass index, Lp-PLA$_2$ levels in the highest tertile were associated with a hazard ratio (HR) of stroke of 1.93 (95% CI 1.14–3.27).

MONItoring of trends and determinants in CARdiovascular disease (MONICA) Augsburg study

The MONICA study consisted of 4022 individuals sampled at random from a mixed urban/rural area. The study on Lp-PLA$_2$ was based on 934 men, aged 45–46 years, followed up for incident fatal or non-fatal acute myocardial infarction and sudden cardiac death.[23] Lp-PLA$_2$ level was associated with an increase in coronary risk, with an HR of 1.21 (95% CI 1.01–1.45) per SD increase in Lp-PLA$_2$ after adjustment for age, systolic blood pressure, total cholesterol/HDL cholesterol ratio, physical activity, BMI, smoking, diabetes mellitus, alcohol intake, education, and CRP.

Rotterdam Study

The Rotterdam Study is a prospective population-based cohort study comprising 7983 men and women aged ≥55 years. For the present investigation, a case-cohort design was used, with 308 coronary heart disease cases, 110 ischemic stroke cases, and a random cohort of 1820 controls.[24] After adjustment for age, sex, BMI, systolic blood pressure, non-HDL cholesterol, HDL cholesterol, diabetes, smoking, cholesterol-lowering medication, CRP, white blood cell count, and alcohol consumption, the HR of coronary heart disease was 1.20 (95% CI 1.04–1.39) per SD of Lp-PLA$_2$ activity. The association was present over the entire range of cholesterol levels. For ischemic stroke, this HR was 1.24 (95% CI 1.02–1.52).

LP-PLA$_2$ AND INCIDENT CARDIOVASCULAR EVENTS IN PATIENTS WITH CORONARY ARTERY DISEASE

Brilakis et al evaluated the association between Lp-PLA$_2$ level and incidence of major adverse events in 504 patients, aged 26–76 years, undergoing clinically indicated coronary angiography.[25] The most frequent indications for this angiography were acute coronary syndrome, an abnormal nuclear imaging study, and dyspnea upon exertion. Major adverse events were defined as death (including cardiac death), myocardial infarction, coronary revascularization, and stroke. The HR for adverse events, adjusted for age, gender, smoking history, hypertension, total and HDL cholesterol, triglycerides, and log-CRP, was 1.30 (95% CI 1.06–1.59) per SD of Lp-PLA$_2$, showing that Lp-PLA$_2$ was an independent predictor.

LP-PLA$_2$ AND CORONARY ATHEROSCLEROSIS

Several studies have examined the association between Lp-PLA$_2$ and coronary artery disease ascertained by coronary angiography (Table 12.2). Shohet et al did so by means of two case-control studies.[26] First, Lp-PLA$_2$ activity was compared between 72 patients with angiographic evidence of severe coronary atherosclerosis and 72 patients with angiographically normal coronary arteries. Cases and controls were matched for age and sex. Although Lp-PLA$_2$ activity was slightly higher in cases, no significant differences could be demonstrated. To confirm these findings, a second study was undertaken in which 50 men

Table 12.2 Lipoprotein-associated phospholipase A$_2$ (Lp-PLA$_2$) and atherosclerosis

Authors, year	Subjects	Design	Cases	Non-cases	Determinant	Outcome	Association (multivariable adjusted)
Coronary atherosclerosis							
Shohet et al, 1999[26]	Patients undergoing coronary angiography	Case-control	72	72	Lp-PLA$_2$ activity (nmol min^{-1} ml^{-1})	Severe coronary disease (at least one vessel with >75% intraluminal obstruction)	Lp-PLA$_2$ activity not significantly different (P >0.2)
Shohet et al, 1999[26]	Men with documented premature coronary artery disease/apparently healthy controls	Case-control	50	50	Lp-PLA$_2$ activity (nmol min^{-1} ml^{-1})	Coronary artery bypass grafting, coronary angioplasty, angiographic evidence of >75% stenosis of at least one major coronary artery before the age of 60 in men and 65 in women	Lp-PLA$_2$ activity not significantly different
Caslake et al, 2000[27]	Men with stenotic disease on coronary angiography/post-myocardial infarction patients/normal controls	Case-control	48/46	54	Lp-PLA$_2$ level (ng/ml)	Stenotic disease/myocardial infarction	General linear model: Lp-PLA$_2$ level associated with coronary artery disease and post-myocardial infarction status, P = 0.01
Blankenberg et al, 2003[28]	Coronary angiography patients with stable angina pectoris or acute coronary syndrome/healthy control subjects	Case-control	496	477	Lp-PLA$_2$ activity (nmol min^{-1} ml^{-1})	Coronary artery disease (lumen reduction >30%)	OR = 1.8 (95% CI 1.01–3.2) for the highest vs the lowest quartile of Lp-PLA$_2$ activity
Brilakis et al, 2004[25]	Patients undergoing clinically indicated coronary angiography	Case-control	382	122	Lp-PLA$_2$ level (ng/ml)	Coronary artery disease	No independent association

Study	Population	Design			Marker	Outcome	Results
Winkler et al, 2005[29]	Patients hospitalized for coronary angiography	Case-control	2454	694	Lp-PLA$_2$ activity (U/1)	Coronary artery disease	OR = 1.06 (95% CI 0.84–1.34) for highest vs lowest quartile of Lp-PLA$_2$ activity. Non-users of lipid-lowering drugs: OR = 1.85 (95% CI 1.23–2.78) for highest vs lowest quartile of Lp-PLA$_2$ activity
Khuseyinova et al, 2005[30]	Patients with coronary stenosis/controls (occasional blood donors)	Case-control	312	479	Lp-PLA$_2$ level (ng/ml)	Coronary stenosis of ≥50% of luminal diameter	OR 1.84 (95% CI 1.12–2.99) for the highest vs the lowest quartile of Lp-PLA$_2$ level
Iribarren et al, 2005[31]	Men and women aged 18–30 years	Nested case-control	266	266	Lp-PLA$_2$ level (ng/ml) and Lp-PLA$_2$ activity (nmol min^{-1} ml^{-1})	Presence of calcified coronary plaque ascertained by cardiac computed tomography	Highest vs lowest tertile: Lp-PLA$_2$ level, OR = 1.28 (95% CI 1.03–1.60); Lp-PLA$_2$ activity, OR = 1.09 (95% CI 0.84–1.42)

Extracoronary atherosclerosis

Study	Population	Design			Marker	Outcome	Results
Campo et al, 2004[32]	Men and women with primary hypercholesterolemia	Case-control	76	114	Lp-PLA$_2$ activity (U/L)	Intima-media thickness > 1 mm	No association
Santos et al, 2004[33]	Patients referred for lower extremity arterial evaluation	Cross-sectional	247		Lp-PLA$_2$ level (ng/ml)	Ankle-brachial index	Multiple regression model: Lp-PLA$_2$ level associated with ankle-brachial index, $P = 0.05$

CI, Confidence interval; OR, odds ratio.

with documented premature coronary artery disease and apparently healthy controls were matched for LDL cholesterol and for age. Again, although Lp-PLA$_2$ activity was slightly higher in cases, it was not significantly different between cases and controls.

Caslake et al performed a case-control study among 48 male subjects with coronary artery disease ascertained by coronary angiography, 46 male post myocardial infarction patients, and 54 normal age-matched controls.[27] Lp-PLA$_2$ level was found to be associated with stenosis, independent of LDL and HDL cholesterol, smoking, and systolic blood pressure.

Blankenberg et al compared 496 coronary artery disease patients of both sexes suffering from stable angina pectoris or acute coronary syndrome, who had a lumen reduction >30% in at least one major coronary artery, to 477 healthy control subjects.[28] They found that, in the entire population, Lp-PLA$_2$ activity was borderline associated with the presence of coronary artery disease, but the case-control difference seemed mainly present in women. However, when the coronary artery disease patients were divided according to stable or unstable angina, Lp-PLA$_2$ activity appeared elevated in coronary artery disease patients suffering from acute coronary syndrome in both genders, even after controlling for age, BMI, ever smoking, history of hypertension, LDL and HDL cholesterol, and triglycerides. This association strengthened when excluding subjects receiving statin or angiotensin-converting enzyme (ACE) inhibitor therapy, and doing so, there was a gradual increase in Lp-PLA$_2$ activity amongst controls, stable angina pectoris patients, and patients with acute coronary syndrome present in both genders.

In the above-mentioned study of Brilakis et al, in which adverse events were examined in 504 patients undergoing clinically indicated angiography, the association between Lp-PLA$_2$ and angiographic coronary artery disease was also examined.[25] Although Lp-PLA$_2$ levels were higher in patients with more extensive angiographic coronary artery disease, Lp-PLA$_2$ was not independently predictive of angiographic coronary artery disease after adjusting for clinical and lipid variables.

Winkler et al performed a case-control study in 2454 subjects with angiographically confirmed coronary artery disease and in 694 control subjects.[29] Lp-PLA$_2$ activity was not associated with coronary artery disease in these subjects. However, after excluding subjects using lipid-lowering drugs (leaving 1630 subjects), Lp-PLA$_2$ activity was associated with risk of coronary artery disease, with an odds ratio (OR) of 1.85 (95% CI 1.23–2.78) for the highest vs the lowest quartile of Lp-PLA$_2$ activity after adjustment for aspirin, β-blockers, digitalis, age, gender, BMI, smoking, diabetes, hypertension, CRP, fibrinogen, white blood cell count, serum amyloid A, and LDL cholesterol.

Finally, Khuseyinova et al carried out a case-control study using 312 patients with a coronary stenosis of ≥50% of luminal diameter of at least one major coronary artery and 479 controls (occasional blood donors).[30] Mean Lp-PLA$_2$ levels were found to be significantly higher in patients (296.1 ± 122.5 ng/ml; mean ± SD) compared with controls (266.0 ± 109.8 ng/ml) ($P<0.0001$). After adjustment for age, gender, BMI, smoking status, alcohol intake, school education years, hypertension, diabetes, and total and HDL cholesterol, the OR of coronary artery disease was 1.84 (95% CI 1.12–2.99) for the highest vs the lowest quartile of Lp-PLA$_2$ concentration.

A study on the association between Lp-PLA$_2$ and coronary calcification ascertained by computed tomography (CT) was performed by Iribarren et al. It was a nested case-control study among participants of the Coronary Artery Risk Development in Young Adults (CARDIA) study, an ongoing investigation of heart disease risk factors and subclinical coronary artery disease among black and white men and women aged 18–30 years.[31] Cases ($n = 266$) were those with and controls ($n = 266$) those without evidence of calcified coronary plaque assessed by CT. The age-adjusted OR of calcified coronary plaque per SD increment was 1.40 (95% CI 1.17–1.67) and 1.39 (95% CI 1.14–1.70) for Lp-PLA$_2$ mass and activity, respectively. After adjusting for multiple covariates including LDL and HDL cholesterol, triglycerides, and CRP, a statistically significant association remained for Lp-PLA$_2$ level (OR = 1.28; 95% CI 1.03–1.60) but not for activity (OR = 1.09; 95% CI 0.84–1.42). The reason for the differential effect of adjustment may have been the stronger correlation between enzymatic activity and LDL cholesterol ($r = 0.52$) than between enzymatic level and LDL cholesterol ($r = 0.39$).

Lp-PLA$_2$ AND EXTRACORONARY ATHEROSCLEROSIS

Campo et al performed a study among 190 hypercholesterolemic Sicilian individuals, and found no association between Lp-PLA$_2$ activity and carotid intima–media thickness (IMT).[32] Patients with abnormal carotid IMT (>1 mm) had a mean Lp-PLA$_2$ activity of 471.3 U/L, whereas in controls this was 463.7 U/L, the difference not being statistically significant. Only unadjusted values of mean plasma Lp-PLA$_2$ activity for subjects with normal and high carotid IMT were presented in this study. Furthermore, none of the established cardiovascular risk factors was found to be associated with IMT, most probably owing to small sample size.

Santos et al investigated the association between Lp-PLA$_2$ level and ankle-brachial index among 247 patients referred for lower extremity arterial evaluation.[33] In a multiple regression model that included univariate predictors of ankle-brachial index (age, hypertension, smoking, fasting plasma glucose) and statin use, Lp-PLA$_2$ was a borderline-significant predictor of lower ankle-brachial index ($P = 0.05$).

GENETIC POLYMORPHISMS AFFECTING Lp-PLA$_2$

Lp-PLA$_2$ is encoded by a gene located at chromosome 6p12-p21.1. The gene is organized in 12 exons spanning at least 45 kb of DNA sequence.[34] In the Japanese, a point mutation, Val279Phe, has been found in exon 9. This mutation completely abolishes enzymatic activity of Lp-PLA$_2$ in homozygotes, and lowers enzymatic activity in heterozygotes compared to wild type: 27% of the Japanese population was found to be heterozygous for the mutant allele and 4% were homozygous.[34] This mutation has been shown to be associated with ischemic stroke, coronary artery disease, atherosclerosis, and abdominal aortic aneurysm in Japanese,[35–39] and thus these results suggest that Lp-PLA$_2$ may play a protective role in cardiovascular disease. However, the findings of these studies could not be reproduced in a large-scale study in 2819 Japanese patients with myocardial infarction and 2242 Japanese controls.[40]

In White populations, the Val279Phe mutation has not been found. However, several common variants are present. In vitro, the Ala379Val variant resulted in a 2-fold decrease in the affinity of Lp-PLA$_2$ for its substrate PAF, resulting in reduced degradation of PAF.[41] Abuzeid et al performed a European case-control study, which compared 527 post-myocardial infarction men with 566 age-matched controls.[42] Homozygosity for the Val allele was independently associated with lower risk of myocardial infarction. Since the Val allele results in lower Lp-PLA$_2$ activity, this study supported the proatherogenic, causal role of Lp-PLA$_2$ in coronary heart disease. These findings do not concur with the findings of Ninio et al.[43] Using a prospective cohort of 1314 coronary artery disease patients and a group of 485 healthy controls, they found that the Val allele was associated with an increased Lp-PLA$_2$ activity. Still, the Val allele was associated with a lower risk of future cardiovascular events and appeared less frequent in coronary artery disease cases than in controls. Campo et al examined the Arg92His, Ile198Thr, and Ala379Val variants in 190 hypercholesterolemic Sicilian individuals.[32] They found no associations of these variants with Lp-PLA$_2$ activity, and no associations with carotid IMT >1 mm. In summary, the findings from the genetic studies performed until now appear to be heterogeneous.

DISCUSSION

Recently, a large amount of epidemiologic research has emerged on the association between Lp-PLA$_2$ and cardiovascular disease, overall suggesting an independent, proatherogenic role for Lp-PLA$_2$ in cardiovascular disease. Several issues remain to be further addressed.

The first issue is whether the effect of Lp-PLA$_2$ on cardiovascular events is truly independent of LDL cholesterol, to which it is bound. The results from WOSCOPS suggested that elevated levels of Lp-PLA$_2$ are a strong risk factor for coronary heart disease that is independent of LDL cholesterol. However, in the WHS, after adjusting for LDL cholesterol, the effect of Lp-PLA$_2$ was minimal and no longer statistically significant. A clear reason for the discrepancy of the results from the WHS with the results from WOSCOPS could not be found. Use of hormone replacement therapy in the WHS may have played a part; however, this was not likely, since prevalence of use did not differ among cases and controls, and no effect modification owing to this factor was found. Furthermore, statistical power may have been low in the WHS, owing to small sample size (123 cases and 123 controls). Finally, the authors suggested the

possibility that the predictive value of Lp-PLA$_2$ may be limited to subjects with overt hyperlipidemia, as used in WOSCOPS. However, studies that followed also found associations between Lp-PLA$_2$ and cardiovascular disease in non-hyperlipidemic subjects. The ARIC study results showed that, in individuals with low LDL cholesterol, elevated Lp-PLA$_2$ was associated with a significantly higher risk for incident coronary heart disease, even after multivariable adjustment. In the total number of individuals, however, the association was not independent of LDL cholesterol. Differing results between this study and the two above-mentioned studies were suggested to be attributable to the markedly different study populations that were used. What followed was the MONICA study, again showing an independent association between Lp-PLA$_2$ and coronary events. Since the average total cholesterol level in the MONICA study was lower than in WOSCOPS but higher than in ARIC, this study suggested that Lp-PLA$_2$ has the ability to predict coronary events across all levels of total cholesterol. The Rotterdam Study provided further evidence for this, by finding associations independent of cholesterol, as did the study by Brilakis et al. Overall, most findings seem to support an independent role for Lp-PLA$_2$ in cardiovascular risk prediction.

Another issue is whether the effect of Lp-PLA$_2$ on cardiovascular events is exerted through atherosclerosis, or whether other mechanisms may contribute. With regard to Lp-PLA$_2$ and coronary atherosclerosis, the studies by Caslake et al, Blankenberg et al, Winkler et al, and Khuseyinova et al suggest independent associations, implying that Lp-PLA$_2$ indeed exerts its effect through atherosclerosis. However, the study by Brilakis et al does not show an independent association with coronary atherosclerosis, although in the same study Lp-PLA$_2$ was independently associated with cardiovascular events. An explanation for the discordance between the association of Lp-PLA$_2$ with angiographic coronary artery disease and the association with adverse events in this study might be the concept that molecules that regulate inflammation will not necessarily correlate with plaque burden measures, and may represent other characteristics than atherosclerotic mass, such as the inflammatory activity within plaques or the degree of plaque destabilization and ongoing ulceration or thrombosis. This study raises the question whether Lp-PLA$_2$ truly measures the extent of atherosclerosis, or whether it may be a marker of vulnerable plaque activity, which is further supported by the fact that Lp-PLA$_2$ is strongly expressed in macrophages within the fibrous cap of rupture-prone lesions.[5] To answer this, further investigation is required. The same issue has been raised with regard to CRP, which, in spite of its ability to predict cardiovascular events, does not seem to correlate equally well with atherosclerosis.[44]

Lp-PLA$_2$ has been suggested to have both proatherogenic and antiatherogenic properties. In humans, given that high levels of Lp-PLA$_2$ are associated with cardiovascular events, evidence is building up that the proatherogenic properties of Lp-PLA$_2$ outweigh the antiatherogenic properties. Until now, genetic research appears to yield inconclusive results with regard to this matter. The issue may be further resolved by research using Lp-PLA$_2$ inhibitors. Potent Lp-PLA$_2$ inhibitors have already been discovered[10] and tested for their ability to lower enzyme activity in plasma and at vascular sites.[45] In the future, randomized controlled trials using these compounds may demonstrate the consequences of reducing Lp-PLA$_2$ activity.

The final issue that needs to be investigated is a potential gender difference. The results from the WHS were not in agreement with studies showing an independent association between Lp-PLA$_2$ and cardiovascular events, possibly due to gender differences. Lp-PLA$_2$ has been found to be higher in men than in women.[21,24,25]

Furthermore, animal models have shown that estrogen decreases Lp-PLA$_2$ activity,[46] and Lp-PLA$_2$ levels are higher in women not taking hormone replacement therapy than among women taking hormone replacement therapy.[20] Further research regarding Lp-PLA$_2$ in populations stratified by gender, and also by other traditional risk factors such as age, is therefore supported.

In summary, studies regarding incident cardiovascular events suggest an independent, proatherogenic role for Lp-PLA$_2$. Studies on coronary atherosclerosis seem to lean in the same direction. With regard to extracoronary atherosclerosis, less research has been performed. Genetic studies have yielded heterogeneous results so far. In the future, trials using Lp-PLA$_2$ inhibitors may provide more insight into the mechanisms of action of Lp-PLA$_2$ and its usefulness for cardiovascular risk reduction.

REFERENCES

1. Libby P, Ridker PM, Maseri A. Inflammation and atherosclerosis. Circulation 2002; 105:1135–43.
2. Danesh J, Wheeler JG, Hirschfield GM et al. C-reactive protein and other circulating markers of inflammation in the prediction of coronary heart disease. N Engl J Med 2004; 350:1387–97.
3. Danesh J, Lewington S, Thompson SG et al; Fibrinogen Studies Collaboration. Plasma fibrinogen level and the risk of major cardiovascular diseases and nonvascular mortality: an individual participant meta-analysis. JAMA 2005; 294:1799–1809.
4. Tjoelker LW, Wilder C, Eberhardt C et al. Anti-inflammatory properties of a platelet-activating factor acetylhydrolase. Nature 1995; 374:549–53.
5. Kolodgie F, Burke A, Taye A et al. Lipoprotein-associated phospholipase A$_2$ is highly expressed in macrophages of coronary lesions prone to rupture. Circulation 2004; 110:246–7.
6. Karasawa K, Harada A, Satoh N, Inoue K, Setaka M. Plasma platelet activating factor-acetylhydrolase (PAF-AH). Prog Lipid Res 2003; 42:93–114.
7. Sudhir K. Clinical review: lipoprotein-associated phospholipase A$_2$, a novel inflammatory biomarker and independent risk predictor for cardiovascular disease. J Clin Endocrinol Metab 2005; 90:3100–5.
8. MacPhee CH, Moores KE, Boyd HF et al. Lipoprotein-associated phospholipase A$_2$, platelet-activating factor acetylhydrolase, generates two

bioactive products during the oxidation of low-density lipoprotein: use of a novel inhibitor. Biochem J 1999; 338(Pt 2):479–87.

9. Macphee CH, Nelson JJ. An evolving story of lipoprotein-associated phospholipase A2 in atherosclerosis and cardiovascular risk prediction. Eur Heart J 2005; 26:107–9.

10. Zalewski A, Macphee C. Role of lipoprotein-associated phospholipase A_2 in atherosclerosis: biology, epidemiology, and possible therapeutic target. Arterioscler Thromb Vasc Biol 2005; 25:923–31.

11. Ostermann G, Ruhling K, Zabel-Langhennig R et al. Plasma from atherosclerotic patients exerts an increased degradation of platelet-activating factor. Thromb Res 1987; 47:279–85.

12. Satoh K, Imaizumi T, Kawamura Y et al. Activity of platelet-activating factor (PAF) acetylhydrolase in plasma from patients with ischemic cerebrovascular disease. Prostaglandins 1988; 35:685–98.

13. Ostermann G, Lang A, Holtz H et al. The degradation of platelet-activating factor in serum and its discriminative value in atherosclerotic patients. Thromb Res 1988; 52:529–40.

14. Graham RM, Stephens CJ, Sturm MJ, Taylor RR. Plasma platelet-activating factor degradation in patients with severe coronary artery disease. Clin Sci (Lond) 1992; 82:535–41.

15. Yoshida H, Satoh K, Imaizumi T et al. Platelet-activating factor acetylhydrolase activity in red blood cell-stroma from patients with cerebral thrombosis. Acta Neurol Scand 1992; 86:199–203.

16. Satoh K, Yoshida H, Imaizumi T, Takamatsu S, Mizuno S. Platelet-activating factor acetylhydrolase in plasma lipoproteins from patients with ischemic stroke. Stroke 1992; 23:1090–2.

17. Stephens CJ, Graham RM, Sturm MJ, Richardson M, Taylor RR. Variation in plasma platelet-activating factor degradation and serum lipids after acute myocardial infarction. Coron Artery Dis 1993; 4:187–93.

18. Winkler K, Abletshauser C, Friedrich I et al. Fluvastatin slow-release lowers platelet-activating factor acetyl hydrolase activity: a placebo-controlled trial in patients with type 2 diabetes. J Clin Endocrinol Metab 2004; 89:1153–9.

19. Packard CJ, O'Reilly DS, Caslake MJ et al. Lipoprotein-associated phospholipase A_2 as an independent predictor of coronary heart disease. West of Scotland Coronary Prevention Study Group. N Engl J Med 2000; 343:1148–55.

20. Blake GJ, Dada N, Fox JC, Manson JE, Ridker PM. A prospective evaluation of lipoprotein-associated phospholipase A(2) levels and the risk of future cardiovascular events in women. J Am Coll Cardiol 2001; 38:1302–6.

21. Ballantyne CM, Hoogeveen RC, Bang H et al. Lipoprotein-associated phospholipase A_2, high-sensitivity C-reactive protein, and risk for incident coronary heart disease in middle-aged men and women in the Atherosclerosis Risk in Communities (ARIC) study. Circulation 2004; 109:837–42.

22. Ballantyne CM, Hoogeveen RC, Bang H et al. Lipoprotein-associated phospholipase A_2, high-sensitivity C-reactive protein, and risk for incident ischemic stroke in middle-aged men and women in the Atherosclerosis Risk in Communities (ARIC) Study. Arch Intern Med 2005; 28:2479–84.

23. Koenig W, Khuseyinova N, Lowel H, Trischler G, Meisinger C. Lipoprotein-associated phospholipase A_2 adds to risk prediction of incident coronary events by C-reactive protein in apparently healthy middle-aged men from the general population: results from the 14-year follow-up of a large cohort from southern Germany. Circulation 2004; 110:1903–8.

24. Oei HH, van der Meer IM, Hofman A et al. Lipoprotein-associated phospholipase A_2 activity is associated with risk of coronary heart disease and ischemic stroke: the Rotterdam Study. Circulation 2005; 111:570–5.

25. Brilakis ES, McConnell JP, Lennon RJ et al. Association of lipoprotein-associated phospholipase A_2 levels with coronary artery disease risk factors, angiographic coronary artery disease, and major adverse events at follow-up. Eur Heart J 2005; 26:137–44.

26. Shohet RV, Anwar A, Johnston JM, Cohen JC. Plasma platelet-activating factor acetylhydrolase activity is not associated with premature coronary atherosclerosis. Am J Cardiol 1999; 83:109–11, A8–9.

27. Caslake MJ, Packard CJ, Suckling KE et al. Lipoprotein-associated phospholipase A(2), platelet-activating factor acetylhydrolase: a potential new risk factor for coronary artery disease. Atherosclerosis 2000; 150:413–19.

28. Blankenberg S, Stengel D, Rupprecht HJ et al. Plasma PAF-acetylhydrolase in patients with coronary artery disease: results of a cross-sectional analysis. J Lipid Res 2003; 44:1381–6.

29. Winkler K, Winkelmann BR, Scharnagl H et al. Platelet-activating factor acetylhydrolase activity indicates angiographic coronary artery disease independently of systemic inflammation and other risk factors: the Ludwigshafen Risk and Cardiovascular Health Study. Circulation 2005; 111:980–7.

30. Khuseyinova N, Imhof A, Rothenbacher D et al. Association between Lp-PLA$_2$ and coronary artery disease: focus on its relationship with lipoproteins and markers of inflammation and hemostasis. Atherosclerosis 2005; 182:181–8.

31. Iribarren C, Gross MD, Darbinian JA et al. Association of lipoprotein-associated phospholipase A_2 mass and activity with calcified coronary plaque in young adults: the CARDIA study. Arterioscler Thromb Vasc Biol 2005; 25:216–21.

32. Campo S, Sardo MA, Bitto A et al. Platelet-activating factor acetylhydrolase is not associated with carotid intima-media thickness in hypercholesterolemic Sicilian individuals. Clin Chem 2004; 50:2077–82.

33. Santos S, Rooke TW, Bailey KR, McConnell JP, Kullo IJ. Relation of markers of inflammation (C-reactive protein, white blood cell count, and lipoprotein-associated phospholipase A$_2$) to the ankle-brachial index. Vasc Med 2004; 9:171–6.

34. Stafforini DM, Satoh K, Atkinson DL et al. Platelet-activating factor acetylhydrolase deficiency. A missense mutation near the active site of an antiinflammatory phospholipase. J Clin Invest 1996; 97:2784–91.

35. Hiramoto M, Yoshida H, Imaizumi T, Yoshimizu N, Satoh K. A mutation in plasma platelet-activating factor acetylhydrolase (Val279→Phe) is a genetic risk factor for stroke. Stroke 1997; 28:2417–20.

36. Yamada Y, Ichihara S, Fujimura T, Yokota M. Identification of the G994→T missense in exon 9 of the plasma platelet-activating factor acetylhydrolase gene as an independent risk factor for coronary artery disease in Japanese men. Metabolism 1998; 47:177–81.

37. Yamada Y, Yoshida H, Ichihara S et al. Correlations between plasma platelet-activating factor acetylhydrolase (PAF-AH) activity and PAF-AH genotype, age, and atherosclerosis in a Japanese population. Atherosclerosis 2000; 150:209–16.

38. Unno N, Nakamura T, Kaneko H et al. Plasma platelet-activating factor acetylhydrolase deficiency is associated with atherosclerotic occlusive disease in Japan. J Vasc Surg 2000; 32:263–7.

39. Unno N, Nakamura T, Mitsuoka H et al. Association of a G994→T missense mutation in the plasma platelet-activating factor acetylhydrolase gene with risk of abdominal aortic aneurysm in Japanese. Ann Surg 2002; 235:297–302.

40. Yamada Y, Izawa H, Ichihara S et al. Prediction of the risk of myocardial infarction from polymorphisms in candidate genes. N Engl J Med 2002; 347:1916–23.

41. Kruse S, Mao XQ, Heinzmann A et al. The Ile198Thr and Ala379Val variants of plasmatic PAF-acetylhydrolase impair catalytic activities and are associated with atopy and asthma. Am J Hum Genet 2000; 66:1522–30.

42. Abuzeid AM, Hawe E, Humphries SE, Talmud PJ. Association between the Ala379Val variant of the lipoprotein associated phospholipase A$_2$ and risk of myocardial infarction in the north and south of Europe. Atherosclerosis 2003; 168:283–8.

43. Ninio E, Tregouet D, Carrier JL et al. Platelet-activating factor-acetylhydrolase and PAF-receptor gene haplotypes in relation to future cardiovascular event in patients with coronary artery disease. Hum Mol Genet 2004; 13:1341–51.

44. Pearson TA, Mensah GA, Alexander RW et al. Markers of inflammation and cardiovascular disease: application to clinical and public health practice: A statement for healthcare professionals from the Centers for Disease Control and Prevention and the American Heart Association. Circulation 2003; 107:499–511.

45. Johnson A, Zalewski A, Janmohamed S et al. Lipoprotein-associated phospholipase A$_2$ (Lp-PLA$_2$) activity, an emerging CV risk marker, can be inhibited in atherosclerotic lesions and plasma by novel pharmacologic intervention: the results of a multi-center clinical study. Circulation 2004; 110:590.

46. Miyaura S, Maki N, Byrd W, Johnston JM. The hormonal regulation of platelet-activating factor acetylhydrolase activity in plasma. Lipids 1991; 26:1015–20.

SECTION III

Invasive imaging

Angiography and the vulnerable plaque

13

John A Ambrose and Cezar S Staniloae

INTRODUCTION

Caleb Hillier Parry, in his *Inquiry into the Symptoms and Causes of the Syncope Anginosa, Commonly Called Angina Pectoris, Illustrated by Dissections* (1799), recounts the classical anecdote in which, during the course of an autopsy, he discovered something hard and gritty in the coronary arteries. He noted that the vessels had hardened, or ossified, and later in the same book he states that, 'a principal cause of the syncope anginosa is to be looked for in disordered coronary arteries.'

Rudolf Virchow's 1856 analysis pointed out one of the first descriptions of atheroma, as a product of an inflammatory process within the intima. He also described the 'reactive fibrosis induced by proliferating connective tissue cells within the intima'.

Plaque rupture was reported for the first time during the autopsy of Bertel Thorvaldsen, the neoclassical Danish artist who died of sudden cardiac death in the Royal Theater in Copenhagen in 1844. On autopsy, his death was attributed to the rupture of an atherosclerotic plaque in the left coronary artery. It was stated that the vessel wall contained 'several atheromatous plaques, one of which quite clearly had ulcerated, pouring the atheromatous mass into the arterial lumen'.[1]

Rupture of so-called vulnerable or unstable atherosclerotic lesions is responsible for a significant proportion of myocardial infarctions (MIs) and strokes.

However, timely identification of such plaques prior to the acute event, in order to allow for aggressive local and/or systemic therapy, remains problematic. In order to address this problem, there is a need to develop techniques that can image the cellular, biochemical, and molecular components that typify the vulnerable plaque. To date, angiography has been the method of choice for detecting these problematic arterial lesions. However, this diagnostic technique does not provide insight into the disease state within the artery, and often fails to detect those lesions prone to thrombosis.

The purpose of this chapter is to summarize the current knowledge regarding the utility of angiography as a diagnostic tool for the detection of the vulnerable plaque.

RELATIONSHIP BETWEEN PLAQUE VULNERABILITY, ANGIOGRAPHIC OBSTRUCTION, AND ACUTE EVENTS

For the purposes of this chapter, the term *vulnerable plaque* (VP) will be used to describe plaques prone to disruption and/or thrombosis. This description situates the VP at the center of the clinical and pathologic spectrum of atherosclerotic disease, between the stable plaque, which is unlikely to progress to acute coronary syndromes (ACSs), and the destabilized or thrombosed plaque, which has already been disrupted or formed a

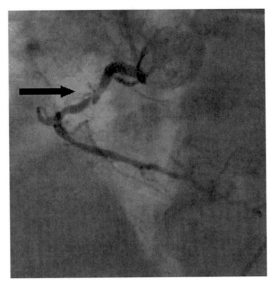

Figure 13.1 Angiographic view of a recently ruptured plaque (arrow) in the right coronary artery.

thrombus, and is the immediate cause of most ACS (Figure 13.1).

A series of landmark angiographic studies in the mid 1980s demonstrated that nearly two-thirds of all MIs originate at atherosclerotic lesions that lack hemodynamic significance.[2-6] The authors of these studies followed two trends: they either compared angiograms of patients who initially had stable coronary syndromes and went on to develop ACS, or they compared angiograms of patients with ACS who underwent follow-up studies. While severely stenotic lesions were routinely found on angiography after an acute event (thrombosed or unstable plaque), analyzing these lesions as an indicator of stenosis severity before the event is misleading. These lesions detected after the event contain significant thrombus that is not necessarily just acute[7] and the underlying atherosclerotic plaque is probably distorted by the plaque rupture. Thus, analysis of serial angiographic studies before and after an acute event is a better way of analyzing the degree of angiographic stenosis severity of the culprit

plaque before the event rather than just measuring stenosis severity immediately after the event.

Based on the findings of these original studies showing that MIs usually originate from non-significant lesions and as supported by future data, four variables have been identified as potential angiographic predictors of future events. They are the location of the plaque, the severity of stenosis, plaque morphology, and the geometry of the plaque.

LOCATION OF THE PLAQUE

Clinical observations reported that the majority of occlusive thromboses leading to acute coronary syndromes are clustered within the proximal portions of the major epicardial arteries. To investigate this hypothesis, numerous studies have attempted to map the portions of the coronary tree at highest risk for future events.

Gotsman et al[8] evaluated the angiographic appearance of the coronary arteries in 308 patients with ST-elevation myocardial infarction (STEMI) who received high-dose intravenous thrombolytic therapy. Coronary angiography was performed in this study 1 week after the admission. The majority of stenoses were proximal and related to bifurcations. These patients differed from a comparable, previously studied, control series of 302 patients with chronic stable angina pectoris who had more extensive disease; these stenoses were also located proximally and at bifurcations, but were more widely distributed in the coronary tree (Figure 13.2).

More recently, Gibson and colleagues used the angiographic data from four large trials on STEMI and measured the distance from the coronary ostia to the end of the culprit lesions. In 75% of the 1914 patients evaluated, the culprit lesions were located within the first 60 mm. The median distance from the vessel ostium to the end

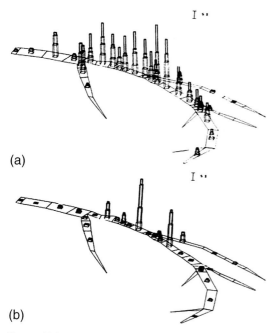

(a)

(b)

Figure 13.2 Angiographic location of coronary lesions in patients with stable angina (a), and patients with acute coronary syndromes (b). (Adapted after Gotsman et al.[8])

of the culprit lesion was 43 mm (mean 50 ± 34), and the relative distance from the vessel ostium to the end of the lesion was 29% (mean 33 ± 17%) of the total culprit artery length.[9]

Wang et al[10] examined the geographical distribution of occlusive thromboses throughout the coronary tree and demonstrated that such occlusions are clustered within the proximal portions of the major epicardial arteries. This group reported the first detailed study of the spatial distribution of coronary thromboses causing STEMI and suggested that these thromboses were highly clustered in discrete coronary segments within the proximal portions of large epicardial vessels (Figure 13.3). Furthermore, the finding of a lack of uniform distribution across the major epicardial vessels suggested a propensity for plaque erosion or rupture to occur in certain high-frequency regions within the coronary tree. These hot spots tend toward the proximal vessel, especially

in the left anterior descending artery (LAD) coronary artery. Half of the thromboses occurred within the first 25 mm of the vessel in the LAD and circumflex distribution, and within the first 45 mm of the right coronary artery (RCA). There was also a preferential distribution of the infarcts within the coronary tree, with the majority of thromboses occurring in the RCA (41%), followed by the LAD (39%).

Based on this evidence, it is believed that the proximal arterial tree is more susceptible to thrombosis and symptomatic acute coronary events than the more distal vessels. Therefore, coronary angiography could potentially be a useful tool in selecting plaques at future risk, simply based on their anatomic location.

PERCENT DIAMETER STENOSIS

The significance of arterial narrowing has been debated practically from the early days of coronary angiography. The initial belief was that the more severe a stenosis, the higher the likelihood of future coronary events. This was confirmed by serial angiographic studies which indicated that the more obstructive a plaque is, the more frequently it progressed to coronary occlusion[11] and/or gave rise to MI.[5] A different concept had been proposed by the studies of Ambrose et al[2] and Little et al.[3] These authors were the first to show that non-obstructive plaques were more likely to lead to acute coronary events, than the more advanced stenoses.

One of the early studies, the Coronary Artery Surgery Study (CASS), prospectively evaluated 2938 non-bypassed coronary segments in 298 patients.[11] Of 2161, 430, 258, and 89 segments narrowed <5%, 5–49%, 50–80%, and 81–95% at baseline, respectively, 0.7%, 2.3%, 10.1%, and 23.6%, respectively, became occluded during the 5-year follow-up period. Although an individual severe stenosis became occluded more frequently than did an individual less-severe stenosis, the less-obstructive

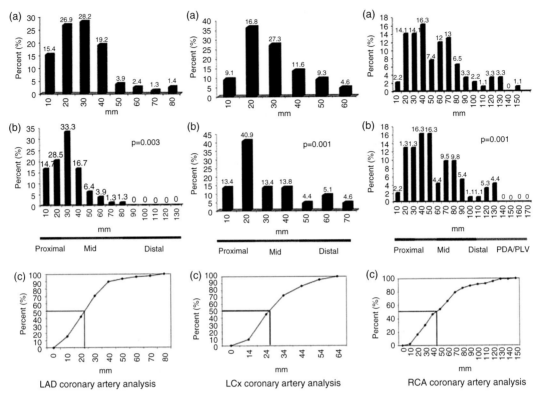

Figure 13.3 Coronary artery spatial distribution of acute myocardial infarction occlusions. (a) Ostium analysis of acute coronary occlusions. (b) Normalized segmental analysis of acute coronary occlusions. (c) Cumulative distribution curve demonstrates the cumulative frequency of thrombotic locations from ostium of left anterior descending coronary artery (LAD), LCx, left circumflex artery; RCA, right coronary artery; POA, posterior descending artery; PLV, posterolateral ventricular artery. (Adapted after Wang et al.[10])

plaques (<80% stenosis at baseline) gave rise to more occlusions than did the severely obstructive plaques (52 vs 21) because of their much greater number (Figure 13.4). Unfortunately, in that paper, no clinical data were included. It is unclear how many occlusions led to acute clinical events.

It is now generally accepted that coronary occlusion and myocardial infarction appear to most frequently evolve from mild to moderate stenoses, as initially reported by Ambrose et al[2] and Little et al[3] and later confirmed by others.[5,12] This has given rise to the notion that less-obstructive plaques may be more susceptible to rupture than larger plaques.[3,12] The smaller plaques, however, could be most dangerous

just because of their greater number, since they by far outnumber the severely obstructive plaques.[5,11] However, it must be appreciated that these mild to moderate lesions, leading to acute myocardial infarction (AMI), are not necessarily small plaques. Postmortem analysis indicates these are well-developed plaques, usually eccentric but with a preserved lumen.[13,14] Positive arterial remodeling, first described by Glagov et al,[15] is generally found at the site of acute lesions based on pathologic or intravascular ultrasound (IVUS) data.[16] Schoenhagen et al performed IVUS before coronary intervention and described the pattern of remodeling at the culprit lesion site in patients with stable vs unstable coronary syndromes.[16] They demonstrated

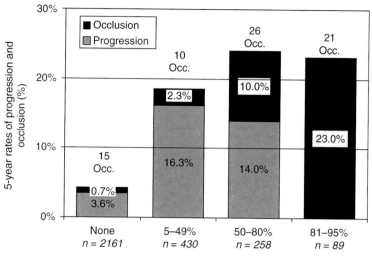

Figure 13.4 Five-year rates of progression and occlusion of coronary lesions relative to baseline stenosis severity. (Adapted after Alderman et al.[11])

a clear relationship between the direction and extent of arterial remodeling and clinical presentation of patients with coronary artery disease. Target lesion sites in patients with ACS more frequently exhibited positive remodeling and a large plaque area, whereas patients with a stable clinical presentation more frequently showed negative remodeling and a smaller plaque area.

There are other data supporting the concept that the less than severe stenosis is the usual precursor of acute events. Kolodgie et al[17] reported that thin-cap fibroatheromas (TCFAs) – the most frequent underlying plaque leading to STEMI – found at autopsy are usually only moderately stenotic. Analyzing pressure-fixed coronary arteries, over 80% of these TCFAs had <75% cross-sectional area luminal narrowing (≤50% diameter stenosis), whereas the mean cross-sectional area was only 60%.

A more recent retrospective cohort angiographic study was performed to determine the rate and features of clinical plaque progression.[18] The 3747 PCI (percutaneous coronary intervention) patients, enrolled consecutively, at multiple centers, in the National Heart, Lung, and Blood Institute Dynamic Registry were reviewed. Two hundred and sixteen (5.8%) of them required additional non-target lesion PCI for clinical plaque progression at 1 year. Fifty-nine percent presented with new unstable angina, and 9.3% presented with non-fatal MI.

Of the 216 patients requiring non-target lesion PCI, angiograms from 157 (72.7%) were available for independent evaluation. The lesion requiring non-target PCI was observed in a different coronary artery in 95 patients (61%), whereas 62 patients (39%) had progression in the same artery but in a separate segment (>5 mm) from the original PCI. The mean stenosis of the progressed lesion was 41.8 ± 20.8% at the initial angiogram and 83.9 ± 13.9% at the time of the second angiogram, with a mean increase in stenosis severity of 42.1 ± 21.9%. The majority of lesions requiring subsequent PCI were <50% in severity at the time of the initial PCI (95/157, 60.5%), whereas only 21 of 157 (13.4%) lesions were >70% in severity at the time of the initial angiogram.

Can one conclude anything about the importance of stenosis severity as a predictor of a future MI? Although considered a 'rudimentary' approach to predicting plaque vulnerability, stenosis severity assessment by coronary angiography, in our opinion, is not a reliable way of signaling potential sites of future coronary events. Under certain circumstances, the more severe the lesion, the less likely it may lead to AMI if it acutely closes off. This is probably true in chronic lesions, as acute total coronary occlusion will be silent or only accelerate angina since collaterals should protect against MI. However, an acutely progressing lesion in an unstable patient is not safe from infarction if the vessel totally occludes. Thus, percent diameter stenosis, in and of itself, is probably not a reliable indicator of the risk of future clinical instability.

PLAQUE MORPHOLOGY

The relationship between the angiographic morphology of coronary plaques and their histologic appearance was first described by Levin and Fallon, in 1982.[19] They correlated the postmortem coronary angiographic morphology with histologic sections of 73 localized subtotal coronary artery stenoses (50–99% reduction of luminal diameter) to determine whether complicated or uncomplicated atherosclerotic lesions could be detected angiographically. Lesions were divided into two types, according to angiographic morphology: type I stenoses had smooth borders, an hourglass configuration, and no intraluminal lucencies; type II stenoses had irregular borders or intraluminal lucencies. Histologic sections were also divided into two types: 'uncomplicated' stenoses had fatty or fibrous plaques with intact intimal surfaces and no superimposed thrombus; 'complicated' stenoses manifested plaque rupture, plaque hemorrhage, superimposed partially occluding thrombus, or recanalized thrombus. Among the 35 lesions with type I angiographic morphology, four (11.4%) were complicated lesions histologically. Among the 38 stenoses showing type II

angiographic morphology, 30 (78.9%) were complicated lesions. This was one of the first studies to conclude that angiography may have a role in detecting complicated stenoses on the basis of irregular borders or intraluminal lucencies. Coronary stenoses characterized angiographically by irregular borders or intraluminal lucencies were considered the clinically more dangerous 'complicated' type.

These data were clinically confirmed by Ambrose et al, who correlated the eccentric, irregular (complex) culprit lesion on angiography with an acute presentation of either unstable angina or non-Q MI. In a series of papers, this lesion was found in 50–70% of the culprit lesion in these syndromes and in <20% of stable presentations.[20–22]

One of the first attempts to describe the relationship between plaque morphology and clinical presentation was made by these investigators in 1985.[20] In 110 patients with either stable or unstable angina, the morphology of coronary artery lesions was qualitatively assessed at angiography. Each obstruction reducing the luminal diameter of the vessel by ≥50% was categorized into one of the following four groups:

- concentric (symmetric narrowing)
- type I eccentric (asymmetric narrowing with smooth borders and a broad neck)
- type II eccentric (asymmetric with a narrow neck or irregular borders, or both)
- multiple irregular coronary narrowings in series.

For the entire group, type II eccentric lesions were significantly more frequent in the 63 patients with unstable angina ($P < 0.001$), whereas concentric and type I eccentric lesions were seen more frequently in the 47 patients with stable angina ($P < 0.05$). The authors concluded that type II eccentric lesions are frequent in patients with unstable angina and probably represent ruptured atherosclerotic plaques or partially occlusive thrombi, or both. These findings were confirmed in subsequent postmortem and clinical angiographic studies.[6,13,14]

Recently, using angioscopy, Waxman and colleagues evaluated the value of Ambrose's angiographic coronary lesion types to predict the presence of disrupted plaques and thrombus.[23] Angioscopy was performed before angioplasty in 60 patients with various coronary syndromes and culprit lesions that were not totally occlusive. Lesions were classified angiographically according to Ambrose's criteria as concentric, type I and II eccentric, and multiple irregularities, or as complex or non-complex, and then compared with the corresponding angioscopic findings. Disruption and/or thrombus were seen in 17 of 19 type II eccentric lesions and 21 of 23 angiographically complex lesions and had the highest positive predictive value to detect complicated atherosclerotic plaques (type II eccentric lesions, positive predictive value 89%; complex lesions, 91%). The authors concluded that Ambrose's type II eccentric stenoses and angiographically complex lesions are strongly associated with disrupted plaques and/or thrombus, as assessed by angioscopy, and represent unstable

plaque substrates. All of these data suggest that the complex lesion seen on angiography is a specific indicator of plaque rupture and/or intracoronary thrombus except perhaps in a heavily calcified vessel. However, its sensitivity is probably only no better than moderate given the inherent limitations of angiography to visualize only the lumen of the vessel and the presence of other confounding variables such as limited resolution, inadequate views, overlying branches, and lesion haziness that tend to obscure the diagnosis (Figure 13.5).

Although the angiographic appearance of a disrupted or thrombotic lesion had been described, the predictive value of such angiographic markers had to be determined. Chester et al[24] studied 222 patients with chronic stable angina who were on a waiting list for single-vessel PCI of an unoccluded lesion and underwent repeat angiography immediately before the procedure. At first angiography, there were 52 unheralded complex target lesions (23%) and 170 smooth target stenoses (77%). At follow-up, 14% of the complex lesions had progressed compared with only 4% of the smooth lesions ($P < 0.02$). The authors concluded that, in this study, complex stenoses were 4.2 times more

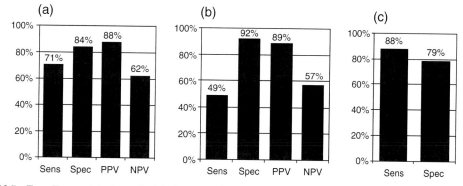

Figure 13.5 Type II eccentric (complex) lesions correlation with clinical presentation (a), angioscopic evidence of plaque disruption (b), and/or intracoronary thrombus and histology (c). (a) Percent with unstable angina. (From Ambrose et al.[20]) (b) Percent with plaque disruption and/or intracoronary thrombus (ICT) on angioscopy. (From Waxman et al.[23]) (c) Irregular stenosis on postmortem angiography with 'complicated' histology. (From Levin and Fallon.[19]) Sens, sensitivity; Spec, specificity; PPV, positive predictive value; NPV, negative predictive value.

likely to progress than smooth stenoses. Thus, if untreated with PCI, complex lesions are prone to progression. Whereas these data were published prior to the use of more potent antiplatelet and statin therapy, they tell us of the potential danger of these lesions.

That complex lesions on angiography indicate a worse prognosis was also suggested by Goldstein et al.[25] These authors found multiple complex plaques on angiography in 39.5% of patients presenting with AMI. Those with multiple complex lesions were more likely to undergo repeat or a second percutaneous intervention (in the non-infarct lesion) or coronary bypass surgery on follow-up than patients with a single complex lesion.

GEOMETRY OF PLAQUE

The geometry of the atherosclerotic plaque has been postulated to play a significant role in the biology of plaque progression, as well as in plaque vulnerability. It is thought that plaque configuration is dynamically influenced by both the longitudinal flexion and the circumferential cyclic bend of the coronary arteries.

The coronary arteries, particularly the LAD coronary artery, tethered to the surface of the beating heart, undergo cyclic longitudinal deformations by axial bending (flexion) and stretching. Angiographically, the angle of flexion was recently found to correlate with subsequent lesion progression, but the coefficient of correlation was low.[26] Like circumferential bending, a sudden accentuated longitudinal flexion may trigger plaque disruption, whereas long-term cyclic flexion may fatigue and weaken the plaque.[26]

The normal compliant arteries accommodate a cyclic diastolic–systolic change in lumen diameter of about 10%.[27] This change becomes smaller with age and during atherogenesis because of the increase in stiffness.[28] Generally, concentric plaques do not change as much as eccentric plaques during the cardiac cycle. The latter typically bend at their edges, i.e. at the junction between the stiff plaque and the more compliant plaque-free vessel wall. Also, changes in vascular tone cause bending of eccentric plaques at their edges. Cyclic bending may, in the long term, weaken these points, leading to unprovoked 'spontaneous' fatigue disruption, whereas a sudden accentuated bending may trigger rupture of a weakened cap. Therefore, the geometry of the plaque could potentially influence the rapidity of plaque progression, as well as the occurrence of an acute coronary syndrome.

Ledru and colleagues[29] looked at the geometry of atheromatous plaques in an attempt to identify predictors of future myocardial infarction. They compared angiograms from patients before and after the MI. The culprit lesions, leading to future MIs, were more symmetrical and had steeper outflow angles than the controls. Their findings suggest a potential role of the continuous cyclic bending of the coronary arteries during the cardiac cycle. However, these calculations appear too cumbersome to be of great value in a prospective evaluation to identify lesions likely to progress to an acute coronary syndrome.

LIMITATIONS OF ANGIOGRAPHY IN DETECTING VULNERABLE PLAQUE

Coronary angiography may reveal advanced lesions, plaque disruption, luminal thrombosis, and calcification, but other qualitative features of the underlying plaque cannot be assessed by this imaging technique. Visualization of the vessel wall and the plaque itself rather than the lumen is necessary for the identification of early lesions and vulnerable plaques at high risk of becoming culprits. Nevertheless, coronary angiography remains the main tool in evaluating the coronary arteries in the current clinical practice, and one should be able to use it to its advantage in the attempt to predict future plaques at risk. In the near future, newer non-invasive imaging modalities such as multislice computed tomography (CT) and magnetic resonance imaging (MRI) will limit the importance of invasive coronary angiography as a diagnostic tool and also allow for characterization of the vessel wall.[30] Already routinely utilized in many centers, multislice CT is changing the role of invasive angiography more towards therapy and less towards diagnosis.

In spite of the major limitations of the existing studies looking at the role of invasive angiography in predicting future vulnerable plaques, one might use variables such as plaque location and morphology as a basic tool to determine the management of atherosclerotic plaques. Prospective clinical trials designed to look at the natural history of different angiographic types of atherosclerotic plaques are required to answer definitively the question about the role of angiography in the diagnosis of the vulnerable plaque.

CONCLUSIONS

Coronary angiography can identify destabilized/unstable plaque. Complex lesion morphology is mildly to moderately sensitive but highly specific for the presence of plaque disruption and/or thrombus.

Angiography is inherently incapable of identifying most vulnerable high-risk plaques, as the potential for destabilization of these plaques involves non-angiographically detectable abnormalities of the vessel wall. However, in some cases, a moderately stenotic, irregular-appearing stenosis on angiography in a clinically stable patient (? proximal location and/or at a branch point) may be a predictor of subsequent acute events, as this probably represents an already destabilized plaque that is presently quiescent. This should be prospectively validated. Natural history

studies assessing the positive predictive value (PPV) of angiographic variables, including the above as well as other imaging modalities, are in progress.

REFERENCES

1. Society minutes. Dahlerup, 1844:214–18.
2. Ambrose JA, Tannenbaum MA, Alexopoulos D et al. Angiographic progression of coronary artery disease and the development of myocardial infarction. J Am Coll Cardiol 1988; 12:56–62.
3. Little WC, Constantinescu M, Applegate RJ et al. Can coronary angiography predict the site of a subsequent myocardial infarction in patients with mild-to-moderate coronary artery disease? Circulation 1988; 78:1157–66.
4. Hackett D, Davies G, Maseri A. Pre-existing coronary stenoses in patients with first myocardial infarction are not necessarily severe. Eur Heart J 1988; 9: 1317–23.
5. Giroud D, Li JM, Urban P, Meier B, Rutishauer W. Relation of the site of acute myocardial infarction to the most severe coronary arterial stenosis at prior angiography. Am J Cardiol 1992; 69:729–32.
6. Lichtlen PR, Nikutta P, Jost S et al. Anatomical progression of coronary artery disease in humans as seen by prospective, repeated, quantitated coronary angiography. Relation to clinical events and risk factors. The INTACT Study Group. Circulation 1992; 86:828–38.
7. Rittersma SZ, van der Wal AC, Koch KT et al. Plaque instability frequently occurs days or weeks before occlusive coronary thrombosis: a pathological thrombectomy study in primary percutaneous coronary intervention. Circulation 2005; 111:1160–5.
8. Gotsman M, Rosenheck S, Nassar H et al. Angiographic findings in the coronary arteries after thrombolysis in acute myocardial infarction. Am J Cardiol 1992; 70:715–23.
9. Gibson CM, Kirtane AJ, Murphy SA et al. Distance from the coronary ostium to the culprit lesion in acute ST-elevation myocardial infarction and its implications regarding the potential prevention of proximal plaque rupture. J Thromb Thrombolysis 2003; 15:189–96.
10. Wang JC, Normand SL, Mauri L, Kuntz RE. Coronary artery spatial distribution of acute myocardial infarction occlusions. Circulation 2004; 110:278–84.
11. Alderman EL, Corley SD, Fisher LD et al. Five-year angiographic follow-up of factors associated with progression of coronary artery disease in the Coronary Artery Surgery Study (CASS). CASS Participating Investigators and Staff. J Am Coll Cardiol 1993; 22:1141–54.
12. Nobuyoshi M, Tanaka M, Nosaka H et al. Progression of coronary atherosclerosis: is coronary spasm

related to progression? J Am Coll Cardiol 1991; 18: 904–10.

13. Virmani R, Kolodgie FD, Burke AP, Farb A, Schwartz SM. Lessons from sudden coronary death: a comprehensive morphological classification scheme for atherosclerotic lesions. Arterioscler Thromb Vasc Biol 2000; 20:1262–75.

14. Burke AP, Farb A, Malcom GT et al. Plaque rupture and sudden death related to exertion in men with coronary artery disease. JAMA 1999; 281:921–6.

15. Glagov S, Weisenberg E, Zarins CK, Stankunavicius R, Kolettis GJ. Compensatory enlargement of human atherosclerotic coronary arteries. N Engl J Med 1987; 316:1371–5.

16. Schoenhagen P, Ziada KM, Kapadia SR et al. Extent and direction of arterial remodeling in stable versus unstable coronary syndromes: an intravascular ultrasound study. Circulation 2000; 101:598–603.

17. Kolodgie FD, Virmani R, Burke AP et al. Pathologic assessment of the vulnerable human coronary plaque. Heart 2004; 90:1385–91.

18. Glaser R, Selzer F, Faxon DP et al. Clinical progression of incidental, asymptomatic lesions discovered during culprit vessel coronary intervention. Circulation 2005; 111:143–9.

19. Levin DC, Fallon JT. Significance of the angiographic morphology of localized coronary stenoses: histopathologic correlations. Circulation 1982; 66:316–20.

20. Ambrose JA, Winters SL, Stern A et al. Angiographic morphology and the pathogenesis of unstable angina pectoris. J Am Coll Cardiol 1985; 5:609–16.

21. Ambrose JA, Winters SL, Arora RR et al. Coronary angiographic morphology in myocardial infarction: a link between the pathogenesis of unstable angina and myocardial infarction. J Am Coll Cardiol 1985; 6:1233–8.

22. Ambrose JA, Dangas G. Unstable angina: current concepts of pathogenesis and treatment. Arch Intern Med 2000; 160:25–37.

23. Waxman S, Mittleman MA, Zarich SW et al. Plaque disruption and thrombus in Ambrose's angiographic coronary lesion types. Am J Cardiol 2003; 92:16–20.

24. Chester MR, Chen L, Kaski JC. The natural history of unheralded complex coronary plaques. J Am Coll Cardiol 1996; 28:604–8.

25. Goldstein JA, Demetriou D, Grines CL et al. Multiple complex coronary plaques in patients with acute myocardial infarction. N Engl J Med 2000; 343: 915–22.

26. Stein PD, Hamid MS, Shivkumar K et al. Effects of cyclic flexion of coronary arteries on progression of atherosclerosis. Am J Cardiol 1994; 73:431–7.

27. Lee RT, Kamm RD. Vascular mechanics for the cardiologist. J Am Coll Cardiol 1994; 23:1289–95.

28. Alfonso F, Macaya C, Goicolea J et al. Determinants of coronary compliance in patients with coronary artery disease: an intravascular ultrasound study. J Am Coll Cardiol 1994; 23:879–84.

29. Ledru F, Theroux P, Lesperance J et al. Geometric features of coronary artery lesions favoring acute occlusion and myocardial infarction: a quantitative angiographic study. J Am Coll Cardiol 1999; 33: 1353–61.

30. Viles-Gonzalez JF, Poon M, Sanz J et al. In vivo 16-slice, multidetector-row computed tomography for the assessment of experimental atherosclerosis: comparison with magnetic resonance imaging and histopathology. Circulation 2004; 110:1467–72.

Imaging the vulnerable plaque by ultrasound

14

Ehtisham Mahmud and Anthony N DeMaria

INTRODUCTION

In the early stages of disease, atherosclerosis is characterized by lipid-laden plaque accumulation in the arterial vasculature, whereas in later stages this is often replaced by fibrosis and calcification. Vulnerable plaque has come to be defined as an atherosclerotic plaque prone to disruption and/or thrombosis. The non-invasive and invasive ultrasound imaging modalities that have been used to identify vulnerable plaques include intravascular ultrasound (IVUS), transcutaneous ultrasound to visualize carotid arteries, and contrast echocardiography. Of these, carotid artery ultrasound is well established as a technique to diagnose and monitor early and progressive atherosclerosis. Recently, ultrasound plaque characterization has enabled the identification of lesions more prone to embolization during carotid stenting.[1] Although transthoracic echocardiography has been used to visualize large epicardial coronary arteries, visualization of coronary plaque is limited by this technique. Miniaturization of ultrasound transducers and positioning them at the tip of small-diameter catheters has made IVUS possible. When an IVUS catheter is placed in a coronary artery, an ultrasound beam is directed perpendicular to the course of the vessel and steered either electronically or mechanically throughout its 360° circumference. An image of cross-sectional arterial anatomy is obtained,[2] and in normal arteries these images depict a sharp, bright endothelial/lumen border, a clear sonolucent media, and an echo-dense adventitia.[3]

Plaque constitutes thickening of the intimal–medial layers of the vessel wall. Plaque morphology may be characterized by ultrasound according to the intensity of the signals recorded: soft (gray) echoes, very high-intensity (bright) echoes which usually create distal shadowing, and echoes of increased but intermediate intensity. These ultrasound features correspond to usual tissue components, calcification, and fibrosis respectively.[4] In addition, echolucent or signal-free zones have been found to represent lipid accumulations.[5–8] Plaques can be circumferential and occupy the entire perimeter of a vessel, or be eccentric and occupy only a portion of the vessel circumference.

Atherosclerotic lesions often result in an expansion of the overall vessel to accommodate plaque without encroaching upon the lumen, a process termed positive remodeling.[9] Furthermore, ruptures or ulcerations of lesions can also be detected with ultrasound, typically seen with IVUS in culprit coronary arteries responsible for acute coronary syndromes (ACS).[10] As compared with angiography, which evaluates the vessel lumen and thereby assesses atherosclerosis only indirectly, ultrasound has the advantage of directly visualizing plaque within the vessel wall. Thus, an ultrasound examination can detect and localize plaque, characterize it as hypoechoic, fibrous, or calcified, and determine whether it is ulcerated or manifests positive expansile remodeling.

UNSTABLE CORONARY PLAQUES: PREVALENCE

Angiographic and angioscopic studies

Data on the prevalence of unstable plaques obtained by angiography and angioscopy in patients undergoing cardiac catheterization have corroborated earlier pathologic studies[11] showing that patients, especially ones presenting with ACS, often have multiple complex and disrupted coronary plaques. In an angiographic study, Goldstein et al[12] demonstrated that ~60% of patients presenting with acute myocardial infarction have a single complex plaque, whereas ~40% of patients have multiple complex coronary plaques and this finding portends a worse 1-year prognosis. The finding of multiple plaques with vulnerable characteristics throughout the coronary vasculature by angiography is also consistent with angioscopic data showing that ~90% of culprit lesions are yellow and histologically associated with vulnerable characteristics.[13] Interestingly, follow-up angioscopic studies suggest that complete plaque healing, manifested by neointimal coverage of the disrupted plaque and resolution of thrombus, occurs only in a minority of such lesions (at 13 months follow-up)[14] but lipid-lowering therapy with atorvastatin reduces the yellow score of such lesions, compared with a control group.[15]

Intravascular ultrasound studies

IVUS has also been used to examine plaque prevalence. In recent studies, IVUS evaluation of the three major coronary arteries in patients with ACS has detected a 25% prevalence of multiple ruptured coronary plaques.[16] This is probably an underestimate, as IVUS is limited in its ability to adequately image plaque erosion and overlying thrombus, which may obscure ruptured plaques. In addition, some plaque ruptures may have occurred at bifurcation points and branch vessels that were not imaged in most studies. In a small study of 24 patients (72 arteries) with troponin-positive ACS, Rioufol et al[17] demonstrated a prevalence of two ruptured plaques (range 0–6) per patient, with 37.5% of patients having plaque rupture at the presumed culprit lesion whereas 79% of patients also had ruptured plaques in non-culprit arteries. In a larger study of 235 patients, Hong et al[18] demonstrated that although plaque rupture in the infarct-related vessel occurs in 66% of acute myocardial infarction (AMI) patients and 27% of stable angina patients, multiple plaque ruptures occur in 20% of AMI and 6% of stable angina patients. Tanaka et al[19] performed a similar study in patients with ACS and showed that 47% of culprit lesions had plaque rupture and that 24% of patients had plaque rupture in more than one coronary artery. The difference in the prevalence of plaque rupture in these studies also reflects differences in the patient population, selection bias in IVUS imaging, and the retrospective nature of some studies. However, these data are consistent with other IVUS studies demonstrating culprit lesion plaques having more vulnerable characteristics, including greater plaque burden, positive remodeling, and presence of thrombus, than non-culprit plaques in patients with ACS.[20,21]

The pattern of calcification is also different in patients with ACS and plaque rupture. ACS patients have less overall calcification and a larger number of small, discrete calcium deposits (often present as spotty superficial and/or deep calcium deposits) than patients with stable angina.[22–24] Regardless of the presence of various anatomic features of a vulnerable plaque, 50% of ruptured plaques heal in response to medical therapy without a significant change in plaque dimension,[25] a feature previously documented in pathologic studies that showed multiple layers of plaque rupture and healing within the same area.[26]

PLAQUE CHARACTERIZATION BY SURFACE ULTRASOUND

Surface ultrasound has been effectively utilized to quantify carotid arterial wall thickening, which has also proven to be a strong indicator of the presence of coronary artery disease (CAD).[27,28] Furthermore, there is a significant correlation between carotid and coronary plaque vulnerability,[29,30] with plaque echogenicity assessed by ultrasound with integrated backscatter (IBS) predicting lipid content of plaques.[31,32] Echolucent plaques with low IBS values have been shown to be macrophage-rich plaques[33] and to be associated with lipid-rich vulnerable lesions.[34] The presence of echolucent carotid plaques, as detected by IBS analysis, has also been shown to predict cardiovascular events in patients with CAD,[29] whereas treatment with pravastatin, in non-hypercholesterolemic patients with CAD, results in a reduction in carotid plaque echogenicity without a change in plaque volume, indicating plaque stabilization[35] (Figure 14.1).

Box 14.1 IVUS characteristics associated with culprit lesions
1. Echolucent core
2. Eccentricity
3. Positive remodeling
4. Ulceration
5. Thrombosis
6. Calcification

PLAQUE CHARACTERIZATION BY INTRAVASCULAR ULTRASOUND

Volumetric analysis of IVUS images can accurately quantitate atheroma volume and is useful in assessing plaque regression and progression in trials of lipid-lowering agents.[36] Three-dimensional (3D) reconstruction allows morphologic assessment of lesions but is not as useful in detecting clinically relevant plaque characteristics such as lipid content. Initially, to identify vulnerable plaque by IVUS, image characteristics of culprit lesions which had led to ACS were determined (Box 14.1).[10] Although these characteristics were observed with variable frequency, most culprit plaques were consistently hypoechoic, eccentric, positively remodeled, and relatively free of calcification.

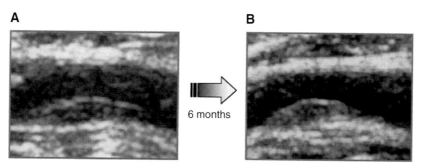

A   **B**   6 months

Figure 14.1 Representative integrated backscatter images of carotid atheroma (cIBS) from baseline to follow-up. (**A**) Carotid atheroma at pretreatment. Values of cIBS and plaque maximum intima–media thickness (IMT_{max}) of this plaque are −17.8 dB and 2.05 mm, respectively. (**B**) The same carotid atheroma post-pravastatin therapy (6 months). Values of calibrated integrated backscatter (cIBS) and plaque IMT_{max} of this plaque are −14.2 dB and 2.10 mm, respectively. (Reprinted with permission from Watanabe et al.[35])

Although the proposed IVUS descriptors of vulnerable plaque seem reasonable, a number of considerations prevent them from being accepted as definitive. First, most studies upon which the descriptors are based have been retrospective, and plaque morphology following an acute event does not provide definitive information regarding morphology prior to the episode. Secondly, the characteristics reported for vulnerable plaque by IVUS have differed from study to study. Thirdly, non-culprit plaques in stable patients have often been found to show the same characteristics associated with vulnerable plaque. Schoenhagen et al[37] found that culprit lesions from patients with ACS were identical in 'vulnerable IVUS characteristics' to lesions observed in patients with stable angina, thereby casting uncertainty upon the ability of IVUS to identify plaques susceptible to rupture, fissure, or erosion. Fourthly, the resolution of IVUS (150–300 µm) is too low to detect thin fibrous caps (50–75 µm), which have been identified as one of the features of vulnerable plaques.

Plaque vulnerability can only be assessed with certainty by serial observations that demonstrate the transition of a lesion from stability to instability. Yamagishi et al[38] examined 114 coronary sites in 106 patients by IVUS during a follow-up period of nearly 22 months. The coronary sites at which an event occurred, and which had been examined previously, were characterized by large, eccentric lesions. The vast majority of these plaques contained shallow echolucent zones, and subsequent studies have verified that positive (outward) remodeling is typically found in culprit lesions. Thus, this IVUS characteristic of an eccentric lesion with echolucent zones in areas of positive expansile remodeling seems the most definitive for vulnerable plaque. In addition, several novel approaches have recently been developed to more precisely define plaque characteristics.

Intravascular ultrasound with integrated backscatter

Three-dimensional IVUS with integrated backscatter (3D-IBS-IVUS) provides more optimal plaque characterization by implementing color coding and integration of sequential 1 mm segments obtained by motorized pullback. Radiofrequency (RF) signals digitized at 2 GHz can be obtained using a conventional 40 MHz IVUS catheter. Subsequent IBS signals can be calculated and color coded, providing a quantitative visual readout. This system uses a conventional IVUS instrument, a digital analog converter, and computer software to identify and quantitate various plaque characteristics. Kawasaki et al[39] recently described the usefulness of 3D-IBS-IVUS in detecting lipid-rich plaques and monitoring their response to lipid-lowering therapy. They evaluated the tissue characteristics of an 18 mm length coronary arterial segment in patients randomized to atorvastatin, pravastatin, or placebo for 6 months. The 6-month 3D-IBS-IVUS images showed a significant reduction in lipid volume and a similar increase in fibrous and mixed lesion volume in response to either statin, but not to placebo (Figures 14.2 and 14.3). These changes were detected despite no significant changes in lumen area, vessel area, plaque area, and diameter stenosis, thus validating the ability of this technique to identify early changes in plaque characteristics prior to geometric plaque regression and suggesting a role for defining plaque stabilization. Sano et al[40] have also demonstrated that vulnerable plaque can be differentiated from stable plaque when plaque morphology is evaluated by IBS during IVUS evaluation of coronary arteries (Figures 14.4 and 14.5).

Wavelet analysis

Wavelet analysis of RF IVUS signals is a novel mathematical model for assessing

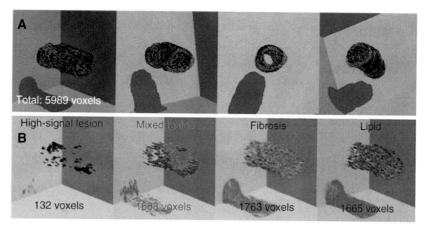

Figure 14.2   **(A)** The three-dimensional (3D) color-coded maps of the coronary arterial plaques constructed by 3D integrated backscatter intravascular ultrasound (3D-IBS-IVUS). **(B)** The 3D color-coded maps of each characteristic. The number of voxels of each tissue characteristic was automatically calculated. (Reprinted with permission from Kawasaki et al.[39])

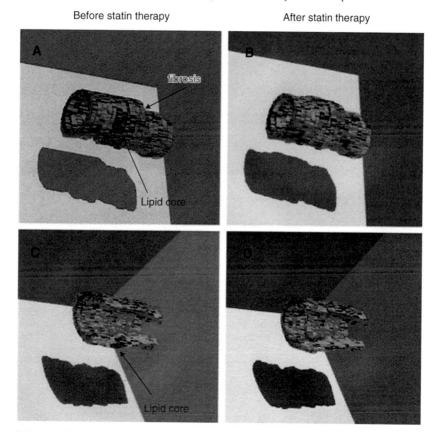

Figure 14.3   Color-coded maps of the coronary arterial plaques constructed by three-dimensional integrated backscatter intravascular ultrasound (3D-IBS-IVUS) imaging at baseline and after statin therapy. **(A)** At baseline. The plaque consists of a large lipid core (blue), which is covered with a fibrous cap (green). **(B)** After statin therapies, the lipid core (blue) decreased and the fibrous area (green) increased. **(C)** Cut-out image of 3D color-coded map at baseline. There was a small lipid core (blue) in the center of the plaque. **(D)** Cut-out image of 3D color-coded map after statin therapy. Note the reduction in the lipid core. Red = high intensity signal; yellow = mixed lesion. (Reprinted with permission from Kawasaki et al.[39])

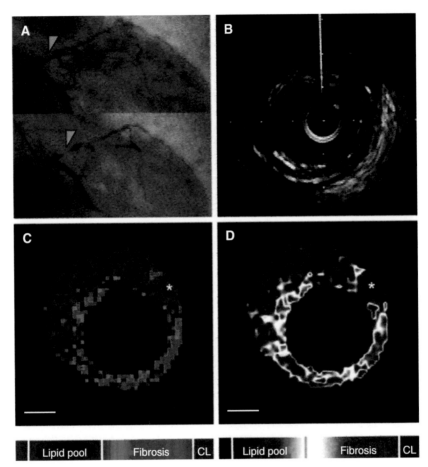

Figure 14.4 Images of the culprit lesion causing acute coronary syndrome. **(A)** Angiography of the left coronary artery. Upper: the arrowhead indicates a lesion in which intravascular ultrasound (IVUS) measurements were recorded at baseline. Lower: the arrowhead indicates the culprit lesion at follow-up. **(B)** Conventional IVUS image of segment indicated by the arrowhead in **A**. **(C)** Integrated backscatter (IB)-IVUS image of Cartesian coordinates, constructed using conventional color gradation, of the segment indicated by the arrowhead in **A**. The asterisk indicates the guidewire artifact. Note the large lipid core (blue) with fibrous cap (green). **(D)** IB-IVUS image of Cartesian coordinates, constructed using another color gradation, of the segment indicated by the arrowhead in **A**. This type of color-coded map illustrates the difference between lipid pool and fibrous tissue. The asterisk indicates the guidewire artifact. Note the large lipid core (blue) with fibrous cap (red or white). CL = calcification. Bar = 1 mm. (Reprinted with permission from Sano et al.[40])

focal differences within arterial walls. Color coding of the wavelet correlation coefficient derived from the RF signal allows detection of changes in the geometrical profile of time-series signals to derive an image of plaque components (Figures 14.6 and 14.7). Using wavelet analysis, Murashige et al[41] showed that lipid-rich plaques, derived from necropsy specimens and subsequently confirmed as such by histology, could be detected with a sensitivity of 83% and specificity of 83% in an in-vitro system. Furthermore, IVUS imaging of coronary arteries in 13 patients showed similar results with confirmation of the presence of lipid-rich components by histology after obtaining tissue by directional atherectomy.

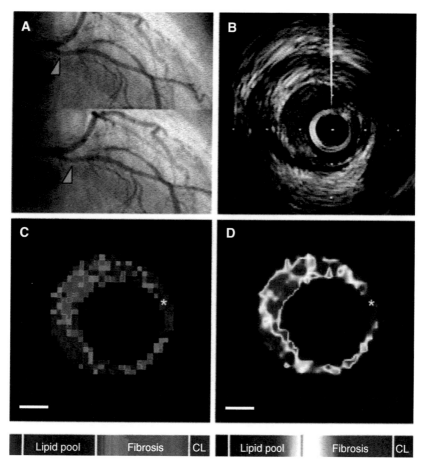

Figure 14.5   Images of the lesion not causing acute coronary syndrome. (**A**) Angiography of the left coronary artery. Upper: the arrowhead indicates a lesion, in which intravascular ultrasound (IVUS) measurements were recorded at baseline. Lower: the arrowhead indicates the segment indicated by the arrowhead at baseline after the follow-up period. (**B**) Conventional IVUS image of the segment indicated by the arrowhead in **A**. (**C**) Integrated backscatter (IB)-IVUS image of Cartesian coordinates, constructed using conventional color gradation, of the segment indicated by the arrowhead in **A**. The asterisk indicates the guidewire artifact. Note the small lipid core (blue) with large fibrous tissue (green). (**D**) IB-IVUS image of Cartesian coordinates, constructed using another color gradation, of the segment indicated by the arrowhead in **A**. The asterisk indicates the guidewire artifact. Note the small lipid core (blue) with large fibrous tissue (red or white). CL = calcification. Bar = 1 mm. (Reprinted with permission from Sano et al.[40])

Virtual histology

Virtual histology applies spectral analysis of the IVUS backscatter RF signal to characterize plaque components based on tissue characteristics such as density, compressibility, concentration of various components, and size. Using quantitative spectral parameters and advanced mathematical techniques to classify plaque composition, this approach has been validated using histologic techniques on ex-vivo coronary specimens to classify lesions as calcified, fibrofatty, calcified-necrotic core, and lipid-rich.[42,43] It enables real-time, 3D vessel cross-sectional and longitudinal views, facilitating visualization of the complete length of the artery and assessing individual plaque components. Although this technique appears

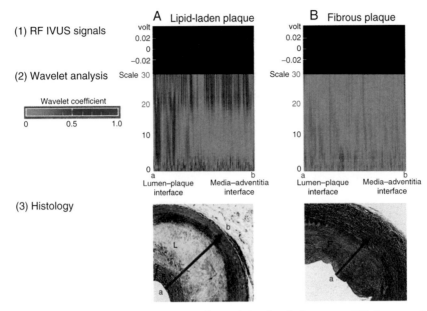

Figure 14.6 Representative examples of in-vitro wavelet analysis of radiofrequency (RF) intravascular ultrasound (IVUS) signals from a lipid-laden plaque **(A)** and from a fibrous plaque without a lipid core **(B)**. The upper panels show RF signals, the middle panels show the results of wavelet analysis, and the lower panels show the histologic specimen of the corresponding arterial cross section with Masson's trichrome. In the time-scale domain color-coded mapping of wavelet analysis, an apparently different pattern of pink area from an RF signal vector of a lipid-laden plaque is observed between scale 20 and scale 30, compared with the fibrous plaque. F = Fibrous area; L = lipid core. (Reprinted with permission from Murashige et al.[41])

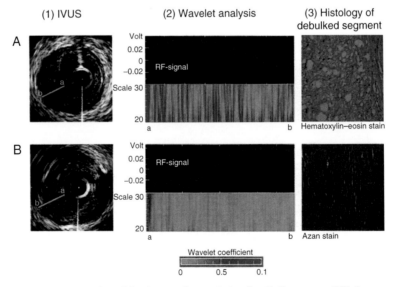

Figure 14.7 Representative examples of in-vivo wavelet analysis of radiofrequency (RF) intravascular ultrasound (IVUS) signals from a lipid-laden plaque **(A)** and from a fibrous plaque without a lipid core **(B)**. The left panels show conventional IVUS images, the middle panels show the results of wavelet analysis, and the right panels show histologic cross sections of the corresponding directional coronary atherectomy specimen with hematoxylin–eosin and Azan stains. A similar pattern of color mapping was observed from the RF signal vector of a lipid-laden plaque, as seen in the in-vitro study. (Reprinted with permission from Murashige et al.[41])

promising and is currently at the forefront of the IVUS approach to plaque characterization, definition of its clinical usefulness awaits ongoing clinical trials.

Optical coherence tomography

This imaging modality is a catheter-based high-resolution imaging technique analogous to ultrasound, except that it utilizes the measurement of reflected infrared light rather than sound. The imaging resolution is in the range of 10–20 µm but is limited by attenuation by blood and weak tissue penetration. However, when optimized, thin-capped fibroatheromas and small lipid collections can be identified.[44] The advantages of this technique include its high resolution, fast data acquisition rate, and ability to combine it with other adjuvant techniques. Ongoing studies will further help identify markers of plaque vulnerability with this technique.

INTRAVASCULAR ULTRASOUND AND TRANSTHORACIC ULTRASOUND WITH TARGETED CONTRAST AGENTS

In recent years, development of new microbubble ultrasound contrast agents and enhanced recording instrumentation has enabled the opacification and visualization not only of the cardiac chambers but also of blood vessels and myocardium.[45]

Myocardial contrast echocardiography can provide visualization of myocardial perfusion following the intravenous injection of a variety of ultrasonic contrast agents. However, the microbubble agents have a finite life span before dissolving, and may be destroyed by the ultrasound energy applied in the process of imaging. In addition, the generalized myocardial and vascular opacification produced by contrast echocardiography may mask uptake of microbubbles by plaque. Therefore, there are a number of challenges to identify vulnerable plaque by contrast echocardiography.

Contrast echo imaging methods to detect vulnerable plaque rely on targeted imaging with the use of a compound (beacon), which on attachment to the target of interest is detectable by the imaging technique. For ultrasound, the beacon that can be detected is the signal from microbubble contrast agents. Assuming that the target is specific for plaque (vulnerable or otherwise), it is not necessary to image the vessel to establish the presence of the target. Thus far, contrast echo has been confined primarily to the identification of white blood cells and endothelial cell surface markers such as adhesion molecules. However, the principles will be the same for identifying specific markers of vulnerable plaque when they are defined.

Because of the above reasons, targeted diagnostic imaging by contrast echocardiography has been achieved by having microbubbles or acoustically reflective liposomes ingested by or attached to the specific target to be visualized.[45,46] Attachment has been achieved either by the inherent properties of the microbubble shell or by attaching specific ligands such as monoclonal antibodies. In experimental models, these microbubbles are injected and, after an appropriate time is allowed for either ingestion or attachment, conventional echocardiographic recordings are obtained. In this manner the bulk of the contrast injected has disappeared and the residua are the microbubbles ingested by or attached to the target.

Although most microbubble ultrasonic contrast agents rapidly transit the capillary bed, some microbubble agents become transiently attached to vessels, particularly venules.[47] Subsequent studies related this prolonged residence within the microcirculation to a negative surface charge on the bubble (usually due to a lipid shell), with subsequent phagocytosis by white blood cells gathered along the surface of the endothelium. The ingestion of microbubbles by leukocytes has been found to be sufficiently avid to enable identification of inflammation such as that encountered following ischemia/reperfusion or transplant rejection in the experimental setting.[48,49]

The detection of white blood cells associated with plaque inflammation as a marker of vulnerable plaque would present a serious challenge. However, an alternate approach consists of using microbubble contrast to identify leukocyte adhesion molecules such as selectins or integrins which may be up-regulated in vulnerable plaque. Initial in-vitro studies, using either microbubble contrast agents or lipid emulsions to which antibodies to intracellular cell adhesion molecules (ICAMs) had been incorporated, documented the ability of these agents to attach to and be visualized on endothelium in which these molecules had been up-regulated.[50] Subsequently, targeted identification of leukocytes adherent to the endothelium of venules was accomplished by microbubbles to which phosphatidylcholine was incorporated into the lipid shell. Microbubbles to which ligands to ICAM-1 have been incorporated have also been utilized to visualize transplant rejection in the experimental setting.[51] Thus, exploiting both shell characteristics and incorporated ligands to specific targets, microbubbles have been found to be capable of identifying white blood cells as well as adhesion molecules.[46,52]

A number of challenges exist to the detection of vulnerable plaque by targeted echocardiographic contrast imaging. It requires a minimum concentration of microbubbles at the target site, and the ultrasonic signal transmitted must be capable of generating a sufficiently strong signal from the tethered/ingested microbubbles. Finally, one must be able to distinguish the resident microbubbles from both circulating microbubbles and from ultrasonic signals generated by the blood–intimal border. Thus, targets must be chosen which are present in sufficient quantity to attract an adequate number of microbubbles per target to be detected by external ultrasonic imaging. Given these constraints, it is likely that targeted imaging by contrast echocardiography may find detecting vulnerable plaque in the carotid arteries, or in the coronary arteries in conjunction with IVUS, as its initial clinical application. Contrast echocardiography offers the opportunity to detect vulnerable plaque by non-invasive imaging, but presents significant challenges to the recording of microbubbles tethered to specific sites. Nevertheless, the safety, repeatability of recording, portability, and cost-effectiveness of ultrasound provide a substantial incentive to develop approaches utilizing this modality for the identification of vulnerable plaque.

CONCLUSIONS

Currently, intravascular, surface, and transthoracic ultrasonic techniques for the detection of vulnerable plaque must be considered as either not established or experimental. However, recent advances suggest that plaque characterization with a variety of techniques may be feasible. Ultimately, clinical trials will determine whether ultrasound approaches may identify vulnerable plaques or result in new algorithms in patient care.

REFERENCES

1. Biasi GM, Froio A, Diethrich EB et al. Carotid plaque echolucency increases the risk of stroke in carotid stenting: the Imaging in Carotid Angioplasty and Risk of Stroke (ICAROS) study. Circulation 2004; 110:756–62.
2. Mintz GS, Nissen SE, Anderson WD et al. American College of Cardiology Clinical Expert Consensus Document on Standards for Acquisition, Measurement and Reporting of Intravascular Ultrasound Studies (IVUS) 13. A report of the American College of Cardiology Task Force on Clinical Expert Consensus Documents developed in collaboration with the European Society of Cardiology endorsed by the

Society of Cardiac Angiography and Interventions. J Am Coll Cardiol 2001; 37:1478–92.

3. Nishimura RA, Edwards WD, Warnes CA et al. Intravascular ultrasound imaging: in vitro validation and pathologic correlation. J Am Coll Cardiol 1990; 16:145–54.

4. Kimura BJ, Bhargava V, DeMaria AN. Value and limitations of intravascular ultrasound imaging in characterizing coronary atherosclerotic plaque. Am Heart J 1995; 130:386–96.

5. Gronholdt ML. Ultrasound and lipoproteins as predictors of lipid-rich, rupture-prone plaques in the carotid artery. Arterioscler Thromb Vasc Biol 1999; 19:2–13.

6. Prati F, Arbustini E, Labellarte A et al. Correlation between high frequency intravascular ultrasound and histomorphology in human coronary arteries. Heart 2001; 85:567–70.

7. Wickline SA. Plaque characterization: surrogate markers or the real thing? J Am Coll Cardiol 2004; 43:1185–7.

8. Honda O, Sugiyama S, Kugiyama K et al. Echolucent carotid plaques predict future coronary events in patients with coronary artery disease. J Am Coll Cardiol 2004; 43:1177–84.

9. Glagov S, Weisenberg E, Zarins CK, Stankunavicius R, Kolettis GJ. Compensatory enlargement of human atherosclerotic coronary arteries. N Engl J Med 1987; 316:1371–5.

10. Maehara A, Mintz GS, Bui AB et al. Morphologic and angiographic features of coronary plaque rupture detected by intravascular ultrasound. J Am Coll Cardiol 2002; 40:904–10.

11. Davies MJ, Thomas A. Thrombosis and acute coronary-artery lesions in sudden cardiac ischemic death. N Engl J Med 1984; 310:1137–40.

12. Goldstein JA, Demetriou D, Grines CL et al. Multiple complex coronary plaques in patients with acute myocardial infarction. N Engl J Med 2000; 343:915–22.

13. Asakura M, Ueda Y, Yamaguchi O et al. Extensive development of vulnerable plaques as a pan-coronary process in patients with myocardial infarction: an angioscopic study. J Am Coll Cardiol 2001; 37:1284–8.

14. Takano M, Inami S, Ishibashi F et al. Angioscopic follow-up study of coronary ruptured plaques in non-culprit lesions. J Am Coll Cardiol 2005; 45:652–8.

15. Takano M, Mizuno K, Yokoyama S et al. Changes in coronary plaque color and morphology by lipid-lowering therapy with atorvastatin: serial evaluation by coronary angioscopy. J Am Coll Cardiol 2003; 42:680–6.

16. Libby P. Act local, act global: inflammation and the multiplicity of "vulnerable" coronary plaques. J Am Coll Cardiol 2005; 45:1600–2.

17. Rioufol G, Finet G, Ginon I et al. Multiple atherosclerotic plaque rupture in acute coronary syndrome: a three-vessel intravascular ultrasound study. Circulation 2002; 106:804–8.

18. Hong MK, Mintz GS, Lee CW et al. Comparison of coronary plaque rupture between stable angina and acute myocardial infarction: a three-vessel intravascular ultrasound study in 235 patients. Circulation 2004; 110:928–33.

19. Tanaka A, Shimada K, Sano T et al. Multiple plaque rupture and C-reactive protein in acute myocardial infarction. J Am Coll Cardiol 2005; 45:1594–9.

20. Fujii K, Kobayashi Y, Mintz GS et al. Intravascular ultrasound assessment of ulcerated ruptured plaques: a comparison of culprit and nonculprit lesions of patients with acute coronary syndromes and lesions in patients without acute coronary syndromes. Circulation 2003; 108:2473–8.

21. Kotani JI, Mintz GS, Castagna MT et al. Intravascular ultrasound analysis of infarct-related and non-infarct-related arteries in patients who presented with an acute myocardial infarction. Circulation 2003; 107: 2889–93.

22. Beckman JA, Ganz J, Creager MA, Ganz P, Kinlay S. Relationship of clinical presentation and calcification of culprit coronary artery stenoses. Arterioscler Thromb Vasc Biol 2001; 21:1618–22.

23. Ehara S, Kobayashi Y, Yoshiyama M et al. Spotty calcification typifies the culprit plaque in patients with acute myocardial infarction: an intravascular ultrasound study. Circulation 2004; 110:3424–9.

24. Fujii K, Carlier S, Mintz GS et al. Intravascular ultrasound study of patterns of calcium in ruptured coronary plaques. Am J Cardiol 2005; 96:352–7.

25. Rioufol G, Gilard M, Finet G et al. Evolution of spontaneous atherosclerotic plaque rupture with medical therapy. Long-term follow-up with intravascular ultrasound. Circulation 2004; 110:2875–80.

26. Burke AP, Kolodgie FD, Farb A et al. Healed plaque ruptures and sudden coronary death: evidence that subclinical rupture has a role in plaque progression. Circulation 2001; 103:934–40.

27. Bots ML, Hoes AW, Koudstaal PJ, Hofman A, Grobbee DE. Common carotid intima–media thickness and risk of stroke and myocardial infarction: the Rotterdam study. Circulation 1997; 96:1432–7.

28. Nichols WW, Pepine CJ, O'Rourke MF. Carotid-artery intima and media thickness as a risk factor for myocardial infarction and stroke. N Engl J Med 1999; 340:1762–3.

29. Honda O, Sugiyama S, Kugiyama K et al. Echolucent carotid plaques predict future coronary events in patients with coronary artery disease. J Am Coll Cardiol 2004; 43:1177–84.

30. Lombardo A, Biasucci LM, Lanza GA et al. Inflammation as a possible link between coronary and carotid plaque instability. Circulation 2004; 109: 3158–63.

31. Takiuchi S, Rakugi H, Honda K et al. Quantitative ultrasonic tissue characterization can identify high-risk

atherosclerotic alteration in human carotid arteries. Circulation 2000; 102:766–70.

32. Rossi M, Cupisti A, Perrone L, Santoro G. Carotid ultrasound backscatter analysis in hypertensive and in healthy subjects. Ultrasound Med Biol 2002; 28:1123–8.

33. Gronholdt ML, Nordestgaard BG, Bentzon J et al. Macrophages are associated with lipid-rich carotid artery plaques, echolucency on B-mode imaging, and elevated plasma lipid levels. J Vasc Surg 2002; 35:137–45.

34. Waki H, Masuyama T, Mori H et al. Ultrasonic tissue characterization of the atherosclerotic carotid artery: histological correlates of carotid integrated backscatter. Circ J 2003; 67:1013–16.

35. Watanabe K, Sugiyama S, Kugiyama K et al. Stabilization of carotid atheroma assessed by quantitative ultrasound analysis in nonhypercholesterolemic patients with coronary artery disease. J Am Coll Cardiol 2005; 46:2022–30.

36. Nissen SE, Tuzcu EM, Schoenhagen P et al. Effect of intensive compared with moderate lipid-lowering therapy on progression of coronary atherosclerosis: a randomized controlled trial. JAMA 2004; 291: 1071–80.

37. Schoenhagen P, Stone GW, Nissen SE et al. Coronary plaque morphology and frequency of ulceration distant from culprit lesions in patients with unstable and stable presentation. Arterioscler Thromb Vasc Biol 2003; 23:1895–900.

38. Yamagishi M, Terashima M, Awano K et al. Morphology of vulnerable coronary plaque: insights from follow-up of patients examined by intravascular ultrasound before an acute coronary syndrome. J Am Coll Cardiol 2000; 35:106–11.

39. Kawasaki M, Sano K, Okubo M et al. Volumetric quantitative analysis of tissue characteristics of coronary plaques after statin therapy using three-dimensional integrated backscatter intravascular ultrasound. J Am Coll Cardiol 2005; 45:1946–53.

40. Sano K, Kawasaki M, Ishihara Y et al. Assessment of vulnerable plaques causing acute coronary syndrome using integrated backscatter intravascular ultrasound. J Am Coll Cardiol 2006; 47:734–41.

41. Murashige A, Hiro T, Fujii T et al. Detection of lipid-laden atherosclerotic plaque by wavelet analysis of radiofrequency intravascular ultrasound signals: in

vitro validation and preliminary in vivo application. J Am Coll Cardiol 2005; 45:1954–60.

42. Nair A, Kuban BD, Obuchowski N, Vince DG. Assessing spectral algorithms to predict atherosclerotic plaque composition with normalized and raw intravascular ultrasound data. Ultrasound Med Biol 2001; 27:1319–31.

43. Nair A, Kuban BD, Tuzcu EM et al. Coronary plaque classification with intravascular ultrasound radiofrequency data analysis. Circulation 2002; 106:2200–6.

44. Stamper D, Weissman NJ, Brezinski M. Plaque characterization with optical coherence tomography. J Am Coll Cardiol 2006; 47(8 Suppl):C69–79.

45. Lindner JR, Song J, Xu F et al. Noninvasive ultrasound imaging of inflammation using microbubbles targeted to activated leukocytes. Circulation 2000; 102:2745–50.

46. Hamilton AJ, Huang SL, Warnick D et al. Intravascular ultrasound molecular imaging of atheroma components in vivo. J Am Coll Cardiol 2004; 43:453–60.

47. Yasu T, Schmid-Schonbein GW, Cotter B, DeMaria AN. Flow dynamics of QW7437, a new dodecafluoropentane ultrasound contrast agent, in the microcirculation: microvascular mechanisms for persistent tissue echo enhancement. J Am Coll Cardiol 1999; 34:578–86.

48. Christiansen JP, Leong-Poi H, Klibanov AL, Kaul S, Lindner JR. Noninvasive imaging of myocardial reperfusion injury using leukocyte-targeted contrast echocardiography. Circulation 2002; 105:1764–7.

49. Weller GE, Lu E, Csikari MM et al. Ultrasound imaging of acute cardiac transplant rejection with microbubbles targeted to intercellular adhesion molecule-1. Circulation 2003; 108:218–24.

50. Villanueva FS, Jankowski RJ, Klibanov S et al. Microbubbles targeted to intercellular adhesion molecule-1 bind to activated coronary artery endothelial cells. Circulation 1998; 98:1–5.

51. Weller GE, Lu E, Csikari MM et al. Ultrasound imaging of acute cardiac transplant rejection with microbubbles targeted to intercellular adhesion molecule-1. Circulation 2003; 108:218–24.

52. Kaul S, Lindner JR. Visualizing coronary atherosclerosis in vivo: thinking big, imaging small. J Am Coll Cardiol 2004; 43:461–3.

Intravascular palpography for vulnerable plaque assessment

15

Johannes A Schaar, Anton FW van der Steen, Frits Mastik, and Patrick W Serruys

INTRODUCTION

For the detection of vulnerable plaque, it is not only important to measure the composition and geometry of the plaques but also the response of the tissue on the pulsating force applied by the blood pressure. The plaque is supposed to be rupture-prone, if the cap is unable to withstand the stress applied on it. All the stress that is applied on the plaque by the blood pressure is concentrated in the cap, since the lipid pool is unable to withstand forces on it.[1,2] This leads to a higher stress in a thin cap compared with a thicker cap. Furthermore, the strength of the cap is affected by inflammation: fibrous caps with inflammation by macrophages were locally weakened.[3] Therefore, the strength of a cap seems to be a more important parameter than the thickness of the cap.

Intravascular palpography is based on intravascular ultrasound (IVUS), which is the only commercially available clinical technique providing real-time cross-sectional imaging of the coronary artery.[4] Using IVUS, detailed information on the coronary wall and plaque can be obtained. Furthermore, calcified and non-calcified plaque components can be identified. However, the sensitivity to identify fatty plaque components remains low.[5,6] Recent radiofrequency (RF)-based tissue identification strategies appear to have a better performance.[6,7] With palpography, the local strain of the tissue is obtained. This strain is directly related to the mechanical properties. It is well known that the mechanical properties of fibrous and fatty plaque components are different,[8-10] and therefore palpography has the potential to differentiate between different plaque components. An even more promising feature of palpography is the detection of high stress regions. Using computer simulations, concentrations of circumferential tensile stress were more frequently found in unstable plaque than in stable plaques.[2,11] A local increase in circumferential stress in tissue is directly related to an increase of radial strain.

INTRAVASCULAR PALPOGRAPHY

Ophir and colleagues[12,13] developed an imaging technique called elastography that was based on tissue deformation. The rate of deformation (strain) of the tissue is directly related to the mechanical properties. The tissue under inspection is deformed and the strain between pairs of ultrasound signals before and after deformation is determined.[14] For intravascular purposes, the compression can be obtained from the pressure difference in the artery. Additionally, well-controlled deformation is possible by using a compliant intravascular balloon.[15]

The principle of intravascular elastography is illustrated in Figure 15.1. An ultrasound image of a human coronary artery is acquired at an intracoronary pressure. A second acquisition at a slightly lower pressure (approx 5 mmHg) is performed. The strain is determined by correlating the signals of the two

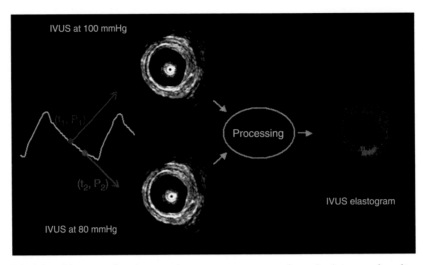

Figure 15.1   Principle of intravascular elastography measurement procedure. An intravascular ultrasound (IVUS) echogram is acquired with a low (P$_2$) and a high (P$_1$) intraluminal pressure. Using cross-correlation analysis on the high-frequency radiofrequency (RF) data, the radial strain in the tissue is determined. This information is plotted as an additional image to the IVUS echogram. In this example, an eccentric soft lesion is visible between 6 and 12 o'clock in the elastogram, where this lesion cannot be identified from the IVUS echogram.

IVUS echograms. The elastogram (image of the radial strain) is plotted as a complementary image to the IVUS echogram. The elastogram shows the presence of an eccentric region, with increased strain values at the shoulders of the eccentric plaque. Since the acting force is applied on the lumen boundaries, a surface-based assessment of the mechanical properties was developed. This robust technique is easier to interpret and is called palpography. Palpography derives mechanical information on the surface of the plaque, where the rupture may happen. This information is colour-coded and superimposed on the IVUS echogram.

PLAQUE CHARACTERIZATION

Elastographic experiments were performed in excised human coronary ($n = 4$) and femoral ($n = 9$) arteries.[16] Data were acquired at room temperature at intraluminal pressures of 80 and 100 mmHg. Coronary arteries were measured using a solid-state 20 MHz array catheter

(Volcano, Rancho Cordova, CA, USA). Femoral arteries were investigated using a single-element 30 MHz catheter (Du-MED/EndoSonics, Rijswijk, the Netherlands). The RF data were stored. The processing is done off-line. The visualized segments were stained for the presence of collagen, smooth muscle cells (SMCs), and macrophages. Matching of elastographic data and histology was performed using the IVUS echogram. The cross sections were segmented in regions ($n = 125$) based on the strain value on the elastogram. The dominant plaque types in these regions (fibrous, fibrofatty, or fatty) were obtained from histology and correlated with the average strain and echo intensity.

Mean strain values of 0.27%, 0.45%, and 0.60% were found for fibrous, fibrofatty, and fatty plaque components, respectively. The strain for the three plaque types as determined by histology differed significantly ($P = 0.0002$). This difference was independent of the type of artery (coronary or femoral) and was mainly evident between fibrous and fatty tissue ($P = 0.0004$).

The plaque types did not reveal echo-intensity differences in the IVUS echogram ($P = 0.992$). Conversion of the strain into Young's modulus values resulted in 493 kPa, 296 kPa, and 222 kPa for fibrous, fibrofatty, and fatty plaques, respectively. Although these values are higher than values measured by Lee et al,[17] the ratio between fibrous and fatty material is similar. Since fibrous and fatty tissue demonstrated a different strain value, and high strain values were often co-localized with increased concentrations of macrophages, these results reveal the potential of identification of the vulnerable plaque features.

VULNERABLE PLAQUE DETECTION

Although plaque vulnerability is associated with the plaque composition, detection of a lipid or fibrous composition does not directly warrant identification of the vulnerable plaque. Therefore, a study to evaluate the predictive power of palpography to identify the vulnerable plaque was performed.[18]

Diseased coronary arteries ($n = 24$) were measured in vitro. Elastographic data were acquired at intracoronary pressures of 80 and 100 mmHg using a standard IVUS catheter (Volcano, Rancho Cordova, CA, USA). After the ultrasound experiments, the cross sections were stained for collagen and fat, SMCs, and macrophages. In histology, a vulnerable plaque was defined as a lesion with a large atheroma (>40%), a thin fibrous cap with moderate to heavy infiltration of macrophages. A plaque was considered vulnerable in elastography when a high strain region was present at the lumen–plaque boundary that was surrounded by low strain values. Using this definition, the instability of the region is assessed.

Figure 15.2 shows a typical example of a vulnerable plaque. High strain regions are present at 6 and 12 o'clock and these regions are surrounded by low strain values. These regions correspond to the shoulders of this eccentric plaque. The histology reveals a large lipid pool (absence of collagen and SMCs) that is covered by a thin fibrous cap. The cap lacks collagen at the shoulder regions. Inflammation by macrophages is found in the lipid pool and in the cap.

In 24 diseased coronary arteries, we studied 54 cross sections. In histology, 26 vulnerable plaques and 28 non-vulnerable plaques were found; elastography was positive in 23 cases but negative in 3 cases. Non-vulnerable plaques were seen by histology in 28 cases and detected by elastography in 25 cases but were falsely diagnosed as positive in three cases, resulting in a sensitivity of 88% and a specificity of 89% for detecting vulnerable plaques.

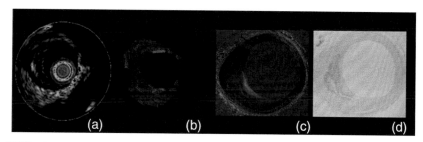

Figure 15.2 IVUS echogram (a) and elastogram (b) with corresponding histology of a coronary artery with a vulnerable plaque. The echogram reveals an eccentric plaque between 6 and 12 o'clock. The elastogram shows high strain regions (yellow) at the shoulders of the plaque surrounded by low strain values (blue). The histology reveals a plaque with a typical vulnerable appearance: a thin cap with a lack of collagen (c) at the shoulders, a large atheroma, and heavy infiltration of macrophages (d).

Linear regression showed high correlation between the strain in caps and the amount of macrophages ($P < 0.006$), and an inverse relationship between the amount of SMCs and strain ($P < 0.0001$). Plaques that are declared vulnerable in elastography have a thinner cap than non-vulnerable plaques ($P < 0.0001$).[18]

IN-VIVO VALIDATION

IVUS elastography was validated in vivo using an atherosclerotic Yucatan minipig.[19] External iliac and femoral arteries were made atherosclerotic by endothelial Fogarty denudation and subsequent atherosclerotic diet for the duration of 7 months. Balloon dilation was performed in the femoral arteries and the diet was discontinued. Before termination, 6 weeks after balloon dilation and discontinuation of the diet, data were acquired in the external iliac and femoral artery in 6 Yucatan pigs. In total, 20 cross sections were investigated with a 20 MHz Visions catheter (Volcano, Rancho Cordova, CA, USA). The tissue was strained by the pulsatile blood pressure. Two frames acquired at end diastole with a pressure differential of about 4 mmHg were taken to determine the elastograms.

After the ultrasound experiments and before dissection, an X-ray was used to identify the arterial segments that had been investigated by ultrasound. The specimens were frozen in liquid nitrogen. The cross sections (7 μm) were stained for collagen (picrosirius red and polarized light) and macrophages (alcalic phosphatase). Plaques were classified as absent, early fibrous lesion, early fatty lesion, or as advanced fibrous plaque. The mean strain in these plaques and normal cross sections was determined to assess the tissue characterization properties of the technique. Furthermore, the deformability of the acquisition was correlated with the presence of fat and macrophages. The deformability was characterized by the presence of a high strain region (strain is higher than 1%) at the lumen vessel wall boundary.

Strains were similar in the plaque-free arterial wall and the early and advanced fibrous plaques. Univariate analysis of variance revealed significantly higher strain values in cross sections with early fatty lesions than in fibrous plaques ($P = 0.02$) independently of the presence of macrophages. Although a higher strain value was found in plaques with macrophages than in plaques without macrophages, this difference was not significant after correction for fatty components. However, the presence of a high strain region had a high sensitivity (92%) and specificity (92%) to identify the presence of macrophages. Therefore, it was concluded that the tissue type dominates the mean strain value. Localized high strain values are related to local phenomena such as inflammation.

CLINICAL STUDIES

Preliminary acquisitions were performed in patients during percutaneous transluminal coronary angioplasty (PTCA) procedures.[20] Data were acquired in patients ($n = 12$) with an echoapparatus (InVision, Volcano, Rancho Cordova, CA) equipped with an analog RF output that was interfaced to a Signatec digitizer (Signatec, Inc., Corona, CA). To obtain the RF data, the machine worked in ChromaFlo mode, resulting in images of 64 angles with unfocused ultrasound data. The systemic pressure was used to strain the tissue. This strain was determined using cross-correlation analysis of sequential frames. A likelihood function was determined to obtain the frames with minimal motion of the catheter in the lumen, since motion of the catheter prevents reliable strain estimation. Minimal motion was observed near end diastole. Reproducible strain estimates were obtained within one pressure cycle and over several pressure cycles.

Validation of the results was limited to the information provided by the echogram. Strain in calcified material (0.20%) was lower (*P* <0.001) than in non-calcified tissue (0.51%).

High-resolution elastograms were acquired using an echoapparatus (InVision, Volcano, Rancho Cordova, CA).[21] The beam-formed image mode (512 angles) ultrasound digital RF data (f_c = 20 MHz) were acquired with a PC-based acquisition system. Frames acquired at end-diastole with a pressure difference of about 5 mmHg were taken to determine the elastograms.

The palpogram of a patient with unstable angina pectoris reveals high strain values in the plaque, with very high strain values (up to 2%) at the shoulders of this plaque (Figure 15.3). This geometry and strain distribution was also found in the in-vitro studies. The corresponding histology revealed in in-vitro studies a plaque with a large lipid core covered from the blood by a thin cap. Calcified material, as identified from the echogram, shows strain values of 0-0.2%.

THREE-DIMENSIONAL PALPOGRAPHY

In the previous studies, elastograms revealed information on a two-dimensional (2D) cross section. However, the distribution of the strain in the three-dimensional (3D) geometry of an artery is an important tool to identify the presence of high strain spots, the amount and the distribution. In particular, since the correlation between plaque vulnerability and parameters provided by the echogram is low,[5,6] selection of cross sections based on the IVUS echogram introduces selection bias and increases the chance of missing the vulnerable part. Additionally, during longitudinal monitoring of patients, it is

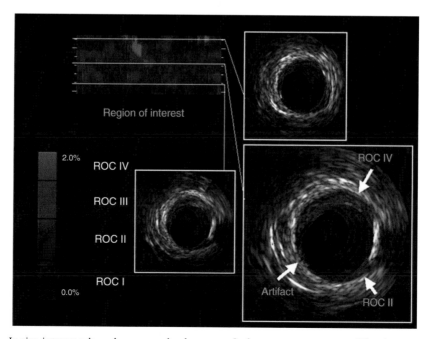

Figure 15.3 In-vivo intravascular echogram and palpogram of a human coronary artery. The elastogram reveals that the plaque has soft edges with adjacent hard (calcified) tissue. Plaque deformability was scored according to the Rotterdam classification (ROC), in which ROC I and IV indicate low (0–0.6%) and very high (>1.2%) deformation, respectively, by strain.

extremely difficult to come back to the same spot after some months. Therefore, an acquisition method of obtaining strain information on the full 3D coronary artery was developed. Since the rupture of a plaque occurs in the superficial area of the plaque, the elastic information on the surface is displayed as a palpogram.

In palpography, out-of-plane motion is considered as one of the main sources for decorrelation of the signals and thus decreases the quality of the strain estimate.[22,23] Therefore, for palpographic acquisitions, the position of the transducer is kept as stable as possible and only motion in the direction of the beam is allowed. As a consequence, it is unlikely that valid intravascular strain palpograms can be obtained while performing a continuous pullback of the catheter. However, if the pullback speed is slow and the strain is determined using two subsequent frames, the motion introduced by the pullback is minimal. Furthermore, it is known that, owing to the contraction of the heart, in diastole, the catheter will move distally in the coronary artery if it is kept at a steady position. Therefore, performing a pullback will decrease out-of-plane motion in this phase of the heart cycle. Since elastography uses data acquired in the diastolic phase, performing a pullback and thus obtaining 3D data seems feasible.

Preliminary experiments in rabbit aortas revealed that 3D palpography is feasible in vivo. Despite the introduction of out-of-plane motion by the continuous pullback of the catheter, the similarity between successive frames acquired in the diastolic phase is high enough to calculate several palpograms per heart cycle. By combining these palpograms, one compound palpogram per heart cycle is determined.[24] In a recent study in humans, 3D palpograms were derived from continuous IVUS pullbacks of entire coronary arteries. Patients ($n = 55$) were classified by clinical presentation as having stable angina, unstable angina, or acute myocardial infarction (AMI). In every patient, one coronary artery was scanned (culprit vessel in stable and unstable angina, non-culprit vessel in AMI), and the number of deformable plaques assessed. Stable angina patients had significantly fewer deformable plaques per vessel (0.6 ± 0.6) than did unstable angina patients ($P < 0.0019$) (1.6 ± 0.7) or AMI patients ($P < 0.0001$) (2.0 ± 0.7). Levels of C-reactive protein (CRP) were positively correlated with the number of mechanically deformable plaques ($R^2 = 0.65$, $P < 0.0001$).[25]

Strain measurements give an indication of the mechanical properties of the plaque, without taking into account the shear forces that may be responsible for activation of biologic processes which induce instabilities. Assessment of shear stress is feasible by obtaining high-resolution reconstruction of 3D coronary lumen and wall morphology using a combination of angiography and IVUS.[26] Briefly, a biplane angiogram of a sheath-based IVUS catheter taken at end diastole allows reconstruction of the 3D pullback trajectory of the catheter. Combining this path with lumen and wall information derived from IVUS images that are successively acquired during catheter pullback at end diastole gives accurate 3D lumen and wall reconstruction with resolution determined by IVUS. Filling the 3D lumen space with high-resolution 3D grit allows calculation of the detailed blood velocity profile in the lumen.[27] For this purpose, absolute flow and blood viscosity need to be provided as boundary conditions. From the blood velocity profile, local wall shear stress on the endothelium can be accurately calculated. Wall shear stress is the frictional force, normalized to surface area, that is induced by the blood passing the wall. Although from a mechanical point of view shear stress is of a very small magnitude compared with blood pressure-induced tensile stress, it has a profound influence on vascular biology[28] and explains the localization of atherosclerotic plaque in the presence of systemic risk factors.[29] Many of these biologic processes, including inflammation, thrombogenicity, vessel remodeling, intimal thickening or regression, and SMC proliferation, also influence the stability of the vulnerable plaque. Therefore, the assessment of shear stress in combination with strain measurement will reveal significant pathophysiologic aspects of plaque vulnerability.

CONCLUSIONS

Both in-vitro and in-vivo studies have revealed that the strain is higher in fatty than in fibrous plaques. Additionally, the presence of a high strain region has a high sensitivity and specificity to detect the vulnerable plaque. High strain spots correlate with clinical symptoms and inflammation markers. The presence of a high strain spot that is surrounded by low strain has a high predictive power to identify the rupture-prone plaque in vitro with high sensitivity and specificity. Intravascular palpography is a technique that assesses the local strain of the vessel wall and plaque, and can therefore be applied in patients to assess the vulnerability of plaques. Three-dimensional palpography allows the identification of weak spots over the full length of a coronary artery. A prospective study in patients that correlates clinical events with the distribution of these weak spots is currently being performed. Since palpography only requires ultrasound data sets that are acquired at different levels of intraluminal pressure, it can be realized using conventional clinically used catheters.

SUMMARY

Palpography assesses the local mechanical properties of tissue using its deformation caused by the intraluminal pressure. The technique was validated in vitro using diseased human coronary and femoral arteries. In particular, a highly significant difference in strain ($P = 0.0012$) was found between fibrous and fatty tissue. Additionally, the predictive value of identifying the vulnerable plaque was investigated. A high strain region at the lumen vessel wall boundary has an 88% sensitivity and 89% specificity for identifying these plaques.

In vivo, the technique was validated in an atherosclerotic Yucatan minipig animal model. This study also revealed higher strain values in fatty than fibrous plaques ($P < 0.001$). The presence of a high strain region at the lumen–plaque interface has a high predictive value for identifying macrophages. Patient studies revealed high strain values (1–2%) in non-calcified plaques. Calcified material shows low strain values (0–0.2%). With the development of 3D elastography, identification of weak spots over the full length of a coronary artery has become available. Patients with myocardial infarction or unstable angina have more high strain spots in their coronary arteries than patients with stable angina.

In conclusion, intravascular palpography is a unique tool for assessing lesion composition and vulnerability. Three-dimensional palpography provides a technique that may develop into a clinically available tool for decision making to treat hemodynamically non-significant lesions by identifying vulnerable plaques.

ACKNOWLEDGMENTS

This work was supported by the Dutch Technology Foundation (STW) and the Netherlands Organization for Scientific Research (NWO), the Dutch Heart Foundation (NHS), and, the German Heart Foundation (DHS).

REFERENCES

1. Loree HM, Kamm RD, Stringfellow RG et al. Effects of fibrous cap thickness on peak circumferential stress in model atherosclerotic vessels. Circ Res 1992; 71:850–8.

2. Richardson PD, Davies MJ, Born GVR. Influence of plaque configuration and stress distribution on fissuring of coronary atherosclerotic plaques. Lancet 1989; 21:941–4.

3. Lendon CL, Davies MJ, Born GVR et al. Atherosclerotic plaque caps are locally weakened when macrophage density is increased. Atherosclerosis 1991; 87:87–90.

4. Mintz GS, Nissen SE, Anderson WD et al. ACC Clinical Expert Consensus Document on Standards for Acquisition, Measurement and Reporting of Intravascular Ultrasound Studies (IVUS). A report of the American College of Cardiology Task Force on Clinical Expert Consensus Documents. J Am Coll Cardiol 2001; 37:1478–92.

5. Prati F, Arbustini E, Labellarte A et al. Correlation between high frequency intravascular ultrasound and histomorphology in human coronary arteries. Heart 2001; 85:567–70.

6. Komiyama N, Berry G, Kolz M et al. Tissue characterization of atherosclerotic plaques by intravascular ultrasound radiofrequency signal analysis: an in vitro study of human coronary arteries. Am Heart J 2000; 140:565–74.

7. Hiro T, Fujii T, Yasumoto K et al. Detection of fibrous cap in atherosclerotic plaque by intravascular ultrasound by use of color mapping of angle-dependent echo-intensity variation. Circulation 2001; 103: 1206–11.

8. Loree HM, Tobias BJ, Gibson LJ et al. Mechanical properties of model atherosclerotic lesion lipid pools. Arterioscler Thromb 1994; 14:230–4.

9. Loree HM, Grodzinsky AJ, Park SY, Gibson LJ, Lee RT. Static circumferential tangential modulus of human atherosclerotic tissue. J Biomech 1994; 27:195–204.

10. Lee RT, Richardson G, Loree HM et al. Prediction of mechanical properties of human atherosclerotic tissue by high-frequency intravascular ultrasound imaging. Arterioscler Thromb 1992; 12:1–5.

11. Cheng GC, Loree HM, Kamm RD et al. Distribution of circumferential stress in ruptured and stable atherosclerotic lesions. A structural analysis with histopathological correlation. Circulation 1993; 87:1179–87.

12. Céspedes EI, Ophir J, Ponnekanti H et al. Elastography: elasticity imaging using ultrasound with application to muscle and breast in vivo. Ultrason Imaging 1993; 17:73–88.

13. Ophir J, Céspedes EI, Ponnekanti H et al. Elastography: a method for imaging the elasticity in biological tissues. Ultrason Imaging 1991; 13:111–34.

14. Céspedes EI, Huang Y, Ophir J et al. Methods for estimation of subsample time delays of digitized echo signals. Ultrason Imaging 1995; 17:142–71.

15. Sarvazyan AP, Emelianov SY, Skovorada AR. Intracavity device for elasticity imaging. US patent; 1993.

16. de Korte CL, Pasterkamp G, van der Steen AF, Woutman HA, Bom N. Characterization of plaque components using intravascular ultrasound elastography in human femoral and coronary arteries in vitro. Circulation 2000; 102:617–23.

17. Lee RT, Richardson G, Loree HM et al. Prediction of mechanical properties of human atherosclerotic tissue by high-frequency intravascular ultrasound imaging. Arterioscler Thromb 1992; 12:1–5.

18. Schaar JA, de Korte CL, Mastik F et al. Characterizing vulnerable plaque features with intravascular elastography. Circulation 2003; 108:2636–41.

19. de Korte CL, Sierevogel M, Mastik F et al. Identification of atherosclerotic plaque components with intravascular ultrasound elastography in vivo: a Yucatan pig study. Circulation 2002; 105:1627–30.

20. de Korte CL, Carlier SG, Mastik F et al. Morphological and mechanical information of coronary arteries obtained with intravascular elastography: feasibility study in vivo. Eur Heart J 2002; 23:405–13.

21. de Korte CL, Doyley MM, Carlier SG et al. High resolution IVUS elastography in patients. In: IEEE Ultrasonics Symposium, Puerto Rico, USA; 2000: 1767–70.

22. Konofagou E, Ophir J. A new elastographic method for estimation and imaging of lateral displacements, lateral strains, corrected axial strains and Poisson's ratios in tissues. Ultrasound Med Biol 1998; 24:1183–99.

23. Kallel F, Ophir J. Three dimensional tissue motion and its effect on image noise in elastography. IEEE Trans UFFC 1997; 44:1286–96.

24. Doyley M, Mastik F, de Korte CL et al. Advancing intravascular ultrasonic palpation toward clinical applications. Ultrasound Med Biol 2001; 27:1471–80.

25. Schaar JA, Regar E, Mastik F et al. Incidence of high-strain patterns in human coronary arteries: assessment with three-dimensional intravascular palpography and correlation with clinical presentation. Circulation 2004; 109:2716–19.

26. Slager CJ, Wentzel JJ, Schuurbiers JC et al. True 3-dimensional reconstruction of coronary arteries in patients by fusion of angiography and IVUS (ANGUS) and its quantitative validation. Circulation 2000; 102:511–16.

27. Thury A, Wentzel JJ, Schuurbiers JC et al. Prominent role of tensile stress in propagation of a dissection after coronary stenting: computational fluid dynamic analysis on true 3d-reconstructed segment. Circulation 2001; 104:E53–4.

28. Malek AM, Alper SL, Izumo S. Hemodynamic shear stress and its role in atherosclerosis. JAMA 1999; 282:2035–42.

29. Asakura T, Karino T. Flow patterns and spatial distribution of atherosclerotic lesions in human coronary arteries. Circ Res 1990; 66:1045–66.

Diffuse reflectance near-infrared spectroscopy as a clinical technique to detect high-risk atherosclerotic plaques

16

*Pavan K Cheruvu, Pedro R Moreno, Barbara J Marshik, and James E Muller**

INTRODUCTION

Extensive efforts have been made to apply the well-established technique of near-infrared (NIR) spectroscopy for the identification of the composition of coronary artery plaques. It is anticipated that knowledge of plaque composition, which NIR is well-suited to provide, will provide an index of plaque vulnerability. This chapter will focus on diffuse reflectance NIR spectroscopy; Raman NIR spectroscopy and nuclear magnetic resonance spectroscopy have been the subject of a prior review by others.[1]

THE POSITION OF NEAR-INFRARED LIGHT IN THE ELECTROMAGNETIC SPECTRUM

The electromagnetic spectrum includes light or radiation with wavelengths that may be as small as 10^{-14} m or as large as 104 m (Figure 16.1). Many portions of the electromagnetic spectrum, such as γ-rays, X-rays, ultraviolet, infrared, microwaves, and radio waves (which include AM and

FM frequencies), have been utilized to create valuable medical and non-medical devices. The NIR range consists of light of wavelength ranging from 700 to 2500 nm. A useful feature of light in this wavelength range is that it can penetrate several millimeters into tissue, and is absorbed and scattered by different chemicals very selectively. This makes it possible to perform spectroscopic analysis to identify chemical composition of the tissue.

Definition of spectroscopy

Spectroscopy is the science of measurement of the amount of electromagnetic radiation that is absorbed or emitted by molecules or their atoms as they move from one energy level to another. When a molecule is exposed to infrared radiation (of which NIR is a subset) the molecule absorbs a portion of the light at frequencies that may induce twisting, bending, rotating, and vibrating of atoms within the molecule. A key feature of the infrared transition is that the molecule must have a non-zero dipole moment in order for the transition to occur. For this reason linear diatomic molecules such as N_2 and H_2 are not active in the infrared region, while HCl and the functional carbonyl group C=O have very strong signals.

16*Pedro R Moreno, James E Muller, and Pavan K Cheruvu have financial interest in InfraReDx, Inc., a company developing near-infrared spectroscopy to detect vulnerable plaques.

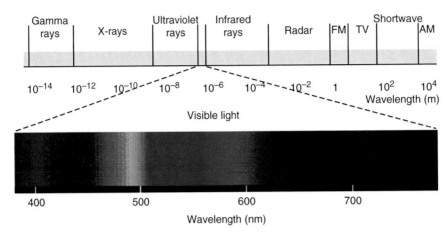

Figure 16.1 Electromagnetic spectrum. Specific wavelength scales are given for each form of light, from γ-rays to audio/radio light (see text for details). (Reproduced with permission from PE Kaiser. www.yorku.ca/eye/how-to.htm5. Peter K Kaiser either owns the intellectual property rights in the underlying HTML, text, audio clips, video clips, and other content that is made available to you on our website, or has obtained the permission of the owner of the intellectual property in such content to use the content on our website.)

A spectrometer measures the frequencies of the radiation that are absorbed by the molecule as a function of wavelength. The resulting graph of frequencies (plotted along the x-axis) vs absorbance (y-axis) is termed a spectrum. The shape and position of the peaks of the spectrum are directly correlated to the characteristic absorbancies of each of the functional chemical groups within the component. The magnitude of the absorption is related to the concentration of the species within the material being analyzed and is attenuated by the amount of light that is scattered and absorbed by the material (extinction coefficient).

Understanding the interaction between photons and tissue is crucial for a variety of diagnostic and therapeutic biomedical applications of spectroscopy, which vary depending upon the wavelength of the incident light and the intrinsic optical characteristics of tissue. Combinations of carbon–hydrogen and/or carbon–oxygen functional groups, water, and other components in tissue result in characteristic absorbance patterns for that particular tissue. The presence or absence of specific frequencies is the basis of sample identification and tissue characterization. Figure 16.2 shows the NIR absorbance spectra from a human aortic atherosclerotic plaque.

INTERACTIONS BETWEEN LIGHT AND TISSUE EVALUATED BY DIFFUSE REFLECTANCE NEAR-INFRARED SPECTROSCOPY

When light meets an interface between two media, photons are either absorbed by the new medium, scattered, or transmitted through it. Light that is not absorbed will penetrate a portion of the sample. As it progresses, it may change directions, or scatter, as it encounters another medium or particle boundary. This light scattering is a result of reflection, refraction, and random diffraction at the surfaces of the various media and particles encountered. As the light continues through the sample some is absorbed while the rest continues to be scattered randomly. This process produces diffusely reflected light. Scattering and absorption occur simultaneously until the light emerges back at the entry point

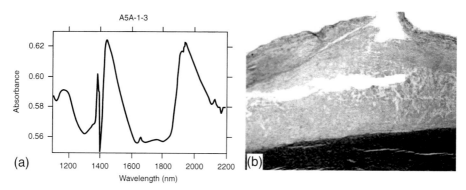

A5A-1-3

Figure 16.2 Near-infrared spectra collected from an atheromatous, lipid-rich aortic plaque. (a) Near-infrared absorbance tracing from spectra collected with a Bran + Luebbe (Hamburg, Germany) InfraAlyzer 500 spectrophotometer. Absorbance values were collected from the 1100–2200 nm wavelength window at 10 nm intervals. (b) Lipid-rich aortic plaque (Elastic Trichrome staining). The spike at 1400 nm is an instrumentation artifact. (Spectra obtained at Dr Lodder's spectroscopy lab at the University of Kentucky, Lexington, KY, USA.)

attenuated due to all the interactions with the medium (Figure 16.3).

Diffuse reflectance NIR spectroscopy is the analysis of the frequencies of the multiply scattered and absorbed photons of molecules excited by NIR light in the energy range of 700–2500 nm. The resulting NIR spectrograph contains absorbance bands resulting from the harmonic overtones and combinations of the fundamental vibrational and stretching bands in the mid infrared region. While absorbance intensities in the NIR region are only about 1/100 the intensity of those fundamental bands, most organic compounds still have a measurable spectrum that can be identified in the NIR region. Even though the spectral features are less intense and broader in the NIR region than the mid infrared, the application of multivariate mathematical techniques such as principal component regression analysis upon the NIR spectral signals combined with the known chemical information of the system[2] has promoted the use of the NIR region as the premier region for quantitative and qualitative analysis of the chemical composition of specimens.[3] This method of analysis, termed chemometrics, has flourished due to the ever-increasing

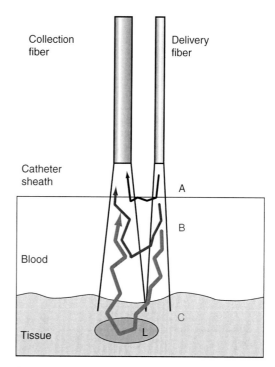

Figure 16.3 Diagram of the path of light from the catheter and back. As the near-infrared light leaves the delivery fiber and interacts with tissue, some photons are absorbed and some are scattered or reflected by the catheter to the collection fiber in the catheter sheath (A). Blood particles (B) and tissue (C) photons may be reflected. The most valuable photons are those that interact with the lipid pool (L) within the tissue and are reflected back to the catheter fiber.

computational power of computers along with the ease of sampling in the NIR region.

Photons in the NIR region penetrate into tissue relatively well, providing simultaneous, multicomponent, non-destructive chemical analysis of biologic tissue with acquisition times less than 1 second.[4] No sample preparation is required and physical and biologic properties, as well as molecular information, can be derived from the spectra. As a result, diffuse reflectance NIR spectroscopy has been successfully employed to quantify systemic and cerebral oxygenation, and to identify multiple plasma constituents, including glucose, total protein, triglycerides, cholesterol, urea, creatinine, uric acid, and human metalloproteins.[5–9] In the NIR wavelength region, hemoglobin – the main chromophore in the visible region – has relatively low absorbance, making diffuse reflectance NIR an attractive technique for the evaluation of plaque composition through blood.

NEAR-INFRARED ATHEROSCLEROTIC PLAQUE CHARACTERIZATION

Atherosclerotic plaque characterization using diffuse reflectance NIR was initially performed by Lodder and Cassis at the University of Kentucky using a novel NIR fiberoptic probe in the hypercholesterolemic rabbit more than a decade ago.[9] A vectorized three-dimensional cellular automaton-based algorithm using the quantile bootstrap error-adjusted single-sample theory (BEAST) technique was developed to analyze the spectra in hyperspace. An NIR color imaging system was then constructed on an IBM 3090-600J parallel vector supercomputer and displayed on an IBM RS 6000 workstation. Figure 16.4 shows an example of color-reconstructed images from aortas with and without low-density lipoprotein (LDL) accumulation.[9]

Analysis of plaque composition by diffuse reflectance NIR spectroscopy in humans was performed by Dempsey et al on carotid plaques exposed at the time of surgery.[3] After surgical exposure of the carotid bifurcation, NIR spectra were obtained from the plaque prior to endarterectomy. After surgery, the excised plaque was examined by a pathologist and frozen in liquid nitrogen for in-vitro NIR scanning followed by validation of lipoprotein composition by ultracentrifugation and gel electrophoresis. Figure 16.5 shows a probability density contour map of the NIR spectra, showing regions of lipoprotein content as well as normal tissue (see Figure 16.5 legend for details).

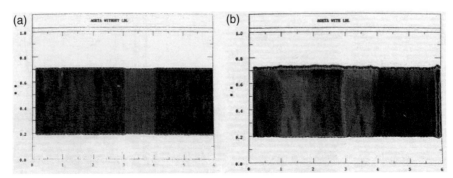

Figure 16.4 Low-density lipoprotein (LDL) reconstructed color images from near-infrared diffuse reflectance spectra analyzed using the quantile bootstrap error-adjusted single-sample theory (BEAST) technique. (a) Normal rabbit aorta; (b) LDL-rich aorta from a hypercholesterolemic rabbit. (Reproduced with permission from Cassis and Loder.[9])

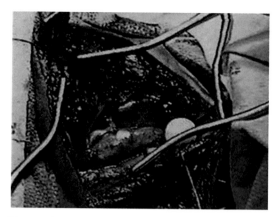

Figure 16.5 A visible light image of a human carotid bifurcation exposed during endarterectomy. The target artery is located at about 8 o'clock relative to the white sterile reflectance standard. The top two reflectors in the black reflectance standard are the surgical lights, which are equipped with cold filters and emit little NIR light. The two smaller reflections are the tungsten sources for the NIR camera. Images are collected at each wavelength with the NIR sources on and off to enable correction for sample blackbody emission in the NIR and for other light sources in the room. (Picture and legend reproduced with permission from Dempsey et al.[3])

Near-infrared spectra of high-risk atherosclerotic plaques

Our group (while at the University of Kentucky) collected spectra from 199 ex-vivo human aortic samples using an InfraAlyzer 500 spectrophotometer and compared the results with histologic findings associated with high-risk atherosclerotic plaques. A chemometric algorithm of principal component regression was used to construct a prediction model using 50% of the samples as a calibration set, and the others as a validation set to predict high-risk features as determined by histology. Sensitivity and specificity as determined by the NIR method were 90% and 93% for lipid pool, 77% and 93% for thin cap, and 84% and 91% for inflammatory cells, respectively.[10] These findings were consistent with data obtained by Jarros et al in their study using human aortic plaque tissue.[11] They found a high correlation coefficient of 0.96 between

the cholesterol content determined by NIR spectroscopy and that determined by reversed-phase, high-pressure liquid chromatography. In addition, Wang et al also found a high correlation between direct ex-vivo measurements of lipid/protein ratios in human carotid plaques and results obtained using an NIR spectrometer fitted with a fiberoptic probe.[12] The same promising results have also been obtained by our group in studying human coronary autopsy specimens ex-vivo.[13] However, in all of the experiments listed above involving human tissue measurements the results were obtained without the presence of blood, which would be encountered in the clinical setting. In most cases the tissue samples had been frozen or even fixed in formalin or paraffin prior to the acquisition of the NIR spectra.

Simulating in-vivo detection of vulnerable plaques in an ex-vivo setting

A significant challenge for detection of vulnerable plaques in patients is the development of an ex-vivo method that will simulate in-vivo performance. Our group (InfraReDx, Inc.) has used human autopsy material to develop algorithms that discriminate high-risk atheromas from all other tissue types (such as fibrotic, calcific, and normal) in ex-vivo conditions. We elected to use fresh human ex-vivo tissue because it has the same variety of chemical composition and morphology as in-vivo tissue. To more accurately replicate the in-vivo situation, the studies were performed through varying depths of blood. Even though the absorbance of hemoglobin from the bloodstream is low within some portions of the NIR wavelength region, the absorbance of water severely affects other NIR regions. The presence of red blood cells is also another contributing factor that strongly affects the NIR spectra due to the scatter of the incident light as it penetrates and bounces off the cell or other particles within the bloodstream.

A FOSS NIRSystems (Hamburg, Germany) Model 6500 equipped with a 1 cm fiberoptic probe (SmartProbe™) was used to acquire NIR spectra of 751 specimens from 78 fresh human aortic tissue samples. Specimens were pinned to a $5 \times 5 \times 0.5$ cm black rubber sheet and then immersed in bovine blood pre-warmed to $37 \pm 1°C$. NIR spectra were subsequently acquired at various probe-to-tissue separations of 0.0, 0.25, 0.5, 1.0, 1.5, 2.0, 2.5, and 3.0 mm with blood intervening (Figure 16.6) to simulate the

variability of the proximity of a probe within the blood vessel and the vessel walls. Specimens were then classified by histology into normal, lipid-rich, fibrotic, and calcific tissue, as shown in Figure 16.7. The solid lines demonstrating the spectra recorded near the surface of the tissue reveal visible differences between the various types of plaques. As the probe-to-tissue separation was increased, the NIR signal over plaques and normal tissue looked much more like the spectrum of blood, as seen by the overlapping signals of the dashed lines showing measurements taken at 3.0 mm from the sample in Figure 16.8. However, the application

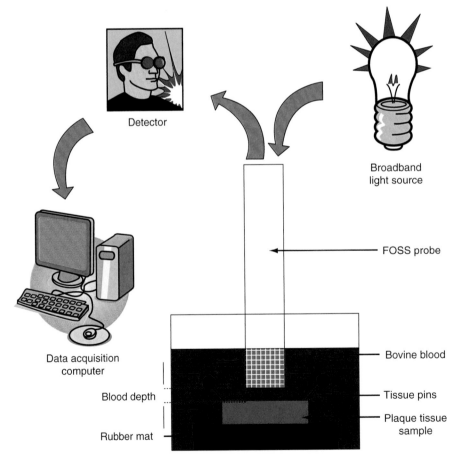

Figure 16.6 FOSS fiberoptic probe configuration used for NIR analysis of human aortic tissue conducted through varying depths of blood. The FOSS probe was connected to a micrometer fixed to the z-axis staging for moving the probe up and down.

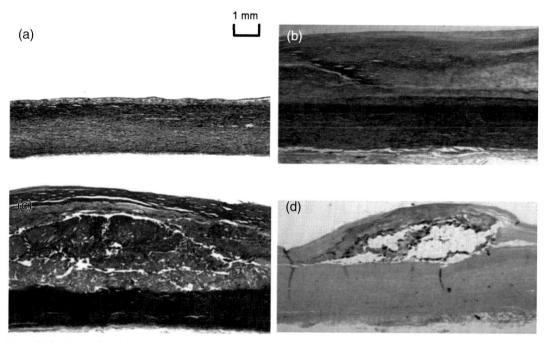

Figure 16.7 Examples of the classifications used in the human aortic tissue NIR study with the FOSS probe. The probe illumination spot was estimated as 1.0 cm. Normal tissue (a), large lipid pool with a thick fibrous cap (b), large fibrotic plaque (c), and large calcific plaque (d).

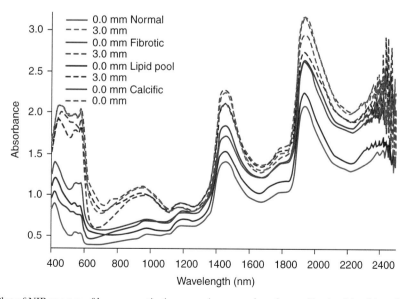

Figure 16.8 Plot of NIR spectra of human aortic tissue specimens under a layer of bovine blood just above the sample (solid lines – 0.0 mm), and at 3.0 mm above the sample (dashed lines). The normal specimens are plotted in magenta, the fibrotic in green, the lipid pool in blue, and the calcific in orange. Differences between spectra of various tissue types become less visible in the presence of 3 mm of blood.

of chemometric methods can extract differences that are not identifiable by simple visual inspection.

The chemometric method of partial least-squares discriminate analysis (PLS-DA) fortified with bootstrapping[14] was used to create a discrimination model that distinguishes the plaques containing large lipid pools regardless of plaque cap thickness from all of the other tissue types. The PLS-DA method creates a mathematical model based upon the spectral information from the two separate populations for which discernment is sought. The specimens used to build and test the discrimination algorithm for each of the types of plaques were selected by maximizing the amount of one constituent (lipid pool, fibrotic, or calcific tissue) over all of the others. In the initial study a discrimination threshold was set to distinguish tissue samples containing mainly lipid pool from those containing mainly fibrotic tissue (Figure 16.9). The best model separating the lipid pool samples from the fibrotic samples was used to produce a blinded discrimination of lipid pool against other plaque tissue compositions (normal, calcific, and fibrotic), also shown in Figure 16.9.

Several discrimination models were built and tested. The separation of the resultant prediction scores of the lipid pool samples shown as sensitivity (SENS) from all other tissue types (fibrotic, calcific, and normal) expressed as specificity (SPEC), using the best discrimination model, is displayed in Figure 16.10 at varying probe-to-tissue separations (blood depth) from 0.0 mm up to 3.0 mm. Table 16.1 summarizes the actual prediction values expressed as sensitivity of the model to identify the lipid pool samples as lipid pools and as specificity of the model to discriminate all other tissue types from those containing mainly lipid pool. As seen in the results, the PLS-DA model was able to distinguish between

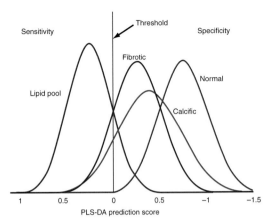

Figure 16.9 Plot of the distributions of the populations used to build and test the partial least-squares discriminate analysis (PLD-DA) prediction algorithm. The model assigns a score from 1 to −1.5 for each NIR spectrum for all four types of atherosclerotic tissue studied. The separation of scores between the lipid pool samples (green) was maximized with respect to the fibrotic samples (blue) and a threshold for predictions was then applied (red line). The distributions of the resultant predictions for the discrimination of the other populations for calcific samples (magenta) and normal samples (orange) are also displayed. Values to the left of the model threshold line (red line) indicate a prediction that the sample contains lipid pool and indicate the method sensitivity. Values to the right of the line indicate a prediction that the sample contains no lipid pool and indicate the method specificity.

lipid pool and other tissue samples through up to 3 mm of blood with at least 86% sensitivity and 72% specificity.

This study proved that an algorithm can be developed that is insensitive to blood thickness using NIR spectra of both diseased and normal samples of fresh human tissue through blood correlated to histology.[15] A study conducted using coronary artery tissue from autopsied human hearts produced similar results. This was a critical development for the use of an in-vivo diagnostic tool, since the data indicate that it is possible to acquire spectral information from a catheter regardless of its position within the coronary artery without requiring flushing or stopping of the blood flow.

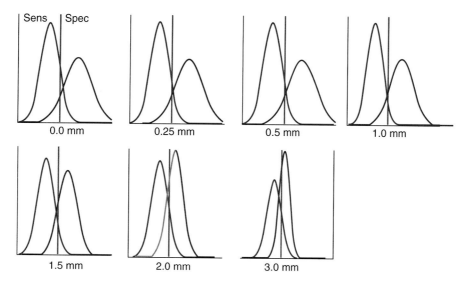

Figure 16.10   Plot of the distribution of the PLS-DA prediction scores (*x*-axis) as a function of sensitivity (SENS) of the lipid pool (green line) vs specificity (SPEC) with respect to all other tissue types (blue line) as a function of the probe-to-tissue separation in varying blood depths ranging from 0.0 mm up to 3.0 mm.

In-vivo catheter-based vulnerable plaque system

An in-vivo coronary catheter has been developed and used to measure intra-coronary NIR spectra in living patients (InfraReDx, Inc., Burlington, MA). Initial safety studies were successfully performed in the coronary arteries of six normal swine using an over-the-wire, 3.2 Fr, NIR-catheter (MedVenture, Louisville, KY). Microscopic histologic evaluation showed no evidence of dissection, thrombus, or perforation in any of the coronary vessels studied.

In 2005, InfraReDx, Inc. developed an ultrafast, tunable laser that enabled an in-vivo NIR coronary catheter to largely overcome the problems of intracoronary analysis: cardiac motion, visibility through blood, rotational scanning, and low signal-to-noise ratios. The system was tested that year in four swine with a genetic mutation strongly leading to swine familial hyper-cholesterolemia. The coronary arteries of these animals had extensive atheroscle-rotic plaques, with features similar to those of humans, including large lipid pools with thin caps.

Four diseased and one normal swine were investigated with the InfraReDx device by a team led by Dr Erling Falk and Dr Stephane Carlier. NIR measurements

Table 16.1   PLS-DA lipid pool model (SENS) predicted against all other tissue types (SPEC) as a function of probe-to-tissue distances with blood intervening

	0 mm	0.25 mm	0.5 mm	1.0 mm	1.5 mm	2.0 mm	2.5 mm	3.0 mm
SENS (%)	86	92	92	94	92	83	81	86
SPEC (%)	88	87	87	90	87	85	77	72

PLS-DA, partial least-squares discriminate analysis; SENS, sensitivity; SPEC, specificity.

were taken in-vivo, and again after excision of the artery from the euthanized pig. To simulate taken in-vivo physiologic conditions ex-vivo, coronary artery samples were pressure-perfused with blood collected from each animal for the NIR ex-vivo analysis. The samples were then sent for histologic analysis.

Excellent quality spectra were obtained. There was good reproducibility of NIR signals during repeat in-vivo pullbacks in the same artery shown and during repeat studies with different catheters. Comparison with intravascular ultrasound (IVUS) showed that NIR signals originated in areas of plaque as determined by IVUS; however, not all areas that IVUS indicated as plaque showed signs of being lipid-rich areas in the NIR analysis. Subsequent preliminary analysis on one artery for which histology is available, however, showed that areas indicating lipid-rich plaques by NIR detected in the ex-vivo scans corresponded to lipid-rich areas by histologic analysis.

In August and September of 2005, InfraReDx initiated and completed a feasibility trial of scanning NIR spectroscopy in 10 patients with stable angina pectoris undergoing percutaneous coronary intervention (PCI). The studies were led by Dr Sergio Waxman at the Lahey Clinic in Burlington, MA, and Dr James Goldstein at the Beaumont Hospital in Detroit, MI. The system, which is similar in use to that of IVUS, demonstrated the expected safety and ease of use. An analysis of special features in the coronary artery wall noted that the signals were different from those obtained from blood alone. In one patient, an area of concentrated lipid-rich signals was noted (Figure 16.11).[16] While tissue was not available for comparison, it was noted that the lesions shared spatial features such as degrees of arc, lesion length, and lesion center as analyzed by both NIR and IVUS.

In another study using the same scanning NIR spectroscopy system and catheter,

Dr Philippe L'Allier and Dr Jean-Claude Tardif of the Montreal Heart Institute have now obtained signals in patients with acute coronary artery syndromes. Preliminary analysis of these data indicates that spectra of excellent quality have been obtained, and lipid-rich areas have been identified. Ongoing clinical and autopsy studies will clarify the significance and value of these signals for detection of lipid-rich and presumably vulnerable plaque.

THE FUTURE OF NEAR-INFRARED SPECTROSCOPY FOR VULNERABLE PLAQUE

The results to date indicate that the well-established technique of NIR spectroscopy can be successfully performed in the human coronary artery through blood, despite coronary motion. Additional studies are needed to develop algorithms in autopsy specimens to characterize the range of spectral information that can be expected in in-vivo patients.

Long-term studies are needed to determine if sites that are identified as lipid-rich areas, and/or inflamed by NIR spectroscopy, carry an increased risk of causing a coronary event. In the immediate future, the ability of the technique to identify lipid-rich or inflamed plaques might be utilized to identify a high-risk group post PCI. Such a group could then be randomized to a novel antiatherosclerotic agent or standard care. The NIR screening would decrease the sample size needed for such a study.

In addition, there has been considerable discussion of the value of stenting intermediate lesions that are not producing ischemia (40–60% stenosis), with the expectation that stenting would increase fibrous cap thickness.[17] Because drug-eluting stents offer promise for the treatment of such high-risk plaques,[18,19] a randomized clinical trial of the treatment is being planned. In this trial, NIR

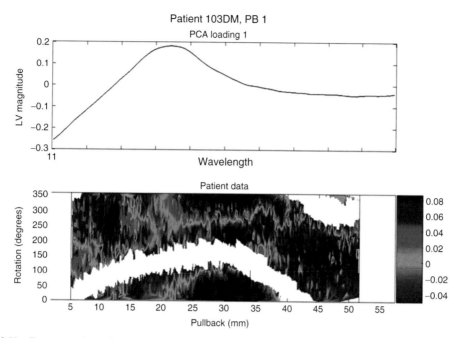

Figure 16.11 Demonstration of spectral findings in the left anterior descending (LAD) coronary artery of a patient with stable angina pectoris (unpublished data, on file InfraReDx, Inc.). A spectral scan of the LAD was performed during PCI. An analysis was performed of all spectra to determine the shapes – principal components analysis (PCA) – that contribute to the spectra obtained in each data point as the catheter scanned the artery. The graph in the top of the figure shows a shape of biologic interest that contributed to the individual spectra in varying degrees. The shape was not detected in a sample of blood only. The bottom graph shows the amount of that shape that was detected at each pixel as the catheter was pulled back (x-axis) and rotated (y-axis) within the coronary artery. The white areas indicate locations from which the shadow created by the guide wire was removed. While interpretation of the spectral findings is not yet complete, and a validated algorithm has not yet been applied to the data, the display shows the ability to obtain relevant NIR signals from the coronary artery of a patient despite the presence of cardiac motion and flowing blood.

spectroscopy has been proposed as a technique to identify the lipid-rich intermediate stenoses that would be expected to be more likely to rupture and cause events than the fibrotic plaques. The standard care arm of the trial would offer the needed natural history data and the stenting arm would test the hypothesis that a treatment of plaque vulnerability is effective.

REFERENCES

1. Moreno PR, Muller JE. Identification of high-risk atherosclerotic plaques: a survey of spectroscopic methods. Curr Opin Cardiol 2002; 17:638–47.
2. De Maesschalck R, Estienne F, Verdú-Andrés J et al. The development of calibration models for spectroscopic data using principal component regression. Internet J Chem 1999; 2:19.
3. Dempsey RJ, Davis DG, Buice RG et al. Biological and medical applications of near-infrared spectroscopy. Appl Spectroscopy 1996; 50:18A–34A.
4. McKinley BA, Marvin RG, Cocanour CS et al. Tissue hemoglobin O_2 saturation during resuscitation of traumatic shock monitored using near infrared spectrometry. J Trauma 2000; 48:637–42.
5. Spielman AJ, Zhang G, Yang C et al. Intracerebral hemodynamics probed by near infrared spectroscopy in the transition between wakefulness and sleep. Brain Res 2000; 866:313–25.
6. Gabriely I, Wozniak R, Mevorach M et al. Transcutaneous glucose measurement using near-infrared spectroscopy during hypoglycemia. Diabetes Care 1999; 12:2026–32.
7. Shaw RA, Kotowich S, Leroux M et al. Multianalyte serum analysis using mid-infrared spectroscopy. Ann Clin Biochem 1998; 35:624–32.
8. Shaw RA, Mansfield JR, Kupriyanov VV et al. In vivo optical/near-infrared spectroscopy and imaging of metalloproteins. J Inorg Biochem 2000; 79:285–93.

9. Cassis LA, Lodder RA. Near-IR imaging of atheromas in living arterial tissue. Anal Chem 1993; 65:1247–56.

10. Moreno PR, Lodder RA, Purushothaman KR et al. Detection of lipid pool, thin fibrous cap, and inflammatory cells in human aortic atherosclerotic plaques by near-infrared spectroscopy. Circulation 2002; 105: 923–7.

11. Jarros W, Neumeister V, Lattke P et al. Determination of cholesterol in atherosclerotic plaques using near infrared diffuse reflection spectroscopy. Atherosclerosis 1999; 147:327–37.

12. Wang J, Geng YJ, Guo B et al. Near-infrared spectroscopic characterization of human advanced atherosclerotic plaques. J Am Coll Cardiol 2002; 39:1305–13.

13. Moreno PR, Eric Ryan S, Hopkins D et al. Identification of lipid-rich plaques in human coronary artery autopsy specimens by near-infrared spectroscopy. J Am Coll Cardiol 2001; 37:1219–90.

14. Martens H, Martens M, eds. Multivariate Analysis of Quality: An Introduction. John Wiley and Sons, 2000.

15. Marshik B, Tan H, Tang J et al. Discrimination of lipid-rich plaques in human aorta specimens with NIR spectroscopy through blood. Am J Cardiol 2002; 90:129H.

16. Caplan JD, Waxman S, Nesto RW, Muller JE. Near infrared spectroscopy for detection of vulnerable coronary artery plaques. JACC 2006; 42:92–6.

17. Moreno PR, Kilpatrick D, Purushothaman KR, Coleman L, O'Connor WN. Stenting vulnerable plaque improves fibrous cap thickness and reduces lipid content: understanding alternatives for plaque stabilization. Am J Cardiol 2002; 90:50H

18. Echeverri D, Purushothaman KR, Moreno PR. Evaluating vascular healing after metallic, polymer, beta-estradiol and everolimus-eluting stents on thin cap fibroatheroma: strut per strut analysis. Vulnerable Plaque Meeting Symposium Proceedings, March 2003.

19. Echeverri D, Purushothaman KR, Moreno PR. Fibrous cap rupture after metallic, beta-estradiol and everolimus eluting stents on thin cap fibroatheroma: potential implications for stent deployment in high-risk, non-stenotic plaques. Vulnerable Plaque Meeting Symposium Proceedings, March 2003.

Optical coherence tomography   17

Evelyn Regar and Ik-Kyung Jang

INTRODUCTION

Every year over one million people in the United State suffer an acute myocardial infarction. Spontaneous rupture or erosion of atherosclerotic plaques with subsequent thrombosis is the most frequent underlying cause of acute coronary syndromes. Autopsy studies have identified several histologic characteristics of plaques that are prone to disruption, so-called vulnerable plaques. Pathologic characteristics of these vulnerable plaques are (1) a thin fibrous cap (<65 μm); (2) a large lipid pool; and (3) activated inflammatory cells, such as monocytes, macrophages, form cells, lymphocytes, and neutrophils, near the fibrous cap.[1–4]

To date, a variety of diagnostic tools to detect structural abnormalities in vulnerable plaques have been developed. Intravascular optical coherence tomography (OCT) is a recently developed optical imaging technique that provides high-resolution, cross-sectional images of tissue in situ.[5] OCT originates from early work on white-light interferometry and optical coherence-domain reflectometry (OCDR). OCDR is a one-dimensional optical ranging technique that uses short coherence length light and interferometric detection[6] that was evolved for finding faults in fiberoptic cables and network components.[7] Its potential for medical application was soon recognized.[8,9] Researchers at the Massachusetts Institute of Technology extended the technique of OCDR and developed *optical coherence tomography* in the early 1990s as a *two-dimensional*, tomographic imaging modality in biologic systems.[10] The second dimension of the two-dimensional image was created by a physical translation or rotation of a fiberoptic probe. Since then, improvements of the light source, the interferometer, and beam scanning optics have been continuously pursued.[11–13]

Today – similar to intravascular ultrasound (IVUS) – intracoronary OCT allows for real-time imaging of the arterial wall but offers 10 times higher resolution and, thus, the possibility of detecting thin fibrous caps. An overview on image resolution of different diagnostic techniques is given in Table 17.1.[14]

This chapter gives an overview on currently available OCT technology for intracoronary application and summarizes the line of investigation with respect to vascular plaque characterization.

THE PRINCIPLE

The principle is analogous to pulse–echo ultrasound imaging; however, light is used rather than sound to create the image. Low coherent near-infrared light is emitted by a superluminescent diode. A wavelength around 1300 nm is used since it minimizes the energy absorption in the light beam caused by protein, water, hemoglobin, and lipids. The light waves are reflected by the internal microstructures within biologic tissues as a result of their differing optical indices. The echo time delay of reflected

Table 17.1   Comparison of invasive diagnostic modalities

Technology	Resolution	Fibrous cap	Lipid core	Inflammation	Calcium	Thrombus	Detection
IVUS	100 μm	+	+	−	+++	+	Plaque morphology and structure
Angioscopy	100 μm	+	++	−	−	+++	Plaque surface visualization
OCT	10 μm	+++	+++	++	+++	+	Detailed morphology, including macrophages
Thermography	500 μm	−	−	+++	−	−	Surface temperature
Spectroscopy	−	+	++	++	++	−	Chemical and tissue characteristics
Intravascular MRI	160 μm	+	++	+	++	+	Plaque morphology and structure

IVUS, intravascular ultrasound; OCT, optical coherence tomography; MRI, magnetic resonance imaging. Adapted from Low et al.[15]

light waves is determined by an interferometer. The angular position of the imaged line is varied and converted into a two-dimensional spatial image. The intensity of the reflected light waves is translated into an intensity map and encoded using a gray or false color scale (Figure 17.1).[15]

INTRAVASCULAR OPTICAL COHERENCE TOMOGRAPHY SYSTEMS

Intravascular OCT has been introduced with the Massachusetts General Hospital (MGH) OCT system and with a commercially available OCT system (LightLab Imaging, Boston, MA).

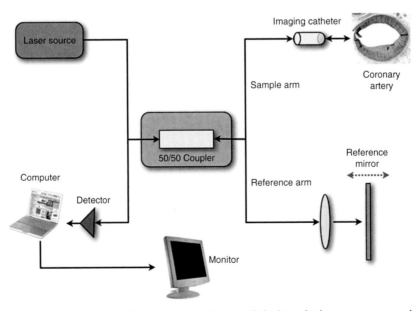

Figure 17.1   Schematic of OCT system. The pulse of low coherence light from the laser source passes through a beam splitter: half the beam is sent to the tissue sample and the other half to a reference moving mirror. Constructive interference from the reflected signals is used to create images.

MGH OCT System

The optical source power is 5 mW, centered at 1300 nm, with a bandwidth of 70 nm, giving an axial resolution of 10 μm. A high-speed phase control delay line is used for coherence gating and is capable of performing 2000 axial scans per second. Images are acquired at either 8 frames per second (500 angular pixels × 250 radial pixels) or 4 frames per second (250 angular pixels × 250 radial pixels). OCT images are displayed in real time using an inverse gray-scale lookup table and are digitally stored.

A commercially available 3.2 Fr IVUS catheter was modified by replacing a core with an optical fiber. This catheter consisted of a single-mode optical fiber within a wound stainless steel cable. At the distal tip of fiber, a gradient index lens and a microprism are used to produce a focused output beam that propagates transversely to the catheter axis.[16] The transverse resolution provided by the distal optics was 25 μm. The mechanical properties of this catheter were tested in porcine experiments and were found to be comparable to those of the 3.2 Fr IVUS catheter.[17] The proximal end design was similar to those described in previous publications.[11,16] The stainless steel cable that carried the fiber and the focusing optics were cemented to an FC fiberoptic connector that could be attached to and detached from the rotating end of the rotational coupler. The coupler consisted of two gradient index lens collimators separated by an air gap precisely aligned to ensure maximal throughput. A stabilized electric motor is used to spin the rotating end of the coupler (4–8 Hz) with the catheter through a belt drive. The rotating coupler, the motor, and the drive are enclosed in a compact (12 cm × 5 cm) handheld unit compatible with the requirements of the cardiology suite.

LightLab OCT System

The system uses advanced fiberoptic interferometers coupled with a mid-IR (1320 nm), low-power (8 mW), broad-bandwidth, light source. It is capable of imaging in real time using video scanning rates of up to 30 frames per second. The system hardware is divided into four major components:

- *The OCT imaging engine* (Figure 17.2a) emits and receives the infrared signals. The light source is housed in the engine, along with the interferometer and the detection circuitry. The detected signal is sent to the computer.
- *The computer controller* further processes the OCT information and converts it to a displayable format. It also controls the optical engine, the probe interface unit, and stores the images.
- *The probe interface unit* is the location where the imaging catheter plugs into the system. It provides the motor drive that spins the imaging core to create the circular image and allows the cardiologist to control the imaging procedure (Figure 17.2b).
- *The catheter system* consists of two components: the 0.019 inch *imaging wire* directs the infrared light into the tissue and returns the reflected light back to the optical engine. It contains the imaging core (diameter = 0.006 inch) that consists of the optical fiber, the lenses, and the turning prism. The proximal end of the catheter has a chamber that captures the imaging core and allows it to move along the catheter axis to perform an 'automated pullback'. The outside of the imaging catheter is stationary with respect to the vessel wall. The imaging core is rotated and translated inside of the external catheter sheath. *The balloon-delivery catheter* consists of a soft balloon with an imaging wire lumen. It is inflated at low pressures (0.5 atm) to interrupt the blood flow and used to

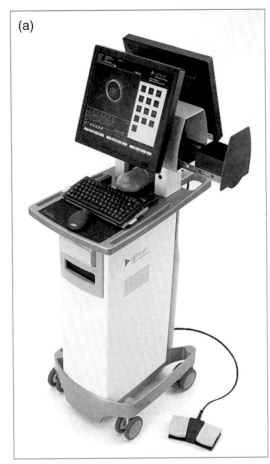

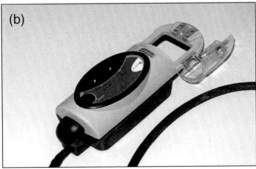

Figure 17.2 The LightLab OCT imaging system (LightLab Imaging, Boston, MA). The system is composed of (a) the imaging console, containing the OCT imaging engine and the computer controller, and (b) the probe interface unit, allowing for automated pullback.

deliver a modest amount of Ringer's lactate or saline flush to the imaging location during image acquisition.

OPTICAL COHERENCE TOMOGRAPHY FOR PLAQUE CHARACTERIZATION

In-vitro OCT imaging of human arteries

The first OCT imaging of a human coronary artery in vitro was described by Huang and coworkers in 1991, proving the concept that OCT is able to image non-transparent tissue.[10]

OCT morphometry, plaque characterization, and thickness of fibrous cap

The accuracy of OCT morphometry was studied in postmortem coronaries of 18 individuals who died of non-cardiac causes:[18] 54 coronary segments were randomly selected. The thickness of the intima and the thickness of the intima plus media (IMT) were measured. The OCT images had good contrast of the layers of the vessel wall, which clearly delineated the intima and media. By OCT, the intima was identified as the signal-rich layer nearest the lumen. The intima plus media was defined as the distance from the internal border of the signal-rich layer nearest the lumen to the outer border of the signal-poor middle layer. Measured by histology, the intimal thickness ranged from 0.10 to 0.89 mm (mean = 0.29 mm) and the IMT from 0.21 to 1.20 mm (mean = 0.56 mm). There was very good agreement between OCT and histologic examination for both: intimal thickness ($y = 0.85x + 0.06$, $r = 0.98$, $P < 0.001$, mean difference by Bland–Altman 0.01 ± 0.04 mm) and IMT ($y = 0.87x + 0.08$, $r = 0.95$, $P < 0.001$, mean difference $= -0.01 \pm 0.07$ mm). Furthermore, the OCT measurements showed low inter- and intraobserver variability (intimal thickness $= 0.01 \pm 0.01$ mm intraobserver, −0.01 ± 0.02 mm interobserver difference; IMT = −0.01 ± 0.02 mm intraobserver, 0.01 ± 0.03 mm interobserver difference).

Comparison studies between OCT and histology have established OCT criteria for different plaque types.[17,19–21] The MGH group studied OCT images of 357 atherosclerotic arterial segments, comprising 162 aortas, 105 carotid bulbs, and 90 coronary arteries from 90 cadavers (48 male and 42 female, mean age = 74.5 ± 13.2 years), and correlated them with histology in order to assess accuracy of objective OCT image criteria for atherosclerotic plaque characterization in vitro. The degree of agreement between histopathologic diagnosis and the results obtained by OCT readers and the OCT interobserver and intraobserver variability were quantified by the k test of concordance.[22] OCT image criteria for three types of plaque, fibrous plaque, fibrocalcific plaque, and lipid-rich plaque, were formulated by analysis of a subset ($n = 50$) of arterial segments. Calcification within the plaques was identified by the presence of well-delineated, signal-poor regions with sharp borders (Figure 17.3). Lipid pools were identified by the presence of signal-poor regions with diffuse borders. Fibrous tissue was identified by the presence of homogeneous, signal-rich regions. Independent validation of OCT image criteria by two OCT readers for the remaining segments ($n = 307$) demonstrated a sensitivity and specificity of 71–79% and 97–98% for fibrous plaques, 95–96% and 97% for fibrocalcific plaques, and 90–94% and 90–92% for lipid-rich plaques, respectively (overall agreement, $k = 0.83$–0.84). The interobserver and intraobserver reliabilities of OCT assessment were high (k values of 0.88 and 0.91, respectively).

Fibrous caps were measured by OCT (30–450 μm), and cap thickness correlated well with histology in the 10 specimens. There was a high degree of correlation between the two measurements ($r = 0.98$).

Quantification of macrophage content in atherosclerotic plaques

OCT images of 26 lipid-rich atherosclerotic arterial segments (19 aortas and 7 carotid bulbs) obtained at autopsy were correlated with histology in order to evaluate the potential of OCT for identifying macrophages in fibrous caps.[23] Cap macrophage density was quantified morphometrically by immunoperoxidase staining with CD68 and smooth muscle actin and compared with the standard deviation of the OCT signal intensity at corresponding locations (Figure 17.4). There was a high degree of positive correlation between OCT and histologic measurements of fibrous cap macrophage density ($r = 0.84$, $P < 0.0001$) and a negative correlation between OCT and histologic measurements of smooth muscle actin density ($r = -0.56$, $P < 0.005$). A range of OCT signal normalized standard deviation thresholds (6.15–6.35%) yielded 100% sensitivity and specificity for identifying caps containing >10% CD68 staining. The results of this in-vitro study suggest that the high contrast and resolution of OCT enables the quantification of macrophages within fibrous caps and this technology may be suited for identifying vulnerable plaques in living patients.

IN-VIVO OCT IMAGING OF SWINE CORONARY ARTERIES

Normal coronary arteries, intimal dissections, and stents were imaged in five swine with OCT and compared with IVUS.[17] In the normal coronary arteries, visualization of all the layers of the vessel wall was achieved with a saline flush, including the intima, which was not identified by IVUS. Following dissections, detailed layered structures including intimal flaps, intimal defects, and disruption of the medial wall

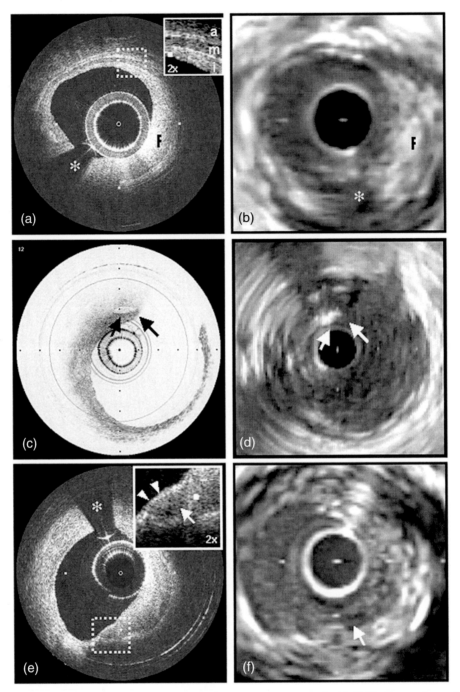

Figure 17.3 In-vivo OCT images of various coronary plaque types as compared with IVUS: fibrous plaque (a, b), calcific plaque (c, d), and lipid-rich plaque (e, f). (a) From 9 o'clock to 2 o'clock, the three-layer structure of a typical plaque is shown (inset): intima (i), media (m), and adventitia (a). From 2 o'clock to 9 o'clock, a homogeneous, signal-rich pattern consistent with a fibrous plaque (F), which is partially obscured by guidewire artifact (*) is shown. (b) The corresponding IVUS image. (c) A signal-poor region surrounded by sharp borders represents a calcific plaque. The exact area of the calcific plaque is clearly delineated (arrows). (d) On the corresponding IVUS image, calcium is easily identified. However, the structure in front of the calcium deposit is obscured due to the strong signal and the structure behind the calcium is not seen due to backshadow artifact. (e) A signal-poor region (arrow in inset) surrounded by diffuse borders and separated by a signal-rich layer (arrowheads in inset) is consistent with a lipid-rich plaque. (f) The corresponding IVUS image suggests a superficial echolucent region. (Adapted from Jang et al.[21])

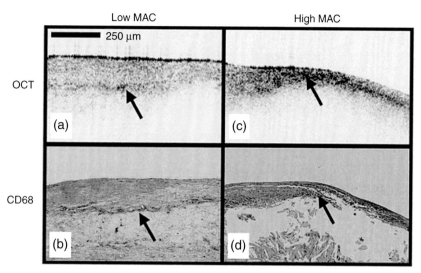

Figure 17.4 Low and high magnification of OCT and corresponding histology images. (a) and (c) OCT imaging with macrophages showing as areas of high-intensity signal beneath the intima. (b) and (d) Corresponding histology for (a) and (c) (CD68 immunoperoxidase). Macrophage accumulation is indicated by arrows. (Adapted from Tearney et al.[23])

were visualized by OCT. IVUS failed to show clear evidence of intimal and medial disruption.

Furthermore, in stented arteries, the microanatomic relationships between stent struts and the vessel walls were clearly identified by OCT. The superior OCT detail resolution in stent assessment has been confirmed by other postmortem[24] or in-vivo human observations. OCT allows for direct measurement of acute stent recoil,[25] the visualization of very thin neointimal layers in drug-eluting stents,[26,27] and, possibly, the visualization of portions of the neovascular bed.[28]

IN-VIVO OCT IMAGING OF HUMAN CORONARY ARTERIES

Comparison with IVUS

The first OCT study in living patients was reported in 2002.[21] In this study, a total of 17 IVUS and OCT image pairs in 10 patients were compared and the feasibility and the ability of intravascular OCT

were evaluated. In order to remove blood from the field of view and allow clear visualization of the vessel wall, OCT images were recorded during intermittent 8–10 ml saline flushes through the guide catheter. Axial resolution measured 13.3 ± 3 µm with OCT and 98 ± 19 µm with IVUS. All OCT procedures were performed without complications. All fibrous plaques, macrocalcifications, and echolucent regions identified by IVUS were visualized in corresponding OCT images. Intimal hyperplasia and echolucent regions, which may correspond to lipid pools, were identified more frequently by OCT than by IVUS.

OCT findings and clinical syndrome

OCT was used to study characteristics in culprit lesions in patients with various clinical presentations. In Rotterdam, a pilot study was conducted to assess whether morphologic features that have been associated with vulnerable plaque[29] could be visualized during in-vivo investigation by OCT.[30] Twenty-three patients with stable angina pectoris (SAP, $n = 17$), unstable angina pectoris (UAP, $n = 4$) or following ST-elevation myocardial infarction (STEMI, $n = 2$) scheduled for percutaneous coronary intervention (PCI) were included. A continuous OCT pullback (speed 1 mm/s) of the target artery was performed prior to intervention. Off-line OCT analysis included plaque characterization according to published literature[24] and assessment of thin-cap fibroatheroma (TCFA). TCFA was defined by OCT as signal-poor lipid/necrotic core, covered by a signal-rich fibrous cap with a cap thickness <0.2 mm and a circumferential extent of >45° vessel circumference in at least five consecutive OCT frames. Mean OCT pullback length was 28.8 ± 12.2 mm. Analysis of the culprit lesion revealed a minimal lumen area of 2.83 ± 0.93 mm^2 with fibrous plaque in 9 lesions ($n = 6$ eccentric, $n = 3$ concentric), plaque with calcification in 8 lesions ($n = 6$ eccentric, $n = 2$ concentric) and fibro-lipid plaque in 4 lesions (3 eccentric, 1 concentric). Two culprit lesions were TCFA, with one showing signs of fissure/rupture and adjacent thrombus (Figure 17.5). Remote from the culprit lesion, but within the culprit vessel,

7 TFCA were observed in 6 patients ($n = 3$ UAP, $n = 2$ following STEMI, $n = 1$ SAP). The fibrous cap thickness was 0.19 ± 0.05 mm, the circumferential extent $103 \pm 49°$. This pilot study demonstrated that intravascular OCT could detect in-vivo morphologic features that have been associated with plaque vulnerability by retrospective pathologic examination. Within the coronary artery, the occurrence of TCFA can be observed as a culprit lesion as well as remote from a culprit lesion.

At the MGH, a larger study enrolling 57 patients was conducted: 20 patients following acute STEMI, 20 patients with NSTEACS (NSTEMI and unstable angina), and 17 patients with SAP.[31] All subjects underwent coronary angiography and concurrent OCT imaging of culprit and non-culprit plaque prior to any intervention. Lipid-rich plaque was defined as lipid occupying ≥2 quadrants of the cross-sectional area and TCFA by lipid-rich plaque with a fibrous cap thickness ≤65 µm. Lipid-rich plaque was observed in 90% of STEMI patients, 75% of NSTEACS patients, and 59% of SAP patients ($P = 0.09$). There were no significant differences between the frequency of TCFA ($P = 0.172$) or the fibrous cap thickness ($P = 0.38$) between subjects with STEMI and NSTEACS. The frequency of plaque rupture or the presence of thrombus, however, was not significantly different.

The significant association between TCFA, fibrous cap attenuation, and the patients who presented with unstable coronary syndromes is in keeping with the findings of the autopsy studies that have provided the foundation for our current understanding of the role of plaque disruption in acute coronary events. This study reinforces the importance of fibrous cap thickness as a measure of plaque vulnerability and demonstrates the advantage of the high resolution provided by OCT.

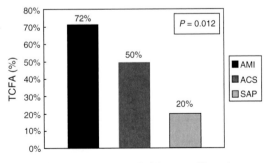

Figure 17.5 Prevalence of thin cap fibroatheroma (TCFA), defined by lipid-rich plaque (≥2 quadrants) and fibrous cap thickness <65 µm. TCFA was observed in 72% of the patients with acute myocardial infarction (AMI), in 50% of patients with acute coronary syndromes (ACS), and in 20% of patients with stable angina pectoris (SAP) ($P = 0.012$).

In-vivo macrophage concentration and distribution

Macrophage concentration was evaluated in 49 patients (19 STEMI, 19 NSTEACS, 11 SAP), both within the culprit plaque and within non-culprit lesions in the same coronary artery:[32] 119 lipid-rich plaques (76 culprit, 43 remote) and 41 fibrous plaques were evaluated. Macrophage densities in lipid-rich plaques varied significantly among the three clinical groups ($P < 0.001$) with a higher macrophage concentration in the acute coronary syndrome (ACS) patients than in the patients with SAP ($P = 0.002$). Consistent with their common pathophysiology, there was no difference in the macrophage densities between the two groups of ACS patients ($P = 0.38$). In line with the concept of pan-arterial inflammation, macrophage densities at both culprit and remote sites within each clinical group were similar. Likewise, within the same patient ($n = 15$), macrophage density at remote sites correlated significantly with that of culprit sites. Macrophage infiltration was not confined to just lipid-rich plaque; a significantly higher macrophage density was seen in fibrous plaques in the unstable coronary group.

In patients with STEMI and NSTEACS, the relationship of focal macrophage density in the fibrous cap to the site of plaque cap rupture was evaluated by analyzing culprit lipid-rich plaques that demonstrated clear evidence of plaque rupture ($n = 6$; 2 STEMI, 4 NSTEACS). For each rupture site, the macrophage density within a 250 μm segment at the point of disruption was analyzed and compared to that of the remainder of the fibrous cap. There was a significantly higher macrophage density at the rupture site than at the adjacent non-ruptured cap within the same image. Furthermore, macrophage density at rupture sites was significantly greater than that of all non-ruptured culprit sites in the combined STEMI and ACS groups ($6.95 \pm 1.6\%$, $5.75 \pm 1.8\%$; $P = 0.04$).

To further evaluate the relevance of focal macrophage infiltration of the fibrous cap, the spatial location of macrophages within the cap of lipid-rich plaques was examined to determine if proximity to the endothelial surface was related to the clinical syndrome. Receiver operating curves for the prediction of an unstable coronary syndrome were constructed for the macrophage densities in the superficial and subsurface layers of the fibrous cap. At culprit sites, the area under the curve (AUC) for superficial macrophage density was significantly better than subsurface macrophage density at predicting an unstable presentation (AUC 0.79 ± 0.06 vs 0.69 ± 0.07, respectively; $P = 0.035$). This was not found to be the case in plaques at remote sites, suggesting that macrophage content at the surface of culprit but not remote lesions was predictive of an acute coronary event. It is possible therefore that OCT-based evaluation of superficial macrophage content could provide us with a new parameter for assessing individual plaque vulnerability.

Mechanical properties of the coronary artery wall

In the combination study with OCT and IVUS, the relationships between the plaque characterization and distensibility, index of mechanical property in vessel wall, were investigated.[33] At the 29 non-culprit lesions with 30–50% stenosis on coronary angiogram, ECG-gated IVUS images were obtained to calculate systolic and diastolic external elastic membrane (EEM) area and lumen cross-sectional area (CSA). Distensibility index was calculated as

$$\Delta \text{ lumen CSA}/(\text{lumen CSA in diastole} \times \Delta P) \times 10^3 \ (\text{mmHg}^{-1})$$

where Δ lumen CSA is the difference between systolic and diastolic lumen CSA and ΔP is the difference between systolic and diastolic intracoronary pressure. Plaque morphology was classified as lipid-rich plaque ($n = 7$), mixed plaque ($n = 6$), or fibrous plaque ($n = 16$) according to OCT criteria. Distensibility index was significantly higher in lipid-rich plaques than in other plaque types ($P < 0.005$). The results of this study suggest that plaques with high distensibility might be one of the mechanical characteristics in the vulnerable plaques.

SAFETY

The applied energies in intravascular OCT are relatively low (output power in the range of 5.0–8.0 mW) and are not considered to cause functional or structural damage to the tissue.

Thus, safety issues seem mainly to concern OCT catheter design and the extent of ischemia caused by flow obstruction from the catheter itself and the displacement of blood. Representative safety data for intravascular OCT are not yet available, as there is only preliminary clinical experience in a small number of patients. In the Rotterdam series, the most frequent complications were transient electrocardiographic changes indicative for ischemia (58%) and chest pain (38%). These data match well with large IVUS registries that reported transient coronary ischemia caused by the imaging catheter in 67% and by angina in 22% of patients.[34]

LIMITATIONS

Optical imaging in non-transparent biologic tissues is, in general, a difficult problem, primarily due to the scattering of the tissue. In coronary arteries, blood (namely red blood cells) represents that non-transparent tissue causing multiple scattering and substantial signal attenuation. As a consequence, blood must be displaced during OCT imaging. This can be accomplished in several ways, e.g. by saline infusion through the guiding catheter, limiting of blood flow by a percutaneous transluminal coronary angioplasty or a soft balloon, or continuous flushing during imaging by a dedicated OCT catheter design. These approaches have different advantages; however, all of them may cause and are limited by ischemia in the territory of the artery under study. Special techniques such as index matching[35] may reduce ischemia in the future.

Another limitation is the relatively low penetration depth of OCT that restricts in-vivo imaging to small to medium-sized coronary arteries (up to a lumen diameter of 4.0 mm) or to the visualization of the luminal vessel surface.

A second-generation OCT, optical frequency domain imaging (OFDI), is being evaluated at MGH.[36] This new platform can potentially overcome all current limitations of OCT such as lack of scanning capability and limited penetration depth.

FUTURE ROLE OF OPTICAL COHERENCE TOMOGRAPHY

Today, a considerable body of evidence from in-vitro, preclinical, and clinical studies has been generated showing that intravascular OCT is able to visualize features of vulnerable plaque in living patients. One important goal will be the performance of a long-term follow-up study to evaluate the clinical significance and natural history of such OCT findings.

Identification of vulnerable plaques might lead to a therapeutic strategy specifically designed for a given patient to prevent ACS, such as sudden cardiac death. OCT might be useful to monitor structural changes in response to genetic, pharmacologic, or other forms of intervention. Finally, with its high resolution, this imaging modality may prove helpful to optimize PCI.

REFERENCES

1. Falk E, Shah PK, Fuster V. Coronary plaque disruption. Circulation 1995; 92:657–71.
2. Davies MJ. Detecting vulnerable coronary plaques. Lancet 1996; 347:1422–3.
3. Virmani R, Kolodgie FD, Burke AP, Farb A, Schwartz SM. Lessons from sudden coronary death: a comprehensive morphological classification scheme for atherosclerotic lesions. Arterioscler Thromb Vasc Biol 2000; 20:1262–75.
4. Naruko T, Ueda M, Haze K, van der Wal AC et al. Neutrophil infiltration of culprit lesions in acute coronary syndromes. Circulation 2002; 106:2894–900.
5. Boppart SA, Bouma BE, Pitris C et al. In vivo cellular optical coherence tomography imaging. Nat Med 1998; 4:861–5.
6. Youngquist R, Carr S, Daries DEN. Optical coherence-domain reflectometry: A new optical evaluation technique. Opt Lett 1987; 12:158–60.
7. Takada K, Yokohama I, Chida K, Noda J. New measurement system for fault location in optical waveguide devices based on an interferometric technique. Appl Opt 1987; 26:1603–6.
8. Fercher AF, Mengedoht K, Werner W. Eye-length measurement by interferometry with partially coherent light. Opt Lett 1988; 13:186–8.
9. Huang D, Wang JP, Lin CP, Puliafito CA, Fujimoto JG. Micron-resolution ranging of cornea anterior-chamber by optical reflectometry. Lasers Surg Med 1991; 11:419–25.
10. Huang D, Swanson E, Lin C et al. Optical coherence tomography. Science 1991; 254:1178–81.
11. Tearney GJ, Brezinski ME, Bouma BE et al. In vivo endoscopic optical biopsy with optical coherence tomography. Science 1997; 276:2037–9.
12. Fujimoto JG, Bouma B, Tearney GJ et al. New technology for high-speed and high-resolution optical coherence tomography. Ann NY Acad Sci 1998; 838:95–107.
13. Schmitt JM. Optical coherence tomography (OPT): a review. IEEE J Select Topics Quantum Electron 1999; 5:1205–15.
14. MacNeill B, Lowe HC, Takano M, Fuster V, Jang IK. Intravascular modalities for detection of vulnerable plaque: current status. Arterioscler Thromb Vasc Biol 2003; 23:1333–42.
15. Low AF, Tearney GJ, Bouma BE, Jang IK. Technology insight: optical coherence tomography – current status and future development. Nat Clin Pract Cardiovasc Med 2006; 3:154–62.
16. Tearney G, Boppart S. Scanning single-mode fiber optic catheter-endoscope for optical coherence tomography. Opt Lett 1996; 21:1–3.
17. Tearney GJ, Jang IK, Kang DH et al. Porcine coronary imaging in vivo by optical coherence tomography. Acta Cardiol 2000; 55:233–7.
18. Kume T, Akasaka T, Kawamoto T et al. Assessment of coronary intima–media thickness by optical coherence tomography: comparison with intravascular ultrasound. Circ J 2005; 69:903–7.
19. Brezinski ME, Tearney GJ, Bouma BE et al. Imaging of coronary artery microstructure (in vitro) with optical coherence tomography. Am J Cardiol 1996; 77:92–3.
20. Brezinski ME, Tearney GJ, Bouma BE et al. Optical coherence tomography for optical biopsy. Properties and demonstration of vascular pathology. Circulation 1996; 93:1206–13.
21. Jang IK, Bouma BE, Kang DH et al. Visualization of coronary atherosclerotic plaques in patients using optical coherence tomography: comparison with intravascular ultrasound. J Am Coll Cardiol 2002; 39:604–9.
22. Yabushita H, Bouma BE, Houser SL et al. Characterization of human atherosclerosis by optical coherence tomography. Circulation 2002; 106:1640–5.
23. Tearney GJ, Yabushita H, Houser SL et al. Quantification of macrophage content in atherosclerotic plaques by optical coherence tomography. Circulation 2003; 107:113–19.
24. Kume T, Akasaka T, Kawamoto T et al. Visualization of neointima formation by optical coherence tomography. Int Heart J 2005; 46:1133–6.
25. Regar E, Schaar J, Serruys P. Images in cardiology. Acute recoil in sirolimus eluting stent: real time, in vivo assessment with optical coherence tomography. Heart 2006; 92:123.
26. Grube E, Gerckens U, Buellesfeld L, Fitzgerald PJ. Images in cardiovascular medicine. Intracoronary imaging with optical coherence tomography: a new high-resolution technology providing striking visualization in the coronary artery. Circulation 2002; 106: 2409–10.
27. Buellesfeld L, Lim V, Gerckens U, Mueller R, Grube E. Comparative endoluminal visualization of TAXUS crush-stenting at 9 months follow-up by intravascular ultrasound and optical coherence tomography. Z Kardiol 2005; 94:690–4.
28. Regar E, van Beusekom HM, van der Giessen WJ, Serruys PW. Images in cardiovascular medicine. Optical coherence tomography findings at 5-year follow-up after coronary stent implantation. Circulation 2005; 112:e345–6.
29. Schaar JA, Muller JE, Falk E et al. Terminology for high-risk and vulnerable coronary artery plaques. Report of a meeting on the vulnerable plaque, June 17 and 18, 2003, Santorini, Greece. Eur Heart J 2004; 25:1077–82.
30. Regar E, Schaar J, McFadden E et al. Real-time, high resolution optical coherence tomography (OCT) – a potential tool to detect features of vulnerable plaque in-vivo? Eur Heart J 2005 abstract 3677.
31. Jang IK, Tearney G, MacNeill B et al. In vivo characterization of coronary atherosclerotic plaque by use of optical coherence tomography. Circulation 2005; 111:1551–5.

32. MacNeill BD, Jang IK, Bouma BE et al. Focal and multi-focal plaque macrophage distributions in patients with acute and stable presentations of coronary artery disease. J Am Coll Cardiol 2004; 44:972–9.

33. MacNeill B, Shaw J, Yabushita H et al. Lipid rich plaques display greater vessel distensibility than fibrous plaques: a combined optical coherence tomography and intravascular ultrasound study. Circulation 2002; abstract 3237.

34. Hausmann D, Erbel R, Alibelli-Chemarin MJ et al. The safety of intracoronary ultrasound. A multicenter survey of 2207 examinations. Circulation 1995; 91:623–30.

35. Brezinski M, Saunders K, Jesser C, Li X, Fujimoto J. Index matching to improve optical coherence tomography imaging through blood. Circulation 2001; 103:1999–2003.

36. Yun S, Tearney G, de Boer J, Iftimia N, Bouma B. High-speed optical frequency-domain imaging. Optics Express 2003; 11:2953–63.

Virtual histology 18

Hector M Garcia-Garcia, Neville Kukreja, and Patrick W Serruys

INTRODUCTION

Angiography has for decades been the gold standard to assess the morphology and severity of atherosclerotic lesions in the coronary tree. Nevertheless, quantitative angiographic measurements can be deceptive, since this technique only allows the assessment of the shape of the lumen.[1] Indeed, coronary angiography as a standard for the assessment of coronary artery disease has two major limitations: first, visual assessment of stenosis severity has high intraobserver and interobserver variabilities; secondly, there is a clear discrepancy between the appearance of the opacified vascular lumen and the actual degree of atherosclerosis. The common finding of mild diffuse disease that involves the whole length of the opacified coronary tree, without a remnant disease-free reference segment, makes the lumen appear as if it was an atherosclerosis-free area. Although quantitative coronary assessment (QCA) has reduced the visual error, it is known that at the site identified by QCA as the proximal boundary of the lesion, there may exist a 50% area stenosis when such a segment is analyzed by intravascular ultrasound (IVUS).[2] Thus, IVUS is the gold standard for evaluation of coronary plaque, lumen, and vessel dimensions; it provides an accurate, reproducible, real-time, tomographic assessment of the vessel wall.[3–5] However, although visual interpretation of gray-scale IVUS can characterize plaque composition, particularly calcification, it cannot reliably differentiate lipid-rich from fibrous plaque.[4] In contrast, IVUS radiofrequency (RF) data analysis (IVUS virtual histology or IVUS-VH) can accurately characterize four tissue types in atherosclerotic plaques.

TECHNICAL ASPECTS OF THE TECHNIQUE

IVUS gray-scale imaging is formed by the envelope (amplitude) of the RF signal, discarding a considerable amount of information lying beneath and between the peaks of the RF signal. The amplitude of the RF data might sometimes be similar between different tissues, leading to misinterpretation of gray-scale imaging. Nevertheless, the frequency and power of the RF signal commonly differs between tissues, regardless of the eventual similarities of the amplitude (Figure 18.1). Spectral analysis of the RF data (IVUS-VH, Volcano Corporation, Rancho Cordova, CA, USA) evaluates different spectral parameters of the RF data (*y*-intercept, minimum power, maximum power, mid-band power, frequency at minimum power, frequency at maximum power, slope, etc.) to construct tissue maps that classify plaque into four major components.

VALIDATION OF THE TECHNIQUE

In preliminary ex-vivo studies, four histologic plaque components (fibrous, fibro-lipidic, necrotic core, and calcium) were

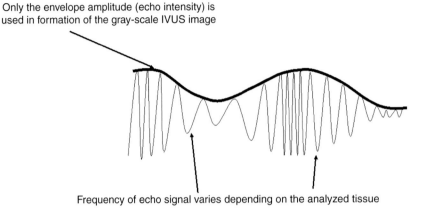

Only the envelope amplitude (echo intensity) is
used in formation of the gray-scale IVUS image

Frequency of echo signal varies depending on the analyzed tissue

Figure 18.1 Intravascular ultrasound (IVUS) gray-scale imaging is formed by the envelope (amplitude) of the radiofrequency (RF) signal, discarding a considerable amount of information lying beneath and between the peaks of the RF signal. The frequency of a tissue may differ, despite having the same amplitude.

correlated with a specific spectrum of the RF signal.[6] These different plaque components were assigned color codes: calcified (dense calcium), fibrous (fibrotic), fibrolipidic (fibrofatty), and necrotic core regions were labeled white, green, greenish-yellow and red, respectively (Figure 18.2). This approach has led to a significant increase in the sensitivity and specificity of IVUS to characterize plaque, particularly lipid deposits. Indeed, the sensitivity of gray-scale imaging to detect lipid deposits was reported to be as low as 46%, whereas the predictive accuracy of IVUS-VH to detect necrotic core areas is 86%.[6,7]

Furthermore, recent improvements in the classification tree have led to a further enhancement in the accuracy of the technique, which has been evaluated using atherectomy samples, reaching a sensitivity of 67.3% and specificity of 92.9% for detecting necrotic core[8] (Table 18.1).

IVUS-VH data are currently acquired using a commercially available phased-array (64 elements) catheter (Eagle Eye™ 20 MHz catheter, Volcano Corporation, Rancho Cordova, CA, USA). Using an automated pullback device, the transducer is withdrawn at a continuous speed of 0.5 mm/s until the ostium.

IVUS-VH acquisition is ECG-gated at the R-wave peaks using a dedicated console (Volcano Corporation, Rancho Cordova, CA, USA).

IVUS-VH analysis

IVUS B-mode images are reconstructed from the RF data by customized software, and contour detection is performed on cross-sectional areas using semi-automatic contour detection software to provide a quantitative geometrical and compositional output (IvusLab 4.4, Volcano Corporation, Rancho Cordova, CA, USA). Due to the unreliability of manual calibration,[9] the RF data are normalized using a technique known as 'Blind Deconvolution', an iterative algorithm that deconvolves the catheter transfer function from the backscatter, thus accounting for catheter-to-catheter variability.[10]

THIN-CAP FIBROATHEROMA DETECTION

It has been established that unheralded acute coronary syndromes (ACS) are common initial manifestations of coronary atherosclerosis and that most such events

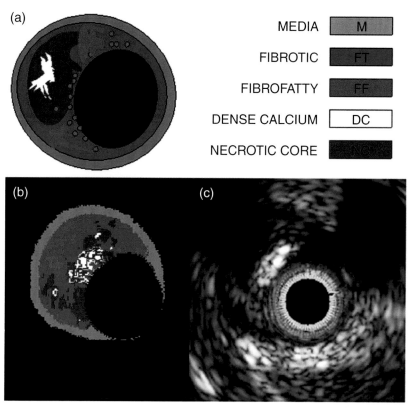

MEDIA   M

FIBROTIC   FT

FIBROFATTY   FF

DENSE CALCIUM   DC

NECROTIC CORE   NC

Figure 18.2   (a) A cartoon of an intravascular ultrasound (IVUS)-derived thin cap fibroatheroma. Notice that the cap is infiltrated by macrophages (small yellow circles), information that is not provided by virtual histology (VH). This panel also contains the color code of VH. (b) An IVUS cross-sectional area reconstructed from backscattered signals, which has a confluent pool of necrotic core in direct contact with the lumen, suggesting a thin cap fibroatheroma. (c) The corresponding IVUS gray-scale cross-sectional area.

arise from sites with non-flow-limiting coronary atherosclerosis.[11,12] Postmortem studies suggested that plaque composition is a crucial determinant of the propensity of atherosclerotic lesions to rupture. Recently, a study including a large series of victims of sudden cardiac death suggested that ruptured thin-cap fibro-atheroma (TCFA) lesions were the precip-itating factor of 60% of acute coronary thrombi. Furthermore, 70% of those patients had other TCFAs in their coro-nary tree that had not ruptured.[13] A large (avascular, hypocellular, lipid-rich) necrotic core, a thin fibrous cap with inflammatory infiltration and paucity of smooth muscle cells, and the presence of expansive (pos-itive) remodeling have been identified as the major criteria to define TCFA lesions.[14-18]

Detection of these non-obstructive, lipid-rich, high-risk plaques may have an impor-tant impact on the prevention of acute myocardial infarction and sudden death.

We recently evaluated the incidence of IVUS-derived thin-cap fibroatheroma (IDTCFA) in coronary artery segments with non-significant lesions on angiogra-phy using IVUS-VH.[19] In this study, two experienced, independent IVUS analysts defined IDTCFA as a lesion fulfilling the following criteria in at least three consec-utive cross-sectional areas: (1) necrotic core ≥10% without evident overlying fibrous tissue and (2) percent obstruction ≥40%. In this study, 62% of patients had

Table 18.1 Validation of IVUS virtual histology

Plaque component	Ex-vivo pressure-fixed (2002) Predictive accuracy (%)	In vivo post-atherectomy (2006) Sensitivity (%)	Specificity (%)	Predictive accuracy (%)	Ex-vivo pressure-fixed (2006) Sensitivity (%)	Specificity (%)	Predictive accuracy (%)
Fibrous tissue	79.7	86	90.5	87.1	83.9	98.8	92.9
Fibrofatty	81.2	79.3	100	87.1	86.9	95	93.4
Necrotic core	85.5	67.3	92.9	88.3	97.1	93.8	94.3
Dense calcium	92.8	50	98.9	96.5	97.8	99.7	99.3

at least one IDTCFA in the interrogated vessels. ACS patients had a significantly higher incidence of IDTCFA than stable patients: 3.0 (interquartile range 0.0, 5.0) IDTCFA/coronary vs 1.0 (interquartile range 0.0, 2.8) IDTCFA/coronary, $P = 0.018$. Of note, no relation was found between patient characteristics and the presence of IDTCFA. Finally, a clear clustering pattern was seen along the coronaries, with 66 (66.7%) IDTCFA located in the first 20 mm, whereas further along the vessels the incidence was significantly lower (33, 33.3%, $P = 0.008$).[19] Such distribution of the IDTCFA was in line with previous ex-vivo and clinical studies, with a clear clustering pattern from the ostium, thus supporting the finding of non-uniform distribution of vulnerable plaques along the coronary tree.[20,21]

The significantly higher prevalence of IDTCFA in non-culprit coronaries of patients presenting with an ACS supports the theory that holds ACS as a multifocal process. Of note, the mean plaque atheroma volume and the mean necrotic core areas of the IDTCFAs detected by IVUS-VH were also similar to previously reported histopathologic data (55.9% vs 59.6% and 19% vs 23%, respectively).[22]

It is worth mentioning that, although the most accepted threshold to define a cap as 'thin' has previously been set at <65 µm, this was based on postmortem studies.[23] Extrapolation of such criteria to in-vivo studies requires caution. It is well established that tissue shrinkage occurs during tissue fixation.[24] Shrinkage (particularly of collagen tissue, the main component of fibrous caps) of up to 60%, 15%, and 80% can occur during critical point drying, freeze drying, and air drying, respectively.[25] Furthermore, postmortem contraction of arteries is an additional confounding factor.[26] It is likely therefore, that the threshold used to define a thin cap in-vivo should be higher than 65 µm. Since the axial resolution of IVUS-VH is 246 µm, we assumed that the absence of visible fibrous tissue overlying a necrotic core suggested a cap thickness of below 246 µm and used the absence of such tissue to define a thin fibrous cap.[27] Finally, it is noteworthy that a number of important ex-vivo studies have used a higher (> 200 µm) threshold.[17,28,29] Indeed, one of these studies identified a mean cap thickness of 260 µm and 360 µm for 'vulnerable' and 'non-vulnerable' plaques, respectively.[29] For all the aforementioned reasons, we believe that IVUS-VH is able to detect thin caps.

POSITIVE REMODELING DETECTION

Expansive remodeling of coronary vessels was originally deemed a beneficial compensatory effect that counterbalanced the axial progressive growth of the vessel wall to preserve the lumen dimensions.[30] However, several studies have shown increased levels of inflammatory markers, larger necrotic cores, and pronounced medial thinning in positive remodeled vessels, which are all factors related to the tendency of plaques to undergo rupture.[31–34] Overall, this has led the experts to confer positive remodeling a major importance in the vulnerability triad.[14]

Precise contour detection of the external elastic membrane (vessel area) is pivotal to estimate the presence and pattern of remodeling. Owing to the high penetration of 20 MHz catheters, IVUS-VH can accurately assess vessel size and, therefore, provided that plaques are not heavily calcified, estimate the degree and type of remodeling. This was recently demonstrated in vivo, where we found a significant positive relationship between relative necrotic core content and the remodeling index ($r = 0.83$, $P < 0.0001$). Moreover, fibrous tissue was inversely correlated to the remodeling index ($r = -0.45$, $P = 0.003$).[34]

Likewise, lesions with positive remodeling presented significantly larger necrotic core percentages than lesions with no remodeling or negative remodeling

$(22.1 \pm 6.3\%$ vs $15.1 \pm 7.6\%$ vs $6.6 \pm 6.9\%$, $P < 0.0001$). Conversely, negative remodeling lesions tended to show larger fibrous tissue percentages than lesions with no remodeling and positive remodeling $(68.6 \pm 13.7\%$ vs $62.9 \pm 9.5\%$ vs $58.1 \pm 12.9\%$, $P = 0.13$).

COMBINING OPTICAL COHERENCE TOMOGRAPHY AND IVUS-VH

It is clear that the optimal tool to assess the presence of the major criteria that define TCFA would be a tool that combines the superior axial resolution of OCT with the accurate plaque characterization and deep penetration of IVUS-VH. Unfortunately, such a tool has not yet been developed. Instead, intensive efforts are being made to overcome the weaknesses of both techniques. In the meantime, we are currently assessing in vivo the agreement between both techniques to characterize plaques. Using side-branches as landmarks and with the aid of longitudinal and cross-sectional views, matching of cross sections is feasible.

Our preliminary experience shows a high agreement among the techniques towards the detection of fibrous, fibrocalcific, and necrotic core regions (Figure 18.3).

Despite major advances in the management and diagnosis of patients with coronary artery disease, a large number of victims who are apparently healthy die suddenly without prior symptoms.[35,36] Most of these events are related to plaque rupture and subsequent thrombotic occlusion at the site of non-flow-limiting atherosclerotic lesions in epicardial coronary arteries.[11,12] In addition, silent plaque rupture and subsequent wound healing accelerate plaque growth and are a more frequent feature in arteries with less-severe luminal narrowing.[37] The prospective detection of TCFA lesions may have a major impact on the prevention of acute myocardial infarction and sudden death. Both OCT and IVUS-VH have demonstrated the ability to identify in-vivo surrogates of TCFA. Nevertheless, prospective studies are needed in order to evaluate the prognostic value of such findings in natural history studies.

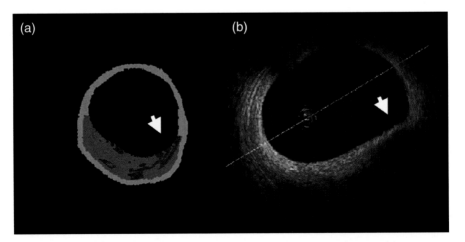

Figure 18.3   This patient was studied with (a) intravascular ultrasound virtual histology (IVUS-VH) and (b) optical coherence tomography (OCT): (a) IVUS-VH shows a pool of necrotic core (red) in direct contact with the lumen (arrow). (b) OCT shows a thin-cap fibroatheroma (arrow) overlying a pool of necrotic core.

COMBINING PALPOGRAPHY AND IVUS-VH

Both palpography and VH use IVUS radiofrequency analysis (RFA) and are acquired in the same IVUS pullback. Specifically, IVUS palpography is a technique that allows the assessment of local mechanical tissue properties.[29,38,39] This technique has shown a high sensitivity and specificity to detect vulnerable plaques in vitro.[29] Indeed, a strong inverse relation was found between cap thickness and strain.[29,40] In parallel, spectral analysis of the IVUS RF data (IVUS-VH) is emerging as a tool to assess plaque morphology and composition.[6,8] This combined imaging assessment might allow a more accurate and complete characterization in vivo of allegedly high-risk plaques. Thereby, it may offer the opportunity to truly identify the number of high-risk plaques in vivo.

The relationship between mechanical and compositional properties of coronary atherosclerosis has not been fully elucidated. In this respect, our group has previously studied the relationship between them, analyzing 123 matched cross-sectional areas (CSAs) from two different transducers (20 MHz and 30 MHz) of the same vessel. In this preliminary study, the mean strain value was higher in CSAs with necrotic core in contact with the lumen (NCCL) than in CSAs with no NCCL (1.03 ± 0.5 vs 0.86 ± 0.4, $P = 0.06$). The sensitivity, specificity, positive predictive value, and negative predictive value of IVUS-VH to detect high strain were 75.0%, 44.4%, 56.3%, and 65.1% respectively.[41]

We are currently working to further explore in vivo the relation between mechanical (palpography) and compositional (IVUS-VH) features of coronary atherosclerotic plaques and the potential to identify high-risk plaques in vivo, specifically IDTCFAs with high strain and positive remodeling in patients with ACS using a single IVUS pullback in each of the three major coronary vessels (Figure 18.4).

CONCLUSIONS

To date, there is no single isolated marker of vulnerability that can accurately and precisely identify atherosclerotic plaques at risk of rupture. On the contrary, it seems that the in-vivo simultaneous assessment of acknowledged high-risk atherosclerotic plaque characteristics may improve the accuracy to reliably identify vulnerable plaques.

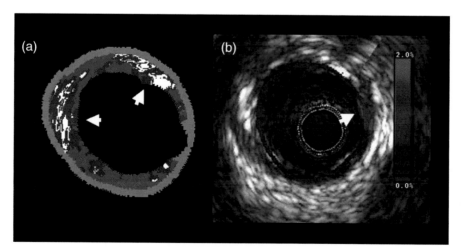

Figure 18.4   This patient was studied with (a) intravascular ultrasound virtual histology (IVUS-VH) and palpography (b). (a) IVUS-VH shows two pools of necrotic core (red) in direct contact with the lumen (arrows). (b) Palpography shows a high strain (ROC III) next to a pool of necrotic core with microcalcifications in contact with the lumen (arrow).

For the first time, numerous high-risk characteristics can be assessed simultaneously by means of IVUS RF analysis (combining IVUS-VH and palpography).

REFERENCES

1. Topol EJ, Nissen SE. Our preoccupation with coronary luminology. The dissociation between clinical and angiographic findings in ischemic heart disease. Circulation 1995; 92:2333–42.

2. Escaned J, Baptista J, Di Mario C et al. Significance of automated stenosis detection during quantitative angiography. Insights gained from intracoronary ultrasound imaging. Circulation 1996; 94:966–72.

3. Tobis JM, Mallery JA, Gessert J et al. Intravascular ultrasound cross-sectional arterial imaging before and after balloon angioplasty in vitro. Circulation 1989; 80:873–82.

4. Potkin BN, Bartorelli AL, Gessert JM et al. Coronary artery imaging with intravascular high-frequency ultrasound. Circulation 1990; 81:1575–85.

5. Nishimura RA, Edwards WD, Warnes CA et al. Intravascular ultrasound imaging: in vitro validation and pathologic correlation. J Am Coll Cardiol 1990; 16:145–54.

6. Nair A, Kuban BD, Tuzcu EM et al. Coronary plaque classification with intravascular ultrasound radiofrequency data analysis. Circulation 2002; 106:2200–6.

7. Peters RJ, Kok WE, Havenith MG et al. Histopathologic validation of intracoronary ultrasound imaging. J Am Soc Echocardiogr 1994; 7:230–41.

8. Nasu K, Tsuchikane E, Katoh O et al. Accuracy of in vivo coronary plaque morphology assessment: a validation study of in vivo virtual histology compared with in vitro histopathology. J Am Coll Cardiol 2006; 47:2405–12.

9. Rodriguez-Granillo GA, Aoki J, Ong AT et al. Methodological considerations and approach to cross-technique comparisons using in vivo coronary plaque characterization based on intravascular ultrasound radiofrequency data analysis: insights from the Integrated Biomarker and Imaging Study (IBIS). Int J Cardiovasc Intervent 2005; 7:52–8.

10. Kåresen K. Deconvolution of sparse spike trains by iterated window maximization. IEEE Trans Signal Process 1997; 45:1173–83.

11. Ambrose JA, Tannenbaum MA, Alexopoulos D et al. Angiographic progression of coronary artery disease and the development of myocardial infarction. J Am Coll Cardiol 1988; 12:56–62.

12. Little WC, Constantinescu M, Applegate RJ et al. Can coronary angiography predict the site of a subsequent myocardial infarction in patients with mild-to-moderate coronary artery disease? Circulation 1988; 78:1157–66.

13. Farb A, Burke AP, Tang AL et al. Coronary plaque erosion without rupture into a lipid core. A frequent cause of coronary thrombosis in sudden coronary death. Circulation 1996; 93:1354–63.

14. Schaar JA, Muller JE, Falk E et al. Terminology for high-risk and vulnerable coronary artery plaques. Report of a meeting on the vulnerable plaque, June 17 and 18, 2003, Santorini, Greece. Eur Heart J 2004; 25:1077–82.

15. Davies MJ, Richardson PD, Woolf N, Katz DR, Mann J. Risk of thrombosis in human atherosclerotic plaques: role of extracellular lipid, macrophage, and smooth muscle cell content. Br Heart J 1993; 69:377–81.

16. Gertz SD, Roberts WC. Hemodynamic shear force in rupture of coronary arterial atherosclerotic plaques. Am J Cardiol 1990; 66:1368–72.

17. Felton CV, Crook D, Davies MJ, Oliver MF. Relation of plaque lipid composition and morphology to the stability of human aortic plaques. Arterioscler Thromb Vasc Biol 1997; 17:1337–45.

18. Virmani R, Kolodgie FD, Burke AP, Farb A, Schwartz SM. Lessons from sudden coronary death: a comprehensive morphological classification scheme for atherosclerotic lesions. Arterioscler Thromb Vasc Biol 2000; 20:1262–75.

19. Rodriguez-Granillo GA Garcia-Garcia HM, McFadden E et al. In vivo intravascular ultrasound-derived thin-cap fibroatheroma detection using ultrasound radiofrequency data analysis. J Am Coll Cardiol 2005; 46:2038–42.

20. Kolodgie FD, Burke AP, Farb A et al. The thin-cap fibroatheroma: a type of vulnerable plaque: the major precursor lesion to acute coronary syndromes. Curr Opin Cardiol 2001; 16:285–92.

21. Wang JC, Normand SL, Mauri L, Kuntz RE. Coronary artery spatial distribution of acute myocardial infarction occlusions. Circulation 2004; 110:278–84.

22. Virmani R, Burke AP, Kolodgie FD, Farb A. Vulnerable plaque: the pathology of unstable coronary lesions. J Interv Cardiol 2002; 15:439–46.

23. Burke AP, Farb A, Malcom GT et al. Coronary risk factors and plaque morphology in men with coronary disease who died suddenly. N Engl J Med 1997; 336:1276–82.

24. Kääb MJ, Nötzli HP, Clark J, Gwynn AP. A critical appraise of the effects of fixation, dehydration and embedding of cell volume. In: Revel JP, Barnard T, Haggis GH, eds. The Science of Biological Specimen Preparation for Microscopy and Microanalysis. Scanning Electron Microscopy. Chicago, IL: AMF O'Hare, 1984:61–70.

25. Boyde A, Bailey E, Jones S, Tamarin A. Dimensional changes during specimen preparation for scanning electron microscopy. Scanning Electron Microscopy 1977; I:507–18.

26. Fishbein MC, Siegel RJ. How big are coronary atherosclerotic plaques that rupture? Circulation 1996; 94:2662–6.

27. Nair A CD, Vince DG. Regularized autoregressive analysis of intravascular ultrasound data: improvement

in spatial accuracy of plaque tissue maps. IEEE Trans Ultrasonics, Ferroelectrics, and Frequency Control 2004; 51:420–31.

28. Mann JM, Davies MJ. Vulnerable plaque. Relation of characteristics to degree of stenosis in human coronary arteries. Circulation 1996; 94:928–31.

29. Schaar JA, De Korte CL, Mastik F et al. Characterizing vulnerable plaque features with intravascular elastography. Circulation 2003; 108:2636–41.

30. Glagov S, Weisenberg E, Zarins CK, Stankunavicius R, Kolettis GJ. Compensatory enlargement of human atherosclerotic coronary arteries. N Engl J Med 1987; 316:1371–5.

31. Pasterkamp G, Schoneveld AH, van der Wal AC et al. Relation of arterial geometry to luminal narrowing and histologic markers for plaque vulnerability: the remodeling paradox. J Am Coll Cardiol 1998; 32:655–62.

32. Varnava AM, Mills PG, Davies MJ. Relationship between coronary artery remodeling and plaque vulnerability. Circulation 2002; 105:939–43.

33. Burke AP, Kolodgie FD, Farb A, Weber D, Virmani R. Morphological predictors of arterial remodeling in coronary atherosclerosis. Circulation 2002; 105:297–303.

34. Rodriguez-Granillo GA, Serruys PW, Garcia-Garcia HM et al. Coronary artery remodelling is related to plaque composition. Heart 2006; 92:388–91.

35. Kannel WB, Doyle JT, McNamara PM, Quickenton P, Gordon T. Precursors of sudden coronary death. Factors related to the incidence of sudden death. Circulation 1975; 51:606–13.

36. Falk E, Shah PK, Fuster V. Coronary plaque disruption. Circulation 1995; 92:657–71.

37. Burke AP, Kolodgie FD, Farb A et al. Healed plaque ruptures and sudden coronary death: evidence that subclinical rupture has a role in plaque progression. Circulation 2001; 103:934–40.

38. Schaar JA, Regar E, Mastik F et al. Incidence of high-strain patterns in human coronary arteries: assessment with three-dimensional intravascular palpography and correlation with clinical presentation. Circulation 2004; 109:2716–19.

39. Van Mieghem CA, McFadden EP, de Feyter PJ et al. Noninvasive detection of subclinical coronary atherosclerosis coupled with assessment of changes in plaque characteristics using novel invasive imaging modalities: the Integrated Biomarker and Imaging Study (IBIS). J Am Coll Cardiol 2006; 47:1134–42.

40. Loree HM, Kamm RD, Stringfellow RG, Lee RT. Effects of fibrous cap thickness on peak circumferential stress in model atherosclerotic vessels. Circ Res 1992; 71:850–8.

41. Rodriguez-Granillo GA, Garcia-Garcia HM, Valgimigli M et al. In vivo relationship between compositional and mechanical imaging of coronary arteries. Insights from intravascular ultrasound radiofrequency data analysis. Am Heart J 2006; 151:1025 e1–6.

Shear stress and the vulnerable plaque   19

*Jolanda J Wentzel, Frank JH Gijsen, Rob Krams, Rini de Crom,
Caroline Cheng, Harald C Groen, Alina G van der Giessen,
Anton FW van der Steen, and Patrick W Serruys*

INTRODUCTION

Atherosclerosis is the main cause of death in Western societies.[1] Myocardial infarction or stroke is, in the majority of cases, caused by rupture or erosion of an atherosclerotic plaque, in either the coronary or carotid circulation. Often, people are unaware of their risk for cardiovascular events, because plaques prone to rupture do not necessarily limit the blood flow and thus do not cause any symptoms. These plaques, called vulnerable plaques, are characterized by their specific morphology and composition: a large lipid pool covered by a thin fibrous cap (<65 μm)[2] infiltrated by macrophages[3] and expansive remodeling.[2,4] In the presence of risk factors, which are systemic in nature, atherosclerotic plaques develop predominantly at specific locations in the arterial tree, including bifurcations and inner curves of arteries.[5] As these predilection sites are associated with deviations of the normal velocity field, flow-induced shear stress, acting on the endothelial cells (ECs), has been recognized as a key player in plaque localization and plaque growth.[6–9] The influence of shear stress on the generation and destabilization of vulnerable plaques is discussed in this chapter.

DEFINITION OF SHEAR STRESS

Vessel wall shear stress is the (tangential) drag force induced by blood flow through a vessel acting on the inner vascular wall (Figure 19.1a). Shear stress is defined as force per area and its dimension equals that of pressure, i.e. N/m^2 or Pa. An older, frequently used unit for shear stress is $dyne/cm^2$ and relates to Pa according to 1 Pa = 10 $dyne/cm^2$. Shear stress on the vascular wall can be calculated from the local shear rate ($\dot{\gamma}$; s^{-1}) × blood viscosity (μ; Pa·s). Shear rate (Figure 19.1b) is the spatial blood velocity gradient ([m/s]/m). Especially near the vessel wall, large velocity gradients between adjacent fluid layers exist and, as a consequence, the shear stress is there at its highest value. In a simple straight tube the Hagen–Poisseuille formula (shear stress = $4\mu Q/\pi R^3$, where μ is the viscosity, Q is the flow, and R is the tube radius) can be applied for steady laminar viscous flow.[10] In biology, normal shear stress values differ per vessel type, location, and age.[11] For instance, for human coronary arteries the average shear stress is 0.68 ± 0.2 Pa in healthy segments,[12] 1.15 ± 0.21 Pa in carotid arteries,[13] and 0.48 ± 0.15 Pa in brachial arteries.[13] In more detail, spatial differences in shear stress were observed close to side branches, in inner curves of arteries, and in the bulb of the carotid artery.[9,14]

ROLE OF SHEAR STRESS IN VASCULAR BIOLOGY

Extensive studies in search of the specific shear stress conditions that predict plaque

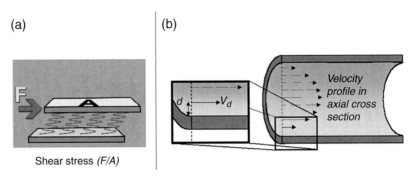

Figure 19.1   (a) Illustration of the induced shear stress by a force acting along a surface. (b) Wall shear stress exerted by the blood flow is determined by the shear rate at the wall multiplied by viscosity. Over a small distance from the wall, velocity increases linearly with distance, and wall shear rate nearly equals velocity difference divided by distance. A, area; d, distance; F, force; V_d, velocity.[40]

location have mainly identified low shear stress levels and oscillatory shear stress to be atherogenic. The effects of low shear stress and oscillatory shear stress on the pathology of the vascular wall have been extensively studied in vitro using cultured ECs. Exposure of these cultures to high shear stress levels (>1.5 Pa) induced the expression of atheroprotective genes with antioxidant properties, such as endothelial nitric oxide synthase (eNOS),[15] cyclo-oxygenase-1 (COX-1),[16] C-natriuretic protein (CNP),[16] hemoxygenase I (HO-I),[17] NAD(P)H:quinone oxidoreductase (NQO-1),[17] and glutathione S-transferase.[18] Furthermore, high shear stress decreased expression levels of atherogenic genes such as endothelin-1 (ET-1).[19] In contrast, low shear stress levels induced the expression of adhesion factors that are associated with inflammation such as vascular cell adhesion molecule-1 (VCAM-1)[20] and intercellular adhesion molecule (ICAM-1).[21] It also increases the endothelial uptake of oxidized low-density lipoprotein (oxLDL) by up-regulation of the expression of the lectin-like oxLDL receptor (LOX-1)[22] on the ECs. Furthermore, low shear stress stimulated vascular smooth muscle cell (VSMC) migration and proliferation by inducing the expression of platelet-derived growth

factor (PDGF) and vascular endothelial growth factor (VEGF), whereas the expression of atheroprotective genes (e.g. eNOS and antioxidants) is reduced. Oscillatory shear stress also induced expression of atherogenic genes, such as ET-1[23] and matrix metalloproteinase 9 (MMP-9),[24] while down-regulating the expression of atheroprotective genes such as endothelial transforming growth factor-β_1 (TGF-β_1).[25] It has also recently been shown to up-regulate the expression of bone morphogenic protein-4 (BMP-4), a member of the TGF-β family of cytokines, which was associated with increased ICAM-1 expression through a nuclear factor-kappa B (NF-κB)-dependent (inflammatory transcription factor) mechanism.[26] From these distinct gene expression profiles obtained in vitro, high shear stress is supposed to be atheroprotective, and low and oscillatory shear stress to be atherogenic.

Indeed, in-vivo findings on gene expression linked to presumed shear stress conditions confirm these in-vitro data. In a normal porcine aortic arch (disturbed flow pattern) the expression and activity of endothelial protein kinase C (PKC), an important family of regulatory proteins, was increased when compared with the descending thoracic aorta (undisturbed flow).[27] Furthermore, it was shown that altered shear stress can prime the endothelium to respond to proatherosclerotic stimuli through up-regulation of NF-κB[28] and up-regulation of ICAM-1 and VCAM-1[29] in vascular regions exposed to disturbed blood flow in a mouse model. The laminar flow with normal shear stress levels promoted an anti-inflammatory and antioxidative expression profile, acting through promoter elements identified as shear stress responsive elements (SSREs), antioxidant responsive elements (AREs), and peroxisome proliferator-activated receptor (PPAR) γ-responsive elements.[28] Conversely, low shear stress triggered adhesion of leukocytes to activated endothelium through enhanced expression of ICAM-1, VCAM-1, and E-selectin. Furthermore, using a unique in-vivo shear stress altering device,[30,31] we recently found chemokine up-regulation of monocyte chemoattractant protein-1 (MCP-1), the mouse homolog of interleukin-8 (IL-8), interferon-γ-inducible protein-10 (IP-10), and fractalkine under low shear stress conditions in an ApoE[−/−] mouse carotid artery. Up-regulation of the chemokines MCP-1 and IL-8 was also identified in the vessel segments subjected to oscillatory shear stress. High expression levels of chemokines attract different inflammatory cell types into the vessel wall and trigger the development of atherosclerosis. Another important consequence of wall shear stress is its influence on endothelial permeability. In-vivo measurements showed higher (albumin) permeability at low and oscillatory shear stress regions compared with high shear stress regions in both porcine aortas[32] and iliac arteries.[33]

These findings may explain the specific and local accumulation of (immunocompetent) cells and molecules at predilection sites and provide important insight for the role of shear stress in the development of pathologies in the vessel wall.

ROLE OF SHEAR STRESS IN THE GENERATION OF THE VULNERABLE PLAQUE

Observations in humans

Already at birth, shear stress-related predilection sites for atherosclerosis show a focal and eccentric increase in intimal thickness.[34] Although these sites are inevitably related to atherosclerosis-prone sites in later life, these adaptive intimal thickenings are not the heralds of atheromas, but are the effect of a physiologic adaptive process to mechanical stimuli.[35] Stary[36] showed, based on a histologic study of coronary arteries in children and young adults, that in 38% of the infants younger than 2 years old fatty streaks were already found. These lesions were even more frequently found (in 69% of the cases) in children at the age of puberty, and the lesions already contained fatty droplets. Although these lesions were capable of regressing and disappearing in atheroprotective conditions,[37] they tended to develop into atheromas with a lipid core and were frequently found at similar sites where severe atherosclerosis in adults usually occur.[34] The fatty streaks and early lesions were observed near bifurcations and, more specifically, the low shear stress regions along the outer wall of the bifurcations were affected.[6] In the Pathobiological Determinants of Atherosclerosis in Youth (PDAY) study, approximately 3000 arteries of young individuals were collected and analyzed.[38] The results from this study showed that the fatty streaks in coronary arteries appeared 5–10 years later than they did in the aorta, and that the fatty lesions were precursors of the more advanced or 'raised' lesions. In the third decade, the raised streaks were already characterized by abundant cellular infiltration and vascularization. The results from this study also clearly showed the focal distribution of these lesions: both fatty streaks and raised lesions were predominantly present at the myocardial part of the arterial circumference, where low shear stresses prevailed (Figure 19.2).

Once fatty streaks develop into raised lesions, they trigger a shear stress-related mechanism called vascular remodeling.[39] Glagov et al observed that human coronary arteries enlarge during plaque build-up and thereby preserve normal lumen dimensions until relative plaque area roughly occupies 40% of the vessel area.[39] Since plaques are usually eccentric, it was proposed that the plaque-free wall controls lumen dimensions during vascular (compensatory) remodeling by responding to the rise in shear stress when the plaque intrudes into the lumen.[39,40] An alternative explanation for lumen preservation was plaque retraction and wall expansion at the site of the plaque. This process could be mediated by atrophy of the underlying media and enzymatic destruction of plaque matrix and, indeed, can also induce significant outward remodeling.[41] Findings from intracoronary ultrasound studies[42,43] showed that eccentric plaques have more outward

remodeling than concentric plaques, suggesting that the remaining plaque-free wall, not the circumferential extension of plaque, stimulated outward remodeling. As a consequence of lumen preservation, the shear stress distribution that was present in the healthy artery was maintained, including the unfavorable eccentric low shear stress conditions. This shear stress environment allows continuous plaque growth from fatty streaks to complex lesions and might explain the frequent observation of American Heart Association type IV large focal and eccentric lipid-laden atherosclerotic vulnerable plaques in mildly stenosed coronary arteries.[44]

Observations in mouse models

After a period of using large animals for research on atherosclerosis, the mouse model has become more popular for studying progression and interventions for this disease,[45–49] including the research on vulnerable plaque generation and destabilization. An apolipoprotein E (ApoE) deficiency combined with a

Figure 19.2 Maps of prevalence of fatty streaks and raised lesions in male human right coronary arteries for four different age categories, ranging from 15–34 years. Note the focal distribution of the fatty streaks and the raised lesions in the central part of each map: this region corresponds to the inner curve of the right coronary artery where low shear stress can be expected.[38]

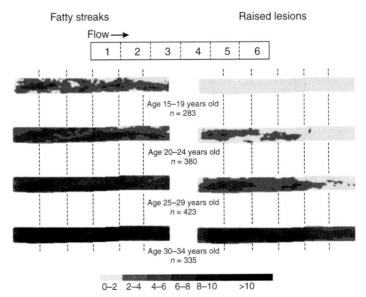

Western diet results in complex vulnerable plaques in the mice. Mice having additional genes knocked out develop vulnerable plaques in a shorter period of time. Vulnerable plaques are only observed at certain locations in the arterial bed: at or near branching sites.[50–52] The best-studied branch is the brachiocephalic trunk, showing a vulnerable plaque phenotype with, in the majority of the cases, plaque rupture.[50–52] At present, the mechanism responsible for the development of vulnerable plaques at or near side branches, like the brachiocephalic trunk, is unknown. It has been postulated that disturbances of the normal velocity field might be the underlying cause. Indeed, at the first 150 μm from the branching side vulnerable plaques are observed, where the velocity field is expected not to be fully developed. This usually occurs at a distance 3–5 times the diameter of the blood vessel, i.e. after approximately 300–500 μm for most aortic branches in mice. Until now, it was unknown whether low shear stress or oscillating shear stress was responsible for the generation of vulnerable plaques.

We therefore developed a method of changing the normal pulsatile velocity field in straight vessel segments, such as the common carotid artery, to a pulsatile velocity field with low, high, and oscillating mean velocities by placing a cone-shaped device (cast) around the vessel.[30,31] As a result, a relatively low shear stress region upstream, a high shear stress inside, and an oscillating shear stress field downstream of the cast is introduced (Figure 19.3a). After feeding ApoE[−/−] mice a Western diet for 9 weeks, atherosclerotic plaques are found in the low and oscillatory shear stress regions, confirming other findings.[50–52] However, only in the low shear stress regions was a vulnerable plaque phenotype observed, comprising a thin fibrous cap, abundant presence of macrophages, low content of VSMCs, and a lipid-rich core (Figure 19.3b). These data indicate that low shear stress – and not oscillatory shear stress – is important for vulnerable plaque generation. The model was shown to be reproducible and illustrates the importance of hemodynamics in the transformation of simple plaques to complex plaques.

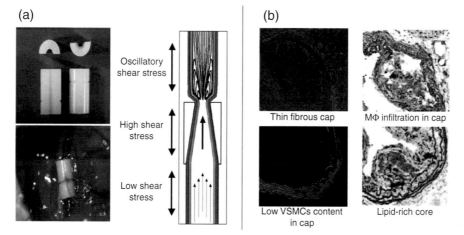

Figure 19.3   (a) The newly developed device was placed around the carotid artery of a mouse to create low, high, and oscillatory shear stress regions. (b) Representative sections showing the composition of the plaques found in the low shear stress region proximal to the device in the carotid artery of an ApoE[−/−] mouse after 9 weeks of Western diet.[94]

DESTABILIZATION OF THE VULNERABLE PLAQUE

The role of inflammation

During the last decade, inflammation has been recognized as a key component of atherogenesis.[53] In a landmark review, Ross even termed atherosclerosis an inflammatory disease.[54] Obviously, other factors are involved as well. Notably, lipid accumulation is another key player in the process. Therefore, Steinberg called inflammation and hypercholesterolemia 'partners in crime'.[55]

In the advanced stages of atherosclerosis, lipid-filled macrophages (foam cells) die and leave a necrotic core[53–55] with a fibrous cap. If the cap of the plaque is thin and poor in collagen and VSMCs,[56,57] it becomes vulnerable. Both foam cells and T cells produce proinflammatory cytokines that inhibit the proliferation and extracellular matrix production of VSMCs. However, the inflammatory process is controlled by a balance between subsets of T cells (Th1/Th2 paradigm).[58–61] Microvessels that develop into the lesions are sources for intraplaque hemorrhages which contribute to the inflammation process and lesion instability.[53,62,63] In addition, similar activities are attributed to mast cells that have been found in lesions, which secrete chymase and tumor necrosis factor-α (TNF-α).[64] Degradation of collagen and other extracellular matrix components leads to further weakening of the cap. MMPs are capable of such breakdown and have been the subject of intense research. MMPs constitute a family of more than 20 members, including collagenases (MMP-1, -8, and -13), gelatinases (MMP-2 and -9), and stromelysins (MMP-3).[65] Various cell types in atherosclerotic lesions, including monocytes/macrophages and VSMCs, produce MMPs. Several MMPs have been shown to be expressed to higher levels in human atherosclerotic lesions than in normal media, in particular in the macrophage-rich shoulder regions.[53,65] In addition, higher MMP activity was demonstrated by in-situ zymography.[66] It has been shown in in-vitro studies that inflammatory mediators, including IL-1, TNF-α, and CD40 ligand, increase MMP expression by vascular cells.

The role of shear stress

During the advanced stages of the atherosclerotic process, plaques start to encroach into the lumen, eventually causing lumen narrowing. As a consequence, the locally acting shear stress at the endothelium will change from low (Figure 19.4a) to high at the upstream side of the plaque

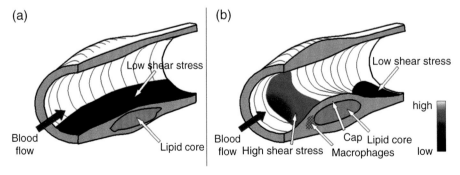

Figure 19.4 Change in shear stress distribution at the upstream side of the plaque from low shear stress (a) to high shear stress (b) caused by the formation of a lumen-encroaching plaque with lipid core, cap, and macrophages, including outward vessel wall remodeling.

(Figure 19.4b). The question is raised of what is the consequence of the shear stress increase on the underlying plaque composition and possibly for the local plaque vulnerability.[40] Because plaque ruptures or ulcers are frequently observed at the upstream side of the plaque,[67–69] it was suggested that shear stress mechanically induce rupture of the cap.[70] This seems very unlikely, since, even in the presence of 75% stenosis, the shear stress remains several orders of magnitude lower than the tensile stress induced by the blood pressure pulse. However, shear stress induces major biologic effects in ECs that might affect the crucial balance between cap-enforcing matrix synthesis by synthetic VSMCs and matrix breakdown by MMPs produced by macrophages.[71,72]

At the upstream side of a stenosis, shear stress is maximally enhanced compared to the situation without lumen narrowing (see Figure 19.4). There is a large body of evidence that ECs excellently adapt to modifications in their biochemical and biomechanical environment by changing their phenotype,[23,73–79] such that high shear stress induces an antiproliferative and anti-inflammatory and antithrombotic action of the endothelium. The increase in shear stress upstream of a plaque, caused by lumen narrowing, could induce a similar action in ECs covering the top of a plaque, as corroborated by the data of Tricot et al, who showed less apoptosis at the upstream than the downstream side of the plaque.[80] Even in an inflammatory or oxidative environment, ECs in vitro were shown to be sensitive to changes in shear stress, which counteracted endothelial apoptosis induced by either oxidative stress, oxLDL, or TNF-α.[81] Increased shear stress has been shown to induce regression of graft hyperplasia in baboons.[82] Likewise, the increased shear stress at the upstream side of the plaque might induce regression of the fibrous cap,[83] which is attributed to cell apoptosis[84] and matrix degradation.

It has been suggested that high shear stress-induced tissue regression due to VSMC apoptosis is mediated by nitric oxide (NO) production. Experiments blocking NO, however, did not prove its necessity in the process of tissue regression.[84] Nonetheless, the up-regulation of eNOS during those experiments still strongly suggests a contribution of NO.[84] The role of NO in inducing apoptosis of VSMCs is complex. In an inflammatory environment, VSMCs change from contractile into synthetic phenotypes; they may sustain their synthetic state by expression of inducible nitric oxide synthase (iNOS) and its high-output delivery of NO.[85] When high shear stress stimulates ECs to counteract inflammation, such as by up-regulation and activation of TGF-β,[86] this could result in inhibition of the expression and activity of iNOS in VSMCs.[87] Therefore, VSMCs that stop producing NO themselves may respond to the relatively high amount of NO produced by the endothelium, which is stimulated by high shear stress. NO can up-regulate surface Fas, a receptor for apoptosis, on VSMCs and the corresponding death factor, surface Fas-Ligand (Fas-L), on macrophages.[88] The Fas/Fas-L interaction induces cell–cell proximity-dependent VSMC apoptosis.[88] Special attention should be paid to the protection of NO against oxidation. It is known that NO is oxidized by superoxide anions, which diffuse from the lipid core to the luminal surface. The oxidation could be prevented by superoxide dismutase (SOD) scavenging the superoxide anions.[89] SOD is produced

- intracellular, by the endothelium, stimulated by high shear stress[77]
- extracellular, by the VSMC, stimulated by NO.[90]

In the previously mentioned hyperplasia experiments in baboons,[82] shear stress-induced regression of the extracellular proteoglycan matrix was explained by the

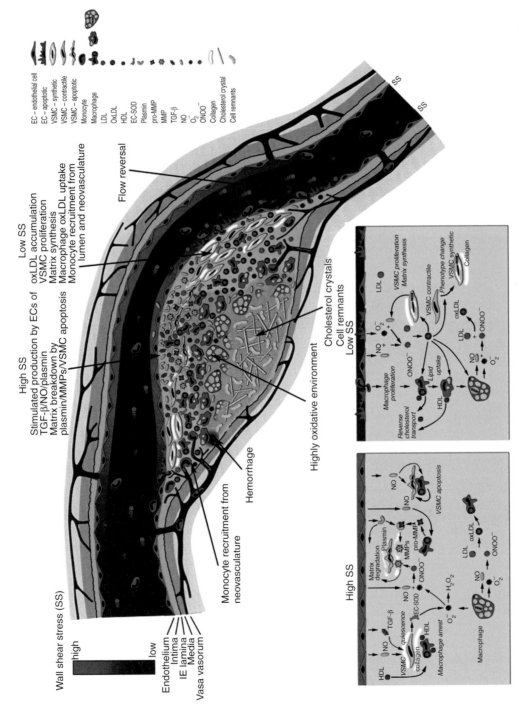

Figure 19.5   Proposed shear stress-related mechanisms that influence the composition of a vulnerable plaque. ECs, endothelial cells; EC-SOD, extracellular superoxide dismutase; H_2O_2, hydrogen peroxide; HDL, high-density lipoprotein; iNOS, inducible nitric oxide; LDL, low-density lipoprotein; MMPs, matrix metalloproteinases; NO, nitric oxide; O_2^-, superoxide; ONOO$^-$, peroxynitrite; oxLDL, oxidized low-density lipoprotein; pro-MMP, pro-matrix metalloproteinase; SS, shear stress; TGF-β, tissue growth factor-β; VSMC, vascular smooth muscle cell. (Adapted from Slager et al.[95])

high shear stress-stimulated endothelial production of serine proteinases, including urokinase and plasmin.[91] Plasmin production in the ECs on top of a fibrous cap of a vulnerable plaque could, in addition, activate pro-MMPs (1, 3, 9, 10 and 13), which are secreted by the abundantly present macrophages,[92] stimulating the breakdown of the fibrous cap.

Another possible mechanism through which the cap could destabilize is via activation of gelatinases (MMP-2 and -9) by peroxynitrite.[93] Peroxynitrite could be available if the SOD does not scavenge all the superoxide anions, which can then react with NO, or because of its production by uncoupled eNOS. Figure 19.5 (lower left panel) summarizes the molecular mechanisms involved in cap weakening and thinning.

REFERENCES

1. Mackay J, Mensah GA. The Atlas of Disease and Stroke. Geneva, Switzerland: World Health Organization; 2004.

2. Burke AP, Farb A, Malcom GT et al. Coronary risk factors and plaque morphology in men with coronary disease who died suddenly. N Engl J Med 1997; 336:1276–82.

3. Moreno P, Falk E, Palacios I et al. Macrophage infiltration in acute coronary syndromes. Implications for plaque rupture. Circulation 1994; 90:775–8.

4. Pasterkamp G, Schoneveld AH, van der Wal AC et al. Relation of arterial geometry to luminal narrowing and histologic markers for plaque vulnerability: the remodeling paradox. J Am Coll Cardiol 1998; 32:655–62.

5. VanderLaan PA, Reardon CA, Getz GS. Site specificity of atherosclerosis: site-selective responses to atherosclerotic modulators. Arterioscler Thromb Vasc Biol 2004; 24:12–22.

6. Zarins CK, Giddens DP, Bharadvaj BK et al. Carotid bifurcation atherosclerosis. Quantitative correlation of plaque localization with flow velocity profiles and wall shear stress. Circ Res 1983; 53:502–14.

7. Gnasso A, Irace C, Carallo C et al. In vivo association between low wall shear stress and plaque in subjects with asymmetrical carotid atherosclerosis. Stroke 1997; 28:993–8.

8. Stone PH, Coskun AU, Kinlay S et al. Effect of endothelial shear stress on the progression of coronary artery disease, vascular remodeling, and in-stent restenosis in humans: in vivo 6-month follow-up study. Circulation 2003; 108:438–44.

9. Krams R, Wentzel J, Oomen J et al. Evaluation of endothelial shear stress and 3D geometry as factors determining the development of atherosclerosis and remodeling in human coronary arteries in vivo. Combining 3D reconstruction from angiography and IVUS (ANGUS) with computational fluid dynamics. Arterioscler Thromb Vasc Biol 1997; 17:2061–5.

10. Fox RW, McDonald AT. Introduction to Fluid Mechanics, 4th edn. Chichester, UK: John Wiley & Sons, 1992.

11. Samijo SK, Willigers JM, Barkhuysen R et al. Wall shear stress in the human common carotid artery as function of age and gender. Cardiovasc Res 1998; 39:515–22.

12. Doriot PA, Dorsaz PA, Dorsaz L et al. In-vivo measurements of wall shear stress in human coronary arteries. Coron Artery Dis 2000; 11:495–502.

13. Dammers R, Stifft F, Tordoir JHM et al. Shear stress depends on vascular territory: comparison between common carotid and brachial artery. J Appl Physiol 2003; 94:485–9.

14. Ku DN, Giddens DP, Zarins CK, Glagov S. Pulsatile flow and atherosclerosis in the human carotid bifurcation. Positive correlation between plaque location and low oscillating shear stress. Arteriosclerosis 1985; 5:293–302.

15. Harrison DG, Sayegh H, Ohara Y, Inoue N, Venema RC. Regulation of expression of the endothelial cell nitric oxide synthase. Clin Exp Pharmacol Physiol 1996; 23:251–5.

16. Okahara K, Sun B, Kambayashi J. Upregulation of prostacyclin synthesis-related gene expression by shear stress in vascular endothelial cells. Arterioscler Thromb Vasc Biol 1998; 18:1922–6.

17. Chen Z, Milner TE, Wang X, Srinivas S, Nelson JS. Optical Doppler tomography: imaging in vivo blood flow dynamics following pharmacological intervention and photodynamic therapy. Photochem Photobiol 1998; 67:56.

18. Chen XL, Varner SE, Rao AS et al. Laminar flow induction of antioxidant response element-mediated genes in endothelial cells. A novel anti-inflammatory mechanism. J Biol Chem 2003; 278:703–11.

19. Malek AM, Greene AL, Izumo S. Regulation of endothelin 1 gene by fluid shear stress is transcriptionally mediated and independent of protein kinase C and cAMP. Proc Natl Acad Sci USA 1993; 90:5999–6003.

20. Mohan S, Mohan N, Valente AJ, Sprague EA. Regulation of low shear flow-induced HAEC VCAM-1 expression and monocyte adhesion. Am J Physiol 1999; 276:C1100–7.

21. Houston P, Dickson MC, Ludbrook V et al. Fluid shear stress induction of the tissue factor promoter in vitro and in vivo is mediated by Egr-1. Arterioscler Thromb Vasc Biol 1999; 19:281–9.

22. Murase T, Kume N, Korenaga R et al. Fluid shear stress transcriptionally induces lectin-like oxidized

LDL receptor-1 in vascular endothelial cells. Circ Res 1998; 83:328–33.

23. Ziegler T, Bouzourene K, Harrison V, Brunner H, Hayoz D. Influence of oscillatory and unidirectional flow environments on the expression of endothelin and nitric oxide synthase in cultured endothelial cells. Arterioscler Thromb Vasc Biol 1998; 18:686–92.

24. Magid R, Murphy TJ, Galis ZS. Expression of matrix metalloproteinase-9 in endothelial cells is differentially regulated by shear stress. Role of c-Myc. J Biol Chem 2003; 278:32994–9.

25. Lum RM, Wiley LM, Barakat AI. Influence of different forms of fluid shear stress on vascular endothelial TGF-beta1 mRNA expression. Int J Mol Med 2000; 5:635–41.

26. Sorescu GP, Sykes M, Weiss D et al. Bone morphogenic protein 4 produced in endothelial cells by oscillatory shear stress stimulates an inflammatory response. J Biol Chem 2003; 278:31128–35.

27. Magid R, Davies PF. Endothelial protein kinase C isoform identity and differential activity of PKCzeta in an athero-susceptible region of porcine aorta. Circ Res 2005; 97:443–9.

28. Tzima E, Irani-Tehrani M, Kiosses WB et al. A mechanosensory complex that mediates the endothelial cell response to fluid shear stress. Nature 2005; 437:426–31.

29. Nakashima Y, Raines EW, Plump AS, Breslow JL, Ross R. Upregulation of VCAM-1 and ICAM-1 at atherosclerosis-prone sites on the endothelium in the ApoE-deficient mouse. Arterioscler Thromb Vasc Biol 1998; 18:842–51.

30. Cheng C, van Haperen R, de Waard M et al. Shear stress affects the intracellular distribution of eNOS: direct demonstration by a novel in vivo technique. Blood 2005; 106:3691–8.

31. Cheng C, de Crom R, van Haperen R et al. The role of shear stress in atherosclerosis: action through gene expression and inflammation? Cell Biochem Biophys 2004; 41:279–94.

32. Himburg HA, Grzybowski DM, Hazel AL et al. Spatial comparison between wall shear stress measures and porcine arterial endothelial permeability. Am J Physiol Heart Circ Physiol 2004; 286:H1916–22.

33. LaMack JA, Himburg HA, Li XM, Friedman MH. Interaction of wall shear stress magnitude and gradient in the prediction of arterial macromolecular permeability. Ann Biomed Eng 2005; 33:457–64.

34. Stary HC. Evolution and progression of atherosclerotic lesions in coronary arteries of children and young adults. Arteriosclerosis 1989; 9:I19–32.

35. Stary HC, Chandler AB, Glagov S et al. A definition of initial, fatty streak, and intermediate lesions of atherosclerosis. A report from the Committee on Vascular Lesions of the Council on Arteriosclerosis, American Heart Association. Circulation 1994; 89:2462–78.

36. Stary HC. Lipid and macrophage accumulations in arteries of children and the development of atherosclerosis. Am J Clin Nutr 2000; 72:1297S-1306S.

37. Stary HC. Atlas of Atherosclerosis Progression and Regression. New York: Parthenon; 1999.

38. McGill HC Jr, McMahan CA, Herderick EE et al. Effects of coronary heart disease risk factors on atherosclerosis of selected regions of the aorta and right coronary artery. PDAY Research Group. Pathobiological Determinants of Atherosclerosis in Youth. Arterioscler Thromb Vasc Biol 2000; 20:836–45.

39. Glagov S, Weisenberg E, Zarins CK, Stankunavicius R, Kolettis GJ. Compensatory enlargement of human atherosclerotic coronary arteries. N Engl J Med 1987; 316:1371–5.

40. Slager CJ, Wentzel JJ, Gijsen FJ et al. The role of shear stress in the generation of rupture-prone vulnerable plaques. Nat Clin Pract Cardiovasc Med 2005; 2:401–7.

41. Bentzon JF, Pasterkamp G, Falk E. Expansive remodeling is a response of the plaque-related vessel wall in aortic roots of ApoE-deficient mice: an experiment of nature. Arterioscler Thromb Vasc Biol 2003; 23:257–62.

42. Ito K, Higashikata T, Hanatani A et al. Effect of disease eccentricity on compensatory remodeling of coronary arteries: evidence from intravascular ultrasound before interventions. Int J Cardiol 2002; 86:99–105.

43. von Birgelen C, Mintz GS, de Vrey EA et al. Atherosclerotic coronary lesions with inadequate compensatory enlargement have smaller plaque and vessel volumes: observations with three dimensional intravascular ultrasound in vivo. Heart 1998; 79:137–42.

44. Fuster V, Stein B, Ambrose JA et al. Atherosclerotic plaque rupture and thrombosis; evolving concepts. Circulation 1990; 82:II-47–II-59.

45. Aikawa M, Rabkin E, Okada Y et al. Lipid lowering by diet reduces matrix metalloproteinase activity and increases collagen content of rabbit atheroma: a potential mechanism of lesion stabilization. Circulation 1998; 97:2433–44.

46. Fukumoto Y, Libby P, Rabkin E et al. Statins alter smooth muscle cell accumulation and collagen content in established atheroma of Watanabe heritable hyperlipidemic rabbits. Circulation 2001; 103:993–9.

47. Madjid M, Naghavi M, Malik BA et al. Thermal detection of vulnerable plaque. Am J Cardiol 2002; 90:36L–39L.

48. Tsimikas S. Noninvasive imaging of oxidized low-density lipoprotein in atherosclerotic plaques with tagged oxidation-specific antibodies. Am J Cardiol 2002; 90:22L–27L.

49. Chen J, Tung CH, Mahmood U et al. In vivo imaging of proteolytic activity in atherosclerosis. Circulation 2002; 105:2766–71.

50. Naghavi M, Libby P, Falk E et al. From vulnerable plaque to vulnerable patient: a call for new definitions and risk assessment strategies: Part I. Circulation 2003; 108:1664–72.

51. Naghavi M, Libby P, Falk E et al. From vulnerable plaque to vulnerable patient: a call for new definitions and risk assessment strategies: Part II. Circulation 2003; 108:1772–8.

52. Williams H, Johnson JL, Carson KG, Jackson CL. Characteristics of intact and ruptured atherosclerotic plaques in brachiocephalic arteries of apolipoprotein E knockout mice. Arterioscler Thromb Vasc Biol 2002; 22:788–92.

53. Libby P. Inflammation in atherosclerosis. Nature 2002; 420:868–874.

54. Ross R. Atherosclerosis – an inflammatory disease. N Engl J Med 1999; 340:115–26.

55. Steinberg D. Atherogenesis in perspective: hypercholesterolemia and inflammation as partners in crime. Nat Med 2002; 8:1211–17.

56. Virmani R, Burke AP, Kolodgie FD, Farb A. Pathology of the thin-cap fibroatheroma: a type of vulnerable plaque. J Interv Cardiol 2003; 16:267–72.

57. Aikawa M, Libby P. The vulnerable atherosclerotic plaque: pathogenesis and therapeutic approach. Cardiovasc Pathol 2004; 13:125–38.

58. Daugherty A, Rateri DL. T lymphocytes in atherosclerosis: the yin-yang of Th1 and Th2 influence on lesion formation. Circ Res 2002; 90:1039–40.

59. Huber SA, Sakkinen P, David C, Newell MK, Tracy RP. T helper-cell phenotype regulates atherosclerosis in mice under conditions of mild hypercholesterolemia. Circulation 2001; 103:2610–16.

60. Laurat E, Poirier B, Tupin E et al. In vivo downregulation of T helper cell 1 immune responses reduces atherogenesis in apolipoprotein E-knockout mice. Circulation 2001; 104:197–202.

61. Zhou X, Paulsson G, Stemme S, Hansson GK. Hypercholesterolemia is associated with a T helper (Th) 1/Th2 switch of the autoimmune response in atherosclerotic apo E-knockout mice. J Clin Invest 1998; 101:1717–25.

62. Kolodgie FD, Gold HK, Burke AP et al. Intraplaque hemorrhage and progression of coronary atheroma. N Engl J Med 2003; 349:2316–25.

63. Virmani R, Kolodgie FD, Burke AP et al. Atherosclerotic plaque progression and vulnerability to rupture: angiogenesis as a source of intraplaque hemorrhage. Arterioscler Thromb Vasc Biol 2005; 25:2054–61.

64. Lindstedt KA, Kovanen PT. Mast cells in vulnerable coronary plaques: potential mechanisms linking mast cell activation to plaque erosion and rupture. Curr Opin Lipidol 2004; 15:567–73.

65. Newby AC. Dual role of matrix metalloproteinases (matrixins) in intimal thickening and atherosclerotic plaque rupture. Physiol Rev 2005; 85:1–31.

66. Galis ZS, Sukhova GK, Lark MW, Libby P. Increased expression of matrix metalloproteinases and matrix degrading activity in vulnerable regions of human atherosclerotic plaques. J Clin Invest 1994; 94: 2493–503.

67. Dirksen MT, van der Wal AC, van den Berg FM, van der Loos CM, Becker AE. Distribution of inflammatory cells in atherosclerotic plaques relates to the direction of flow. Circulation 1998; 98:2000–3.

68. Lovett JK, Rothwell PM. Site of carotid plaque ulceration in relation to direction of blood flow: an angiographic and pathological study. Cerebrovasc Dis 2003; 16:369–75.

69. Fujii K, Kobayashi Y, Mintz GS et al. Intravascular ultrasound assessment of ulcerated ruptured plaques: a comparison of culprit and nonculprit lesions of patients with acute coronary syndromes and lesions in patients without acute coronary syndromes. Circulation 2003; 108:2473–8.

70. Gertz SD, Roberts WC. Hemodynamic shear force in rupture of coronary arterial atherosclerotic plaques. Am J Cardiol 1990; 66:1368–72.

71. van der Wal AC, Becker AE, van der Loos CM, Das PK. Site of intimal rupture or erosion of thrombosed coronary atherosclerotic plaques is characterized by an inflammatory process irrespective of the dominant plaque morphology. Circulation 1994; 89:36–44.

72. Libby P. Molecular bases of the acute coronary syndromes. Circulation 1995; 91:2844–50.

73. Topper JN, Cai J, Falb D, Gimbrone MA Jr. Identification of vascular endothelial genes differentially responsive to fluid mechanical stimuli: cyclooxygenase-2, manganese superoxide dismutase, and endothelial cell nitric oxide synthase are selectively up-regulated by steady laminar shear stress. Proc Natl Acad Sci USA 1996; 93:10417–22.

74. Resnick N, Gimbrone MA Jr. Hemodynamic forces are complex regulators of endothelial gene expression. FASEB J 1995; 9:874–82.

75. Cheng C, van Haperen R, de Waard M et al. Shear stress affects the intracellular distribution of eNOS: direct demonstration by a novel in vivo technique. Blood 2005; 106:3691–8.

76. Malek AM, Alper SL, Izumo S. Hemodynamic shear stress and its role in atherosclerosis. JAMA 1999; 282:2035–42.

77. Inoue N, Ramasamy S, Fukai T, Nerem RM, Harrison DG. Shear stress modulates expression of Cu/Zn superoxide dismutase in human aortic endothelial cells. Circ Res 1996; 79:32–7.

78. Nerem RM, Alexander RW, Chappell DC et al. The study of the influence of flow on vascular endothelial biology. Am J Med Sci 1998; 316:169–75.

79. Ando J, Tsuboi H, Korenaga R et al. Down-regulation of vascular adhesion molecule-1 by fluid shear stress in cultured mouse endothelial cells. Ann NY Acad Sci 1995; 748:148–56; discussion 156–7.

80. Tricot O, Mallat Z, Heymes C et al. Relation between endothelial cell apoptosis and blood flow direction in human atherosclerotic plaques. Circulation 2000; 101:2450–3.

81. Dimmeler S, Hermann C, Galle J, Zeiher AM. Upregulation of superoxide dismutase and nitric oxide synthase mediates the apoptotic-suppressive effects of shear stress on endothelial cells. Arterioscler Thromb Vasc Biol 1999; 19:656–64.

82. Mattsson EJ, Kohler TR, Vergel SM, Clowes AW. Increased blood flow induces regression of intimal hyperplasia. Arterioscler Thromb Vasc Biol 1997; 17:2245–9.

83. Clowes AW, Berceli SA. Mechanisms of vascular atrophy and fibrous cap disruption. Ann NY Acad Sci 2000; 902:153–61; discussion 161–2.

84. Berceli SA, Davies MG, Kenagy RD, Clowes AW. Flow-induced neointimal regression in baboon polytetra-fluoroethylene grafts is associated with decreased cell proliferation and increased apoptosis. J Vasc Surg 2002; 36:1248–55.

85. Lincoln TM, Dey N, Sellak H. Invited review: cGMP-dependent protein kinase signaling mechanisms in smooth muscle: from the regulation of tone to gene expression. J Appl Physiol 2001; 91:1421–30.

86. Cucina A, Sterpetti AV, Borrelli V et al. Shear stress induces transforming growth factor-beta 1 release by arterial endothelial cells. Surgery 1998; 123:212–17.

87. Lopez Farre A, Mosquera JR, Sanchez de Miguel L et al. Endothelial cells inhibit NO generation by vascular smooth muscle cells. Role of transforming growth factor-beta. Arterioscler Thromb Vasc Biol 1996; 16:1263–8.

88. Boyle JJ, Weissberg PL, Bennett MR. Human macrophage-induced vascular smooth muscle cell apoptosis requires NO enhancement of Fas/Fas-L interactions. Arterioscler Thromb Vasc Biol 2002; 22:1624–30.

89. Cromheeke KM, Kockx MM, De Meyer GR et al. Inducible nitric oxide synthase colocalizes with signs of lipid oxidation/peroxidation in human atherosclerotic plaques. Cardiovasc Res 1999; 43:744–54.

90. Fukai T, Folz RJ, Landmesser U, Harrison DG. Extracellular superoxide dismutase and cardiovascular disease. Cardiovasc Res 2002; 55:239–49.

91. Kenagy RD, Fischer JW, Davies MG et al. Increased plasmin and serine proteinase activity during flow-induced intimal atrophy in baboon PTFE grafts. Arterioscler Thromb Vasc Biol 2002; 22:400–4.

92. Lijnen HR. Plasmin and matrix metalloproteinases in vascular remodeling. Thromb Haemost 2001; 86:324–33.

93. Castier Y, Brandes RP, Leseche G, Tedgui A, Lehoux S. p47phox-dependent NADPH oxidase regulates flow-induced vascular remodeling. Circ Res 2005; 97: 533–40.

94. Cheng C. The sheer stress of shear stress; responses of the vascular wall to a haemodynamic force. Dissertation, Erasmus MC, 2006.

95. Slager CJ, Wentzel JJ, Gijsen FJ et al. The role of shear stress in the destabilization of vulnerable plaques and related therapeutic implications. Nat Clin Pract Cardiovasc Med 2005; 2:456–64.

Vasa vasorum and vulnerable plaques

20

Mario Gössl and Amir Lerman

INTRODUCTION

The role of vasa vasorum in atherosclerosis has been speculated upon for over a century,[1-3] with interest waxing and waning but always overshadowed by the flood of literature about the many other factors known to play a role in atherogenesis. The recent development of more sophisticated imaging techniques such as micro-computed tomography (micro CT) in conjunction with molecular biology techniques (such as immunohistochemistry or Western blotting), however, offers the opportunity to analyze the vasa vasorum and their impact on the vascular vessel wall in more detail. Thus, recent research has led to convincing evidence that the abluminal part of the vessel wall, especially the adventitia and the vasa vasorum located there, may play as an important role in atherogenesis as the inner luminal layers of the vessel wall. In particular, vasa vasorum neovascularization in atherosclerosis has become one main focus of investigation within recent years because of its potential role in plaque development, growth, and progression from a stable to an unstable atherosclerotic lesion.

VASA VASORUM ANATOMY AND PHYSIOLOGY

In the past, the detailed study of vasa vasorum anatomy has proven difficult, owing to the lack of appropriate imaging modalities. The development of three-dimensional (3D) micro CT and its implementation into physiologic imaging opened, for the first time, the opportunity of studying the spatial distribution of vasa vasorum, their course within the vessel wall, and their connection and relation to the host vessel.[4] In contrast to histologic techniques, 3D micro CT allows imaging of an intact (i.e. non-dissected) coronary artery and its concomitant veins and, thereby, allows differentiating three types of vasa vasorum by their origin. It has been demonstrated that coronary arteries of pigs and humans contain three types of vasa vasorum (Figure 20.1).[5,6] Arterial vasa vasorum interna originate from the main coronary artery lumen and arborize into the vessel wall; arterial vasa vasorum externa originate from major branches and 'dive back' into the vessel wall; and, finally, venous vasa vasorum drain into concomitant veins. Detailed 3D tree analysis based on micro CT data suggests that vasa vasorum are end arteries and do not form a network as suggested earlier (Figure 20.2).[5,7,8] Nevertheless, there are anastomoses between the two arterial vasa vasorum types, between venous vasa vasorum and also arteriovenous shortcuts.[5]

We have shown recently, using cryogenic micro CT, that arterial vasa vasorum have a significant role in perfusion of the outer coronary vessel wall. After a bolus injection of contrast media, we could demonstrate that contrast was visible within the adventitia at the same time as it was inside the main

Figure 20.1 The three types of vasa vasorum found in the wall coronary arteries. (a) Vasa vascular interna (VVI) originate directly from the aorta's main lumen. (b) Vasa vasorum externa (VVE) originate from major branches deriving from the main coronary lumen and dive back into the coronary vessel wall. (c) Venous vasa vasorum (VVV) develop in the coronary vessel wall and finally drain into branches of concomitant veins. (Reproduced with permission from Gössl et al.[5])

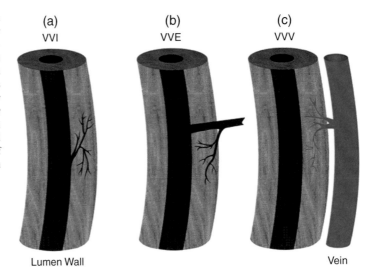

coronary artery lumen. In addition, as contrast media accumulate within the inner layers of the vessel wall, it also resolves within the adventitia over time (Figure 20.3),[9] indicating a significant role of venous vasa vasorum in the drainage of the coronary vessel wall. Hence, the vasa vasorum contains the same blood components and substances as the main lumen, and thus should be regarded as a mature circulation.

Using the detailed micro CT data, we were able to estimate the amount of endothelial exchange surface available within the porcine coronary vessel wall through vasa vasorum. Our data from normal pigs show that about two-thirds of the amount of the main lumen's endothelial surface area is also available within the vessel wall by virtue of the vasa vasorum's endothelium. In hypercholesterolemic animals, this value even increases the endothelial surface of the vasa vasorum equal to that of the main lumen.

Taken together, these data indicate that there is a significant role of arterial and venous vasa vasorum in perfusion and drainage of the coronary vessel wall and that vasa vasorum provide a considerable exchange surface for potentially beneficial as well as harmful circulating substances and mediators within the coronary vessel wall.

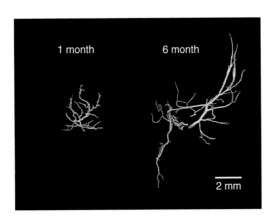

Figure 20.2 Volume rendered micro CT images of two single vasa vasorum from a 1-month-old and a 6-month-old pig. Three-dimensional (3D) micro CT imaging shows nicely that vasa vasorum are end arteries with a tree-like branching structure that grows with age. Fluid dynamic analyses based on this 3D information have demonstrated that vasa vasorum have fluid dynamic characteristics that are comparable to vasculature in general.[5,8] (Reproduced with permission from Gössl et al.[8]).

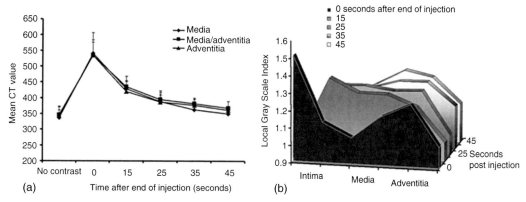

Figure 20.3 (a) Coronary vessel wall perfusion over time. The graph shows that the maximal opacification occurs immediately after complete injection of contrast medium into the lumen (0 second) and shows two peaks: one in the subintimal layer and one in the adventitial layer. This indicates that arterial vasa vasorum play a significant role in the perfusion of the outer layers of the coronary vessel wall, such as diffusion via the endothelium for the subintimal layers. With time, all layers of the coronary vessel wall show a progressive decrease in opacification. (b) Enhancement of the scale more clearly conveys how the 'wave of opacification' moves through the vessel wall from subintima to adventitia, without significant accumulation, which emphasizes the role of venous vasa vasorum in draining the coronary vessel wall. (Reproduced with permission from Gössl et al.[9])

THE ROLE OF VASA VASORUM IN ATHEROSCLEROSIS AND THE DEVELOPMENT OF VULNERABLE PLAQUES

Vasa vasorum neovascularization – a potential entry port into the growing plaque

Experimental studies have demonstrated that the exposure to an atherosclerotic risk factor such as hypercholesterolemia alone leads to an up-regulation of the hypoxia inducible factor 1 alpha (HIF-1α) and the vascular endothelial growth factor (VEGF),[10] which results in vasa vasorum neovascularization prior to the development of an atherosclerotic lesion and even before the development of endothelial dysfunction.[11–13] Conceivably, it has been proposed that vasa vasorum neoangiogenesis serves as a supply system for different substrates – such as oxidized low-density lipoprotein (oxLDL), endothelial progenitor cells, and endothelin – and immunoinflammatory/modulatory cells – neutrophils, T cells, and fibroblasts – into the developing atherosclerotic lesion.[14–16]

If there is a path into the lesion, is there also a way out? Several imaging studies, including our own, confirm that vasa vasorum neovascularization derives mainly from the adventitia (i.e. from vasa vasorum externa and venous vasa vasorum) and less frequently from the main lumen of the host vessel (i.e. vasa vasorum interna, Figures 20.1 and 20.4). Using conventional histologic techniques, it has been difficult to differentiate between arterial and venous vasa vasorum. However, future analysis, using 3D micro CT techniques, may shed light on the differential role of the different types of vasa vasorum in lesion initiation, progression, and stability. Venous venules are known to show earlier neoangiogenesis than arterial vessels;[17,18] hence, it may be speculated that the observed intraplaque angiogenesis is in part due to venous neovascularization growing inward into the vascular wall. The differential role of supply to and drainage from the coronary vessel wall in atherosclerosis is still not defined but needs to be addressed in future studies, especially when treatment

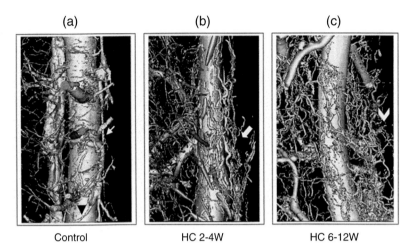

Figure 20.4   Micro CT images of the left anterior descending artery from control animals (Group 1; control (a)) and animals fed a hypercholesterolemic diet for 4 weeks (Group 2; HC2–4W (b)) or for 12 weeks (Group 3; HC6–12W (c)). In Group 1, the spatial pattern of vasa vasorum is characterized by a clear separation into first-order vasa vasorum, running longitudinally (small arrow), and second-order vasa vasorum, running circumferentially (arrowhead). In both Group 2 and Group 3, a network of newly formed vasa vasorum surrounds the host vessel (arrow), predominantly formed by second-order vasa vasorum (open arrow). Reconstruction voxel for illustration 21 μm. (Reproduced with permission from Herrmann et al.[12])

options preventing or reducing plaque angiogenesis are considered.

Results from recent experimental studies on rodent aortas provide strong evidence that vasa vasorum neovascularization correlates with plaque size[19] and that the inhibition of plaque neoangiogenesis reduces plaque progression.[20] The main issue of vasa vasorum neovascularization occurring prior to plaque progression or the progressing plaque producing the angiogenic factors that lead to vasa vasorum neovascularization is still contentious. It may be speculated that vasa vasorum neovascularization initiates atherosclerotic plaque development and leads to plaque progression, although vasa vasorum neovascularization may just be a physiologic response to the increasing nutritional demands of a growing plaque. The answer to all these questions is of high importance, since the future treatment of atherosclerotic disease might need to be more differentiated than it is today.

Based on our basic anatomic and physiologic data described earlier, the avascular portions of the media are virtually 'sandwiched' between two significant endothelial exchange surfaces: the main lumen on the inner side and the vasa vasorum at the outer side (Figure 20.5). It is conceivable that the same proatherogenic processes that occur at the luminal endothelium also take place at the interface of the vasa vasorum endothelium and the outer vessel wall. Thus, the atherogenetic process is 'fed' from two sides, which may lead to a significant potentiation.

There is convincing evidence that vessel wall neovascularization is the main route for the migration and influx of immunocompetent and inflammatory cells and plasma solutes into the atherosclerotic lesion.[14] In addition, several investigators have shown that vasa vasorum endothelial cells express adhesion molecules – vascular cell adhesion molecule (VCAM), intercellular adhesion molecule (ICAM), and E-selectin and CD40, a trimeric, transmembrane protein of the tumor necrosis factor (TNF) family.[16,21] Thus, it may be speculated that vasa vasorum

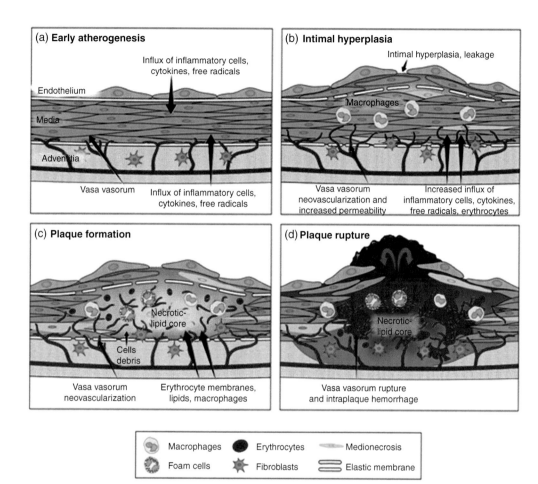

Figure 20.5   (a) Both the main lumen and the vasa vasorum encase the media with an extensive amount of endothelial surface. Thus, in the early stages of atherogenesis, there is influx of inflammatory cells, cytokines, and free radicals into the vessel wall from two sides. (b) Vasa vasorum neovascularization develops, which increases the influx of cellular and acellular proatherogenic components and promotes intimal hyperplasia. (c) In a later stage, a necrotic, lipid-rich core develops, which shows invasion of vasa vasorum and beginning hemorrhage. (d) Vasa vasorum rupture with hemorrhage, the expanding lipid core, and thinning of the fibrous cap lead to plaque rupture with the well-known consequence of occlusive coronary artery disease. That way, early and ongoing vasa vasorum neovascularization may promote plaque growth, expansion of the necrotic core, and finally plaque rupture.

neovascularization may even be more responsible for the delivery of harmful cellular and acellular components than diffusion through the main lumen's endothelium. Moreover, the newly formed vasa vasorum within atherosclerotic lesions show altered interendothelial cell contacts that allow extravascular leakage, which probably further enhances the effect of neovascularization-induced migration and influx.[22]

Vasa vasorum and plaque instability – new hypotheses derived from human pathology and experimental observations

Although we do not know whether vasa vasorum are initiating or promoting atherogenesis, it is widely accepted that complicated atherosclerotic lesions are associated with significant vasa vasorum neovascularization. Moreover, the rupture of vasa vasorum and subsequent intraplaque hemorrhage has been hypothesized to be a possible factor in the pathogenesis of plaque fissuring and plaque rupture for many years (see Figure 20.5[2,3,23]). However, the precise mechanism by which vasa vasorum rupture contributes to the progression of a stable to an unstable vulnerable plaque is not clear. Kolodgie et al have demonstrated an association between intraplaque hemorrhage (conceivably through ruptured vasa vasorum), an increase in the size of the necrotic core, and lesion instability.[24] Their studies on a large series of human coronary plaques from sudden coronary death victims show that the accumulation of erythrocyte membranes causes an increase in the levels of free cholesterol and an excessive recruitment of macrophages within the plaque. Thus, intraplaque hemorrhage increases the size of the necrotic core and serves as an inflammatory stimulus, further enhancing the transition of a stable to an unstable vulnerable plaque. Indeed, intraplaque hemorrhage has been shown to occur more frequently in ruptured than in more stable lesions in the human aorta.[25]

Several investigators have shown that intraplaque neovascularization alone, without the direct evidence of intraplaque hemorrhage, was associated with inflammatory cell infiltration and lipid deposition.[26] Furthermore, intraplaque neovascularization is also associated with clinical presentation. Depré et al reported that an increasing severity of the unstable angina score was associated with increasing prevalence of neovessels within human coronary plaque fragments.[27,28]

Several reports found a correlation between the amount of plaque neovascularization and plaque stability. Sun et al showed that unstable coronary atherosclerotic plaques (defined as plaques containing a lipid core of more than 40% of plaque area) showed more intraplaque neovascularization than stable lesions.[29]

Recent pathology studies of human unstable lesions have demonstrated that intraplaque hemorrhage and plaque rupture are associated with an increased vasa vasorum density. Mofidi et al showed in a carotid endarterectomy specimen a significantly higher microvessel count in hemorrhagic (>50% hemorrhage), unstable lesions, and symptomatic patients.[30]

Likewise, McCarthy et al showed that symptomatic carotid plaques showed more neovessels compared with asymptomatic plaques, and that plaque hemorrhage and rupture was associated with intraplaque neovascularization.[31] It has been shown that intraplaque microvessels mainly derive from adventitial vasa vasorum.[32] However, as indicated earlier, it has not yet been clarified if the intraplaque neovessels consist of arterial or venous vasa vasorum or both. Ongoing micro CT analysis may elucidate this question and thereby may lead to a therapeutic approach to prevent the transition from a stable to an unstable vulnerable plaque and thus possibly prevent acute vascular syndromes.

Preliminary micro CT studies suggest that the location of a vulnerable plaque may be determined by the spatial distribution of vasa vasorum along the longitudinal axis of a coronary artery.[33] Wang et al have demonstrated that occlusive coronary lesions leading to a ST-elevation myocardial infarction are predominately located in the proximal portions of coronary arteries.[34] In addition, intravascular ultrasound (IVUS) studies have shown that the size of the ulcerated ruptured coronary plaque is bigger the more proximal it is located within the coronary artery.[35] This concept is further supported by the observation of Hong et al, who demonstrated that the site of plaque rupture in patients with acute and stable coronary syndromes is mainly located within the proximal portion of the left anterior descending coronary artery (LAD) and the right coronary artery (RCA).[36] Based on previous reports about the association of vasa vasorum neovascularization and vulnerable plaques, one can hypothesize that the distribution of vasa vasorum neovascularization must therefore be pronounced in proximal parts of coronary arteries.

Vasa vasorum are differentially expressed in different vascular beds of experimental animals and humans,[6,37] with the highest vasa vasorum density in coronary arteries and the lowest in the internal mammary arteries. Thus, it may be speculated that the inherent density of vasa vasorum of a vascular bed may determine its propensity to develop symptomatic atherosclerotic plaques and may also explain the differential expression of atherosclerosis in different vascular beds.

Animal models of plaque rupturing

To our knowledge it has not yet been possible to develop an animal model that reliably simulates human coronary plaque rupturing. In order to approach this difficult task, the majority of investigators use the aortas of knockout rodents to study atherosclerosis and the role of neovascularization in its progression and complications. Although these models are more convenient than large animal models like the pig and mimic plaque growth and human atherosclerotic disease very well, rodents are not a good model to study the role of vasa vasorum. Rodents actually are lacking vasa vasorum, since their aortas have a very thin vessel wall that does not need vasa vasorum supply or drainage (critical depth theory by Geringer[38] and Wolinsky[39]). The periaortic vessels (erroneously called vasa vasorum) are mainly aortic intercostal branches. During plaque growth, sprouts of these intercostal arteries enter the progressing atherosclerotic lesion, which is recognized as increased plaque neovascularization,[19] but in how far this model is comparable to the complex anatomy and structure of the human coronary vessel

wall and its vasa vasorum is not known. To mimic human atherosclerotic disease and its complications as closely as possible, future investigations will have to address a way to create risk-factor induced, complex atherosclerotic lesions in large animals (pigs, monkeys). This is especially necessary because the transfer of knowledge derived from rodent studies to human disease remains challenging. Angiogenic and antiangiogenic treatment of atherosclerosis has been investigated in various experimental[40–43] and clinical studies,[44,45] but unfortunately the results are inconsistent. According to these studies, both treatments can have either no effect, increase, or even decrease neointima proliferation. Reasons for the wide spectrum of results are the great variety of the atherosclerosis models and vascular beds chosen by the different investigators (e.g. denudation, diet-induced, percutaneous transluminal coronary angioplasty [PTCA], carotids, aortas, femoral arteries), as well as the delivery of treatment and different stages of atherosclerosis at the time of intervention. As a result, there still remains warranted uncertainty about the usefulness of pro- or antiangiogenic treatment in atherosclerosis, and further investigations in large animals are necessary. Plaque or vasa vasorum neoangiogenesis is a complex process with inter- and intra-arterial variability,[46] which makes it necessary to study and probably treat different stages of atherosclerosis and different locations within the coronary artery differentially.

In-vivo imaging of vasa vasorum and potential therapeutic approaches

The analysis of potential mechanisms of plaque rupturing is still based on post-mortem pathologic studies. Hence, identifying the vulnerable plaque by in-vivo imaging is probably one of the most intriguing tasks in the near future. Based on the above, in-vivo visualization of the degree of vasa vasorum neovascularization within a plaque may help to identify a rupture-prone plaque earlier and may eventually lead to specific treatments using vasa vasorum as a therapeutic target. Recent developments in high-resolution IVUS algorithms show promising results regarding imaging of vasa vasorum in human coronary arteries in vivo after injection of echo contrast.[47] However, future studies have to show feasibility in a routine clinical setting. Other imaging modalities, such as cardiac computed tomography (CT) or cardiac magnetic resonance tomography (MRT), do not yet provide the resolution needed to resolve vasa vasorum within the coronary vessel wall. Future studies will have to show whether an indirect quantification of vasa vasorum density and neovascularization, respectively, will be possible through the quantification of coronary vessel wall contrast accumulation. In addition, it has yet to be proven in a prospective study if identifying atherosclerotic lesions with high vasa vasorum neovascularization is associated with an increased incidence of plaque rupture and morbidity and mortality, respectively.

The deployment of antiproliferative drug-eluting stents (DES) has been shown to be superior to previous treatments of coronary artery stenoses. It may be speculated that the implantation pressure as well as the effect of the eluting drug itself may have an impact on vasa vasorum perfusion and neovascularization. However, neither acute nor chronic effects have yet been investigated in a detailed systematic fashion. In addition, because of vasa vasorum anatomy (vasa vasorum externa originate from major branches; see Figure 20.1), treatment of a major coronary artery branch may have an indirect effect on the main coronary artery. The implantation pressure may occlude a vasa vasorum externa that supplies the main artery (and originates from that major branch), or the eluting drug may penetrate into the wall of the main artery via such a vasa vasorum externa, thus affecting an area that was originally not intended to be treated. Thus, the deployment of anti-inflammatory/antiangiogenic DES – bare-metal or resolvable stents[48] – into advanced atherosclerotic lesions with significant vasa vasorum neovascularization may not only inhibit plaque progression and restenosis locally but also lead to a therapeutic effect elsewhere along the coronary artery tree. Indeed, it has been suggested recently that drugs eluting from DES may reach downstream portions of the coronary artery by diffusion and through the vasa vasorum channels within the vessel wall.[49] This concept may warrant further investigation, since it may help to explain unexpected effects of DES on coronary atherosclerosis and endothelial function.

SUMMARY AND CONCLUSIONS

Vasa vasorum, arterial and venous, play a significant role in perfusion and drainage of the coronary vessel wall and there is growing evidence that growth of an atherosclerotic lesion is associated with significant neovascularization of leaky and friable vasa vasorum, possibly leading to vasa vasorum rupture and subsequent plaque hemorrhage. Recent studies provide the first evidence that these processes may further accelerate plaque vulnerability and eventually lead to plaque rupture. Future studies have to further elucidate this mechanism and show if vasa vasorum may become a therapeutic target for plaque stabilization.

REFERENCES

1. Koester W. Enarteritis and arteritis. Berl Klin Wochenschr 1876; 13:454–5.
2. Patterson JC. The reaction of the arterial wall to intramural hemorrhage. In: Symposium of Atherosclerosis. Washington, DC: National Academy of Sciences; 1954.
3. Winternitz MC, Thomas RM, Le Compte PM. Thrombosis. In: Thomas CC, ed. The Biology of

Atherosclerosis. Sprinfield, Illinois: Charles C Thomas; 1938:94–103.

4. Jorgensen SM, Demirkaya O, Ritman EL. Three-dimensional imaging of vasculature and parenchyma in intact rodent organs with X-ray micro-CT. Am J Physiol 1998; 275(3 Pt 2):H1103–14.

5. Gössl M, Rosol M, Malyar NM et al. Functional anatomy and hemodynamic characteristics of vasa vasorum in the walls of porcine coronary arteries. Anat Rec A Discov Mol Cell Evol Biol 2003; 272(2): 526–37.

6. Galili O, Sattler KJ, Lerman LO, Lerman A. Vasa vasorum density of human coronary arteries in different stages of atherosclerosis. J Am Coll Cardiol 2005; 45(3):437A.

7. Gössl M, Malyar NM, Rosol M, Beighley PE, Ritman EL. Impact of coronary vasa vasorum functional structure on coronary vessel wall perfusion distribution. Am J Physiol Heart Circ Physiol 2003; 285(5):H2019–26.

8. Gössl M, Zamir M, Ritman EL. Vasa vasorum growth in the coronary arteries of newborn pigs. Anat Embryol 2004; 208(5):351–7.

9. Gössl M, Beighley PE, Malyar NM, Ritman EL. Transendothelial solute transport in the coronary vessel wall: role of vasa vasorum: - a study with cryostatic micro-CT. Am J Physiol Heart Circ Physiol 2004; 287(5):H2346–51.

10. Zhu XY, Rodriguez-Porcel M, Bentley MD et al. Antioxidant intervention attenuates myocardial neovascularization in hypercholesterolemia. Circulation 2004; 109(17):2109–15.

11. Kwon HM, Sangiorgi G, Ritman EL et al. Enhanced coronary vasa vasorum neovascularization in experimental hypercholesterolemia. J Clin Invest 1998; 101(8):1551–6.

12. Herrmann J, Lerman LO, Rodriguez-Porcel M et al. Coronary vasa vasorum neovascularization precedes epicardial endothelial dysfunction in experimental hypercholesterolemia. Cardiovasc Res 2001; 51(4): 762–6.

13. Herrmann J, Best PJ, Ritman EL et al. Chronic endothelin receptor antagonism prevents coronary vasa vasorum neovascularization in experimental hypercholesterolemia. J Am Coll Cardiol 2002; 39(9):1555–61.

14. Bobryshev YV, Lord RS. Mapping of vascular dendritic cells in atherosclerotic arteries suggests their involvement in local immune-inflammatory reactions. Cardiovasc Res 1998; 37(3):799–810.

15. O'Brien KD, Allen MD, McDonald TO et al. Vascular cell adhesion molecule-1 is expressed in human coronary atherosclerotic plaques. Implications for the mode of progression of advanced coronary atherosclerosis. J Clin Invest 1993; 92(2):945–51.

16. O'Brien KD, McDonald TO, Chait A, Allen MD, Alpers CE. Neovascular expression of E-selectin, intercellular adhesion molecule-1, and vascular cell adhesion molecule-1 in human atherosclerosis and their relation to intimal leukocyte content. Circulation 1996; 93(4):672–82.

17. Vaupel P, Kallinowski F, Okunieff P. Blood flow, oxygen and nutrient supply, and metabolic microenvironment of human tumors: a review. Cancer Res 1989; 49(23):6449–65.

18. Shubik P. Vascularization of tumors: a review. J Cancer Res Clin Oncol 1982; 103(3):211–26.

19. Langheinrich AC, Michniewicz A, Sedding DG et al. Correlation of vasa vasorum neovascularization and plaque progression in aortas of apolipoprotein E(−/−)/low-density lipoprotein(−/−) double knock-out mice. Arterioscler Thromb Vasc Biol 2005; 26(2):347–52.

20. Moulton KS, Vakili K, Zurakowski D et al. Inhibition of plaque neovascularization reduces macrophage accumulation and progression of advanced atherosclerosis. Proc Natl Acad Sci USA 2003; 100(8):4736–41.

21. de Boer OJ, van der Wal AC, Teeling P, Becker AE. Leucocyte recruitment in rupture prone regions of lipid-rich plaques: a prominent role for neovascularization? Cardiovasc Res 1999; 41(2):443–9.

22. Bobryshev YV, Cherian SM, Inder SJ, Lord RS. Neovascular expression of VE-cadherin in human atherosclerotic arteries and its relation to intimal inflammation. Cardiovasc Res 1999; 43(4):1003–17.

23. Wartman WB. Occlusion of the coronary arteries by hemorrhage into their walls. Am Heart J 1938; 15:459–70.

24. Kolodgie FD, Gold HK, Burke AP et al. Intraplaque hemorrhage and progression of coronary atheroma. N Engl J Med 2003; 349(24):2316–25.

25. Moreno PR, Purushothaman KR, Fuster V et al. Plaque neovascularization is increased in ruptured atherosclerotic lesions of human aorta: implications for plaque vulnerability. Circulation 2004; 110(14):2032–8.

26. Juan-Babot JO, Martinez-Gonzalez J, Berrozpe M, Badimon L. [Neovascularization in human coronary arteries with lesions of different severity]. Rev Esp Cardiol 2003; 56(10):978–86. [in Spanish]

27. Depŕe C, Havaux X, Wijns W. Neovascularization in human coronary atherosclerotic lesions. Cathet Cardiovasc Diagn 1996; 39(3):215–20.

28. Depŕe C, Wijns W, Robert AM, Renkin JP, Havaux X. Pathology of unstable plaque: correlation with the clinical severity of acute coronary syndromes. J Am Coll Cardiol 1997; 30(3):694–702.

29. Sun L, Wei LX, Shi HY et al. [Angiogenesis in coronary atherosclerotic plaques and its relationship to plaque stabilization]. Zhonghua Bing Li Xue Za Zhi 2003; 32(5):427–31. [in Chinese]

30. Mofidi R, Crotty TB, McCarthy P et al. Association between plaque instability, angiogenesis and symptomatic carotid occlusive disease. Br J Surg 2001; 88(7):945–50.

31. McCarthy MJ, Loftus IM, Thompson MM et al. Angiogenesis and the atherosclerotic carotid plaque: an association between symptomatology and plaque morphology. J Vasc Surg 1999; 30(2):261–8.

32. Kumamoto M, Nakashima Y, Sueishi K. Intimal neo-vascularization in human coronary atherosclerosis: its origin and pathophysiological significance. Hum Pathol 1995; 26(4):450–6.

33. Gossi M, Versari D, Mannheim D, Ritman EL, Lerman LO, Lerman A. Increased spatial vasa vasorum density in the proximal LAD in hypercholesterolemia. Implications for vulnerable plaque development. Atherosclerosis 2006.

34. Wang JC, Normand SL, Mauri L, Kuntz RE. Coronary artery spatial distribution of acute myocardial infarction occlusions. Circulation 2004; 110(3):278–84.

35. Gössl M, von Birgelen C, Mintz GS et al. Volumetric assessment of ulcerated ruptured coronary plaques with three-dimensional intravascular ultrasound in vivo. Am J Cardiol 2003; 91(8):992–6, A7.

36. Hong MK, Mintz GS, Lee CW et al. The site of plaque rupture in native coronary arteries: a three-vessel intravascular ultrasound analysis. J Am Coll Cardiol 2005; 46(2):261–5.

37. Galili O, Herrmann J, Woodrum J et al. Adventitial vasa vasorum heterogeneity among different vascular beds. J Vasc Surg 2004; 40(3):529–35.

38. Geiringer E. Intimal vascularization and atherosclerosis. J Pathol Bact 1951; 63:201–11.

39. Wolinsky H, Glagov S. Nature of species differences in the medial distribution of aortic vasa vasorum in mammals. Circ Res 1967; 20(4):409–21.

40. Leppänen P, Koota S, Kholov I et al. Gene transfers of vascular endothelial growth factor-A, vascular endothelial growth factor-B, vascular endothelial growth factor-C, and vascular endothelial growth factor-D have no effects on atherosclerosis in hypercholesterolemic low-density lipoprotein-receptor/apolipoprotein B48-deficient mice. Circulation 2005; 112(9):1347–52.

41. Celletti FL, Waugh JM, Amabile PG et al. Vascular endothelial growth factor enhances atherosclerotic plaque progression. Nat Med 2001; 7(4):425–9.

42. Moulton KS, Heller E, Konerding MA et al. Angiogenesis inhibitors endostatin or TNP-470 reduce intimal neovascularization and plaque growth in apolipoprotein E-deficient mice. Circulation 1999; 99(13):1726–32.

43. Khurana R, Zhuang Z, Bhardwaj S et al. Angiogenesis-dependent and independent phases of intimal hyperplasia. Circulation 2004; 110(16):2436–43.

44. Hedman M, Hartikainen J, Syvanne M et al. Safety and feasibility of catheter-based local intracoronary vascular endothelial growth factor gene transfer in the prevention of postangioplasty and in-stent restenosis and in the treatment of chronic myocardial ischemia: phase II results of the Kuopio Angiogenesis Trial (KAT). Circulation 2003; 107(21):2677–83.

45. Henry TD, Annex BH, McKendall GR et al. The VIVA trial: Vascular endothelial growth factor in Ischemia for Vascular Angiogenesis. Circulation 2003; 107(10):1359–65.

46. Galili O, Sattler KJ, Herrmann J et al. Experimental hypercholesterolemia differentially affects adventitial vasa vasorum and vessel structure of the left internal thoracic and coronary arteries. J Thorac Cardiovasc Surg 2005; 129(4):767–72.

47. Carlier S, Kakadiaris IA, Dib N et al. Vasa vasorum imaging: a new window to the clinical detection of vulnerable atherosclerotic plaques. Curr Atheroscler Rep 2005; 7(2):164–9.

48. Eggebrecht H, Rodermann J, Hunold P et al. Images in cardiovascular medicine. Novel magnetic resonance-compatible coronary stent: the absorbable magnesium-alloy stent. Circulation 2005; 112(18):e303–4.

49. Hofma SH, van der Giessen WJ, van Dalen BM et al. Indication of long-term endothelial dysfunction after sirolimus-eluting stent implantation. Eur Heart J 2006; 27(2):166–70.

Intravascular magnetic resonance imaging

21

Robert L Wilensky and David A Halon

USE OF MAGNETIC RESONANCE IMAGING FOR EVALUATION OF ATHEROSCLEROTIC PLAQUE COMPOSITION

Magnetic resonance imaging (MRI) is an excellent diagnostic tool to evaluate arterial wall composition. High-resolution MRI imaging can differentiate between the medial and adventitial layers of the arterial wall and detect intimal thickening at early stages of the atherosclerotic process using multiple contrast protocols.[1] In addition, MRI has been used to discriminate between the collagenous cap and lipid core of atherosclerotic lesions.[2] Yuan and colleagues have developed imaging protocols for plaque tissue characterization using a combination of time-of-flight (TOF), proton-density-weighted (PDW), and T_2- and T_1-weighted scans.[3,4] Several investigative teams have applied MRI and shown its discriminating properties in determining the presence of vascular calcifications, lipid deposits, necrotic cores, and recent hemorrhage, as well as determining fibrous cap thickness, necrotic core size, and fissures within the fibrous cap.[3–8] In combination with local delivery of contrast agents, MRI can also determine the presence of specific cell types while providing important data on the biologic activity of potentially vulnerable lesions – i.e. cap thickness, lipid content, presence of activated macrophages, or tissue factor – and direct objective evidence of response to therapy on a morphologic as well as a functional basis.[7–10] However, MRI has not effectively evaluated coronary artery lesion composition because of inadequate image quality. The degraded image quality is primarily caused by image smearing as a result of cardiac and respiratory motion, the small volume of the typical coronary plaque, and the remote location of the vessels with respect to the scanner. More practical issues include the challenge of integrating traditional MRI scanner studies into a cardiac catheterization laboratory due to procedural complexity, size of the equipment, and high acquisition costs. To provide a solution to these issues, a novel intravascular MRI catheter that does not require the application of external magnetic fields was designed for intravascular interrogation of the arterial wall. This catheter is unencumbered by cardiac motion and holds promise, due to its high resolution and contrast, for the in-vivo evaluation of lipid-rich unstable coronary artery lesions.

PRINCIPLES OF MAGNETIC RESONANCE IMAGING

MRI exploits the differential responses of biologic tissues to an application of electromagnetic radiofrequency (RF) pulses within a strong static magnetic field (B_0).[11] Specifically, MRI is dependent on response signals of protons within the interrogated biologic tissue. After application of the

B_0 field, a net alignment of the proton spins along the direction of the field results. A short RF pulse is then applied, leading to a weak, transient oscillatory magnetic field (B_1) perpendicular to the B_0 field. The proton spins will rotate around the applied transverse B_1 field but once the B_1 field is turned off, the spins return to a rotation about the B_0 field.

Net magnetization of protons in the transverse plane can be detected secondary to the proton spin caused by the oscillatory magnetic field. The absorbed RF energy is released and the excited protons return to their original equilibrium state at a rate determined by spin–lattice relaxation or longitudinal relaxation rate, called T_1. The spins also dephase with a specific relaxation time determined by the spin–spin relaxation time, or T_2. Both T_1 and T_2 relaxation times are dependent on tissue composition and the local spin environment. The signal produced by the relaxing spins is detected with an RF receiver coil. PDW are obtained by reducing the contribution from T_1 and T_2, leaving only the differences in water or lipid proton densities for image contrast. These imaging contrasts (T_1, T_2, and PDW), along with a TOF scan, are used to determine plaque composition.

In addition to the conventional relaxation mechanisms listed above, self-diffusion of molecules can rival or even dominate T_2. The self-diffusion of an excited molecule in an inhomogeneous field will accumulate random phase as it changes positions (and so magnetic field strength) within a tissue, leading to a net dephasing of the region. The random fluctuations of position experienced by the molecule are due to Brownian motion, which is affected primarily by temperature and the molecular environment. The measured self-diffusion of molecules in MRI is referred to as apparent diffusion coefficient (ADC) and the modified T_2 relaxation time as T_2^*.

TECHNICAL PROPERTIES OF THE IVMRI CATHETER (IVMRI)

The IVMRI system is a self-contained MRI probe integrated at the tip of a vascular catheter attached to a portable control unit (Figure 21.1). The IVMRI probe contains all the components necessary for MR analysis, including magnets, an RF transmission and receiver coil, and the electronics for efficient transmission and

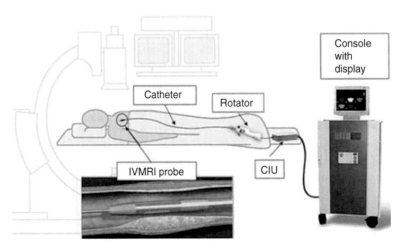

Figure 21.1 Schematic outline of the IVMRI system. The intravascular MRI catheter incorporates miniature magnets and a transmit/receive coil that looks sideways into the arterial wall. The IVMRI catheter is introduced into the artery via a standard guide wire and is connected proximally to the display console by a rotator and a control/interface unit (CIU).

reception of signals. There are no external magnets or coils so that the system can be used within the cardiac catheterization laboratory, not the MR suite. Locally, static magnetic field gradients are generated around the catheter, at the site of measurement, which are responsive to the diffusion properties of the analyzed vascular tissue.

The IVMRI probe is stabilized vis-à-vis the arterial wall using a gentle side balloon and creates a sector-shaped field of view (FOV) that is 2 mm along the vessel by 60° along the circumference, with a radial depth of penetration of 250 μm (Figure 21.2). After completion of data acquisition from each sector, the balloon is deflated and the catheter is rotated by 120° using the rotator to acquire data from the next sector. A new spiral rotator allows the acquisition of data at various angles while pulling back the catheter.

The principles of operation of the IVMRI probe are shown in Figure 21.3. Prior to introduction of the IVMRI catheter, water proton spins point at arbitrary orientations (see Figure 21.3a). When the IVMRI catheter is introduced and the probe is stabilized vis-à-vis the vessel wall, the static magnetic field (B$_0$) causes spins to align with the field direction (see Figure 21.3b). As the static field strength decreases substantially with increasing radial penetration depth into the vessel wall, different measurement depths correspond to different precession frequencies of the protons (see Figure 21.3c). This allows the division of the FOV into measurement zones with a very high radial resolution that is of the order of 100 μm. For acquiring MR data from each zone, a series of transmit RF pulses are applied (see Figure 21.3d). The pulse frequency determines with high accuracy

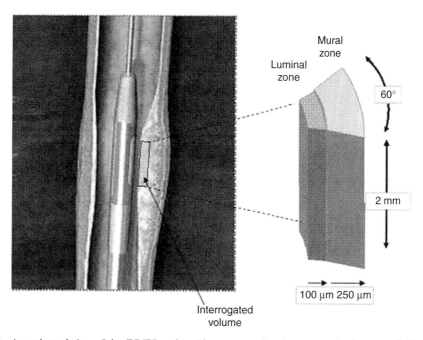

Figure 21.2 An enlarged view of the IVMRI probe with corresponding interrogated volume, or field of view (FOV). The FOV dimensions of the current catheter configuration are 2 mm in the longitudinal axis, 60° radially along the circumference, and 250 μm in depth. The FOV can be internally divided into measurement zones having different depths. The illustration demonstrates two zones: a luminal 0–100 μm zone and a mural 100–250 μm zone.

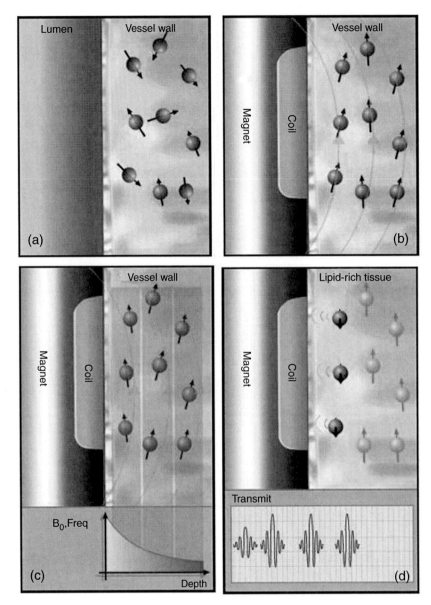

Figure 21.3 (a) Lumen and proton activity within the vessel wall before introduction of the IVMRI catheter. (b) Introduction of the IVMRI catheter induces a net magnetization of the protons in the direction of the static magnetic field (B_0) generated by the magnets in the probe. (c) Static field strength and precession frequency of water proton spins decrease as a function of the depth of penetration. The various fields of view (FOVs) are noted in the shaded regions. (d) The transmission of a series of short RF pulses at preselected frequencies creates excitation of proton spins in the corresponding measurement zone.

which zone is being measured at any given time.

A significant advantage of the IVMRI configuration over conventional MRI is that substantial spatial changes, termed gradients, in the static field can assist in differentiating vascular tissues based on the intrinsic self-diffusion of water protons. The IVMRI catheter has been specifically designed to evaluate with high accuracy the presence of lipid-rich tissue by measuring the ADC of water molecules in the vessel wall. Toussaint et al demonstrated that fibrous and lipid-laden tissue could be differentiated on the basis of ADC measurements.[12] Whereas, the IVMRI probe cannot differentiate between the fibrous cap and the normal medial layer using the current pulse sequence, insofar as they possess similar biophysical properties (i.e. similar water diffusion coefficients), the probe can easily differentiate the lipid-laden necrotic core of thin-cap fibroatheromas from normal and fibrous tissue. The underlying cause for differences in ADC between fibrous and lipid-rich tissues is that in fibrous tissue water molecules self-diffuse with little or no confinement, giving rise to a high ADC, whereas the self-diffusion of water molecules in lipid-rich tissue is confined by large cholesterol molecules, and therefore

gives rise to a low ADC. Using a series of short RF pulses, the IVMRI probe receives a series of corresponding echo signals from each measurement zone. The decay time of the echo amplitude accurately corresponds to the ADC, and therefore to the lipid content, of the measurement zone. Figure 21.4 illustrates the differences between the significant self-diffusion of water protons in fibrous tissue (produces fast echo decay) vs the restricted diffusion in lipid-rich tissue (produces slow decay).

The image obtained by the IVMRI probe is not a reflection of the actual morphology of the plaque but provides a simplified spatial representation of its lipid-rich component. In order to allow 'on-line' interpretation of the lipid composition in each measurement zone, a simple color-coding technique is used. The amplitudes of received echoes are

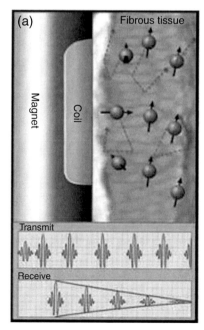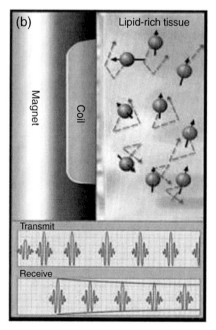

Figure 21.4 The received echo amplitude decay time is dependent on tissue composition. (a) In fibrous tissue, the self-diffusion of the water molecules within the tissue is virtually unrestricted, leading to a fast signal decay. (b) In lipid-rich tissue, the self-diffusion of the water molecules is restricted by the presence of large lipid molecules, which results in a signal decay that is much slower.

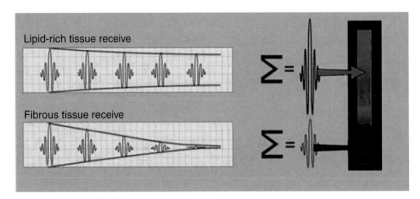

Figure 21.5 Illustration of the color-coding technique: echo amplitudes are summed up to result in accumulated amplitude, which is then normalized to a color scale. Lipid-rich tissue is characterized by slow echo decay (above) and a high accumulated amplitude, which is coded to yellow, whereas fibrous tissue is characterized by fast echo decay (below) and a low accumulated amplitude, which is coded to blue.

summed to present accumulated echo amplitude, as shown in Figure 21.5. The amplitude is then normalized onto a color scale that ranges from blue (completely fibrous tissue) to yellow (lipid-rich tissue).

Color-coded data from each measurement sector are displayed separately with a numerical lipid fraction index (LFI) and

estimated error (Figure 21.6). Depending on the imaging protocol, each sector can display lipid fraction of either one measurement zone (based on the zone depth) or more than one zone. In the section below that will describe clinical results to date, the first part of the protocol was based on measuring two zones per sector, luminal 0–100 μm and mural 100–250 μm,

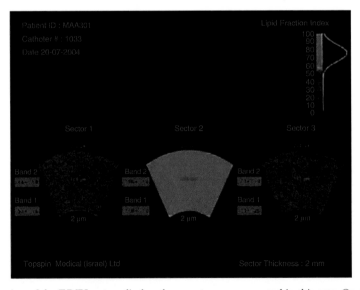

Figure 21.6 Illustration of the IVMRI system display: three sectors are presented in this case. On the left side of each sector (denoted as band) is a numerical result of the lipid fraction index (LFI) in two measurement zones: luminal 0–100 μm and mural 100–250 μm. An estimation of the error is also given. The central sector is entirely yellow (lipid-rich tissue) whereas the left and right sectors are blue (fibrous tissue).

and the second part was based on measuring a single 50–200 μm zone.

Previous histologic studies have shown that thin-cap fibroatheromas, considered 'vulnerable plaques', have a fibrous cap thickness that does not exceed 100 μm.[13] Hence, the IVMRI determinates of a thin-cap fibroatheroma may, with refined catheter configurations in the future, be defined as the presence of an increased lipid fraction (or the relative *absence* of fibrous tissue) in the shallow luminal zone of the FOV. Conversely, the absence of lipid within the superficial FOV may denote a fibrous cap >100 μm observed in more stable lesions. Increased lipid in the deep mural zone, in turn, may indicate the presence of a necrotic core or increased foam cells. Since most thin-cap fibroatheromas have >120° of their circumference affected by a necrotic core and have a mean length of 8–9 mm,[14] sequential IVMRI measurements are obtained in a spiral pattern so that data are obtained from longer arterial segments.

IVMRI technology offers high flexibility to change the imaging protocol and, hence, the tissue parameters measured. In addition to diffusion-weighted imaging, multicontrast MRI such as T_1, T_2, and PDW are potentially obtainable with this catheter. Changing the transmit pulse frequency can change the internal division within the sector-shaped FOV to improve the radial resolution: e.g. the luminal zone can be made thinner than 100 μm, which may improve the classification of fibrous caps into thin vs thick caps.

PRELIMINARY EXPERIMENTS WITH THE IVMRI PROBE

The diagnostic capabilities of the IVMRI probe were initially tested on formalin-fixed carotid endarterectomy plaques obtained from symptomatic and asymptomatic patients. To account for tissue fixation, parallel experiments were performed on unfixed samples. Although formalin fixation, in comparison to fresh unfixed tissue, lowers the tissue's MR signal by 30–50%, the detectable tissue property was not abolished. The tissues were dissected according to the plaque's morphology to allow direct application of the probe to the tissue surface. Both lipid-rich tissue and fibrous tissue were analyzed at multiple loci, with precise registration of the interrogated sites. A pathologist unaware of the IVMRI results reviewed the histologic slides and delineated areas with a high lipid concentration, a low lipid concentration, and the absence of lipids, prior to superposition of the map of analyzed loci. The correlation of IVMRI results vs histologic diagnosis yielded a sensitivity of 90%. Hence, proof of concept was demonstrated, showing that the IVMRI probe was capable of differentiating lipid from fibrous tissue.

In-vivo animal studies

Early in-vivo animal studies were designed to examine specific technical properties of the IVMRI catheter in an in-vivo situation, including the extent of interference with IVMRI recording from the catheter system, the beating heart, and external electronic interference. Following these preliminary studies, a definitive in-vivo safety study was performed in 16 healthy domestic pigs and IVMRI measurements performed. The animals were followed up in two groups for 24 hours and 30 days, respectively. The study results showed the catheter to have mechanical properties and maneuverability suitable for in-vivo use in man, and there was no evidence of significant acute damage or late adverse clinical or histologic effects.

Ex-vivo human studies

Subsequent studies evaluated the functional capacity of the IVMRI catheter in fresh postmortem human aortic samples and coronary arteries. Proximal aortic and coronary samples were obtained within 48 hours of death and evaluated in a saline bath at 37°C. The 16 aortic segments exhibited a variety of atherosclerotic lesions, comprising ulcerated plaques (absence of fibrous cap, $n = 4$), thin-cap fibroatheromas ($n = 2$), thick-cap fibroatheromas ($n = 2$), intimal xanthomas ($n = 2$), and adaptive intimal thickening ($n = 6$). IVMRI results demonstrated a strong correlation with the blinded histologic diagnosis, yielding a correct diagnosis in 15 of 16 samples, with 95% sensitivity and 100% specificity.[15]

Studies were also performed in ex-vivo, in-situ coronary arteries ($n = 18$) from 14 hearts. Moderately stenotic proximal and mid lesions (30–60% in severity) were located by postmortem coronary angiography. The IVMRI catheter was placed within the artery and the exact location, vis-à-vis the lesion, was validated electronically. Following circumferential IVMRI acquisition, the examined arteries were dissected free and the arterial segments were processed for histologic evaluation. The lesions were classified, by histology, using a recently published classification scheme (M): adaptive intimal thickening ($n = 1$), fatty streak (intimal xanthoma, $n = 2$), thick-cap fibroatheroma ($n = 4$), thin-cap fibroatheroma (vulnerable plaque, $n = 3$), ruptured plaque with intraplaque hemorrhage ($n = 1$), plaque hemorrhage ($n = 1$), healed plaque rupture ($n = 1$), and fibrocalcific plaque ($n = 5$). Thin-cap fibroatheromas (vulnerable plaques) were defined as lesions containing necrotic cores and thin (<75 μm) fibrous caps. The IVMRI diagnosis of lesion characteristics correlated with histologic diagnosis in 16 out of the interrogated 18 lesions (89%), with correct assessment of all three thin-cap fibroatheromas.[15] These studies demonstrated that the IVMRI catheter could diagnose the presence of thin-cap fibroatheromas and differentiate potentially vulnerable plaques from stable atherosclerotic lesions in human coronary arteries.

Clinical studies

The first IVMRI clinical study (first-in-man; FIM) was recently completed (N) and the second phase is now in progress. These early clinical studies were designed to demonstrate safety and feasibility of operating the self-contained IVMRI system within the confines of a standard catheterization laboratory. The FIM was a prospective, multicenter study including 29 patients from four centers in Europe. Patients had either stable or unstable coronary artery disease and underwent a clinically indicated diagnostic or interventional procedure. The 5.2F device was introduced through an 8F-guiding catheter to examine a single non-obstructive plaque with a minimal arterial luminal diameter between 2 and 4 mm, within the proximal to mid portion of the left anterior descending (LAD) or right coronary artery (RAC). Since the catheter has an angular view of 60°, a rotation system was used to allow measurements to be recorded at three different sectors following 120° catheter rotation. IVMRI recordings were made at each sector.

The catheter proved to be easily maneuverable and was successfully introduced into all but one artery. The angiographic appearance of the catheter during clinical studies is shown in Figure 21.7, together with representative IVMRI findings. IVMRI data could not be obtained in three patients due to calcium deposition and in six patients due to electromechanical interference from guidewire artifacts and surrounding catheter laboratory equipment. The FIM study demonstrated that the IVMRI catheter was safe for use in humans with no catheter-related complications at 30-day follow-up (absence of a composite of cardiac death, myocardial infarction [Q wave and non-Q wave], unstable angina, or subacute thrombosis of the interrogated coronary artery). In addition, the study demonstrated that IVMRI recordings were feasible in the

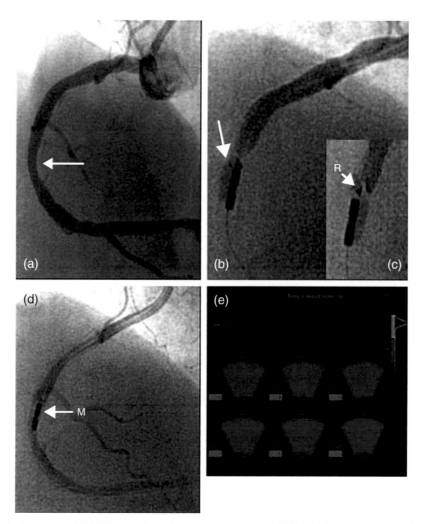

Figure 21.7   Angiograms and IVMRI recording of a right coronary artery (RCA) during interrogation of a non-obstructive coronary lesion. (a) Arrow denotes intermediate lesion in the mid RCA. (b) Angiogram obtained during interrogation of the mid RCA plaque with the IVMRI catheter. The eccentrically placed balloon is inflated (vertical arrow) obstructing passage of contrast distally. (c) The IVMRI catheter interrogating a second angular sector of the same plaque after rotation of the catheter. The balloon is now inflated on the opposite side of the catheter (horizontal arrow). (d) Angiogram made following deflation of the IVMRI catheter balloon showing free passage of the contrast distally. (e) Data recorded from six sectors of the plaque. The sectors were obtained in a spiral fashion (from the distal edge to the proximal edge of the plaque) and are displayed sequentially. All sectors had a pattern consistent with fibrous plaque. M = magnet, R = rotation marker.

catheterization laboratory. On the basis of the ex-vivo studies previously described, plaques were characterized according to the predominant IVMRI pattern as fibrous, fatty streak, or lipid-rich. The plaque lipid fraction in the study population showed a frequency distribution similar to that found in the ex-vivo study of aortic plaques.[16]

The study also revealed unforeseen technical issues related to guide-wire artifacts, external interference from catheter laboratory equipment, and incomplete catheter rotation. These issues were addressed and several technical improvements were introduced into the IVMRI catheter for the second part of the study. Shielding of the guide-wire tube significantly reduced the occurrence of guide-wire artifacts and an improved spiral rotator device was devised to allow sector analysis at multiple points in a spiral manner along the longitudinal axis of the plaque. An increased balloon attachment pressure was implemented in order to resolve cases of incomplete attachment.

The technically improved version of the IVMRI catheter is now being studied using an amended protocol that allows extended data acquisition of up to six sectors at different points along the plaque. In the current study, an intravascular ultrasound (IVUS) pullback is obtained in the study-related vessel in addition to the IVMRI acquisition. By December 2005, 27 patients had been studied, with a significantly improved technical success rate and no catheter-related adverse events reported.

FUTURE DEVELOPMENT PLANS

Development is underway of new-generation IVMRI catheters, with smaller probe diameters that are compatible with standard low-profile guide catheters, increased field of view per sensor, and incorporating multiple sensors acquiring data simultaneously from longer segments. Also, multicontrast techniques, e.g. measurement of inflammation and thrombus characterization based on the same catheter platform, will be studied. This new-generation equipment will be available for larger-scale clinical trials that will obtain further data for initial correlations of the IVMRI findings with clinical data and subsequent clinical events.

REFERENCES

1. Martin AJ, Gotlieb AI, Henkelman RM. High-resolution MR imaging of human arteries. J Magn Reson Imaging 1995; 5:93–100.

2. Toussaint JF, LaMuraglia GM, Southern JF, Fuster V, Kantor HL. Magnetic resonance images lipid, fibrous, calcified, hemorrhagic, and thrombotic components of human atherosclerosis in vivo. Circulation 1996; 94(5):932–8.

3. Yuan C, Mitsumori LM, Beach KW, Maravilla KR. Carotid atherosclerotic plaque: noninvasive MR characterization and identification of vulnerable lesions. Radiology 2001; 221(2):285–99.

4. Cai J, Hatsukami TS, Ferguson MS et al. In-vivo quantitative measurement of intact fibrous cap and lipid-rich necrotic core size in atherosclerotic carotid plaque. Circulation 2005; 112:3437–44.

5. Hatsukami TS, Ross R, Polissar NL, Yuan C. Visualization of fibrous cap thickness and rupture in human atherosclerotic carotid plaque in vivo with high-resolution magnetic resonance imaging. Circulation 2000; 102:959–64.

6. Trivedi RA, U-King-Im JM, Graves MJ et al. MRI-derived measurements of fibrous-cap and lipid-core thickness: the potential for identifying vulnerable carotid plaques in vivo. Neuroradiology 2004; 46:738–43.

7. Yuan C, Kerwin WS, Ferguson MS et al. Contrast-enhanced high resolution MRI for atherosclerotic carotid artery tissue characterization. J Magn Reson Imaging 2002; 15:62–7.

8. Wasserman BA, Smith WI, Trout HH III et al. Carotid artery atherosclerosis: in vivo morphologic characterization with gadolinium-enhanced double-oblique MR imaging – initial results. Radiology 2002; 223:566–73.

9. Zhao XQ, Yuan C, Hatsukami TS et al. Effects of prolonged intensive lipid-lowering therapy on the characteristics of carotid atherosclerotic plaques in vivo by MRI: a case-control study. Arterioscler Thromb Vasc Biol 2001; 21:1623–9.

10. Wilensky RL, Song HK, Ferrari VA. Role of magnetic resonance and intravascular magnetic resonance in the detection of vulnerable plaques. J Am Coll Cardiol 2006; 47 (8 Suppl):C48–56.

11. Balaban RS. Physics of image generation by magnetic resonance. In: Manning WJ, Pennell DJ, eds. Cardiovascular Magnetic Resonance. New York: Churchill Livingstone; 2002.

12. Toussaint JF, Southern JF, Fuster V, Kantor HL. Water diffusion properties of human atherosclerosis and thrombosis measured by pulse field gradient nuclear magnetic resonance. Arterioscler Thromb Vasc Biol 1997; 17:542–6.

13. Schaar JA, Muller JE, Falk E et al. Terminology for high-risk and vulnerable coronary artery plaques. Eur Heart J 2004; 25:1–6.

14. Virmani R, Burke AP, Kolodgie FD, Farb A. Understanding atherosclerotic coronary artery disease: What makes the plaque unstable? Proceedings of the Paris Course on Revascularization (Euro PCR 04), 2004:7–32.

15. Schneiderman J, Wilensky RL, Weiss A et al. Diagnosis of thin fibrous cap atheromas by a self-contained intravascular magnetic resonance imaging probe in *ex-vivo* human aortas and *in-situ* coronary arteries. J Am Coll Cardiol 2005; 45:1961–9.

16. Regar E, Hennen B, Grube E et al. First-in-man application of a self-contained intracoronary magnetic resonance imaging system. A multi-center safety and feasibility trial. Am J Cardiol 2005; 96 (Suppl 7A): 192H.

Intracoronary thermography: basic principles

Anna G ten Have, Frank JH Gijsen, Joland J Wentzel, Cornelis J Slager, Patrick W Serruys, and Anton FW van der Steen

INTRODUCTION

Heart disease is the number one cause of death in the Western world and number two in the non-Western world.[1] Coronary atherosclerosis is by far the most frequent cause of ischemic heart disease,[2] and it can be subdivided into a number of developmental stages. One of these stages involves the vulnerable plaque.

Plaque disruption with superimposed thrombosis is the main cause of events such as the acute coronary syndromes of unstable angina, myocardial infarction, and sudden death.[2] It is suggested that increased plaque heat is a feature of vulnerable plaques.[3] This heat might be caused by increased metabolic activity of inflammatory cells, such as macrophages, or by enzymatic extracellular matrix breakdown. Detection of heat could thus possibly lead to detection of vulnerable plaques.

Since the first publication in the field of vulnerable plaque detection using thermographic methods,[3] many thoughts and results on this detection technique have been published. The temperature differences that were published have decreased over time, but are still of significant value to conclude that thermal heterogeneity exists in vivo. Based on these values, it is worthwhile to continue studying the exact details of the origin and the clinical consequences of this thermal heterogeneity. This chapter aims to explain the basic principles regarding intracoronary thermography. It describes what needs to be measured and which pitfalls arise when measuring temperatures in vivo. In addition, it suggests ways to overcome these problems.

HEAT GENERATION

The mechanism by which heat production of plaques occurs is unknown, as are the resulting heat production values. Most evidence points towards high metabolism of macrophages or other exothermal processes related to macrophages, such as matrix breakdown by matrix metalloproteinases (MMPs). Macrophages are abundantly present in vulnerable plaques, bordering the atheromatous core, and are located in the fibrous cap, especially near the shoulder regions of the cap.[2] Speculations have been made with regard to the processes that are involved in the heat generation. Some of these are described in this section.

MACROPHAGE METABOLISM

The turnover rate for the total adenosine triphosphate (ATP) content of the macrophage in culture is about 10 times per minute, being an order of magnitude higher than a typical mammalian cell,[4] which indicates that macrophages have a high metabolic rate.[5]

Macrophage metabolism, and thus heat generation, can be measured in vitro using microcalorimetry. Heat production values of non-phagocytosing mouse macrophages were shown to be 0.78–6.5 pW per cell, its value decreasing upon increasing cell density.[6] The generated heat was primarily due to glucose metabolism, and glycolysis was a major contributor to the produced heat. Heat production values of alveolar rabbit macrophages grown in a monolayer were 19.4 ± 3.2 pW per cell.[7] Adding 20% homologous rabbit serum to the growth medium increased the heat production to 27.0 ± 2.0 pW per cell. Heat production values of phagocytosing peritoneal mouse macrophages were measured in different experimental conditions.[8] Mean heat production values for resting cells were around 20.6 ± 10.1 and 16.2 ± 3.1 pW per cell. When, for example, lipopolysaccharide-bounded high-density polyethylene particles were phagocytosed, these values could rise up to 92 pW per cell, implying an increase of up to five times the basal value. Whether the heat production values mentioned here are high enough to cause the temperature differences that have been published is currently unknown.

Mechanisms responsible for increased energy consumption

Enzymatic extracellular matrix degradation

Microcalorimetric analysis of bacterial collagenase degradation of porcine pericardium tissues revealed that the heat released during degradation correlates well with the degree of degraded tissue.[9] Therefore, the MMP-related breakdown of extracellular matrix in atherosclerotic plaques might also be an exothermal process. Toutouzas et al[10] have demonstrated that patients with acute coronary syndromes show increased MMP-9 concentration, which was well correlated with temperature differences between the atherosclerotic plaque and the normal vessel wall. Krams et al[11] have correlated temperature heterogeneity to regions of increased MMP-9 activity.

Lipid metabolism

After the uptake of modified lipids by macrophages through various routes of endocytosis, most of the lipids are finally transported into lysosomes, digested therein, and degraded into amino acids and free cholesterol, which is released into the cytosol and further into the extracellular space. In the cytosol, the free cholesterol is trapped in a continued cycle of esterification and hydrolysis, called the cholesterol ester cycle,[12] that wastes ATP.[13] The rate of cholesterol esterification is positively correlated with the cholesterol content of arterial segments from atherosclerotic animals.[14]

Uncoupling proteins

The uncoupling protein-1 (UCP-1), also called thermogenin, is a protein that is found exclusively in brown adipose tissue (BAT) in mammals. Thermogenesis, or heat production, in BAT depends largely on UCP-1 activity.[15] Of the UCP-1 molecule, a number of homologs exist, of which UCP-2 has been speculated to cause the temperature increase in vulnerable plaques.[16] Advanced complicated atherosclerotic plaques have shown a dense infiltration of macrophages, of which a subpopulation strongly expressed UCP-2. The UCP-2-positive macrophages were associated with oxidized lipids, inducible nitric oxide synthase (iNOS), and nitrotyrosine, and a fraction showed apoptosis. Whether UCP-2 acts thermogenic in any tissue is still under debate.[17]

HEAT TRANSFER

Net transfer of thermal energy, or heat transfer, between two objects occurs only when the objects are at different temperatures, and its direction is from a region of higher temperature to a region of lower temperature. This occurs either by conduction, convection, radiation, or by a combination of these depending on the media involved.

Conduction

Conduction is the transfer of heat through a solid or fluid medium due to a temperature gradient by the exchange of molecular kinetic energy during collisions of molecules (Figure 22.1a). Thermal parameters governing this process are the specific heat capacity (how many joules are needed to raise a certain amount of the material 1°C) and the heat conductivity (the amount of joules per second (watts) that pass a certain distance of material driven by a temperature difference of 1°C). Materials can be divided into conductors, e.g. metals, known for their ability to transfer heat fast, and insulators, e.g. air and most plastics, which have low heat conductivity values. Fatty tissue is also known for its insulating properties,[18] so lipid present in the lipid core of a vulnerable plaque is likely to behave as an insulating material and may obstruct the transfer of heat produced by macrophages to its neighborhood.

Convection

Convection is the transfer of heat due to bulk motion of the medium (Figure 22.1b). Heat produced by the vulnerable plaque will be transferred through the wall by means of conduction, as described above. Once the heat has arrived at the lumen wall, it will be transported by the flow of blood. Distal from the heat source, the heat can be transferred back to the lumen wall by conduction. Parameters influencing the blood flow profile, such as curvature of the vessel and presence of a catheter, will result in changes of temperature distribution. Increase of local flow velocity

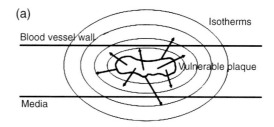

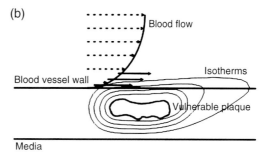

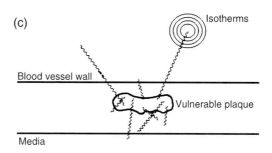

Figure 22.1 Heat transfer by (a) conduction, (b) conduction and convection, and (c) radiation and absorption.

will decrease the temperatures at the lumen wall.[19] In addition, pulsatility might affect the measurement, since pulsating axial velocity produces a pulsating temperature distribution.[20]

Radiation and absorption

Heat transfer due to radiation is energy transfer via electromagnetic waves (Figure 22.1c). Every object radiates electromagnetic waves, the amount and the wavelength depending on the temperature and its emissivity (how well the object radiates compared with a perfectly radiating black body). Heat transfer by radiation does not require a medium. The radiation in its turn may again be absorbed in a medium, which results in local heating. This type of heat transfer is usually neglected in intracoronary thermography. Whether it is correct to neglect radiation depends on, among others, the dimensions of the heat source, with a tendency for larger sources to have a higher radiative emission, and on the emissivity of the heat source.

HEAT DETECTION

Unfortunately, heat production cannot be measured in vivo using calorimetric methods, so other measuring techniques have to be used. One method is measuring temperature. By detecting a higher temperature among a range of so-called background temperatures, one is able to locate a spot of higher heat production in the region.

Temperature can be measured by a variety of methods, using electrical, optical, magnetic, or other types of sensors. Electrical methods include resistance, thermistor, and thermocouple. Some of these have already been applied in the catheters that are currently used for intracoronary thermography.[21–23] Optical methods include infrared detection, liquid crystals,[24] and temperature-dependent fluorescence techniques.[25]

Magnetic resonance thermography is a method using the magnetic properties of molecules.[26] Another method is the use of quartz crystals or microwave thermography.[27] These methods can be divided into either contact or non-contact methods. Contact thermography methods require contact between the thermosensitive material of the device and the lumen wall, whereas non-contact temperature methods can do without such contact.

Heat detection by a contact method occurs by conduction of heat from the luminal wall to the sensor. When the sensor does not approach the wall close enough, however, the sensor area is exposed to surrounding influences and this will influence the measurement. When designing a contact method, one should be extremely cautious, since a vulnerable plaque is easily ruptured. The stress the sensor induces in the lumen wall cannot be too high, in order to prevent adverse events.

Non-contact thermographic methods require an absorptive material, that will absorb the electromagnetic radiation emitted by the medium. The choice of this material is wavelength-dependent. Many materials used for this purpose are sensitive for absorption in the infrared region. Blood is highly absorptive for most electromagnetic waves of these wavelengths, which makes in-vivo detection difficult, since it requires flushing of the artery. Microwave detection could be a better option for in-vivo temperature measurements, since microwaves have greater penetration depth for these wavelengths.

The design of an intracoronary thermography catheter will influence the temperature measurement, both by material choice as well as its geometric design (shape). As the presence of a catheter in an artery will change the flow profile, and the shape of the catheter is of influence on the profile, presence of a catheter will thus influence the temperature reading.

SIMULATIONS

Using numerical simulations, a number of fundamental questions can be answered with respect to intracoronary thermography:

• How is convection of influence on the temperature profile at the lumen wall?
• Is the geometry of the heat source of influence on the temperatures at the lumen wall?
• How does the catheter influence the measured temperature?

In the following subsections we describe the simulations we have performed in an attempt to answer these questions. A simplified geometry was created representing the lumen wall and the tissue surrounding it (Figure 22.2). In this tissue a heat source was embedded and a heat source production value was assigned. The heat source could be extended in the circumferential, longitudinal, and radial directions. Blood flow through the lumen could be simulated. A catheter could be added to the geometry to study the effect of its presence.

Convection

The influence of convection can be studied by comparing the images of the temperature profiles at the lumen wall when no flow exists in the lumen and when a flow is simulated. For these simulations, the longitudinally extended heat source (see Figure 22.2) was used. The results are given in Figure 22.3. It is clear that the flow is of influence on both the maximal temperature at the lumen wall as well as on the shape of the profile. The maximal temperature of 40.7°C when no flow is in the lumen is reduced to 38.8°C when a flow exists in the lumen. The profile when no flow exists in the lumen covers a greater part of the lumen than when a flow exists. In addition, the maximal temperature at the lumen when a flow exists has moved to a location further down on the lumen in the flow direction. The profile is smeared out in the flow direction when a flow exists. The influence of flow can be calculated using the flow influence factor (FIF),[19] which is the ratio between the maximal temperature difference at the lumen wall when no flow exists in the lumen and the maximal temperature difference at the lumen wall when a

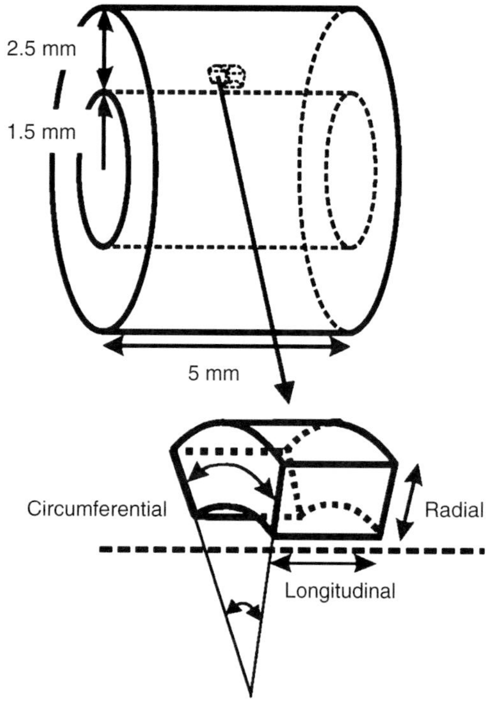

Figure 22.2 Simplified geometry of a vessel and the tissue surrounding it. In the tissue a heat source is embedded, which could be extended in the circumferential, longitudinal, and radial directions.

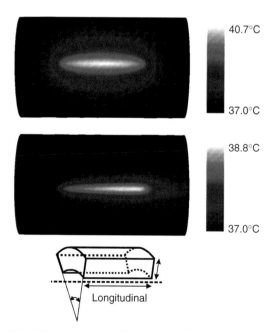

Figure 22.3 Influence of flow. Top, no flow; bottom, flow (parabolic, 53 ml/min). Longitudinally extended heat source volume - 25.1×10^{-3} mm³. Heat source production - 0.4 W/mm³. Cap thickness - 50 μm. Note the different temperature scales.

flow does exist in the lumen. It can be interpreted by how much the measured temperature differences are underestimated when they are measured in the presence of blood flow. In this case, FIF = 2.0. We can conclude that convection has a strong impact by reducing the maximal lumen wall temperature greatly and by limiting the region where this maximal temperature can be measured.

Heat source

The influence of the heat source geometry on the lumen wall temperature profile is shown in Figure 22.4. The top panels of the figure represent the no flow situations; the bottom panels the flow situations. The heat sources considered here all had the same volume, but were extended in different directions, which are depicted under the temperature profiles. The temperature scales differ for the different heat source geometries. The results are given in Table 22.1.

The influence of flow is highest for the circumferentially extended heat source and lowest for the radially extended heat source. This can be explained by the surface of the heat source closest to the lumen, which is largest for the circumferentially and longitudinally extended heat sources, and lowest for the radially extended one. The higher FIF for the circumferential heat source compared with that of the longitudinal heat source can be attributed to the direction of this surface area. In case of the longitudinal heat source, there exists a possibility to exchange the heat that has been taken by the flow from the beginning of heat source back to the heat source. In case of the circumferential heat source, this option does not exist. In conclusion, the shape of the heat source is of influence on the temperature profile on the lumen wall and on the maximal temperature that can be measured.

Catheter

The presence of a catheter influences the temperatures at the lumen wall, as well as the temperature profile. The geometry that was created to study the influence of a catheter in the lumen is depicted in

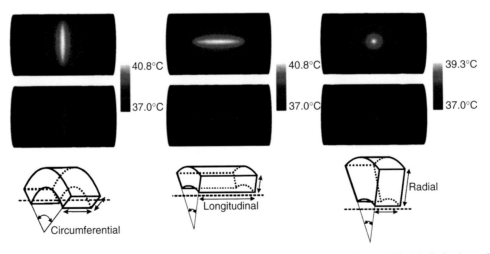

Figure 22.4   Influence of heat source geometry. Top, no flow; bottom, flow (parabolic, 53 ml/min). Left, circumferential; middle, longitudinal; right, radial heat source. Heat source production - 0.4 W/mm³. Cap thickness - 50 μm. Note the different temperature scales.

Table 22.1 Flow influence factor (FIF) for circumferential, longitudinal, and radial heat sources

Heat source	$T_{max\ wall,\ no\ flow}$ (°C)	$T_{max\ wall,\ flow}$ (°C)	FIF
Circumferential	40.8	38.3	3.0
Longitudinal	40.7	38.8	2.0
Radial	39.3	38.8	1.3

Figure 22.5. In Figure 22.6, temperature profiles on the lumen wall are shown when no catheter is present in the lumen (top), when a 1 mm diameter polyurethane catheter contacts the lumen wall (middle), and when a 1 mm diameter nitinol catheter (bottom) contacts the lumen wall. The maximal lumen wall temperature is 37.12°C when no catheter lies in the lumen, whereas these values increase to 37.51°C for the polyurethane catheter and to 37.14°C for the nitinol catheter. The maximal temperature lies on the contact surface of the catheter and the lumen for the polyurethane catheter, but for the nitinol catheter it lies beside the contact surface. This maximum will thus not be detected using the nitinol catheter. This phenomenon is due to the conductive properties of polyurethane and nitinol. The heat conductivity of nitinol is much higher than that of polyurethane. Nitinol thus acts as a conductor and will remove heat from regions of higher temperature to regions of lower temperatures. In this case, the heat is removed from the heat source to the catheter and to the surrounding tissue via the catheter. Polyurethane acts as an insulator, preventing this process. This results in different temperatures on the

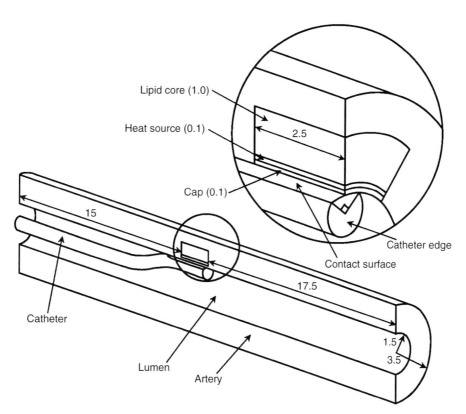

Figure 22.5 Simplified geometry of a vessel and the tissue, surrounding it. In the tissue, a heat source is embedded. A catheter could be modeled in the lumen. Dimension are in mm.

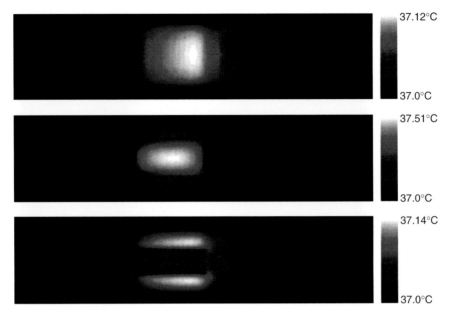

Figure 22.6 Influence of the presence of a catheter and its material. Top, no catheter; middle, polyurethane catheter; bottom, nitinol catheter. All with flow (uniform inflow, 75 ml/min). Heat source production - 5 mW/mm3. Cap thickness - 100 µm. Note the different temperature scales.

contact surfaces of the catheters and the location of the maximal lumen wall temperatures. For optimal detection temperature differences, and thus for vulnerable plaque detection, polyurethane, or any other insulator, is a good choice for intracoronary thermography catheters.

Heat source production

The heat source production values used in these simulations are higher than the heat production values of macrophages that were reported in the literature. For the simulations reported in Figures 22.2 and 22.3, the heat source volume was 25.1×10^{-3} mm^3. This would fit 25 100 macrophages with a volume of $10 \times 10 \times 10$ µm^3. If these macrophages all produce 20 pW, this would result in a heat source production of 0.5 µW. This is 20 000 times lower than the 0.4 W/mm^3 used to obtain the temperature differences depicted in these figures. For Figure 22.4, in which the reported temperatures are lower, a heat source volume of 0.65 mm^3 was used and a heat source production of 5 mW/mm^3. This is still a factor 250 higher than can be fitted with macrophages with identical volume and heat source production, as were used above. It is therefore highly unlikely that the increased metabolism of macrophages alone would have resulted in the temperatures that have been detected in vivo in previous papers. Most probably, other exothermal processes have contributed to these temperatures.

CLINICAL STUDIES IN TERMS OF SIMULATION RESULTS

The electrical sensors, thermistor and thermocouple, are well known and currently applied in intracoronary thermography catheters. These sensors are very sensitive to thermal changes of the object, but will also be affected by thermal changes of the surroundings of the object. Therefore, these sensors need to be well insulated to optimize the detection of local hot spots.

A thermistor needs a current to achieve accurate readings. However, using a current will heat the thermistor, which will influence the measurement and is thus unwanted. A compromise is thus needed. The catheters that are currently in use have electrical sensors that transport the electrical signal from the sensor to the measuring device using metal wires. Metals are known to be very good conductors, so the flow of heat from a hot spot through these wires may significantly lower readout: This is called thermal leakage and should be minimized. In this section, the measuring devices that are used in intracoronary thermography are discussed. The results are discussed in light of the framework presented in the previous sections.

Polyurethane catheters

The hydrofoil catheter that was used in the studies of Stefanadis et al[21,28] and Toutouzas et al[29] is made of a single thermistor embedded in a polyurethane housing. From the results in the previous section, it can be concluded that polyurethane is a very good material for vulnerable plaque detection. The spatial sampling of the lumen wall by this catheter type is very low, since only one thermistor is embedded. Although the sensitivity of this device may be high, its practical utility may be somewhat restricted regarding the necessity of repeated pullbacks at different angular positions, due to the presence of only one thermistor in the catheter.

Nitinol catheters

The catheters that were used for intracoronary thermography that were made out of nitinol are those used by Verheye et al,[22,30] Diamantopoulos et al,[31] Krams et al,[11] and Naghavi et al.[23] From the previous section we know that this material enhances the conductive heat transfer from the heat source to its surroundings, thereby lowering the temperatures on the contact surface.

The diameters of these catheter strands were smaller than the one considered above, so the influence will be smaller than has been suggested above. Nevertheless, the influence still exists. The spatial sampling of these catheters is higher, since four thermistors[11,22,30,31] or five thermocouples[23] are used. This still does not cover the whole lumen wall. The heat source, and thus the vulnerable plaque, can still be missed when a focal heat source is present.

CONCLUSIONS AND RECOMMENDATIONS

Intracoronary thermography is a relatively new method in cardiology. Its further development could be a very important subject in the field of vulnerable plaque detection. However, great variations exist in the temperature differences that have been reported. This makes it difficult to interpret the results and nearly impossible to validate the method. This chapter has covered the basic principles of intracoronary thermography, splitting it up in three components: heat generation, transfer, and detection. Using the principles of physics, literature study, and numerical simulations, these three aspects were clarified.

Heat generation

The data that have been published on this subject show great variation. The last in-vivo studies reported temperature differences that converged to values between 0 and $0.3°C$.[32–35] This makes it plausible that these temperature differences are most likely to be expected in vivo. These temperature differences, though, are hard to reconcile with the heat production values of macrophages that can be found in the literature.[19] It is therefore necessary to quantify more accurately the heat-generating processes in atherosclerotic plaques. To determine the amount of heat that can be generated by atherosclerotic plaques, one would have to isolate fresh atherosclerotic plaque and study it using calorimetric methods. After this, one could isolate different cells, such as macrophages and foam cells, and/or other substances from the atherosclerotic plaque, and subsequently study these selections calorimetrically to determine the exact origin of the heat generation. When a relationship between temperature increases in vulnerable plaques and plaque composition has been determined, the vulnerability of a plaque could be related to temperature measurements.

Heat transfer

Reported results from ex-vivo studies[3,22] should be interpreted with great care. When tissue is removed from a living organism, it will cool down when it is not kept at body temperature. Temperature measurements on this tissue can be interpreted as differences in heat production, but they could represent different cooling rates as well. This has to do with the transfer of heat, which is only possible when temperatures differ.

Given the fact that the temperature differences that have been reported most recently are small, it appears mandatory to exclude external thermal influences during temperature measurements, such as those from heart muscle heat production and cooling of blood in lungs, or to compensate for them. Evidence for such mechanisms may be derived from several studies, since flow of blood influences the lumen wall temperature measurements.[30–32] Furthermore, the location and organization of heat sources are of influence.[19] For these reasons it is recommended to combine intracoronary temperature measurements with both flow measurements and a vessel wall imaging modality.

Heat detection

The catheters that are currently used are based on electrical principles, and need to be insulated very well. Other methods to measure temperature exist (described in the Heat detection main section above) and may prove to be advantageous regarding this matter. Optical equipment, using fiber technology, might be a more appropriate choice for temperature measurement, since optical fibers are bad heat conductors. Combined with heat-sensitive fluorescent coatings or liquid crystal coatings, this equipment might give a whole new direction to the field of intracoronary thermographic measurements. Another method to measure temperatures is by using magnetic resonance,[26] but so far its resolution is not sufficiently high. A great advantage is the non-invasiveness of this method.

All catheters that are currently used for intracoronary thermography, and those that have been described in this chapter, only sparsely sample the vascular wall. The hydrofoil thermistor design measures temperature at one location, leaving most of the circumference of the vascular wall unexplored. The thermistor catheter and the thermocouple basket catheter measuring at four and five locations, respectively, still leave over 2 mm of vascular wall in circumferential direction undetermined. If we assume that macrophage clusters are the heat sources, they may be focal and have sizes <1 mm. For that reason, temperature increases on the vascular wall may be missed and a higher spatial resolution is needed, although the homogeneity of the temperature measurements in the temperatures reported in the latest publications on this subject counteract this argument.

During the cardiac cycle the position of the catheter moves, so it is difficult to ensure contact at the same location during the full cardiac cycle. Measuring during the diastole phase of cardiac cycle could be a solution, but then the measurement needs to be triggered and the thermal response time of the heat transducers must be accordingly short.

Closing remarks

Intracoronary thermography is still in development, despite the number of publications that have already appeared in the literature. A lot of research has already been done, but many questions are still unanswered. What is missing is the answer to the question: 'What are we measuring?' Temperature differences exist in coronary arteries in vivo, but it is unclear what causes them. Is it really a temperature difference due to inflammation that has been measured? And what is the contribution of noise and artifacts? External thermal influences must be investigated. Influences of catheter design must be studied intensively. Changes in temperature due to source differences and flow must be known. All of these, and maybe even more, need to be studied in order to more extensively validate intracoronary thermography and to be able to conclude on the usefulness of the method for vulnerable plaque detection.

ACKNOWLEDGMENTS

The STW is greatly acknowledged for its financial support (grant RPG.5442).

REFERENCES

1. World Health Organization. Global health: today's challenges. In: Campanini B, ed. The World Health Report 2003 – Shaping the Future. Geneva, Switzerland: World Health Organization; 2003:3–22.
2. Falk E, Shah PK, Fuster V. Coronary plaque disruption. Circulation 1995; 92:657–71.
3. Casscells W, Hathorn B, David M et al. Thermal detection of cellular infiltrates in living atherosclerotic plaques: possible implications for plaque rupture and thrombosis. Lancet 1996; 347:1447–51.
4. Alberts B, Bray D, Lewis J et al. Molecular Biology of the Cell, 2nd edn. New York: Garland; 1989.
5. Newsholme P, Newsholme EA. Rates of utilization of glucose, glutamine and oleate and formation of end-products by mouse peritoneal macrophages in culture. Biochem J 1989; 261:211–18.
6. Loike JD, Silverstein SC, Sturtevant JM. Application of differential scanning microcalorimetry to the study of cellular processes: heat production and glucose oxidation of murine macrophages. Proc Natl Acad Sci USA 1981; 78:5958–62.
7. Thoren SA, Monti M, Holma B. Heat conduction microcalorimetry of overall metabolism in rabbit alveolar macrophages in monolayers and in suspensions. Biochim Biophys Acta 1990; 1033:305–10.
8. Charlebois SJ, Daniels AU, Smith RA. Metabolic heat production as a measure of macrophage response to particles from orthopedic implant materials. J Biomed Mater Res 2002; 59:166–75.
9. Sung HW, Chen WY, Tsai CC, Hsu HL. In vitro study of enzymatic degradation of biological tissues fixed by glutaraldehyde or epoxy compound. J Biomater Sci Polym Ed 1997; 8:587–600.
10. Toutouzas K, Stefanadis C, Tsiamis E et al. The temperature of atherosclerotic plaques is correlated with matrix metalloproteinases concentration in patients with acute coronary syndromes. J Am Coll Cardiol 2001; 37:356a.
11. Krams R, Verheye S, van Damme LC et al. In vivo temperature heterogeneity is associated with plaque regions of increased MMP-9 activity. Eur Heart J 2005; 26:2200–5.
12. Takahashi K, Takeya M, Sakashita N. Multifunctional roles of macrophages in the development and progression of atherosclerosis in humans and experimental animals. Med Electron Microsc 2002; 35:179–203.
13. Brown MS, Ho YK, Goldstein JL. The cholesteryl ester cycle in macrophage foam cells. Continual hydrolysis and re-esterification of cytoplasmic cholesteryl esters. J Biol Chem 1980; 255:9344–52.
14. St Clair RW. Cholesteryl ester metabolism in atherosclerotic arterial tissue. Ann NY Acad Sci 1976; 275:228–37.
15. Palou A, Pico C, Bonet ML, Oliver P. The uncoupling protein, thermogenin. Int J Biochem Cell Biol 1998; 30:7–11.
16. Kockx MM, Middelheim A, Knaapen MWM et al. Expression of the uncoupling protein UCP-2 in macrophages of unstable human atherosclerotic plaques. Circulation 2000; 102:12–.
17. Nedergaard J, Cannon B. The 'novel' 'uncoupling' proteins UCP2 and UCP3: what do they really do? Pros and cons for suggested functions. Exp Physiol 2003; 88:65–84.
18. Duck FA. Physical Properties of Tissue. A Comprehensive Reference Book. London: Academic Press; 1990.
19. ten Have AG, Gijsen FJ, Wentzel JJ, Slager CJ, van der Steen AF. Temperature distribution in atherosclerotic coronary arteries: influence of plaque geometry and flow (a numerical study). Phys Med Biol 2004; 49:4447–62.
20. Craciunescu OI, Clegg ST. Pulsatile blood flow effects on temperature distribution and heat transfer in rigid vessels. J Biomech Eng 2001; 123:500–5.
21. Stefanadis C, Diamantopoulos L, Vlachopoulos C et al. Thermal heterogeneity within human atherosclerotic coronary arteries detected in vivo: a new

method of detection by application of a special thermography catheter. Circulation 1999; 99:1965–71.

22. Verheye S, De Meyer GR, Van Langenhove G, Knaapen MW, Kockx MM. In vivo temperature heterogeneity of atherosclerotic plaques is determined by plaque composition. Circulation 2002; 105:1596–601.

23. Naghavi M, Madjid M, Gul K et al. Thermography basket catheter: in vivo measurement of the temperature of atherosclerotic plaques for detection of vulnerable plaques. Catheter Cardiovasc Interv 2003; 59:52–9.

24. Ashforth-Frost S. Quantitative thermal imaging using liquid crystals. Journal of Biomed Optics 1996; 1:18–27.

25. Grattan KTV, Zhang ZY. Fiber Optic Fluorescence Thermometry. London: Chapman & Hall; 1995.

26. Wlodarczyk W, Hentschel M, Wust P et al. Comparison of four magnetic resonance methods for mapping small temperature changes. Phys Med Biol 1999; 44:607–24.

27. Quesson B, de Zwart JA, Moonen CT. Magnetic resonance temperature imaging for guidance of thermotherapy. J Magn Reson Imaging 2000; 12:525–33.

28. Stefanadis C, Toutouzas P. In vivo local thermography of coronary artery atherosclerotic plaques in humans. Ann Intern Med 1998; 129:1079–80.

29. Toutouzas K, Vaina S, Tsiamis E et al. Detection of increased temperature of the culprit lesion after recent myocardial infarction: the favorable effect of statins. Am Heart J 2004; 148:783–8.

30. Verheye S, De Meyer GR, Krams R et al. Intravascular thermography: immediate functional and morphological vascular findings. Eur Heart J 2004; 25:158–65.

31. Diamantopoulos L, Liu X, De Scheerder I et al. The effect of reduced blood-flow on the coronary wall temperature. Are significant lesions suitable for intravascular thermography? Eur Heart J 2003; 24:1788–95.

32. Stefanadis C, Toutouzas K, Tsiamis E et al. Thermal heterogeneity in stable human coronary atherosclerotic plaques is underestimated in vivo: the "cooling effect" of blood flow. J Am Coll Cardiol 2003; 41:403–8.

33. Verheye S, Van Langenhove G, Diamantopoulos L, Serruys PW, Vermeersch P. Temperature heterogeneity is nearly absent in angiographically normal or mild atherosclerotic coronary segments: interim results from a safety study. Am J Cardiol 2002; 90:24h.

34. Schmermund A, Rodermann J, Erbel R. Intracoronary thermography. Herz 2003; 28:505-12.

35. Webster M, Stewart J, Ruygrok P et al. Intracoronary thermography with a multiple thermocouple catheter: initial human experience. Am J Cardiol 2002; 90:24h.

Intracoronary thermography 23

Christodoulos Stefanadis and Konstantinos Toutouzas

INTRODUCTION

Initiated early in life, atherosclerosis is a continuous process that gradually progresses with potentially devastating consequences: atherosclerotic plaque rupture is the most common underlying pathologic mechanism causing acute coronary syndromes. This term refers to the process whereby the endothelial surface of the plaque is disrupted to expose the underlying prothrombotic vessel wall to circulating platelets and coagulation factors.

The underlying pathophysiologic mechanisms resulting in plaque erosion or plaque disruption and subsequent thrombosis[1] include endothelial dysfunction,[2] lipid accumulation,[3] extensive adventitial and intimal neovascularity,[4] and enhanced inflammatory involvement. Several morphologic and immunologic determinants specific for the vulnerable plaque have been reported:

- a large lipid core (≥40% plaque volume) composed of free cholesterol crystals, cholesterol esters, and oxidized lipids impregnated with tissue factor;[5]
- a thin fibrous cap depleted of smooth muscle cells and collagen;[5]
- an outward (positive) remodeling;[6]
- inflammatory cell infiltration of fibrous cap and adventitia (mostly monocyte-macrophages, some activated T cells, and mast cells)
- increased neovascularity.

The terms vulnerable or unstable are now widely used to describe plaques that exhibit such features irrespective of whether rupture has taken place. Coronary angiography, one of the most commonly performed invasive procedures for the illustration of arterial anatomy and luminal narrowing does not provide direct information on plaque composition and plaque burden and plaque changes within the vessel wall. Futhermore, the majority of culprit lesions that produce acute coronary syndromes are not severely stenotic, possibly due to significant positive remodeling, and they do not manifest protective collateral circulation.[6] In addition, the risk of plaque rupture is more closely related to plaque content than plaque size. Therefore, there is an urgent need for techniques that can identify plaques at risk of rupture and creation of acute coronary events.

Numerous imaging modalities (Table 23.1) have evolved to evaluate plaque vulnerability, but no single method currently provides the necessary structural and functional information to identify plaques at risk for rupture. Non-invasive and invasive tools have been developed or are at the stage of development. Imaging modalities such as intravascular ultrasound (IVUS) or optical coherence tomography (OCT) are focused on the assessment of structural characteristics, whereas other diagnostic techniques such as spectroscopy and thermography are directed towards the functional assessment of the plaque. A combined approach capable of evaluating both the morphologic and functional characteristics of the vulnerable plaque may prove to be of higher predictive value than a single imaging method.

Table 23.1 Methods for the evaluation of the vulnerable plaque

Modality	Resolution	Penetration	Fibrous cup	Lipid core	Inflammation	Ca²⁺	Thrombus	Current status
IVUS	100 µm	Good	+	++	−	+++	+	CA
Angioscopy	UK	Poor	+	++	−	−	+++	CA
OCT	10 µm	Poor	+++	+++	+	+++	+	CS
Thermography	0.5 mm	Poor	−	−	+++	−	−	CS
Spectroscopy	NA	Poor	+	++	++	++	−	PCS
Intravascular MRI	160 µm	Good	+	++	++	++	+	PCS

IVUS, intravascular ultrasound; OCT, optical coherence tomography; MRI, magnetic resonance imaging; NA, not applicable; CS, clinical studies; CA, clinically approved for commercial use; PCS, preclinical studies; UK, unknown.
+++ = sensitivity >90%; ++ = sensitivity 80–90%; + = sensitivity 50–80%; − = sensitivity <50%.

IN-VIVO TEMPERATURE MEASUREMENT

The infiltration of the atherosclerotic plaque by inflammatory cells has been recognized as one of the leading causes of both plaque vulnerability and thrombogenicity, resulting in plaque disruption and, subsequently, to an acute coronary syndrome.[7] Activated macrophages are responsible for the uptake of glucose and the consumption of oxygen, which increase the local plaque temperature. By the time the inflammatory cells exhaust their supply of oxygen, anaerobic metabolism ensues, leading to local acidosis.[8] Based on this basic knowledge, thermography has been introduced as a technique for the identification of the vulnerable plaque. Since inflammation has been closely related to increased heat production, temperature elevation in atherosclerotic plaques has been suggested to reflect the intensity of the local inflammatory process. First, ex-vivo carotid artery intimal surface temperature measurements were recorded by Casscells et al; with the revelation of several regions in which the surface temperatures varied, reaching 2.2°C of difference in certain plaques.[9] Moreover, temperature correlated well with inflammatory cell density, most of the cells being macrophages.[9] Plaques with large lipid cores had higher temperatures and lower pH values, whereas calcified plaques had lower temperatures and higher pH values.[10] The introduction of a thermography catheter, which was designed and developed in our institution and is now being manufactured (Epiphany catheter, Medispes SW, ZUG, Switzerland),[11,12] made in-vivo temperature measurements feasible. By now, many different types of catheters have been designed to record the coronary vessel wall temperature in vivo. The thermography basket catheter (Volcano Therapeutics, Inc., Rancho Cordova, CA, USA) consists of a 3F shaft with an expandable and externally controllable basket with built-in thermocouples.[13–15] Another thermography catheter has been developed by Thermocore (Thermocore Medical Systems NV, Merelbeke, Belgium). The over-the-wire catheter consists of a functional end that can be engaged by retracting a covering sheath.[16] Four flexible nitinol strips with four dedicated thermistors are placed at the distal end. Once engaged, the nitinol strips expand, ensuring contact of the thermistor with the endoluminal surface of the vascular wall.[17–19] Naghavi et al, introduced a 4F side-viewing infrared thermography catheter capable of imaging the temperature of the vessel wall with a 180° scope.[20,21] Guidewire-based systems have been also proposed as an alternative method of measuring intra-coronary temperature.[22–24]

In-vivo human clinical studies demon-strated that patients with acute coronary syndrome or recent myocardial infarction have higher temperature difference between the culprit lesion and the proxi-mal healthy vessel wall compared to those with stable angina.[11,25] Furthermore, a very good correlation between inflamma-tory indices with temperature difference has been observed.[26] The latter indirect findings were verified by an ex-vivo exper-imental animal study, which showed that there is a relation between local tempera-ture and local total macrophage mass.[18] Preliminary clinical studies showed a posi-tive correlation between temperature and macrophage infiltration of atherectomy specimens.[22,23,27]

COOLING EFFECT

Although inflammation leads to increased heat release from the atherosclerotic plaque, a discrepancy between the ex-vivo and the in-vivo temperature measurements has been observed.[9,13,17] This may be due to the cooling effect of blood flow.[28] To assess the possible influence of coronary blood flow, temperature measurements were performed during complete inter-ruption of flow. Temperature elevation during vessel occlusion was demonstrated both in patients with stable angina and acute coronary syndrome.[29,30] These results strongly imply that coronary flow has a 'cooling effect' on thermal hetero-geneity, which may lead to underestima-tion of local heat production. To eliminate this shortcoming, especially in intermedi-ate lesions in which attachment of the ther-mistor cannot be ensured, new catheter designs were recently introduced. A balloon-thermography catheter with the thermistor opposite to the inflated balloon facilitates the contact of the thermistor to the plaque. By use of this catheter temperature

elevations up to 59% can be recorded in stable lesions.[31] Moreover, Belardi and co-workers presented their preliminary results with a new basket-catheter with multiple thermistors which can also meas-ure atheromatic plaque temperature dur-ing complete interruption of coronary blood flow. All these devices need to be investigated in a large number of patients in order to draw conclusions regarding their safety and prognostic value.[32]

WIDESPREAD INFLAMMATION

It has been shown that inflammation is not a local phenomenon restricted to the culprit lesion, but especially in patients with acute coronary syndrome, inflamma-tion is widespread throughout the coro-nary arteries.[33–35] In a preliminary study, Webster et al found more than one 'hot' spot in the same vessel.[13] Moreover, recent studies support the concept that plaque instability may not represent a mere random 'vascular accident' but a 'pan-coronary' process due to widespread inflammatory activation.[34,35] Leborgne et al have used the Radi Medical Systems PressureWire (a 0.014 inch wire) to detect temperature heterogeneity in non-culprit vessels.[36] Furthermore, Choi et al proved that it was reliable in detecting vulnerable plaque and predicting unfavorable effects after percutaneous coronary intervention (PCI).[37] We presented increased thermal heterogeneity in non-culprit intermediate lesions, similar to the thermal hetero-geneity of culprit lesions (Figure 23.1). In the same study, patients with acute coro-nary syndromes had increased thermal heterogeneity in both culprit and non-culprit lesions, supporting a pan-coronary inflammatory activation.[38,39] These results provide new insights to support the con-cept of diffuse destabilization of coronary atherosclerotic plaques: although a single lesion is clinically symptomatic, acute coro-nary syndromes are associated with diffuse thermal heterogeneity.

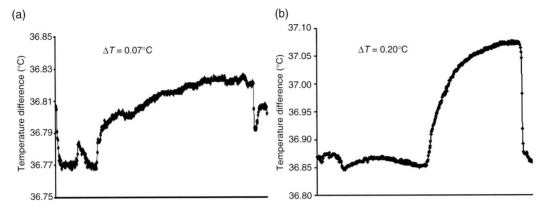

Figure 23.1   (a) An increase of 0.10°C was found in the culprit lesion.(b) An increase of 0.14°C was observed in the non-culprit lesion.

To evaluate whether this widespread coronary inflammation increases blood temperature as blood flows from the coronary arterial tree to the coronary sinus, blood temperature differences were measured between the coronary sinus and the right atrium in patients with symptomatic coronary artery disease. Coronary sinus blood temperature was found to be greater than right atrium blood temperature in patients with angiographically significant lesions, independently of the site of the lesion, as well as the number of coronary arteries with significant lesion, compared with subjects without coronary artery disease.[40,41] Moreover, increased coronary sinus blood temperature, both in patients with significant lesions and in idiopathic dilated cardiomyopathy, was well correlated with C-reactive protein (CRP), which is the most reliable systemic inflammatory marker.[41,42] These findings further support the extensive inflammatory process within the coronary arterial tree in patients with coronary artery disease.

Since non-obstructive lesions may exhibit vulnerability, various diagnostic technologies need to be evaluated, including intracoronary thermography (ICT). In the VIP-1 study, which started in 2006, ICT parameters of the culprit coronary

vessel, clinical outcome, and other components are being correlated to depict a vulnerable plaque or patient and ICT used to define targets for preventive therapies. In 2007, the VIP-2 study will determine the value of ICT by Thermocore catheter in predicting future ischemic events related to non-culprit intermediate lesions and will examine the safety of multiple vessel ICT measurements.

In patients with diabetes mellitus, in particular, inflammation is significantly pronounced and increased infiltration of inflammatory cells is observed in atheromatic lesions of such patients. Using coronary thermography, the local inflammatory involvement in atherosclerotic plaques has been evaluated. Patients with diabetes mellitus suffering from acute coronary syndromes or stable angina show increased local inflammatory involvement compared with non-diabetic patients. Furthermore, diabetic patients receiving statins showed decreased temperature difference than untreated ones, suggesting that statins have a favorable effect in culprit lesions of patients with diabetes.[43]

Increased interest has been shown recently in preventing rather than healing plaque rupture. Thermography has been demonstrated to be effective in evaluating the effect of diet and medications on thermal heterogeneity of atherosclerotic plaques. In a recent study, plaque thickness remained unchanged, but temperature heterogeneity was significantly decreased and paralleled marked histologic loss of macrophages in atheromatic lesions observed after 3 months of cholesterol-lowering treatment.[19] Statins appear to have a pleiotropic effect, beyond their efficiency in cholesterol lowering. It has been demonstrated that thermal heterogeneity was lower in patients treated with statins, independently of the clinical syndrome.[25,44] These findings indicate that aggressive treatment with statins may be essential for further stabilization of the vulnerable atherosclerotic plaque in patients with coronary artery disease, including those planned for PCI, as it has been observed that patients with increased culprit plaque temperature at the time of intervention have a poor prognosis.[45]

CONCLUSION

Plaque rupture is probably the most important mechanism underlying the sudden onset of an acute coronary event. Soft, lipid-rich plaques, heavily infiltrated by macrophages are more prone to rupture. Early detection of the high-risk lesion may lead to the most favorable local or systemic treatment selection that will prevent the sequel of events resulting in acute coronary syndrome. Thermography is a promising method for the functional assessment of vulnerable plaque and has been introduced into clinical practice, with a good predictive value for clinical events in patients with increased temperature in the atherosclerotic plaque.

SUMMARY

Atherosclerosis is a low-grade inflammatory disease resulting in endothelial dysfunction; it is known to predispose to plaque disruption or plaque erosion and subsequent thrombosis. However, the majority of rupture-prone plaques that produce acute coronary syndromes have been shown not to be severely stenotic. Thus, the concept of the 'vulnerable' plaque has recently emerged to explain how quiescent atherosclerotic lesions evolve to cause clinical events. Certain morphologic and immunologic determinants specific for the vulnerable plaque have been reported: a large lipid core ($\geq$40% plaque volume) composed of free cholesterol crystals, cholesterol esters, and oxidized lipids impregnated with tissue factor; a thin fibrous cap depleted of smooth muscle cells and collagen; an outward (positive) remodeling; inflammatory cell infiltration of fibrous cap and adventitia (mostly monocyte-macrophages, some activated T cells, and mast cells) and increased neovascularity. Despite the large amount of information gathered on the morphologic characteristics of remote lesions, there is a lack of studies concerning the functional assessment of non-culprit lesions. Coronary thermography is a technique for functional assessment of coronary atherosclerotic plaques. Several thermography catheter designs have been proposed, with thermistor(s) and wires with thermal sensors at the distal tip. All designs have several advantages and disadvantages and coronary thermography has certain limitations. Nevertheless, we have gained important pathophysiologic and clinical information on the vulnerability of atheromatic plaques.

Increased heat generation has been both experimentally and clinically associated with increased macrophage concentration within the plaque. Furthermore, a correlation of local inflammatory involvement and local heat generation with the peripheral inflammatory markers, such as C-reactive protein, has also been observed. Whether systemic treatment with agents such as statins, or interventional techniques, such as drug-eluting stents, will have an impact on stabilizing vulnerable plaques needs to be determined in future studies.

In conclusion, although there are several techniques for evaluating morphologically atheromatic plaques, thermography is a promising method for the functional assessment of the vulnerable plaque and has been introduced into clinical practice, with a good predictive value for clinical events in patients with increased temperature in the atherosclerotic plaque.

REFERENCES

1. Corti R, Hutter R, Badimon JJ, Fuster V. Evolving concepts in the triad of atherosclerosis, inflammation and thrombosis. J Thromb Thrombolysis 2004; 17:35–44.

2. Celermajer DS. Endothelial dysfunction: does it matter? Is it reversible? J Am Coll Cardiol 1997; 30:325–33.

3. Stary HC, Chandler AB, Dinsmore RE et al. A definition of advanced types of atherosclerotic lesions and a histological classification of atherosclerosis. A report from the Committee on Vascular Lesions of the Council on Arteriosclerosis, American Heart Association. Circulation 1995; 92:1355–74.

4. Shah PK. Mechanisms of plaque vulnerability and rupture. J Am Coll Cardiol 2003; 41:15–22S.

5. Naghavi M, Libby P, Falk E et al. From vulnerable plaque to vulnerable patient: a call for new definitions and risk assessment strategies: Part I. Circulation 2003; 108:1664–72.

6. Glagov S, Weisenberg E, Zarins CK, Stankunavicius R, Kolettis GJ. Compensatory enlargement of human atherosclerotic coronary arteries. N Engl J Med 1987; 316:1371–5.

7. Shah PK. Pathophysiology of coronary thrombosis: role of plaque rupture and plaque erosion. Prog Cardiovasc Dis 2002; 44:357–68.

8. Zarrabi A, Gul K, Willerson JT, Casscells W, Naghavi M. Intravascular thermography: a novel approach for detection of vulnerable plaque. Curr Opin Cardiol 2002; 17:656–62.

9. Casscells W, Hathorn B, David M et al. Thermal detection of cellular infiltrates in living atherosclerotic plaques: possible implications for plaque rupture and thrombosis. Lancet 1996; 347:1447–51.

10. Naghavi M, John R, Naguib S et al. pH Heterogeneity of human and rabbit atherosclerotic plaques; a new insight into detection of vulnerable plaque. Atherosclerosis 2002; 164:27–35.

11. Stefanadis C, Diamantopoulos L, Vlachopoulos C et al. Thermal heterogeneity within human atherosclerotic coronary arteries detected in vivo: a new method of detection by application of a special thermography catheter. Circulation 1999; 99:1965–71.

12. Stefanadis C, Toutouzas P. In vivo local thermography of coronary artery atherosclerotic plaques in humans. Ann Intern Med 1998; 129:1079–80.

13. Webster M, Stewart J, Ruygrok P et al. Intracoronary thermography in stable and unstable coronary disease. Circulation 2002; 106:II657.

14. Naghavi M, Madjid M, Gul K et al. Thermography basket catheter: in vivo measurement of the temperature of atherosclerotic plaques for detection of vulnerable plaques. Catheter Cardiovasc Interv 2003; 59:52–9.

15. Gul K, O'Brien T, Siadaty S et al. Coronary thermosensor basket catheter with thermographic imaging software for thermal detection of vulnerable atherosclerotic plaques. J Am Coll Cardiol 2001; 37:1088–14.

16. Van Langenhove G, Verheye S, Diamantopoulos L, Vermeersch P, Serruys PW. First controlled human intracoronary thermography trial to detect vulnerable plaque. Circulation 2002; 106:II 657.

17. Verheye S, Van Langenhove G, Diamantopoulos L, Serruys PW, Vermeersch P. Temperature heterogeneity is nearly absent in angiographically normal or mild atherosclerotic coronary segments: interim results from a safety study. Am J Cardiol 2002; 90 (Suppl 6A):24H.

18. Verheye S, De Meyer GR, Van Langenhove G, Knaapen MW, Kockx MM. In vivo temperature heterogeneity of atherosclerotic plaques is determined by plaque composition. Circulation 2002; 105:1596–601.

19. Verheye S, De Meyer GR, Krams R et al. Intravascular thermography: immediate functional and morphological vascular findings. Eur Heart J 2004; 25:158–65.

20. Naghavi M, Melling M, Gul K et al. First prototype of a 4 French 180 degree side-viewing infrared fiber optic catheter for thermal imaging of atherosclerotic plaque. J Am Coll Cardiol 2001; 37:3A.

21. Madjid M, Naghavi M, Malik BA et al. Thermal detection of vulnerable plaque. Am J Cardiol 2002; 90: 36–39L.

22. Wainstein MV, Ribeiro JP, Zagaro AJ et al. Coronary plaque thermography: heterogeneity detected by Imetrx Thermocoil Guidewire. Am J Cardiol 2003; 92:5L.

23. Akasaka T, Koyama Y, Neishi Y et al. Increase in plaque temperature reflects macrophage infiltration in coronary stenotic lesions: intracoronary temperature measurement and histological assessment. Circulation 2003; 108:IV373.

24. Courtney BK, Nakamura M, Tsugita R et al. Validation of a thermographic guidewire for endoluminal mapping of atherosclerotic disease: an in vitro study. Catheter Cardiovasc Interv 2004; 62:221–9.

25. Toutouzas K, Vaina S, Tsiamis E et al. Detection of increased temperature of the culprit lesion after recent myocardial infarction: the favorable effect of statins. Am Heart J 2004; 148:783–8.

26. Stefanadis C, Diamantopoulos L, Dernellis J et al. Heat production of atherosclerotic plaques and inflammation assessed by the acute phase proteins in acute coronary syndromes. J Mol Cell Cardiol 2000; 32:43–52.

27. Toutouzas K, Spanos V, Ribichini F et al. Correlation of coronary plaque temperature with inflammatory markers obtained from atherectomy specimens in humans. Am J Cardiol 2003; 92:199L.

28. ten Have AG, Gijsen FJ, Wentzel JJ, Slager CJ, van der Steen AF. Temperature distribution in atherosclerotic coronary arteries: influence of plaque geometry and flow (a numerical study). Phys Med Biol 2004; 49: 4447–62.

29. Stefanadis C, Toutouzas K, Vavuranakis M et al. New balloon-thermography catheter for in vivo temperature measurements in human coronary atherosclerotic plaques: a novel approach for thermography? Catheter Cardiovasc Interv 2003; 58:344–50.

30. Stefanadis C, Toutouzas K, Tsiamis E et al. Thermal heterogeneity in stable human coronary atherosclerotic plaques is underestimated in vivo: the "cooling effect" of blood flow. J Am Coll Cardiol 2003; 41:403–8.

31. Toutouzas K, Drakopoulou M, Stefanadi E, Siasos G, Stefanadis C. Intracoronary thermography: does it help us in clinical decision making? J Interterv Cardiol 2005; 18(6):485–9.

32. Belardi JA, Albertal M, Cura FA et al. Intravascular thermographic assessment in human coronary atherosclerotic plaques by a novel flow-occluding sensing catheter: a safety and feasibility study. J Invasive Cardiol 2005; 17(12):663–6.

33. Cusack MR, Marber MS, Lambiase PD, Bucknall CA, Redwood SR. Systemic inflammation in unstable angina is the result of myocardial necrosis. J Am Coll Cardiol 2002; 39:1917–23.

34. Buffon A, Biasucci LM, Liuzzo G et al. Widespread coronary inflammation in unstable angina. N Engl J Med 2002; 347:5–12.

35. Spagnoli LG, Bonanno E, Mauriello A et al. Multicentric inflammation in epicardial coronary arteries of patients dying of acute myocardial infarction. J Am Coll Cardiol 2002; 40:1579–88.

36. Leborgne L, Dascotte O, Jarry G et al. Multi-vessel coronary plaque temperature heterogeneity in patients with acute coronary syndromes. First study with the Radi Medical System Wire. Circulation 2005; 112(17): 3092.

37. Choi SY, Tahk SJ, Choi BJ et al. Temperature difference of atherosclerotic plaque and normal vessel wall predicts distal embolization after percutaneous coronary stenting. Circulation 2005; 112(17):2918.

38. Drakopoulou M, Toutouzas K, Mitropoulos J et al. Thermal heterogeneity of culprit and non-culprit lesions: widespread inflammation or local inflammatory involvement? Eur Heart J 2004; 25:303.

39. Toutouzas K, Drakopoulou M, Mitropoulos J et al. Elevated plaque temperature in non-culprit de novo atheromatous lesions of patients with acute coronary syndromes. J Am Coll Cardiol 2006; 47(2):301–6.

40. Stefanadis C, Tsiamis E, Vaina S et al. Temperature of the blood in the coronary sinus and right atrium in patients with and without coronary artery disease. Am J Cardiol 2004; 93:207–10.

41. Toutouzas K, Drakopoulou M, Markou V et al. Increased coronary sinus blood temperature: correlation with systemic inflammation. Eur J Clin Invest 2006; 36(4):218–23.

42. Toutouzas K, Stougiannos P, Drakopoulou M et al. Coronary sinus thermography in idiopathic dilated cardiomyopathy: correlation with systemic inflammation and left ventricular contractility. Eur J Heart Fail 2006 May 25 [E pub ahead of print]

43. Toutouzas K, Markou V, Drakopoulou M et al. Increased heat generation from atherosclerotic plaques in patients with type 2 diabetes: an increased local inflammatory activation. Diabetes Care 2005; 28:1656–61.

44. Stefanadis C, Toutouzas K, Vavuranakis M et al. Statin treatment is associated with reduced thermal heterogeneity in human atherosclerotic plaques. Eur Heart J 2002; 23:1664–9.

45. Stefanadis C, Toutouzas K, Tsiamis E et al. Increased local temperature in human coronary atherosclerotic plaques: an independent predictor of clinical outcome in patients undergoing a percutaneous coronary intervention. J Am Coll Cardiol 2001; 37:1277–83.

SECTION IV

Non-invasive imaging

Targeted nanoparticle contrast agents for vascular molecular imaging and therapy

24

Samuel A Wickline, Anne M Neubauer, Patrick Winter,
Shelton Caruthers, and Gregory Lanza

INTRODUCTION

'Molecular imaging' of vascular targets is emerging as a novel approach for specific in-vivo characterization of biomarkers associated with atherosclerosis, inflammation, and vulnerable/unstable plaque. Unlike many other diseases, atherosclerosis and/or vulnerable/unstable plaque are often diagnosed only after an acute, sometimes fatal event. Of the ~700 000 cardiac deaths per year in America, approximately 60% are 'sudden deaths', occurring without any advanced warning of pathology.[1] Predicting if and when a plaque might rupture and cause acute infarction or sudden death is an uncertain business. Atherosclerotic plaques grow in discrete stages, consisting of repeated episodes of rupture, hemorrhage, thrombosis, and healing, leading inevitably to a final rupture event associated with complete vascular obstruction.[2] Exposure of the lipid core, even through a small localized rupture, can induce the clotting cascade through the interaction of serum clotting factors with locally expressed tissue factor.[3] The fibrin matrix and hemorrhagic components are incorporated into the plaque mass and extend the lesion dimension, meaning that even the vulnerable plaque has probably ruptured already (i.e. been unstable or disrupted)

during its life cycle.[4] The accumulation of macrophages as well as other inflammatory cells, which secrete high levels of metalloproteinases (MMPs), also undermines the fibrous cap, potentially exposing the thrombotic lipid core.[5,6] Up-regulation of angiogenesis can lead to erosion of the extracellular matrix and replacement with physically fragile neovascular beds, weakening the fibrous cap and promoting plaque rupture.[7,8] These, and other cellular processes, are suitable targets for molecular imaging and targeted drug therapy.

IMAGING AGENTS AND MODALITIES

Over the next decade, the growth of nanotechnology platforms for molecular imaging and drug delivery will greatly expand the clinical opportunities for cardiovascular molecular imaging.[9–11] Nanotechnology seeks to develop new materials and provide new molecular assemblies on the scale of individual cells or organelles in the range of 5–500 nm. One of the classic original nanoparticulate systems, liposomes (50–700 nm) are uni- or multilamellar vesicles comprising lipid bilayer membranes surrounding an aqueous interior. These agents have now been approved for enhancing the efficacy and safety of drugs such as doxorubicin (e.g. Doxil, ALZA Corporation, Tibotec Therapeutics, NJ). Applications of liposomal technology as molecular imaging agents have been reported for both ultrasound and magnetic resonance imaging (MRI).[12,13]

Nanometer-sized emulsions are chemically distinct from liposomes; they are self-assemble (as oil-in-water)-type mixtures that are stabilized with surfactants to maintain size and shape. Perfluorocarbon core emulsions (200–400 nm) have been used for molecular imaging with MRI, ultrasound, fluorescence, nuclear, and computed tomography (CT) imaging.[9,11,14,15] For example, by incorporating vast numbers of paramagnetic gadolinium complexes (>50 000) onto emulsion particles, the signal enhancement possible for each binding site is magnified dramatically, by a factor of >10^6 over conventional paramagnetic extracellular contrast agents.[16,17] Modified micellar particles such as high-density lipoprotein (HDL) or low-density lipoprotein (LDL) particles have been utilized as molecular imaging agents for MRI.[18,19]

Polymer-based nanoparticles (40–200 nm) support a variety of flexible 'designer approaches' to the development of molecular imaging agents and therapeutic delivery devices.[20] Polymers made from polyhydroxy acids such as the copolymer of poly (lactic acid) (PLA) and poly (D,L-lactide-*co*-glycolide) (PLGA) have been investigated for localized drug and gene delivery. Dendrimers, or cascade polymers, are highly branched polymeric structures that are globular in configuration. Paramagnetic polyamidoamine (PAMAM) and diaminobutane (DAB) dendrimers have been reported for MRI applications.[21,22] The multivalent surfaces of these and other systems contain an array of functional sites that can undergo reactions to add drugs, imaging agents, and targeting ligands.

Metallic particles such as iron oxide nanoparticles (15–60 nm) generally constitute a class of superparamagnetic agents that can be coated with dextran, phospholipids, or other compounds to inhibit aggregation and enhance stability for use as passive or active targeting agents. The iron in MIONs (monocrystalline iron oxide nanoparticles), SPIOs (small particles of iron oxide, 50–500 nm), or USPIOs (ultra-small particles of iron oxide, 10–50 nm) produces strong local disruptions in the magnetic field of MRI scanners, which leads to increased T_2^* relaxation, causing a decrease in image intensity in areas with iron particle accumulation (termed 'susceptibility' effects). These particles exhibit a very long circulating half-life (24+ hours) and have been employed for passive targeted imaging of pathologic inflammatory processes, such as unstable atherosclerotic plaques, by MRI.[23] Alternatively, similar types of particles (e.g. CLIO, or cross-linked iron oxide particles, complexed with retroviral 'tat' protein ligands) have been used for localization and transcellular deposition.[24]

Quantum dots (2–8 nm) are constructed from semiconductor materials (e.g. cadmium selenide) that manifest stable (non-quenching) fluorescent properties at various wavelengths depending on exact composition.[25–27] For use in vivo, they must be coated with materials (polymers) that allow solubilization while also preventing leaching of the toxic heavy metals. Carbon nanotubes and fullerenes (4 nm) have been utilized as particulate systems whose surfaces can also be functionalized for tissue binding.[28] Native fluorescent properties have been reported.[29]

The role of nanoparticles in imaging cardiovascular pathology varies according to the imaging modality. In the case of nuclear (γ/single-proton emission computed tomography [SPECT]) imaging or positron emission tomography (PET) for example, the general approach has been to utilize very small tracer quantities of contrast agents (e.g. radionuclide-labeled antibodies, peptides, or small molecules) rather than to employ large payload particles. For example, folate receptor-targeted polymeric shell cross-linked nanoparticles containing ^{64}Cu have been reported recently for PET imaging of tumors.[30]

Optical imaging with quantum dots that home to vascular endothelial targets have been reported to be useful in identification of selected tissue zipcodes.[25,26] In some cases, multifunctionality has been designed into nanoparticles for combined imaging.[31] Tissue autofluorescence can obscure diagnosis at some wavelengths, although near-infrared wavelengths appear to be useful for enhanced sensitivity and specificity in this regard.[32,33] The lack of larger-scale non-invasive imaging systems for patients is a drawback.

The potential for nanoparticle-based imaging agents for either CT imaging or ultrasound is substantial in view of the large installed base of imaging units worldwide. Because X-ray absorption depends directly on the potency of the material used as contrast agent and exponentially on the thickness of the

layer of material deposited, sensitivity is expected to be only modest for nanoparticles. Nevertheless, lipid emulsion nanoparticles containing radiopaque iodinated triglycerides have been described for passive hepatic targeting,[34] and work is ongoing in the field.[35] An unavoidable drawback for serial use remains the considerable radiation dose.

Ultrasound possesses many advantages such as high throughput, low cost, and excellent patient tolerance but it is more highly operator dependent than other tomographic methods and cannot image all areas of the body. Available ultrasound contrast agents consist of gas-filled microbubbles, and have been developed for targeting vascular epitopes.[34] In the regimen of smaller particles, acoustically active emulsion nanoparticles for both imaging and therapy and reflective liposomes for imaging[36–38] have received the most attention (Figure 24.1). Although ultrasound is exquisitely sensitive for

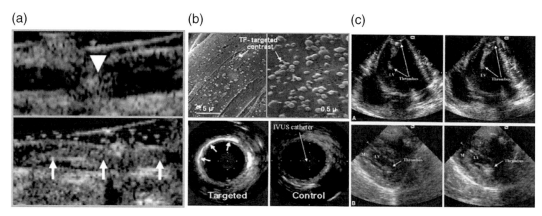

Figure 24.1 Ultrasound molecular imaging with nanoparticles. (a) Fibrin-targeted nanoparticles enhance contrast in thrombi formed in carotid arteries of pigs with use of clinical 7.5 MHz linear array transducers. Top: carotid artery lumen with echogenic anode (arrowhead) to induce fibrin-platelet thrombus that remains invisible at 7.5 MHz. Bottom: after fibrin-targeted nanoparticles bind to thrombus, backscatter augmented throughout and along the extent of the clot (arrows). (Reproduced from Lanza et al,[48] with permission.) (b) Tissue factor (TF) imaging after balloon injury to porcine carotid artery. Top: scanning electron microscopy of TF expression in vitro on smooth muscle cells targeted with nanoparticles containing mAb ligands to TF. Bottom: 30 MHz IVUS (intravascular ultrasound) imaging of TF induced in medial smooth muscle cells by balloon stretch injury. Note contrast enhancement heterogeneously distributed throughout media of vessel, representing binding of TF-targeted nanoparticles (see arrows in targeted site). (Reproduced from Lanza et al,[49] with permission.) (c) Fibrin-targeted echogenic liposomes binding to and enhancing contrast from LV (left ventricle) thrombi in four-chamber and parasternal views (left: pre-injection; right: post-injection). (Reproduced from Hamilton et al,[50] with permission.)

detecting microbubbles, it is less so for nanoparticles because of the size dependency (r^6) and relative incompressibility of liquid particles, which eliminates the use of available harmonic resonance-based imaging techniques typically applied to microbubble detection.

MRI enjoys several advantages over the other modalities, such as high resolution, high anatomic contrast, high signal-to-noise, widespread clinical availability, and lack of ionizing radiation.[11,39] However, the comparatively modest MR contrast enhancement achievable with targeted contrast agents for molecular imaging necessitates the delivery of higher payloads of contrast materials that can be provided by novel nanotechnologies. In the case of T_1-weighted imaging, the surfaces of nanoparticles can be decorated with numerous copies of gadolinium (Gd) chelates (up to 100 000) to achieve the micromolar concentrations required per voxel (Figure 24.2). Imaging with superparamagnetic agents takes advantage of a sufficiency of material that can be packed into the core of the nanoparticle to exert a prominent T_2^* effect, producing a localized signal reduction that can be

detected with potentially greater sensitivity than is possible with paramagnetic agents. Recently, quantitative approaches have been described for molecularly targeted paramagnetic emulsions that allow the computation of a concentration of bound nanoparticles under certain circumstances.[40]

Recent advances in pulse sequences have enabled 'bright spot' detection of iron oxide-based particles. Exploiting the same inherent dipole of magnetic particles that causes signal dropout on typical MR imaging, Cunningham et al[41] and also Stuber et al[42] have illustrated techniques for off-resonance imaging that can instead produce bright signals in regions surrounding the accumulation of particles. Alternatively, the signal generated by the fluorine atoms in the perfluorocarbon core of perfluorocarbon-based nanoparticles has been introduced as a unique bright spot signature for MR molecular imaging.[43,44] Because biologic tissues contain little endogenous fluorine, measurement of the fluorine component of targeted particles has the potential for definitive confirmation of nanoparticle deposition at the site.

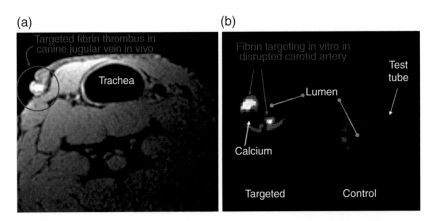

Figure 24.2 Magnetic resonance imaging of thrombi with paramagnetic nanoparticles targeted to fibrin. (a) thrombus formed in vivo in canine jugular vein imaged at 1.5 T. (b) 'Disrupted' carotid endarterectomy specimens incubated with fibrin-targeted nanoparticles binding to small amounts of fibrin at the shoulder regions (yellow arrows) of ruptured plaque cap imaged ex vivo at 1.5 T. (Reproduced from Flacke et al,[16] with permission.)

NANOTECHNOLOGY APPLICATIONS IN CARDIOVASCULAR IMAGING

Imaging

Rupturing atherosclerotic plaques are frequently manifest at various stages in arteries with only modest (40–60%) stenosis,[45] and they remain diagnostically elusive with routine clinical imaging techniques. Serum biomarkers may offer information about the general state of the vasculature but provide no enabling information about the propensity for any given lesion to rupture. Accordingly, one major motivation for molecular imaging is the recognition and localization of telltale molecular elements of unstable or disrupted plaques that might provide a window of opportunity extending from days to weeks or months to intervene before more serious clinical sequelae ensue.[2] A sine qua non of the disrupted plaque is fibrin deposition. Not only is fibrin deposition one of the earliest signs of plaque rupture or erosion but also, along with intraplaque hemorrhage, it forms a considerable part of the core of growing lesions.[46] The diagnosis of disrupted plaque by detecting small deposits of fibrin in erosions or microfractures could allow characterization of a potential 'culprit' lesion before a high-grade stenosis has been formed that is detectable by cardiac catheterization.

The possibility of nanoparticle-targeted fibrin imaging with either ultrasound or paramagnetic MR contrast agents was first demonstrated by Lanza as early as 1996.[37,47] In this case, the ligand comprised an antibody fragment highly specific for certain cross-linked fibrin peptide domains, which can be complexed to the particle either through avidin–biotin linkages, or covalently to the functionalized nanoparticle, as has been shown for tissue factor targeting.[43,48] For ultrasound imaging, thrombi formed in situ in canine carotid arteries were detectable within 30 minutes with commercially available 7.5 MHz linear array imaging transducers (see Figure 24.1a).[47]

Tissue factor is a prothrombotic transmembrane glycoprotein expressed within plaques that is up-regulated following vascular injury or stent placement, and contributes as a mitogen to restenosis.[49] Tissue factor in the core of plaques is exposed during plaque rupture and is the proximate cause of local thrombosis that leads to vessel occlusion or distal embolization. Tissue factor imaging has been demonstrated in vivo for molecular imaging with ultrasound (see Figure 24.1b) and in vitro with MRI.[37,40] In fact, the ability to image tissue factor-targeted paramagnetic nanoparticles bound to smooth muscle cell monolayers in cell culture at 1.5 T attests to the potency of nanoparticle agents that carry 50 000 or more gadolinium chelates.

Echogenic liposomes ('ELIPS'), in contrast to nanoparticles or emulsions, are composed of alternating layers of aqueous fluid and lipid bilayers, which are formulated to produce an ultrasound signal. Hamilton et al used these liposomes to target thrombi (see Figure 24.1c) and various vascular signatures associated with atheroma development in injured vessels of miniswine for intravascular ultrasound (IVUS) imaging.[12,36,50] By targeting intercellular adhesion molecule-1 (ICAM-1), vascular cell adhesion molecule-1 (VCAM-1), fibrin, fibrinogen, and tissue factor, they were able to produce targeted enhancement in the vessel walls 5 minutes after intravenous administration of the liposomes.

For MRI, perfluorocarbon particles loaded with 50 000 to 90 000 Gd atoms per particle yielded a substantial amplification of signal from fibrin clots at 1.5 T both in vitro and in vivo.[11,51] Furthermore, the detection of disrupted plaque was illustrated in actual human carotid endarterectomy specimens obtained from patients symptomatic with transient ischemic attacks, stroke, or bruits (see Figure 24.2b).[16] MR imaging of VCAM-1 has also been reported recently with the use of peptide-targeted superparamagnetic nanoparticles in aortas of cholesterol-fed ApoE null mice by Kelly et al (Figure 24.3).[31]

Phage display methods have been used by EPIX Pharmaceuticals (Cambridge, MA) to produce a peptide ligand specific for fibrin (EP-2104R), which may be useful for imaging thrombi in various body locations such as left atrium, pulmonary arteries, or coronary arteries in experimental preparations.[52–54] It contains four gadolinium–diethylenetriamine pentaacetic acid (Gd–DTPA) chelates per peptide moiety and thus provides signal enhancement on an MR image. Despite the low Gd load per binding site, the excess of fibrin epitopes in fresh or chronic clots allows accumulation of contrast agent concentrations sufficient to achieve micromolar levels of the lanthanide, and thus ready detection of the clot after the signal in the blood pool is sufficiently decreased (1–2 hours).

Whereas fibrin and tissue factor can be utilized to delineate unstable cardiovascular diseases, the $\alpha_v\beta_3$-integrin is a general marker of angiogenesis and plays an important role in a wide variety of disease states, including atherosclerosis[55] and cancer. The $\alpha_v\beta_3$-integrin is a well-characterized heterodimeric adhesion molecule that is widely expressed by endothelial cells, monocytes, fibroblasts, and vascular smooth muscle cells. In particular, $\alpha_v\beta_3$-integrin plays a critical part in smooth muscle cell migration and cellular adhesion,[56,57] both of which are required for the formation of new blood vessels. The $\alpha_v\beta_3$-integrin is expressed on the luminal surface of activated endothelial cells but not on mature quiescent cells.[58] We have demonstrated the utility of $\alpha_v\beta_3$-integrin targeted nanoparticles for the detection

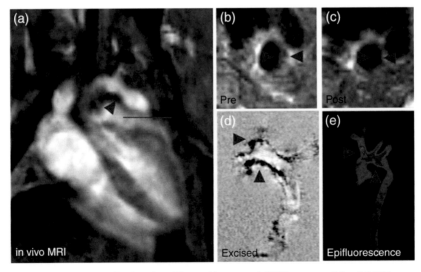

Figure 24.3 VCAM-1 imaging in ApoE −/− mice with peptide-targeted CLIO nanoparticles. (a) 24 hours after injection, MRI signal loss occurs where nanoparticles localize to aortic plaque in vivo (arrowheads). (b) and (c) Before and 24 hours after injection of targeted nanoparticles showing aortic cross sections with signal loss at plaque cap (arrows in (c) after injection correspond to locus (b) before injection). (d) Ex-vivo MRI of signal loss in aorta after nanoparticle binding (arrows). (e) Matched epifluorescent image of dual-function particles containing fluorescent probe labeling tissue VCAM (arrows). (Reproduced from Kelly et al,[31] with permission.)

and characterization of angiogenesis associated with growth factor expression,[59] tumor growth,[60,61] and atherosclerosis.[62]

Angiogenesis plays a critical role in plaque growth and rupture.[63,64] In regions of atherosclerotic lesions, angiogenic vessels proliferate from the vasa vasorum to meet the high metabolic demands of plaque growth.[65,66] Inflammatory cells within the lesion stimulate angiogenesis through local molecular signaling, which in turn promotes neovascular growth, thereby providing an avenue for more inflammatory cells to enter the plaque.[63]

Molecular imaging of expanded vasa vasorum in atherosclerotic lesions in cholesterol-fed rabbits was first demonstrated for MRI by Winter et al with the use of paramagnetic nanoparticles targeted to $\alpha_v\beta_3$-integrin-expressing endothelial cells (Figure 24.4).[62] Animals on a control diet exhibited no increased signal, and background was minimal. Expression of $\alpha_v\beta_3$-integrins in the adventitial layer and beyond was confirmed by co-localized histologic staining of $\alpha_v\beta_3$-integrin and PECAM, a general endothelial marker.

Macrophage imaging has been reported with the use of non-targeted USPIOs, first by Schmitz et al in Watanabe rabbits, and by Reuhm et al in cholesterol-fed atherosclerotic rabbits (Figure 24.5).[23,67] Because macrophages are abundant in plaques throughout the vascular tree, and they are well known to ingest particulate matter, the use of superparamagnetic agents to delineate macrophages and foam cells has been pursued in both animal models and in clinical trials.[68] The demonstration of macrophage targeting in vivo in rabbits required a waiting period of 1–3 days to allow for both passive uptake of sufficient numbers of particles and for bloodstream clearance of the long circulating particles. In general, the susceptibility artifacts produced extended beyond the confines of the plaque macrophages and appeared as

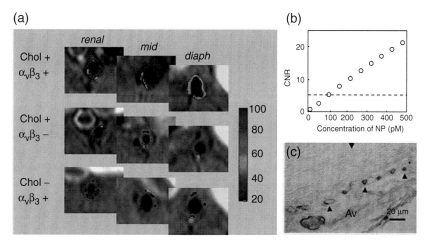

Figure 24.4 Detection of plaque neovascularization in cholesterol-fed (Chol+) rabbits. (a) Aortic cross sections imaged at 1.5 T with $\alpha_v\beta_3$-integrin targeted nanoparticles at level of renal arteries (renal), mid aorta (mid), and diaphragm (diaph). Note heterogeneous distribution in aortic cross sections (false-colored contrast enhancement), but little enhancement in non-targeted rabbits ($\alpha_v\beta_3$-) or rabbits on a standard diet (Chol–). (b) MRI signal modeling illustrates that picomolar (~100 pM) intravoxel concentrations of perfluorocarbon-based paramagnetic nanoparticles (NP) are required to achieve a diagnostic contrast-to-noise (CNR) ratio of ~5 (blue dashed line). (c) Immunochemical staining for $\alpha_v\beta_3$-integrin at the media–adventitia border of aorta segments. Note abundant red-brown vascular segments (arrows) in adventitia (AV). (Reproduced from Winter et al,[62] with permission.)

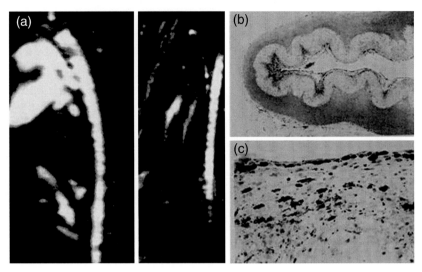

Figure 24.5 Macrophage imaging in cholesterol-fed rabbits with untargeted superparamagnetic nanoparticles. (a) Superparamagnetic iron oxide nanoparticles taken up by plaque macrophages depict atherosclerosis in cholesterol-fed rabbits according to magnetic susceptibility effects ('cold spots') that are seen distributed along the aorta in T_2-weighted images acquired more than 24 hours after injection. (b) and (c) Iron stain of plaque demonstrating uptake of particles by intimal macrophages (blue stain). Low power (upper panel) and higher power (lower panel) histological preparations for iron stains in the aorta are shown. (Reproduced from Ruehm et al,[67] with permission.)

heterogeneously distributed signal voids up and down the aorta.

In similar clinical trials of patients undergoing carotid endarterectomy by Kooi et al and by Trivedi et al, USPIOs accumulated in the macrophages in plaques and were optimally imaged as signal reductions at 24 hours after injection.[69,70] Kooi et al also noted that more contrast change was observed for ruptured than for stable plaques: USPIO-labeled macrophages have been imaged and localized to unstable and ruptured plaques (75% demonstrating uptake), but not in stable lesions (only 7% showing USPIO uptake).[69]

Recently, Fayad's group has reported the development of recombinant paramagnetic HDL-like particles that have been shown to enhance atherosclerotic regions in apolipoprotein E (ApoE)-deficient mice.[18] These particles are formed through the delipidation of normal isolated human HDL particles, followed by reconstitution with phospholipids and addition of a phospholipid-based conjugate of Gd–DTPA (15–20 molecules of gadolinium included in each 9 nm particle) for signal enhancement. Non-selective accumulation in atherosclerosis has been demonstrated.

This group has also demonstrated the use of conventional non-targeted agents such as gadofluorine that appear to preferentially label the fatty cores of plaques.[71] Gadofluorine is a lipophilic chelate of gadolinium (Gd–DO3A derivative) with a fluorinated side-chain that forms 5 nm-sized micelles in aqueous solution. The small size and lipophilic nature of this contrast agent allows it to accumulate in lipid-rich areas of plaque in cholesterol-fed rabbits.

Vessel wall inflammatory biomarkers such as smooth muscle cell $\alpha_v\beta_3$-integrins and matrix components such as collagen III can be imaged, as demonstrated recently by Cyrus et al.[72] The $\alpha_v\beta_3$-integrins

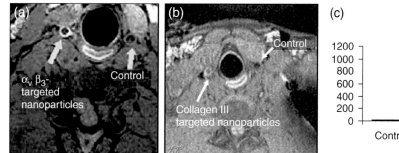
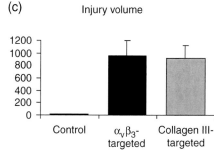

Figure 24.6 Imaging vascular biomarkers associated with acute injury. MR images (T_1-weighted proton MRI at 1.5 T) of carotid arteries of domestic pigs following balloon overstretch injury exposed for 10 minutes locally to paramagnetic nanoparticles covalently coupled to either (a) peptidometics targeted to $\alpha_v\beta_3$-integrin or (b) collagen III F$_{(ab)}$ fragments. (c) Quantitation of injury volume based on molecular imaging of targeted nanoparticles. (Reproduced from Cyrus et al,[72] with permission.)

are present in small quantities on vascular smooth muscle cells but are rapidly up-regulated in response to balloon hyperin-flation injury, and may play a role in the subsequent restenotic response following angioplasty. Figure 24.6 shows that MR three-dimensional molecular imaging with $\alpha_v\beta_3$-integrin- and collagen III-targeted nanoparticles can delineate microfrac-ture patterns of injury after balloon stretch in pigs. This unique technology could per-mit in-situ physiologic characterization of atherosclerotic plaques immediately post injury, which could facilitate individual-ized therapy decisions based on the local immune and inflammatory activity. In addition to pathologic character, the gen-erous distribution and bioavailability of collagen III and $\alpha_v\beta_3$-integrin within the vessel wall permitted the three-dimen-sional geometry and volume of the mural injury to be quantified, which could also be factored into treatment strategies required to preserve post-revascularization patency.

The fluorine component of perfluoro-carbon (PFC)-based nanoparticles might be utilized to advantage for imaging unique signatures of nanoparticle bind-ing. Our group originally demonstrated the concept of targeted nanoparticle fluo-rine imaging at 1.5 or 4.7 T for detection

of experimental thrombi or small fibrin deposits in disrupted human carotid arteries (Figure 24.7) using particles made with perfluorooctyl bromide (PFOB), crown ether (CE), or other PFC core materials.[43,44] We have recently demonstrated the use of rapid steady-state free precession ^{19}F imaging of combined PFOB and CE fibrin-targeted nanoparti-cles on fibrin clots and endaterectomy specimens in vitro at 1.5 T.[73]

Therapeutics

The potential dual use of nanoparticles for both imaging and site-targeted delivery of therapeutic agents to cardiovascular disease offers great promise for individu-alizing therapeutics. As an example of this new paradigm for drug delivery, Lanza et al treated smooth muscle cells in culture with tissue factor-targeted nanoparticles that were loaded with paclitaxel.[15,43] The smooth muscle cells were harvested from pig aorta and constitutively expressed tis-sue factor epitopes in vitro. Binding of the drug-free nanoparticles to the cells yielded no alterations in growth characteristics of the cultured cells. However, when pacli-taxel-loaded nanoparticles were applied to the cells, specific binding elicited a substantial reduction in smooth muscle

(a) (b) (c)

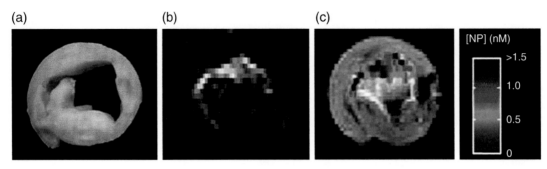

Figure 24.7 Fluorine imaging with fibrin-targeted perfluorocarbon-based nanoparticles. (a) Optical image of an excised human carotid endarterectomy sample shows asymmetrical plaque distribution, with areas of fat deposition (yellow). (b) Matched fluorine projection image at 4.7 T shows heterogeneous binding where fibrin is present on the plaque. (c) Using NMR spectroscopy, the fluorine image can be converted into a false-color map of the nanoparticle binding and coregistered and overlaid on the proton image (in gray scale), corresponding to the intravoxel concentration of nanoparticles bound to fibrin epitopes. Note quantitative false-color mapping scale at right illustrating quantification of signal enhancement as a nanoparticle concentration [NP] expressed in nanomoles (nM). (Reproduced from Morawski et al,[44] with permission.)

cell proliferation. Non-targeted paclitaxel-loaded particles applied to the cells, i.e. no binding of nanoparticles to cells occurred, resulted in normal cell proliferation, indicating that selective targeting may be a requirement for effective drug delivery for these emulsions. Similar behavior has been demonstrated for doxorubicin-containing particles.[43] Recent reports indicate that intravenous delivery of fumagillin-loaded nanoparticles (an antiangiogenic agent) targeted to $\alpha_v\beta_3$-integrin epitopes on vasa vasorum in growing plaques results in marked inhibition of plaque angiogenesis in cholesterol-fed rabbits.[74] Virmani's group has also utilized taxol-containing albumin nanoparticles for limitation of the restenotic response after angioplasty and stent placement in experimental animals.[75]

The unique mechanism of drug delivery for highly lipophilic agents such as paclitaxel contained within emulsions depends on close apposition between the nanoparticle carrier and the targeted cell membrane, and has been described as 'contact facilitated drug delivery'.[43] In contrast to liposomal drug delivery (generally requiring endocytosis), the mechanism of

drug transport in this case involves lipid exchange or lipid mixing between the emulsion vesicle and the targeted cell membrane (Figure 24.8),[76,77] which depends on the extent and frequency of contact between two lipidic surfaces.[43,76,77] The rate of lipid exchange and drug delivery can be greatly increased by the application of clinically safe levels of ultrasound energy that increase the propensity for fusion or enhanced contact between the nanoparticles and the targeted cell membrane by stimulating these interactions between nanoparticles and cell membranes (see Figure 24.8).[77]

In conclusion, the combination of targeted drug delivery and molecular imaging with MRI has the potential to revolutionize the approach to detecting and treating cardiovascular disease. Drug delivery agents that are also quantifiable at the targeted site based on imaging readouts may ultimately permit serial characterization of the molecular epitope expression and confirmation of therapeutic efficacy. Rapid developments in genomics, molecular biology, and nanotechnology are contributing to the multidisciplinary field of molecular imaging, and clinical trials are beginning.

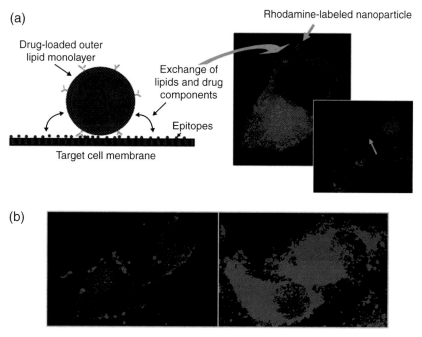

Figure 24.8 Augmenting therapeutics with ultrasound applied to bound targeted nanoparticles. (a) Perfluorocarbon-based nanoparticles can be loaded with lipophilic drug in outer lipid monolayer and delivered to cell by lipid mixing and/or lipid vesicle–cell membrane fusion. As an example, rhodamine-labeled lipids rapidly mix into the cell membrane (see arrow in inset) upon interaction with C32 melanoma cells (cells are transfected with green fluorescent protein [GFP] to label endosomes), then rapidly distribute into the cytoplasm without requiring endocytosis of the intact particles. (b) Ultrasound potentiation of lipid uptake by cells in culture. Left: fluorescein isocyanate (FITC)-labeled nanoparticles targeted to C32 cells demonstrate lipid mixing and fusion of particles and cells, and cytoplasmic delivery (note green distributed in cytoplasm). Right: after 5 min insonification of cells in culture with 2.5 MHz clinical phased array transducer at medium power, a marked increase in cytoplasmic lipid delivery is achieved with no untoward effects on viability of targeted cells. (Reproduced from Crowder et al,[76] with permission.)

REFERENCES

1. Zheng ZJ, Croft JB, Giles WH et al. Sudden cardiac death in the United States, 1989 to 1998. Circulation 2001; 104(18):2158–63.

2. Ojio S, Takatsu H, Tanaka T et al. Considerable time from the onset of plaque rupture and/or thrombi until the onset of acute myocardial infarction in humans: coronary angiographic findings within 1 week before the onset of infarction. Circulation 2000; 102:2063–9.

3. Petit L, Lesnik P, Dachet C, Moreau M, Chapman MJ. Tissue factor pathway inhibitor is expressed by human monocyte-derived macrophages: relationship to tissue factor induction by cholesterol and oxidized LDL. Arterioscler Thromb Vasc Biol 1999; 19: 309–15.

4. Kolodgie FD, Gold HK, Burke AP et al. Intraplaque hemorrhage and progression of coronary atheroma. N Engl J Med 2003; 349(24):2316–25.

5. Newby AC, Zaltsman AB. Fibrous cap formation or destruction – the critical importance of vascular smooth muscle cell proliferation, migration and matrix formation. Cardiovasc Res 1999; 41:345–60.

6. Shah PK. Role of inflammation and metalloproteinases in plaque disruption and thrombosis. Vasc Med 1998; 3:199–206.

7. de Boer OJ, van der Wal AC, Teeling P et al. Leucocyte recruitment in rupture prone regions of lipid-rich plaques: a prominent role for neovascularization? Cardiovasc Res 1999; 41(2):443–9.

8. McCarthy MJ, Loftus IM, Thompson MM et al. Angiogenesis and the atherosclerotic carotid plaque: an association between symptomatology and plaque morphology. J Vasc Surg 1999; 30(2):261–8.

9. Wickline SA, Lanza GM. Molecular imaging, targeted therapeutics, and nanoscience. J Cell Biochem 2002; 39:90–7.

10. Buxton DB, Lee SC, Wickline SA et al. Recommendations of the National Heart, Lung, and

Blood Institute Nanotechnology Working Group. Circulation 2003; 108(22):2737–42.

11. Wickline SA, Lanza GM. Nanotechnology for molecular imaging and targeted therapy. Circulation 2003; 107:1092–5.

12. Demos SM, Alkan-Onyuksel H, Kane BJ et al. In vivo targeting of acoustically reflective liposomes for intravascular and transvascular ultrasonic enhancement. J Am Coll Cardiol 1999; 33(3):867–75.

13. Sipkins DA, Cheresh DA, Kazemi MR et al. Detection of tumor angiogenesis in vivo by alphaVbeta3-targeted magnetic resonance imaging. Nat Med 1998; 4:623–6.

14. Lanza GM, Wickline SA. Targeted ultrasonic contrast agents for molecular imaging and therapy. Curr Probl Cardiol 2003; 28(12):625–53.

15. Lanza GM, Winter P, Caruthers S et al. Novel paramagnetic contrast agents for molecular imaging and targeted drug delivery. Curr Pharm Biotechnol 2004; 5(6):495–507.

16. Flacke S, Fischer S, Scott MJ et al. Novel MRI contrast agent for molecular imaging of fibrin: implications for detecting vulnerable plaques. Circulation 2001; 104:1280–5.

17. Yu X, Caruthers SD, Love SM et al. Rapid and sensitive thrombus detection with a fibrin-targeted nanoparticle MRI contrast agent. Circulation 2001; 104(17):1635.

18. Frias JC, Williams KJ, Fisher EA et al. Recombinant HDL-like nanoparticles: a specific contrast agent for MRI of atherosclerotic plaques. J Am Chem Soc 2004; 126(50):16316–17.

19. Li H, Gray BD, Corbin I et al. MR and fluorescent imaging of low-density lipoprotein receptors. Acad Radiol 2004; 11(11):1251–9.

20. Hawker CJ, Wooley KL. The convergence of synthetic organic and polymer chemistries. Science 2005; 309(5738):1200–5.

21. Kobayashi H, Kawamoto S, Jo SK et al. Macromolecular MRI contrast agents with small dendrimers: pharmacokinetic differences between sizes and cores. Bioconjug Chem 2003; 14(2):388–94.

22. Sato N, Kobayashi H, Hiraga A et al. Pharmacokinetics and enhancement patterns of macromolecular MR contrast agents with various sizes of polyamidoamine dendrimer cores. Magn Reson Med 2001; 46(6):1169–73.

23. Schmitz SA, Coupland SE, Gust R et al. Superparamagnetic iron oxide-enhanced MRI of atherosclerotic plaques in Watanabe hereditable hyperlipidemic rabbits. Invest Radiol 2000; 35(8):460–71.

24. Koch AM, Reynolds F, Merkle HP, Weissleder R, Josephson L. Transport of surface-modified nanoparticles through cell monolayers. Chembiochem 2005; 6(2):337–45.

25. Akerman ME, Chan WC, Laakkonen P et al. Nanocrystal targeting in vivo. Proc Natl Acad Sci USA 2002; 99(20):12617–21.

26. Chen L, Zurita AJ, Ardelt PU et al. Design and validation of a bifunctional ligand display system for receptor targeting. Chem Biol 2004; 11(8):1081–91.

27. Gao X, Nie S. Quantum dot-encoded beads. Methods Mol Biol 2005; 303:61–71.

28. Cherukuri P, Bachilo SM, Litovsky SH et al. Near-infrared fluorescence microscopy of single-walled carbon nanotubes in phagocytic cells. J Am Chem Soc 2004; 126(48):15638–9.

29. Barone PW, Baik S, Heller DA, Strano MS. Near-infrared optical sensors based on single-walled carbon nanotubes. Nat Mater 2005; 4(1):86–92.

30. Rossin R, Pan D, Qi K et al. ^{64}Cu-labeled folate-conjugated shell cross-linked nanoparticles for tumor imaging and radiotherapy: synthesis, radiolabeling, and biologic evaluation. J Nucl Med 2005; 46(7):1210–18.

31. Kelly KA, Allport JR, Tsourkas A et al. Detection of vascular adhesion molecule-1 expression using a novel multimodal nanoparticle. Circ Res 2005; 96(3):327–36.

32. Chen J, Tung C, Mahmood U et al. In vivo imaging of proteolytic activity in atherosclerosis. Circulation 2002; 105:2766–71.

33. Jaffer FA, Tung CH, Wykrzykowska JJ et al. Molecular imaging of factor XIIIa activity in thrombosis using a novel, near-infrared fluorescent contrast agent that covalently links to thrombi. Circulation 2004; 110(2):170–6.

34. Weber SM, Peterson KA, Durkee B et al. Imaging of murine liver tumor using microCT with a hepatocyte-selective contrast agent: accuracy is dependent on adequate contrast enhancement. J Surg Res 2004; 119(1):41–5.

35. Winter PM, Shukla HP, Caruthers SD et al. Molecular imaging of human thrombus with computed tomography. Acad Radiol 2005; 12:S9–13.

36. Hamilton AJ, Huang SL, Warnick D et al. Intravascular ultrasound molecular imaging of atheroma components in vivo. J Am Coll Cardiol 2004; 43(3):453–60.

37. Lanza G, Wickline S. Targeted ultrasonic contrast agents for molecular imaging and therapy. Prog Cardiovasc Dis 2001; 44(1):13–31.

38. Morawski AM, Lanza GA, Wickline SA. Targeted contrast agents for magnetic resonance imaging and ultrasound. Curr Opin Biotechnol 2005; 16(1):89–92.

39. Gupta H, Weissleder R. Targeted contrast agents. Magn Reson Imag Clin N Am 1996; 4:171–84.

40. Morawski AM, Winter PM, Crowder KC et al. Targeted nanoparticles for quantitative imaging of sparse molecular epitopes with MRI. Magn Reson Med 2004; 51(3):480–6.

41. Cunningham CH, Arai T, Yang PC et al. Positive contrast magnetic resonance imaging of cells labeled with magnetic nanoparticles. Magn Reson Med 2005; 53(5):999–1005.

42. Stuber M, Gilson WD, Schaer M et al. Shedding light on the dark spot with IRON: a method that generates

positive contrast in the presence of superparamagnetic nanoparticles. Proc Intl Soc Magn Reson Med 2005; 13:2608.

43. Lanza GM, Yu X, Winter PM et al. Targeted antiproliferative drug delivery to vascular smooth muscle cells with an MRI nanoparticle contrast agent: implications for rational therapy of restenosis. Circulation 2002; 106:2842–7.

44. Morawski AM, Winter PM, Yu X et al. Quantitative "magnetic resonance immunohistochemistry" with ligand-targeted ^{19}F nanoparticles. Magn Reson Med 2004; 52:1255–62.

45. Goldstein JA. Multifocal coronary plaque instability. Prog Cardiovasc Dis 2002; 44:449–54.

46. Constantinides P. Plaque fissuring in human coronary thrombosis. J Atheroscler Res 1966; 6:1–17.

47. Lanza GM, Wallace KD, Scott MJ et al. A novel site-targeted ultrasonic contrast agent with broad biomedical application. Circulation 1996; 95:3334–40.

48. Lanza GM, Abendschein DR, Hall CS et al. In vivo molecular imaging of stretch-induced tissue factor in carotid arteries with ligand-targeted nanoparticles. J Am Soc Echocardiogr 2000; 13(6):608–14.

49. Oltrona L, Speidel CM, Recchia D et al. Inhibition of tissue factor-mediated coagulation markedly attenuates stenosis after balloon-induced arterial injury in minipigs. Circulation 1997; 96(2):646–52.

50. Hamilton A, Huang SL, Warnick D et al. Left ventricular thrombus enhancement after intravenous injection of echogenic immunoliposomes: studies in a new experimental model. Circulation 2002; 105(23): 2772–8.

51. Lanza GM, Trousil RL, Wallace KD et al. In vitro characterization of a novel, tissue-targeted ultrasonic contrast system with acoustic microscopy. J Acoust Soc Am 1998; 104:3665–72.

52. Botnar RM, Buecker A, Wiethoff AJ et al. In vivo magnetic resonance imaging of coronary thrombosis using a fibrin-binding molecular magnetic resonance contrast agent. Circulation 2004; 110(11):1463–6.

53. Spuentrup E, Fausten B, Kinzel S et al. Molecular magnetic resonance imaging of atrial clots in a swine model. Circulation 2005; 112(3):396–9.

54. Spuentrup E, Katoh M, Wiethoff AJ et al. Molecular magnetic resonance imaging of pulmonary emboli with a fibrin-specific contrast agent. Am J Respir Crit Care Med 2005; 172(4):494–500.

55. Kerr JS, Mousa SA, Slee AM. Alpha$_v$beta$_3$ integrin in angiogenesis and restenosis. Drug News Perspect 2001; 14(3):143–50.

56. Bishop GG, McPherson JA, Sanders JM et al. Selective alpha$_v$beta$_3$-receptor blockade reduces macrophage infiltration and restenosis after balloon angioplasty in the atherosclerotic rabbit. Circulation 2001; 103(14):1906–11.

57. Corjay MH, Diamond SM, Schlingmann KL et al. alpha$_v$beta$_3$, alpha$_v$beta$_5$, and osteopontin are coordinately upregulated at early time points in a rabbit

58. Brooks PC, Stromblad S, Klemke R et al. Antiintegrin alpha$_v$beta$_3$ blocks human breast cancer growth and angiogenesis in human skin. J Clin Invest 1995; 96(4):1815–22.

59. Anderson SA, Rader RK, Westlin WF et al. Magnetic resonance contrast enhancement of neovasculature with alpha$_v$beta$_3$-targeted nanoparticles. Magn Reson Med 2000; 44(3):433–9.

60. Winter PM, Caruthers SD, Kassner A et al. Molecular imaging of angiogenesis in nascent Vx-2 rabbit tumors using a novel alpha(nu)beta3-targeted nanoparticle and 1.5 tesla magnetic resonance imaging. Cancer Res 2003; 63(18):5838–43.

61. Schmieder AH, Winter P, Caruthers S et al. Molecular MR imaging of melanoma angiogenesis with $\alpha_v\beta_3$-targeted paramagnetic nanoparticles. Magn Reson Med 2005; 53(3):621–7.

62. Winter PM, Morawski AM, Caruthers SD et al. Molecular imaging of angiogenesis in early-stage atherosclerosis with alpha$_v$beta$_3$-Integrin-targeted nanoparticles. Circulation 2003; 108(18):2270–4.

63. Moulton KS, Heller E, Konerding MA et al. Angiogenesis inhibitors endostatin or TNP-470 reduce intimal neovascularization and plaque growth in apolipoprotien E-deficient mice. Circulation 1999; 99:1653–5.

64. Tenaglia AN, Peters KG, Sketch MH Jr et al. Neovascularization in atherectomy specimens from patients with unstable angina: implications for pathogenesis of unstable angina. Am Heart J 1998; 135(1):10–14.

65. Wilson SH, Hermann J, Lermann LO et al. Simvastatin preserves the structure of coronary adventitial vasa vasorum in experimental hypercholesterolemia independent of lipid lowering. Circulation 2002; 105:415–18.

66. Zhang Y, Cliff WJ, Schoefl GI et al. Immunohistochemical study of intimal microvessels in coronary atherosclerosis. Am J Pathol 1993; 143(1):164–72.

67. Ruehm SG, Corot C, Vogt P, Kolb S, Debatin JF. Magnetic resonance imaging of atherosclerotic plaque with ultrasmall superparamagnetic particles of iron oxide in hyperlipidemic rabbits. Circulation 2001; 103:415–22.

68. Corot C, Petry KG, Trivedi R et al. Macrophage imaging in central nervous system and in carotid atherosclerotic plaque using ultrasmall superparamagnetic iron oxide in magnetic resonance imaging. Invest Radiol 2004; 39(10):619–25.

69. Kooi ME, Cappendijk VC, Cleutjens KB et al. Accumulation of ultrasmall superparamagnetic particles of iron oxide in human atherosclerotic plaques can be detected by in vivo magnetic resonance imaging. Circulation 2003; 107(19):2453–8.

70. Trivedi RA, U-King-Im JM, Graves MJ et al. In vivo detection of macrophages in human carotid

model of neointima formation. J Cell Biochem 1999; 75(3):492–504.

atheroma: temporal dependence of ultrasmall super-paramagnetic particles of iron oxide-enhanced MRI. Stroke 2004; 35:1631–5.

71. Sirol M, Itskovich VV, Mani V et al. Lipid-rich athero-sclerotic plaques detected by gadofluorine-enhanced in vivo magnetic resonance imaging. Circulation 2004; 109(23):2890–6.

72. Cyrus T, Abendschein DR, Caruthers SD et al. MR three-dimensional molecular imaging of intramural biomarkers with targeted nanoparticles. J Cardiovasc Magn Reson 2006; 8(3):535–41.

73. Caruthers SD, Neubauer AM, Hockett F et al. In vitro demonstration using ^{19}F magnetic resonance to aug-ment molecular imaging with paramagnetic nanoparticles at 1.5 Tesla. Invest Radiol 2006; 41(3):305–12.

74. Winter PM, Morawski AM, Caruthers SD et al. Antiangiogenic therapy of early atherosclerosis with paramagnetic alpha$_v$beta$_3$-integrin-targeted fumag-illin nanoparticles. J Am Coll Cardiol 2004; 43(5):322–3A.

75. Kolodgie FD, John M, Khurana C et al. Sustained reduction of in-stent neointimal growth with the use of a novel systemic nanoparticle paclitaxel. Circulation 2002; 106(10):1195–8.

76. Crowder KC, Hughes MS, Marsh JN et al. Sonic acti-vation of molecularly-targeted nanoparticles acceler-ates transmembrane lipid delivery to cancer cells through contact-mediated mechanisms: implications for enhanced local drug delivery. Ultrasound Med Biol 2005; 31(12):1693–700.

77. Crowder KC, Hughes MS, Marsh JN et al. Augmented and selective delivery of liquid perfluo-rocarbon nanoparticles to melanoma cells with non-cavitational ultrasound. Proc IEEE Ultrason Symp 2003; 03CH37476C:532–5.

Nuclear imaging of the vulnerable plaque

25

Sotirios Tsimikas and Jagat Narula

INTRODUCTION

Nuclear imaging is ideally poised to lead the way in detecting vulnerable plaques owing to its ability to image molecular targets. Nuclear imaging approaches have high sensitivity and very good specificity and resolution for imaging subanatomical components of vulnerable plaques. These imaging applications are enhanced in large respect by the ability to radiolabel various targeting agents and deliver them to a target of interest. Potential targets include apoptotic cells and bodies, oxidative species, inflammatory components such as macrophages, scavenger receptors, and metalloproteinases, endothelial cells and their products such as adhesion molecules and LOX-1 receptors, vasa vasorum, and angiogenesis and thrombus components.

In order for a nuclear imaging agent to detect vulnerable plaques, it must have strong specificity for its target, low uptake in adjacent tissues, high target-to-blood ratio, and optimal pharmacokinetics, including rapid uptake in the target and fast blood clearance. It must also provide an accurate assessment of the activity of disease, detect clinically relevant changes, and, ultimately, provide prognostic information that will lead to clinical decision making. This chapter reviews the ability of specific nuclear imaging techniques and approaches in imaging selected targets that may reflect plaque vulnerability and may provide a framework for future research and clinical applications.

TARGETING MACROPHAGES

The presence of macrophages in the subendothelial space, particularly at the shoulder region where the plaque is highly metabolically active, rapidly growing, and expanding radially, is one of the hallmarks of a vulnerable plaque. Activated macrophages are associated with a number of proinflammatory, immunologic, and proatherogenic properties, such as expression of a variety of scavenger receptors, up-regulation of proinflammatory genes, secretion of chemokines and cytokines and collagen-degrading metalloproteinases, and foam cell formation. Activation of macrophages leads to up-regulation of scavenger receptors, which take up oxidized low-density lipoprotein (OxLDL), which is generated in the subendothelial space, in preference to normal LDL. When macrophage/foam cells reach full capacity to take up additional OxLDL, they ultimately either undergo necrosis and release their contents into the lipid pool, further resulting in plaque growth, or undergo apoptosis. Therefore, targeting any of these macrophage processes appears to be a viable approach in detecting vulnerable plaques.

18-Fluorodeoxyglucose with positron emission tomography

18-fluorodeoxyglucose (FDG) is an isomer of glucose whose uptake in tissues is proportional to the metabolic rate of that tissue. FDG uptake is not specific to any tissue/organ and will accumulate in sites of cancer metastases, infection, and inflammation, particularly where there are activated inflammatory cells such as macrophages. It has the ideal property of being a positron emission tomography (PET) isotope which provides high photon flux allowing for quantitation of signal and improved spatial resolution (0.4–0.5 mm) compared with technetium 99m (^{99m}Tc) and other nuclear imaging radiolabels (1.0–1.5 mm).

It was incidentally noted that when FDG-PET scans were performed in patients suspected of having cancer metastases, enhanced FDG uptake was noted in the aorta, carotid, and femoral arteries, in abdominal aortic aneurysms, and in diffuse arteritis.[1,2] In fact, up to 50–80% of scans had evidence of FDG uptake in arteries, and the incidence increased with age and with risk factors, with younger patients having more FDG uptake and less calcification than older patients.[3,4] In studies where FDG-PET images were co-registered with computed tomography (CT) images, only 2–10% of patients had co-localization of FDG uptake and presence of calcification.[4,5] This suggests that calcified plaques are relatively quiescent metabolically and that younger plaques are more metabolically active. This is consistent with studies where FDG-PET uptake correlated with macrophage density both ex vivo[6] and in vivo in hypercholesterolemic rabbits.[7]

Importantly, this work has also been translated to the clinical arena by Rudd et al,[8] who determined with co-registered FDG-PET/CT scans that 8 patients with transient ischemic attacks (TIAs) had 27% ($P = 0.005$) higher uptake in the carotid artery ipsilateral to the TIA compared with the asymptomatic contralateral carotid artery. In addition, they showed that normal carotid arteries had no FDG uptake. Using autoradiography techniques in a separate set of studies, they showed that tritiated deoxyglucose (an isomer of FDG) accumulated at sites of necrotic core.[8] In a follow-up study by the same group, Davies et al[9] imaged 12 patients with recent TIA and a stenotic 'culprit' carotid plaque with co-registered FDG-PET/high-resolution magnetic resonance imaging (MRI). Interestingly, only 7/12 (58%) patients had evidence of increased ipsilateral FDG-PET signal. In 3 of the 5 patients without uptake in the 'culprit' plaque, there was evidence of enhanced FDG-PET uptake in a non-stenotic lesion that could explain the symptoms, including hot spots at sites closely adjacent to the stenotic lesion (Figure 25.1). This strongly suggests that non-stenotic but highly inflamed plaques may cause TIAs and stroke and that FDG-PET imaging may allow identification of vulnerable plaques. Future studies will need to focus on identifying such plaques prior to clinical events.

Limitations of FDG-PET include a limited spatial resolution of ~0.5 mm, which may not allow imaging of small plaques, the need for co-registration of an imaging modality such as MRI or CT, which adds additional time, cost, and, in particular, more radiation exposure – which may be in the range of 3–5 mSv – similar to a chest CT scan. There is also the need for electrocardiographic and respiratory gating and breath-holding to minimize cardiac motion during coronary imaging. In addition, imaging coronary arteries is additionally limited by myocardial uptake of FDG in all metabolically active cells/tissues/organs and it is not yet clear what the true sensitivity and specificity will be for detecting vulnerable plaques. Future areas of research to enhance specificity of imaging plaque components will focus on improving resolution and reducing radiation exposure, enhancing imaging

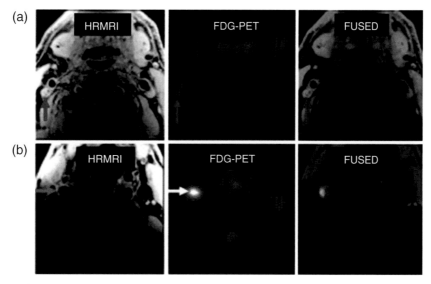

Figure 25.1   High-resolution magnetic resonance imaging (HRMRI) and FDG-PET scans taken from patient 1 after a right carotid territory stroke. (a) Transaxial images taken at the level of the proximal right internal carotid (RIC) artery. There is a large atherosclerotic plaque in the RIC artery causing severe luminal stenosis (green arrow). Despite its size, only low FDG uptake is demonstrated (blue and red arrows). (b) Axial images taken at the level of the proximal common carotid arteries (CCA). The yellow arrow highlights a non-stenotic plaque in the wall of the right CCA. The white arrow points to an area of high FDG uptake, the location of which is confirmed on the fused scan as the right CCA (black arrow). (Reprinted with permission from Davies et al[9].)

protocols, particularly with hybrid techniques, and using more specific targeting agents with PET labels.

Annexin V

During the early stages of macrophage apoptosis, the phospholipid phosphatidylserine (PS) translocates from the inner to the outer leaflet of the cell membrane bilayer. PS is strongly bound by the endogenous protein annexin V, a 35–36 kDa, Ca^{2+}-dependent, phospholipid-binding protein.[10] Annexin V can be labeled with ^{99m}Tc using a hydrazino-nicotinamide (HYNIC) bifunctional agent. ^{99m}Tc-HYNIC-annexin V has a half-life of approximately 24 minutes in humans, allowing rapid clearance of the agent to allow optimal plaque/blood ratios for imaging.[11]

Imaging of non-plaque apoptosis with ^{99m}Tc-HYNIC-annexin V in animal models was initially performed in 1992.[12] Subsequently, autoradiographic studies in hypercholesterolemic rabbits showed that ^{125}I-annexin V accumulated in lesioned areas.[13] More recently, several animal and human studies have shown the feasibility of non-invasively imaging plaques with characteristics of vulnerability. Kolodgie et al[14] first reported that ^{99m}Tc-HYNIC-annexin V accumulated in experimentally produced atherosclerotic lesions in New Zealand White rabbits and could be detected by non-invasive imaging with planar gamma camera imaging. ^{99m}Tc-HYNIC-annexin V uptake was 9.3-fold higher in plaque vs normal areas in the aorta, with a plaque:blood ratio of 3.0 ± 0.37. There was a correlation of ^{99m}Tc-HYNIC-annexin V uptake with macrophage content, advancing lesions, and apoptotic index but not with smooth muscle cell content. Further supporting the role of annexin V in plaque vulnerability, it was shown that following dietary withdrawal of cholesterol or treatment with statin therapy, plaque uptake of ^{99m}Tc-HYNIC-annexin V was significantly reduced (control 0.051% of the injected dose [% ID] vs 0.03% ID in both the diet withdrawal and statin groups, P <0.0001).[15]

Non-invasive imaging of human carotid artery atherosclerosis was performed in 4 patients with TIA with ^{99m}Tc-HYNIC-annexin V 1–3 days prior to carotid endarterectomy.[16] There was evidence of specific accumulation of radiolabel in the carotid artery ipsilateral to the TIA, but no uptake in the contralateral carotid artery. Histologic assessment revealed evidence of macrophage infiltration (15.7% of cells) and morphologic features of unstable plaque, such as plaque hemorrhage (Figure 25.2). In addition to these applications, annexin V may also have a role in detecting ischemia/reperfusion injury,[17] cardiomyopathy, and in tumor imaging.

Future developments may propel annexin V imaging as a potentially clinically useful tool in cardiovascular disease. Confirmatory studies are awaited in larger human populations followed prospectively; enhancement of imaging sensitivity, specificity, and precision; development of PET labels for improved sensitivity and

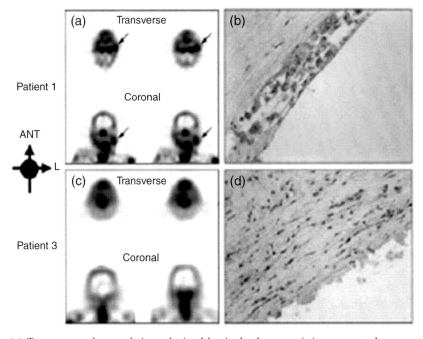

Figure 25.2 (a) Transverse and coronal views obtained by single-photon emission computed tomography (SPECT) in Patient 1, who had a left-sided transient ischemic attack (TIA) 3 days before imaging. Although this patient had clinically significant stenosis of both carotid arteries, uptake of radiolabeled annexin A5 is evident only in the culprit lesion (arrows). (b) Histopathologic analysis of an endarterectomy specimen from Patient 1 (polyclonal rabbit anti-annexin A5 antibody, ×400) shows substantial infiltration of macrophages into the neointima, with extensive binding of annexin A5 (brown). (c) In contrast, SPECT images of Patient 3 who had had a right-sided TIA 3 months before imaging, do not show evidence of annexin A5 uptake in the carotid artery region on either side. Doppler ultrasonography revealed a clinically significant obstructive lesion on the affected side. (d) Histopathologic analysis of an endarterectomy specimen from Patient 3 (polyclonal rabbit anti-annexin A5 antibody, ×400) shows a lesion rich in smooth muscle cells, with negligible binding of annexin A5. ANT, anterior; and L, left. (Reprinted with permission from Kietselaer et al.[16])

resolution; improved pharmacokinetics to reduce liver and kidney uptake; enhanced imaging protocols; and determination of changes in images following therapeutic interventions.[10]

Chemokines and metalloproteinases

Products of macrophages directly influence the inflammatory cascades in atherosclerotic lesions. Macrophages secrete a variety of metalloproteinases (MMPs) such as MMP-1 (collagenase-1), MMP-2 (gelatinase A), MMP-3 (stromelysin-1), and MMP-9 (gelatinase-B), that may degrade the collagen matrix and reduce mechanical stability of plaques, leading to plaque disruption and thrombotic occlusion.[18] MMPs are synthesized by macrophages and released into the atherosclerotic plaque. MMPs are thought to be responsible for collagen degradation, and studies have shown that lipid lowering with diet or statins reduces the expression of MMPs in the vessel wall. Endogenous tissue inhibitors of MMPs (TIMPs) are also present in the vessel wall and regulate the connective tissue breakdown of MMPs. Synthetic analogs of TIMPs have been developed for therapeutic purposes.[19] Recently, they have also been evaluated for in-vivo imaging the presence of MMPs. These compounds have a low molecular weight and are cleared very rapidly (half-life <10 minutes) from the circulation, a significant advantage for nuclear imaging. One such non-specific MMP inhibitor, 123I-HO-CGS 27023A, was shown to specifically image MMPs with PET scintigraphy in cholesterol-fed ApoE$^{-/-}$ mice with carotid artery ligation.[20] There was a 3-fold higher uptake in the ligated carotid artery compared with the contralateral carotid. Further studies in models of vulnerable plaques, such as the innominate artery of ApoE$^{-/-}$ mice, are awaited for confirmation of this potentially exciting approach.

Macrophages also secrete a variety of chemokines such as monocyte chemoattractant protein-1 (MCP-1) and macrophage colony-stimulating factor (M-CSF) that attract, recruit, and maintain monocytes in the vessel wall and induce their differentiation into macrophages.[21] MCP-1 is a 76 amino acid peptide that specifically recruits monocytes to the vessel wall. MCP-1 binds to CCR1 and CCR2 receptors present exclusively on monocytes. ^{125}I-MCP-1 injected into cholesterol-fed rabbits with iliac artery de-endothelialization showed enhanced uptake with autoradiography compared with normal areas (6:1 lesion/normal vessel ratio). The circulating half-life of ^{125}I-MCP-1 was ~10 minutes. As expected, ^{125}I-MCP-1 circulated bound to cells, most probably monocytes, rather than being present free in plasma. A strong correlation was noted between the macrophage content of the lesion and ^{125}I-MCP-1 uptake. Non-invasive imaging studies have not been carried out with this approach.

OXIDIZED LIPID TARGETS

Oxidized LDL (OxLDL) is a generic term that describes a range of oxidized species resulting from a variety of modifications of both the lipid and protein components of LDL that occur when oxygen free radicals react with polyunsaturated fatty acids. Degradation of such fatty acids leads to highly reactive aldehydes and ketones that modify amino groups on lysine groups and other amino acid residues present on both the protein – apolipoprotein B-100 (ApoB) – and lipid phase (i.e. phospholipids) of LDL and other lipoproteins. These modified lipid/protein adducts are not only proatherogenic and proinflammatory but are also recognized as foreign by the immune system and therefore highly immunogenic (reviewed in Tsimikas et al[21]). Circulating OxLDL represents a very small fraction of total LDL (<1%)

that circulates in plasma, since fully oxidized LDL is cleared from the circulation within minutes by the reticuloendothelial system.[22,23] Significant differences exist between OxLDL and LDL and may imply a different pathophysiologic mechanism of cardiovascular risk promotion; OxLDL is a measure of oxidative changes of fatty acids on LDL that result in oxidative damage and immunologic consequences, whereas LDL cholesterol is simply a measure of the cholesterol content of LDL.

OxLDL is not present in normal arteries but is otherwise present in all other lesions, from foam cells to fatty streaks to advanced atheromas, generally in proportion to plaque mass.[24,25] However, highly calcified, fibrotic, or regressing lesions generally contain limited amounts of OxLDL.[26–28] The complex interaction of oxidation, inflammation, and thrombosis leads to atherosclerosis progression and plaque disruption and ultimately to clinical events. Immune mechanisms and inflammatory cells play a central role throughout all these events, resulting in atherosclerotic lesions having many features of a chronic inflammatory disease.[29]

Plasma biomarkers of OxLDL have been recently developed to evaluate patients for cardiovascular risk and prognosis. There is now a wealth of data showing that the circulating OxLDL, measured by a variety of antibodies that actually recognize different and unique epitopes of OxLDL, correlates with the presence, extent, and progression of coronary and peripheral arterial disease.[22] Future work will evaluate whether these plasma OxLDL biomarkers predict cardiovascular events.

The concept of targeting atherosclerotic plaque components was initially proposed in the mid 1980s by Bob Lees and his group, using [125]I- and ^{99m}Tc-labeled LDL in trying to image human carotid arteries.[30,31] Subsequently, several different groups also favored this approach, using different labels without significant success.

This approach, albeit novel, was limited by minimal and slow uptake in lesions, giving a very low target:blood ratio, a long circulation half-life of LDL (up to 2 weeks), and the necessity of isolating autologous LDL. Iuliano et al[32] evaluated autologous radiolabeled malondialdehyde (MDA)-modified LDL (representing an oxidation-specific epitope but the LDL is not actually oxidized) in human carotid artery imaging and showed significantly faster clearance than native LDL, particularly due to uptake by organs rich in reticuloendothelial cells.

In a shift of the paradigm in targeting lipids, our group has studied the feasibility of targeting specific oxidation-specific epitopes, rather than normal lipids, within the atherosclerotic plaque using both murine and human autoantibodies to OxLDL. In a series of experiments we validated the use of the murine monoclonal antibody MDA2, which recognizes MDA-lysine epitopes on LDL and other plaque components, in several animal models of native atherosclerosis including LDLR[-/-] and ApoE[-/-] mice and Watanabe heritable hyperlipidemic rabbits. It was demonstrated that the uptake of ^{125}I-MDA2 in atherosclerotic lesions was proportional to the plaque burden measured by both percent atherosclerotic lesion area and aortic weight.[24,33,34] Furthermore, ^{99m}Tc-MDA2 successfully non-invasively imaged lipid-rich, oxidation-rich plaques (Figure 25.3). Subsequently, in a regression study, LDLR[-/-] mice were fed a high-cholesterol, high-fat diet for 6 months and either continued on this diet (Progression group) or placed back on normal mouse chow (Regression group) for an additional 6 months; each group was then injected with ^{125}I-MDA2. Uptake of ^{125}I-MDA2 was markedly reduced in mouse lesions undergoing atherosclerosis regression and correlated very strongly with measures of plaque stabilization, including reduced macrophage content and increased collagen and smooth muscle cell content

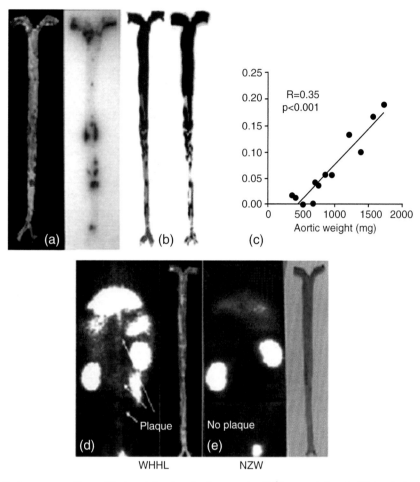

Figure 25.3 En-face preparations of Sudan-stained aortas from an ApoE$^{-/-}$ mouse (a) and a Watanabe heritable hyperlipidemic rabbit (WHHL) (b) injected with ^{125}I-MDA2, respectively. Red color (left panels in a and b) signifies the presence of neutral lipid within the atherosclerotic plaque stained with Sudan IV, and black color (right panels in a and b) in the corresponding autoradiograph signifies the presence of accumulated ^{125}I-MDA2, reflecting the presence of OxLDL. (c) The relationship of ^{125}I-MDA2 uptake and plaque burden as measured by aortic weight. (d) and (e) In-vivo imaging of atherosclerotic WHHL (d) and non-atherosclerotic New Zealand White (NZW) (e) rabbits with ^{99m}Tc-MDA2. (Reprinted with permission from Tsimikas et al.[24,33])

(Figure 25.4).[28] In addition, there was evidence obtained by immunostaining that OxLDL disappeared from the vessel wall following a low-fat diet prior to physical plaque regression, suggesting that this may be a very early mechanism of plaque stabilization.

This series of experiments demonstrated that OxLDL is a viable marker of plaque burden and, more importantly for imaging vulnerable plaque, correlated inversely with measures of atherosclerosis regression. This implies that targeting OxLDL in the vessel wall may reflect both plaque stabilization when OxLDL content is increased and plaque stabilization when OxLDL is removed from the vessel wall. Because MD2 is a murine monoclonal antibody that is not easily applicable to human use owing to potential side effects, we subsequently cloned the first human oxidized LDL antibody, named IK17, which we are now evaluating as a potential human imaging agent.[35]

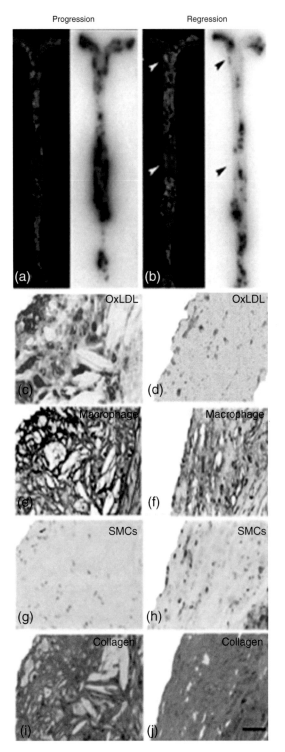

THROMBUS IMAGING

The propensity for thrombus formation is one of the hallmarks of vulnerable plaques.[36] Thrombus formation is often subclinical and may be present for minutes to weeks or even longer prior to an acute coronary syndrome. In fact, pathologic studies have suggested repeated subclinical plaque rupture and healing with superimposed thrombus in many patients ultimately dying of cardiovascular disease.[37] Thrombus imaging in the 1970s was one of the earliest applications of imaging atherosclerotic plaques. Initial attempts at thrombus imaging consisted of radiolabeled autologous platelets, radiolabeled fibrinogen, fibrin, or D-dimer, and radiolabeled antibodies to various components of coagulation, such as to tissue-plasminogen activator, platelets, and fibrinogen. These generally failed because of the non-specific nature of targeting agents, often binding to plasma rather than plaque, minimal uptake in areas of interest, and poor image resolution. More recently, attempts have been made using ^{99m}Tc-labeled antibodies (^{99m}Tc-DMP-444) binding to the glycoprotein IIb/IIIa receptor of platelets.[38] Unfortunately, although these approaches can be shown to work in principle in experimentally produced thrombi,

Figure 25.4 En-face preparation of Sudan-stained mouse aortas (left) and corresponding autoradiographs (right) showing representative examples of intravenously injected ^{125}I-MDA2 distribution in the Progression (a) and Regression (b) groups. Arrowheads depict Sudan-stained areas with diminished ^{125}I-MDA2 uptake. (c)–(j) Examples of immunostained atherosclerotic lesions from LDLR$^{-/-}$ mice from the Progression (c, e, g, i) and Regression (d, f, h, j) groups. Immunostaining was performed for OxLDL, macrophages, smooth muscle cells (SMCs), and collagen. OxLDL and SMCs appear pink/purple, macrophages black, and collagen bright blue. Scale bar = 50 μm. (Reprinted with permission from Torzewski et al.[28])

no data have been generated in spontaneous thrombosis models. Limitations of this approach include the abrupt nature of thrombus formation and resolution, making it a moving target for detection of vulnerable plaques. Future advances will require novel paradigm shifts in detecting clinically relevant thrombus imaging.

FUTURE DIRECTIONS

The field of nuclear cardiology has made significant strides in developing algorithms for imaging vulnerable plaques. FDG-PET and annexin V imaging have already been translated to humans and await larger confirmatory studies in selected patient cohorts. Additional approaches at selectively targeting macrophages, oxidation, and inflammation targets await additional experimental studies and human imaging. Future advances will need to focus on improvement in spatial resolution and image quality, development of novel targeting agents, and evaluation of complementary imaging techniques with anatomic imaging techniques such as CT and MRI. Finally, larger prospective studies are needed to ascertain whether these approaches can provide prognostic information.

ACKNOWLEDGMENTS

Dr Tsimikas is supported in part by the Donald W Reynolds Foundation, Las Vegas, Nevada and NHLBI grant HL-56989 (La Jolla Specialized Center of Research in Molecular Medicine and Atherosclerosis). Dr Narula is supported by NIH/NHLBI R01 HL 078681 and NIH/NHLBI RO1 HL 68657.

REFERENCES

1. Yun M, Yeh D, Araujo LI et al. F-18 FDG uptake in the large arteries: a new observation. Clin Nucl Med 2001; 26:314–19.
2. Tatsumi M, Cohade C, Nakamoto Y, Wahl RL. Fluorodeoxyglucose uptake in the aortic wall at PET/CT: possible finding for active atherosclerosis. Radiology 2003; 229:831–7.
3. Yun M, Jang S, Cucchiara A, Newberg AB, Alavi A. 18F FDG uptake in the large arteries: a correlation study with the atherogenic risk factors. Semin Nucl Med 2002; 32:70–6.
4. Dunphy MP, Freiman A, Larson SM, Strauss HW. Association of vascular 18F-FDG uptake with vascular calcification. J Nucl Med 2005; 46:1278–84.
5. Ben Haim S, Kupzov E, Tamir A, Israel O. Evaluation of 18F-FDG uptake and arterial wall calcifications using 18F-FDG PET/CT. J Nucl Med 2004; 45: 1816–21.
6. Ogawa M, Ishino S, Mukai T et al. (18)F-FDG accumulation in atherosclerotic plaques: immunohistochemical and PET imaging study. J Nucl Med 2004; 45:1245–50.
7. Tawakol A, Migrino RQ, Hoffmann U et al. Noninvasive in vivo measurement of vascular inflammation with F-18 fluorodeoxyglucose positron emission tomography. J Nucl Cardiol 2005; 12:294–301.
8. Rudd JH, Warburton EA, Fryer TD et al. Imaging atherosclerotic plaque inflammation with [18F]-fluorodeoxyglucose positron emission tomography. Circulation 2002; 105:2708–11.
9. Davies JR, Rudd JH, Fryer TD et al. Identification of culprit lesions after transient ischemic attack by combined 18F fluorodeoxyglucose positron-emission tomography and high-resolution magnetic resonance imaging. Stroke 2005; 36:2642–7.
10. Boersma HH, Kietselaer BL, Stolk LML et al. Past, present, and future of annexin A5: from protein discovery to clinical applications. J Nucl Med 2005; 46:2035–50.
11. Kemerink GJ, Liu X, Kieffer D et al. Safety, biodistribution, and dosimetry of ^{99m}Tc-HYNIC-annexin V, a novel human recombinant annexin V for human application. J Nucl Med 2003; 44:947–52.
12. Blankenberg FG, Katsikis PD, Tait JF et al. In vivo detection and imaging of phosphatidylserine expression during programmed cell death. Proc Natl Acad Sci USA 1998; 95:6349–54.
13. Moldovan NI, Moldovan L, Simionescu N. Binding of vascular anticoagulant alpha (annexin V) to the aortic intima of the hypercholesterolemic rabbit. An autoradiographic study. Blood Coagul Fibrinolysis 1994; 5:921–8.
14. Kolodgie FD, Petrov A, Virmani R et al. Targeting of apoptotic macrophages and experimental atheroma with radiolabeled annexin V: a technique with potential for noninvasive imaging of vulnerable plaque. Circulation 2003; 108:3134–9.
15. Hartung D, Sarai M, Petrov A et al. Resolution of apoptosis in atherosclerotic plaque by dietary modification and statin therapy. J Nucl Med 2005; 46:2051–6.
16. Kietselaer BL, Reutelingsperger CP, Heidendal GA et al. Noninvasive detection of plaque instability with use of radiolabeled annexin A5 in patients with

carotid-artery atherosclerosis. N Engl J Med 2004; 350:1472–147a.

17. Murakami Y, Takamatsu H, Taki J et al. 18F-labelled annexin V: a PET tracer for apoptosis imaging. Eur J Nucl Med Mol Imaging 2004; 31:469–74.

18. Aikawa M, Libby P. The vulnerable atherosclerotic plaque: pathogenesis and therapeutic approach. Cardiovasc Pathol 2004; 13:125–38.

19. Kopka K, Breyholz HJ, Wagner S et al. Synthesis and preliminary biological evaluation of new radioiodinated MMP inhibitors for imaging MMP activity in vivo. Nucl Med Biol 2004; 31:257–67.

20. Schafers M, Riemann B, Kopka K et al. Scintigraphic imaging of matrix metalloproteinase activity in the arterial wall in vivo. Circulation 2004; 109:2554–9.

21. Tsimikas S, Glass C, Steinberg D, Witztum JL. Lipoproteins, lipoprotein oxidation and atherogenesis. In: Chien KR, ed. Molecular Basis of Cardiovascular Disease, 2nd edn. A Companion to Braunwald's Heart Disease. Philadelphia, PA: WB Saunders; 2004:385–413.

22. Tsimikas S. Oxidized low-density lipoprotein biomarkers in atherosclerosis. Curr Atheroscler Rep 2006; 8:55–61.

23. Van Berkel TJ, De Rijke YB, Kruijt JK. Different fate in vivo of oxidatively modified low density lipoprotein and acetylated low density lipoprotein in rats. Recognition by various scavenger receptors on Kupffer and endothelial liver cells. J Biol Chem 1991; 266:2282–9.

24. Tsimikas S, Shortal BP, Witztum JL, Palinski W. In vivo uptake of radiolabeled MDA2, an oxidation-specific monoclonal antibody, provides an accurate measure of atherosclerotic lesions rich in oxidized LDL and is highly sensitive to their regression. Arterioscler Thromb Vasc Biol 2000; 20:689–97.

25. Palinski W, Napoli C. The fetal origins of atherosclerosis: maternal hypercholesterolemia, and cholesterol-lowering or antioxidant treatment during pregnancy influence in utero programming and postnatal susceptibility to atherogenesis. FASEB J 2002; 16:1348–60.

26. Crisby M, Nordin-Fredriksson G, Shah PK et al. Pravastatin treatment increases collagen content and decreases lipid content, inflammation, metalloproteinases, and cell death in human carotid plaques:

implications for plaque stabilization. Circulation 2001; 103:926–33.

27. Aikawa M, Sugiyama S, Hill CC et al. Lipid lowering reduces oxidative stress and endothelial cell activation in rabbit atheroma. Circulation 2002; 106:1390–6.

28. Torzewski M, Shaw PX, Han KR et al. Reduced in vivo aortic uptake of radiolabeled oxidation-specific antibodies reflects changes in plaque composition consistent with plaque stabilization. Arterioscler Thromb Vasc Biol 2004; 24:2307–12.

29. Libby P. Inflammation in atherosclerosis. Nature 2002; 420:868–74.

30. Lees RS, Lees AM, Strauss HW. External imaging of human atherosclerosis. J Nucl Med 1983; 24:154–6.

31. Lees AM, Lees RS, Schoen FJ et al. Imaging human atherosclerosis with ^{99m}Tc-labeled low density lipoproteins. Arteriosclerosis 1988; 8:461–70.

32. Iuliano L, Signore A, Vallabajosula S et al. Preparation and biodistribution of 99m technetium labelled oxidized LDL in man. Atherosclerosis 1996; 126:131–41.

33. Tsimikas S, Palinski W, Halpern SE et al. Radiolabeled MDA2, an oxidation-specific, monoclonal antibody, identifies native atherosclerotic lesions in vivo. J Nucl Cardiol 1999; 6:41–53.

34. Tsimikas S, Palinski W, Witztum JL. Circulating autoantibodies to oxidized LDL correlate with arterial accumulation and depletion of oxidized LDL in LDL receptor-deficient mice. Arterioscler Thromb Vasc Biol 2001; 21:95–100.

35. Shaw PX, Hörkkö S, Tsimikas S et al. Human-derived anti-oxidized LDL autoantibody blocks uptake of oxidized LDL by macrophages and localizes to atherosclerotic lesions in vivo. Arterioscler Thromb Vasc Biol 2001; 21:1333–9.

36. Falk E. Pathogenesis of atherosclerosis. J Am Coll Cardiol 2006; 47:C7-C12.

37. Virmani R, Burke AP, Farb A, Kolodgie FD. Pathology of the vulnerable plaque. J Am Coll Cardiol 2006; 47:C13–C18.

38. Mitchel J, Waters D, Lai T et al. Identification of coronary thrombus with a IIb/IIIa platelet inhibitor radiopharmaceutical, technetium-99m DMP-444: A canine model. Circulation 2000; 101:1643–6.

26

Nanoparticle-based targeted delivery of therapeutics and non-invasive imaging of unstable endothelium

Thomas R Porter, Feng Xie, SJ Adelman, and Nicholas Kipshidze

INTRODUCTION

Transluminal coronary angioplasty (percutaneous transluminal coronary angioplasty; PTCA) was introduced in the late 1970s as a non-surgical treatment for obstructive coronary artery disease and blockage due to myocardial infarction (MI). The procedure involves placing a balloon-tipped catheter at the site of occlusion and disrupting and expanding the occluded vessel by inflating the balloon. Although initially successful at removal of the blockage and luminal enlargement, the process also damages the blood vessel wall extensively, including the loss of the endothelial lining. An ensuing response to this severe injury is often enhanced expression of cytokines and growth factors, and subsequently, a rapid acute reclosure and/or a slow progressive reocclusion or restenosis of the vessel. Within the vascular wall, this response typically includes myointimal hyperplasia, proliferation of smooth muscle cells and fibroblasts, connective tissue matrix remodeling, and formation of thrombus. Restenosis, referring to the renarrowing of the vascular lumen following an intervention such as balloon angioplasty, is clinically defined as a >50% loss of the initial luminal diameter gain following the interventional procedure and

has affected anywhere from 25 to 35% of treated patients.[1,2]

Today, standard therapy for MI or other luminal narrowing includes thrombolytics, anticoagulants, and often, interventional procedures such as PTCA. Recently, an advance to the procedure has been the introduction of stents, metallic-based cage/tube-like structures placed into the vessel lumen with PTCA, and the rate of acute reclosure has been minimized. Coronary stents provide luminal scaffolding, eliminating elastic recoil and remodeling which can occur rapidly following an interventional procedure. Unfortunately, however, although the occurrence of acute reclosure was reduced, there was actually no decrease in neointimal hyperplasia, and in fact, the procedure led to an increase in the proliferative component of restenosis and a relatively higher rate of reocclusion and need for reintervention often as early as 3 months to 1 year following the procedure.[3]

Recently, increased success has been achieved against the PTCA-associated neointimal hyperplasia through the invention and development of the drug-eluting stent (DES).[4,5] Drug-coated or impregnated stents deployed within the lumen of the blood vessel have been developed where a given drug is gradually (days to weeks) eluted, diffusing into the proximal vessel wall.[6] Examples of compounds used include inhibitors of mTOR (mammalian target of rapamycin) such as rapamycin (sirolimus, Wyeth-Ayerst Laboratories), a macrolide immunosuppressive agent, as well as chemotherapeutics such as paclitaxel (Taxol, Bristol-Myers Squibb) or actinomycin D. With the recent development of angioplasty combined with DES, such as the CYPHER coronary stent marketed by Johnson & Johnson/Cordis, treatment of the culprit vessel in MI has had a significant advance. Rapamycin (sirolimus), the agent utilized in this first successful DES, is an immune mediator shown to quiet the local immune activation, and also, to reduce or eliminate cellular proliferation. Boston Scientific, with their Taxus/paclitaxel DES, has also shown success. All of these compounds have been shown to inhibit smooth muscle cell proliferation,[7-10] and have reduced the rate of restenosis to the 6–10% range.[11-15] Locally, the drug-eluting stents have been shown to be very effective on the treated lesion, effectively reducing the restenotic process and maintaining patency of the treated vessel over the long term. Their use has changed the paradigm for interventional cardiology and has become the standard of practice in most developed countries.

Despite the advances of DES, a number of critical issues remain in the treatment of cardiovascular disease and the current focus on plaques with the largest stenosis. These concerns include not only the cost to the healthcare systems but also, far more importantly, the true overall benefit to the patient with respect to more serious cardiovascular events. Recent evidence suggests that although treatment of the largest lesion is now successful with PTCA and DES, and that the overall event rate including specifically the need for reintervention within the treated vessel is reduced, the more serious events such as

a second MI have not changed dramatically.[16] In addressing this issue, it has recently been documented in patients undergoing PTCA due to an event with plaque rupture that there was evidence of additional ruptures at sites distal to the culprit or stented lesion. Importantly, it is plaque rupture and exposure and release of underlying procoagulant/thrombotic components that appears to be responsible for most acute cardiovascular events. By utilizing intravascular ultrasound (IVUS) in patients undergoing angioplasty for an infarcted artery, Rioufol et al[17] observed distal rupture sites in at least 80% of patients examined. These ruptures typically occurred in plaques that were less than 50% stenosed, and thus their detection would probably have been overlooked by angiography. This finding suggests that treating the culprit lesion alone (as is accomplished with stent therapy) is not sufficient, and that intervention at multiple active lesion sites will be required to reduce secondary events and mortality.

With respect to costs, approximately 2 million PTCA/stent procedures are performed per year today worldwide, with an estimated cost of over $5 billion for the stents alone (>$3000/stented patient). Unfortunately, the expense of DES is an issue of increasing concern, essentially tripling that of bare metal stents. With multiple stents often implanted into individual patents, this change in clinical practice has had a significant impact on healthcare costs.

Finally, in addition to the issues described above for costs and secondary events, treatment is also lacking for many more at-risk patients who cannot undergo successful angioplasty with stents. These patients, who may have either diffuse, non-stentable lesions, bifurcated lesions, multivessel disease (i.e. diabetics), or those who have failed primary angioplasty with stents, are not benefiting as much from DES, and improved treatments here also remain a clear clinical need.

NEEDS BEYOND PTCA AND RESTENOSIS

Cardiovascular disease and vulnerable plaque

The incidence of atherosclerosis, accompanying acute coronary syndromes (ACS), and, specifically, vulnerable plaque remain significant issues, both medically as well as a considerable cost to the healthcare system. With an estimated 180 million individuals affected at various stages of the disease process, clinically symptomatic disease accounts for approximately 34 million patients worldwide.[18] Nearly 2600 Americans die of cardiovascular disease every day, an average of one death every 34 seconds. This accounted for 38.5% of all deaths or one of every 2.6 deaths in the USA in 2001. Additionally, according to the National Heart, Lung, and Blood Institute (NHLBI), the cost to the USA in 2004 was $368 billion for total cardiovascular disease care. When divided between the interrelated cardiovascular diseases (stroke, coronary artery disease, hypertension, and congestive heart failure), costs for coronary atherosclerosis specifically are the largest.

The need for improved therapies for cardiovascular diseases and the rationale for PTCA therapy is based on the underlying pathology of the disease process. Atherosclerosis has been described as a chronic inflammatory syndrome, a systemic disorder typified by focal lesions throughout the vasculature.[19,20] In the past, plaques have been regarded as being inert and remaining almost unchanged for years. However, work over the past two decades demonstrates that plaques are very active entities, and vulnerable plaques – those with the propensity to crack or rupture and initiate vascular events – are sites of intense inflammatory activity.[21,22]

One of the initial signs of atherosclerotic disease is endothelial dysfunction, characterized as such by an inappropriate constrictive response to normally vasodilatory agents (e.g. acetylcholine).[23–25] Additionally, within the focal lesions of atherosclerotic plaque are sites of increased metabolic activity. These regions differ from non-diseased areas and are characterized by the presence and clustering of immune cells such as macrophages and T cells, along with corresponding expression of signaling molecules such as cytokines, chemokines, and degradative enzymes.[26–28] These disease-fighting components are critical for overall health, but locally they strongly contribute to and direct the atherosclerotic process. Inflammation is a key factor in all three phases of the atherosclerotic process:

- lesion initiation (atherogenesis)
- lesion progression
- rupture and thrombosis.

Specifically, it is through the activities of these immune mediators that rupture of the surface of the lesion occurs, leading to occlusion and cardiovascular events.[29–31] Thus, within the metabolically distinct regions of vascular plaque, targeted local regulation of the activities of these mediators holds considerable promise for future treatments.

It has been recognized recently that rupture and infarctions occur in vessels with plaques that are only mildly to moderately obstructed, more often than not, in vessels less than 50% stenotic on angiography.[32–34] Box 26.1 summarized general characterizations of vulnerable plaque. The concept of vulnerable plaque, characterized by a large lipid core with a high content of inflammatory cells and a thin fibrous cap, has received considerable attention.[22,35,36] These lesions, typically only mildly stenotic, can rupture, and are responsible for most acute coronary thrombosis leading to MI.

Often, in vulnerable patients, there is a large systemic plaque burden with multiple focal regions of vulnerable plaque, and thus a need for therapy at multiple sites

Box 26.1 Characterizations of vulnerable plaque

Background
- Myocardial infarctions occur in regions with <50% stenosis
- Vulnerable plaque: large lipid core, high inflammatory cell content, and thin fibrous cap
- Rupture, leading to most acute coronary thrombosis and MI
- Mortality, ACS, and NSTEMI and STEMI remain high

Success
- Benefit to the culprit lesion and has changed interventional cardiology

Issues
- 2 000 000 PTCA/stent procedures, cost of over $5 billion for the stents alone
- More serious events such as a second MI have not changed significantly
- Evidence of additional ruptures distal to culprit or treated lesion
- Ruptures in plaques <50% stenosed and detection would be missed by angiography
- Treatment lacking for more at-risk patients: diffuse, non-stentable, bifurcated lesions, or multivessel disease (i.e. diabetics)

simultaneously. Mortality here remains high, and short of death, rupture of plaques is associated with significant morbidities, including stable and unstable angina as well as non-ST-elevation myocardial infarction (NSTEMI) and ST-elevation myocardial infarction (STEMI).[37,38] Consequently, vulnerable plaques and vulnerable patients, those having a high systemic total plaque burden, remain of substantial concern (Box 26.1).

Based on this information, there is clearly a need for new, targeted, therapies to quiet the local inflammation within the specific areas of disease of the vascular wall, not solely the largest areas of occlusion, as is addressed with PTCA and DES. Such therapy would be of importance for secondary intervention following an initial event as described above, where there is documentation of multiple sites of rupture, for patients with non-stentable, diffuse, or multivessel disease, and potentially for use as primary prevention in those

patients with documented atherosclerotic disease and elevated immune markers (Box 26.1).

Nanoparticle vehicles

Recently, a new focus has emerged on an approach for the site-selective delivery of therapeutic agents to areas of the injured or dysfunctional vascular wall, including vascular segments at risk for restenosis following percutaneous coronary interventions. The technology is not a stent or device approach, but rather a single intravenous infusion that allows for a targeted delivery of compounds to sites of vascular dysfunction or injury. Components of the technology include a combination of known/approved ultrasound contrast vascular imaging agents complexed with therapeutic agents. Ultrasound contrast agents have been used in diagnostic echocardiology for several decades, and use of such agents has been investigated for the transport and delivery of therapeutic agents, and is well reviewed by Bekeredjian et al.[39]

A number of important properties of these nanoparticles make them ideal as targeted delivery vehicles, including:

- increased adherence to damaged vasculature and endothelium
- ability to non-covalently complex selected compounds
- potentiation of compound uptake by cells or tissue.

The most well-studied system and the focus of the present report is the use of perfluorobutane/dextrose/albumin nanoparticles. Drugs can be incorporated into the microbubbles in a number of different ways, including binding of the drug to the microbubble shell and attachment of site-specific ligands. As perfluorocarbon-filled microbubbles are sufficiently stable for circulating in the vasculature as blood pool agents, they act as carriers of these agents until the site of interest is reached.

Albumin/dextran perfluorobutane gas microbubble carriers (PGMCs)

Albumin-coated gas microbubbles do not adhere to normally functioning endothelium. However, adherence does increase considerably to activated or dysfunctional endothelial cells (ECs) or to extracellular matrix of the disrupted vascular wall, an interaction that could be a marker of endothelial integrity.[40] A second interesting feature of these nanoparticles is the ability to non-covalently complex selected compounds to them, thus allowing for the concentration of the compounds on the particles, and potential for transport with them. Thirdly, these nanoparticles have been demonstrated to be taken up by cells of importance to the diseased vasculature, and, also through a cell membrane fluidizing effect, to enhance the transit of compounds to these cells. Thus, theoretically, delivery of drugs or genes bound to albumin-coated microbubbles could be selectively delivered and concentrated at sites of most therapeutic need.[41,42]

Recent evidence suggests that PGMCs (nanoparticles) can be utilized as local delivery vehicles for compounds to regions of injured or diseased vasculature. These particles are routinely used in Europe, South America, and Asia as ultrasound contrast agents in patients, and have been studied extensively. They are prepared as a liquid suspension of microbubbles containing a blood-insoluble gas by mixing 5% human serum albumin and 5% dextrose with decafluorobutane and briefly sonicating to a consistent size. Once formed, the PGMCs are between 0.1 and 10 µm in diameter, are non-toxic, and are gaseous at body temperature with a diffusion coefficient and blood solubility lower than oxygen or nitrogen. Extensive documentation supports the concept that when injected intravenously, these circulating nanoparticles tend to adhere and are retained preferentially to the denuded or dysfunctional luminal surface of the vascular wall.[40,43,44]

Mechanistically, studies support a role for both the endothelium and for leukocytes in nanoparticle retention. In vitro, images obtained on light microscopy illustrate nanoparticle attachment to the surface of activated neutrophils at 3 minutes and phagocytosis of microbubbles by 15 minutes.[45] At 30 minutes, the bubbles were no longer apparent. Villanueva reported that during pathophysiologic states associated with endothelial dysfunction (ED), microbubbles adhere to disrupted vascular endothelium and that this interaction can be used as a marker of endothelial integrity. In a series of studies exploring retention by cultured ECs, they have found that the particles do not adher to normal confluent ECs. However, upon immune activation with phorbol ester, there was enhanced adherence to the cells, and especially to the extracellular matrix produced and exposed under inflammatory conditions. Within the context of vascular disease, nanoparticle adherence to the dysfunctional endothelium occurs mainly due to destruction of the negatively charged glycocalyx protecting the endothelium and binding of microbubbles to activated leukocytes slowly rolling over the damaged endothelial surface.[44]

Numerous in-vivo studies also support selective adherence of microbubbles to damaged or dysfunctional vasculature. Lindner et al found in vivo that microbubbles quickly attach to activated leukocytes that are adherent to the endothelium after ischemia-reperfusion injury and also during tumor necrosis factor-α (TNF-α)-induced inflammation in the mouse.[46] As studied by intravital microscopy, nanoparticle interactions with the few adherent leukocytes were uncommon when observations were made both early (0–2 minutes) and late (15–17 minutes) after their intravenous infusion in control mice. In contrast, treatment with

TNF-α resulted in a far greater number of microbubble (nanoparticle) interactions with the abundant adherent leukocytes at both time points. Microbubbles attached to the leukocyte surface early after injection, and most appeared to be phagocytosed by 15–17 minutes, at which time freely circulating microbubbles were only occasionally observed. This attachment was ascribed to their β₂-integrin- and complement-mediated binding to activated leukocytes adherent to the vascular wall.

In addition, as shown by Lindner et al[45] using ultrasound imaging, the distribution of PGMCs was affected in models of vascular dysfunction or injury, including the hyperlipidemic and injured pig. In the setting of ED induced by hyperlipidemia, Tsutsui et al[40] found in the pig that retention of intravenously injected albumin microbubbles occurs in the setting of both global and regional ED in large vessels. Microbubbles normally pass freely through large and small vessels but are retained in regions with ED. Intravenous albumin-encapsulated microbubbles were administered in seven pigs while imaging the carotid arteries before and after a 20% intralipid infusion to induce hypertriglyceridemia. The degree of microbubble retention was quantified by measuring endothelial acoustic intensity (AI) by ultrasound after clearance of free-flowing microbubbles, and the arterial diameter responses to acetylcholine were quantified. After induction of hypertriglyceridemia, adherence of the microbubbles was visually evident in all carotid arteries, and endothelial AI increased significantly ($P <0.001$ compared with baseline). The arterial responses to acetylcholine went from vasodilation at baseline to vasoconstriction during hypertriglyceridemia. Endothelial AI also increased in balloon-stretched vessels ($P <0.01$ compared with non-injured vessels) after albumin-encapsulated microbubble injection, with a ring of microbubbles selectively adhering to the injured segment, and scanning electron microscopy confirmed that albumin-coated microbubbles adhered to endothelial cells.

Finally, in a study recently completed exploring the mechanism of adherence, fluorescein isothiocyanate-labeled PGMC (PGMC-FITC) nanoparticles were prepared and infused into C57BL/6J mice 24 hours after wire-induced aortic endothelial injury (TR Porter et al, pers comm, 2006). PGMC-FITC microbubbles were attached to the endothelium of injured-aorta mice (Figure 26.1). The number of microbubbles in the different fields was variable, reflecting the heterogeneous

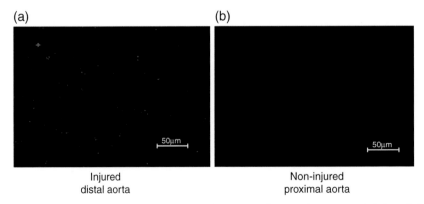

(a)   (b)

Injured
distal aorta

Non-injured
proximal aorta

Figure 26.1   FITC-labeled PESDA microbubbles adhere selectively to the site of mouse aortic injury (left panel). This was not seen in the non-injured proximal aorta of the same mouse (middle panel) or in the injured aorta of a mouse treated with cobra venom factor (right panel) to deplete complement. Scale bar = 50 μm.

pattern of injury caused by the wire. In the non-injured mice, it was reported that there were only isolated PGMC nanoparticles adherent to the aorta-injured endothelium. By quantitative analysis, the number of microbubbles in the injured aorta (31 ± 40 bubbles/field) was significantly higher than in non-injured mice, where only rare bubbles were observed in the proximal non-injured aorta (2 ± 4 bubbles/field; $P < 0.0001$).

Importantly, only rare bubbles were observed in the proximal non-injured aorta, both in the non-CVF (cobra venom factor)-treated (2 ± 4 bubbles/field; $P < 0.001$ vs injured aorta) and in the CVF-treated mice (0 ± 1 bubbles/field; $P < 0.001$ vs injured aorta). Taken together, there is substantial evidence supporting the concept that albumin-containing microbubbles (nanoparticles) can target selectively and be retained in regions of importance to vascular disorders. These regions are characterized by dysfunctional or denuded endothelium where appropriate therapy will have a significant impact on reduction of events. Because these adhered microbubbles retain their acoustic reflectivity, they can be visualized with specialized low mechanical index ultrasound transducers. These transducers have been shown to detect retained albumin microbubbles in the setting of ED produced by either balloon injury (Figure 26.2) or hypertriglyceridemia (Figure 26.3).

DRUGS FOR DELIVERY

A number of therapeutic agents have been explored for incorporation into the nanoparticle delivery vehicle and for efficacy on restenosis. Among the agents chosen are two drugs (sirolimus and paclitaxel) that have previously been demonstrated to be effective on vascular disease, including within the DES paradigm, and a third, antisense to c-myc, with a promising mechanism of action. All three drugs have significant issues (toxicity, stability)

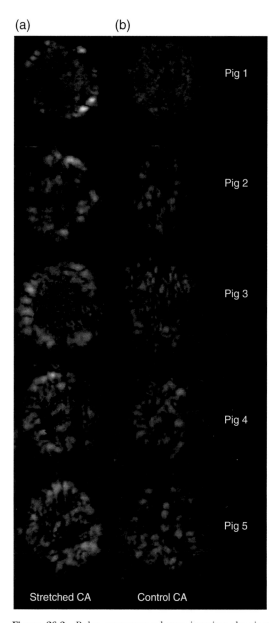

Figure 26.2 Pulse sequence scheme imaging showing microbubble retention to the endothelium in the carotid arteries (CA) submitted to balloon-stretching (a) and absence of retention in the contralateral control vessels (b). In Pig 5 the left CA was initially dissected and the right CA was then submitted to the balloon dilatation and considered for analysis. In this pig, the control demonstrated in the figure is the baseline imaging, before dilatation of the vessel. (Reproduced from Tsutsui et al,[40] with permission.)

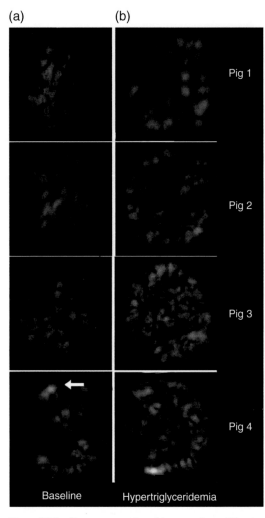

Figure 26.3 Transverse sectional images of carotid arteries obtained with low mechanical index real-time pulse sequence scheme at baseline (a) and during hypertriglyceridemia (b). Note that at baseline there was some adherence of microbubbles to the endothelium only in Pig 4 (arrow) and no adherence in the other pigs. After intralipid infusion we can see microbubbles adherence to the endothelium constituting an echogenic ring around the vessel lumen in all pigs. (Reproduced from Tsutsui et al,[40] with permission.)

upon systemic administration. By combining with the nanoparticle delivery system, with the potential for targeted delivery of these agents to the local site of vascular injury, concerns of systemic liabilities will be minimized. If successful, it is anticipated that this approach will be of benefit

to PTCA, and is reasonable to assume that it can be used in combination with stents (both DES and bare metal) when appropriate. Additionally, the technology has potential for use well beyond PTCA and includes additional indications such as ACS, PAD (peripheral arterial disease), vulnerable plaque, and atherosclerosis.

The feasibility of nanoparticle-mediated site-selective delivery of compounds to injured or dysfunctional regions of the vascular wall has been demonstrated. Recent studies demonstrate that bioactive compounds (i.e. genes, antisense, protein, etc.) as well as small molecules such as sirolimus or paclitaxel can be incorporated into nanoparticles and, with the particles acting as targeting vehicles, be delivered preferentially to sites of vascular injury. As summarized by Feinstein[47] and Bekeredjian et al,[39] preparations of compounds at relatively high concentrations have been incorporated into these nanoparticles using simple and straightforward techniques such as sonication. In addition, as discussed below, studies focused on the delivery of antisense to c-myc or sirolimus undertaken by Kipshidze et al[48] in pigs, or paclitaxel[49] in rabbits, further validate the potential, showing that systemic delivery targeted with PGMC reduced neointimal formation in the porcine coronary restenosis model.

Rapamycin (sirolimus)

Rapamycin is a macrolide antibiotic approved for use as an immunosuppressive agent in the prevention of organ rejection following renal transplantation. Acting through the nuclear cell cycle regulator TOR, the compound has been found to have pleiotropic effects on cellular metabolism and is a novel inhibitor of growth factor- and cytokine-stimulated cell proliferation. Numerous studies have found this compound to be protective against vascular disorders, both in animal models and in patients. As summarized by

Marks,[50] sirolimus has a number of effects of consequence on the processes of restenosis and vascular disease at the molecular level, including the inflammatory response and the proliferative and migratory activity of smooth muscle cells.[51] In-vivo studies have demonstrated the efficacy of rapamycin on vascular disease from a diverse mix of animal models thought to appropriately mimic aspects of human vascular disorders. Initially, Gregory et al[52] demonstrated that rapamycin was a potent inhibitor of the intimal thickening that occurs following balloon injury of the carotid artery in the rat. Subsequent studies by Gallo et al[53] reported that rapamycin significantly reduced the arterial proliferative response after PTCA in the pig. These studies, demonstrating efficacy on induced vascular injury, ultimately led to the development of the CYPHER coronary stent, the first drug (rapamycin)-eluting coronary stent. In addition to induced injury models, Elloso et al[54] and then Basso et al[55] and Waksman et al[56] demonstrated inhibitory effects in the ApoE-deficient mouse model of atherosclerosis by sirolimus on the development and morphology of the plaque, and then, on reduced vascular cholesterol content, and in some of these studies despite an enormous circulating systemic cholesterol load (up to 1300 mg/dl).

In the clinic, the success of the CYPHER-DES for the prevention of restenosis following angioplasty has been well documented.[4,5] By engineering the device to elute rapamycin over a 14-day period,[6] intimal thinking and restenosis formally associated with angioplasty is now reduced to approximately 6% over the long term, and utilization of these drug-eluting devices has brought about a new era in the practice of interventional cardiology. More recently, studies of rapamycin by Ikonen et al[57] in non-human primates have shown lesion inhibition and possibly regression in vascular allograft rejection models, demonstrating efficacy in a severe immune-mediated vascular situation. Finally, clinical studies by Mancini et al[58] and Eisen et al[59] on vasculopathy and also Keogh et al[60] on coronary artery disease undertaken in subjects who have undergone heart transplantation have demonstrated that rapamycin (or analogs) has the ability to maintain patency and potentially reverse stenosis of coronary vessels. Based on the above results, sirolimus would appear to be an ideal candidate as a therapeutic agent for cardiovascular diseases. However, based on its immunosuppressive activity and systemic toxicities, an improved and targeted approach for delivery is required to take full advantage of its potential benefit.

In studies utilizing nanoparticle (PGMC)-based technology in pigs undergoing balloon/stented angioplasty, it has been demonstrated that selective delivery of sirolimus to an injured region of the coronary vasculature could be achieved.[61] In the study by Kipshidze et al, following a single intravenous administration, blood concentrations of sirolimus peaked at 10 minutes and were below the limit of detection after 24 hours. Analysis of balloon-injured coronary vessels showed that sirolimus delivered via PGMCs significantly up-regulates expression of p27, a marker of sirolimus biologic activity, by Western blots in injured areas. Tissue drug concentration from injured arteries showed total sirolimus delivered to the vessel wall at 4 hours was from 169.6 to 240.8 ng per vessel site (note: vessel mass ~40 mg). Drug was homogeneously distributed in the stented areas and in areas adjacent to the stent. Critical to the approach, there was no drug detected in the remote vasculature such as intact coronary or carotid arteries (limit of detection = 0.01 µg/g tissue). Additionally, no drug was detected in injured vessel regions after 72 hours.

As shown in Figure 26.4 and Table 26.1, at 28 days following angioplasty and sirolimus/nanoparticle infusion, there

Table 26.1 Histomorphometry measurements of stented porcine vessels 28 days following implantation of metal stents in treated and control animals

Data at 28 days	Control	Rapamycin	P value
Vessel area (mm²)	9.74 ± 1.26	10.02 ± 2.17	NS
Lumen area (mm²)	3.34 ± 0.72	6.55 ± 2.69	<0.05
Intimal thickness (mm)	0.583 ± 0.207	0.335 ± 0.161	<0.05
IA (mm²)	4.77 ± 1.71	1.84 ± 0.84	<0.001
Media area (mm²)	1.60 ± 0.24	1.62 ± 0.46	NS
Area % occlussion	57.53 ± 13.19	26.13 ± 19.00	<0.05
IS	1.92 ± 0.63	1.75 ± 0.46	NS
IA/IS ratio	2.48 ± 0.67	1.05 ± 0.39	<0.01
Inflammation score	0.67 ± 0.52	0.44 ± 0.13	NS
Intimal vascularity	0.42 ± 0.52	0.38 ± 0.48	NS
Intimal fibrin	0.17 ± 0.14	0.19 ± 0.24	NS
Intimal SMC content	3.00 ± 0.00	3.00 ± 0.00	NS
Adventitial fibrosis	1.17 ± 0.76	0.88 ± 0.25	NS

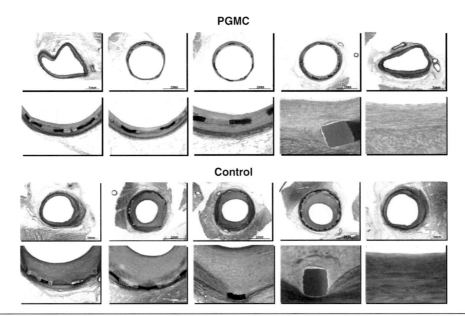

IA, intimal area; IS, injury score; SMC, smooth muscle cell.

was a 40% reduction in neointimal area in treated animals. Control arteries exhibited a substantial neointima consisting mostly of satellite and spindle-shaped cells in a loose extracellular matrix (Figure 26.1). Histopathology showed no difference in endothelialization score, smooth muscle cell (SMC) content, inflammation, or fibrin deposition between groups (Table 26.1). No toxicity or evidence of myocardial damage was seen on gross inspection or after histologic examination of the heart. No thrombosis of treated segments was observed (Figure 26.4).

These studies demonstrated that in the porcine coronary model, site-specific systemic delivery of rapamycin using PGMC resulted in:

- high target vessel tissue concentration of rapamycin
- enhanced local expression of p27
- reduced neointimal formation by 40% at the target site 28 days post procedure.

All these effects provide a solid basis for further preclinical investigation of this novel mode of therapy.

Antisense therapy: antisense for c-myc AVI-4126

Recent advances in gene therapy and molecular biology have enhanced interest in methods of non-invasive or non-systemic delivery of therapeutic agents. However, the clinical applicability of antisense technology has been limited as a result of a relative lack of target specificity, slow uptake across the cell membranes, and rapid intracellular degradation of the oligonucleotide. It has already been demonstrated that perfluorocarbon-filled albumin nanoparticles avidly bind proteins and synthetic oligonucleotides.[48,62,63] In a similar way, these particles can directly take up genetic material, such as plasmids and adenovirus, suggesting a potential for protection of the material and targeted delivery via nanoparticles.

As discussed, restenosis after vascular balloon injury or stent deployment has been shown to result from neointimal hyperplasia due to smooth muscle cell migration and proliferation. The c-myc proto-oncogene is responsible for the regulation of gene expression involved in the process of intimal hyperplasia that leads to restenosis. Synthetic antisense oligonucleotides, such as those to the c-myc proto-oncogene, can bind to the messenger ribonucleic acid (mRNA) and inhibit the synthesis of the proto-oncogenes. Therefore, antisense to c-myc proto-oncogene can prevent its translation into proteins that may be mediators of the pathologic process of restenosis. In testing these hypotheses, the c-myc antisense phosphorodiamidate morpholino oligomer AVI-4126, was bound to PGMCs and injected systemically into pigs and assessed for activity on expression of c-myc in vascular tissue and restenosis after stent implantation.

The effect of the nanoparticle-based systemic delivery of antisense to c-myc on neointimal hyperplasia after 28 days in a swine stent restenosis model was investigated. High-performance liquid chromatography (HPLC) analysis of plasma samples of treated animals showed minimal presence of AVI-4126. However, analysis (HPLC) of stented vessel tissue showed delivery of AVI-4126 at 4 hours. Western blot analysis demonstrated that stent implantation led to activation of the c-myc oncogene. However, when an AVI-4126-loaded stent was implanted, there was significant inhibition of c-myc expression by Western blot analysis of the vessel tissue. Morphometry showed that the neointimal area was significantly reduced in the AVI-4126 PGMC group compared with control (2.63 ± 1.99 vs 4.77 ± 1.71 mm^2, respectively, P <0.05). The quantitative histomorphometry demonstrated a statistically significant reduction of IA (intimal area), and IA normalized to injury score (IA/IS) following treatment. There was also a significant difference in the lumen area between the antisense-treated and the controls; thus, similar to the sirolimus delivery via nanoparticles, systemic targeted delivery of AVI-4126 using PGMC carrier significantly inhibited neointimal formation in the porcine coronary stent model.

Paclitaxel

Paclitaxel, a potent antineoplastic drug, interferes with the assembly of microtubules and thus interferes with cell migration and replication. It has been shown to be effective on mechanisms of restenosis, but as a chemotherapeutic agent with significant systemic toxicities, it is best administered locally for cardiovascular uses. Success has been achieved with local delivery on a DES, which facilitates therapeutic concentrations of the drug without the risk of systemic toxicity.[64] However, paclitaxel-eluting stents in animals cause incomplete healing and, in some instances, a lack of sustained suppression of neointimal growth.[65]

The efficacy of paclitaxel as delivered on an albumin-stabilized systemic delivery nanoparticle for reducing in-stent restenosis was tested in rabbits.[56] New Zealand White rabbits receiving bilateral iliac artery stents were administered paclitaxal as a 10-minute intra-arterial infusion. Pharmacokinetics showed a biphasic profile, with an initial rapid decline in concentration followed by a slower elimination phase. Whole blood concentrations were maximal at 15 minutes after infusion and ranged from 3.0 to 5.0 μmol/L. At 24 and 48 hours, blood levels were approximately 0.1 μmol/L. The total arterial tissue level of paclitaxel in the stented segments at 48 hours was 1.7 ± 0.1 μg/mg of tissue. At 28 days, mean neointimal thickness was reduced, with evidence of delayed healing. The efficacy of a single dose, however, was lost by 90 days. In contrast, a second repeat dose given 28 days after stenting resulted in sustained suppression of neointimal thickness at 90 days and nearly complete neointimal healing. Thus, this formulation of paclitaxel may allow adjustment of dose at the stent treatment site and prove to be a useful adjunct for the clinical prevention of in-stent restenosis.

CONCLUSIONS

Despite important pharmacologic and interventional strategies to treat atherosclerotic vascular disease, it remains a serious clinical problem today. Intravenous microbubbles have been developed which can be used to detect where endothelial dysfunction exists, and which can be targeted to detect inflammatory and prothrombotic mediators on the plaque surface. These same microbubbles can then be used for site-specific delivery of agents that inhibit plaque progression. These novel diagnostic and treatment strategies have the potential to significantly alter patient outcomes in atherosclerotic vascular disease.

REFERENCES

1. Fischman DL, Leon MB, Baim DS et al. A randomized comparison of coronary stent placement and balloon angioplasty in the treatment of coronary artery disease. Stent Restenosis Study Investigators. N Engl J Med 1994; 331:496–501.
2. Serruys PW, de Jaegere P, Kiemeneij F et al. A comparison of balloon-expandable stent implantation with balloon angioplasty in patients with coronary artery disease. Benestent Study Group. N Engl J Med 1994; 331:489–95.
3. Edelman ER, Rogers C. Pathobiologic responses to stenting. Am J Cardiol 1998; 81:4–6E.
4. Morice MC, Serruys PW, Sousa JE et al. A randomized comparison of a sirolimus-eluting stent with a standard stent for coronary revascularization. N Engl J Med 2002; 346:1773–80.
5. Moses JW, Leon MB, Popma JJ et al. Sirolimus-eluting stents versus standard stents in patients with stenosis in a native coronary artery. N Engl J Med 2003; 349:1315–23.
6. Klugherz BD, Llanos G, Lieuallen W et al. Twenty-eight-day efficacy and pharmacokinetics of the sirolimus-eluting stent. Coron Artery Dis 2002; 13(3):183–8.
7. Herdeg C, Oberhoff M, Baumbach A et al. Local paclitaxel delivery for the prevention of restenosis: biological effects and efficacy in vivo. J Am Coll Cardiol 2000; 35(7):1969–76.
8. Suzuki T, Kopia G, Hayashi S et al. Stent-based delivery of sirolimus reduces neointimal formation in a porcine coronary model. Circulation 2001; 104(10):1188–93.
9. Drachman DE, Edelman ER, Seifert P et al. Neointimal thickening after stent delivery of paclitaxel: change in composition and arrest of growth over six months. J Am Coll Cardiol 2000; 36:2325–32.

10. Hiatt BL, Carter AJ, Yeung AC. The drug-eluting stent: is it the Holy Grail? Rev Cardiovasc Med 2001; 2(4):190–6.

11. Morice MC, Serruys PW, Sousa JE et al; RAVEL Study Group. Randomized Study with the Sirolimus-Coated Bx Velocity Balloon-Expandable Stent in the Treatment of Patients with de Novo Native Coronary Artery Lesions. A randomized comparison of a sirolimus-eluting stent with a standard stent for coronary revascularization. N Engl J Med 2002; 346(23): 1773–80.

12. Kipshidze NN, Tsapenko MV, Leon MB, Stone GW, Moses JW. Update on drug-eluting coronary stents. Expert Rev Cardiovasc Ther 2005; 3:953–68.

13. Fajadet J, Morice MC, Bode C, Barragan P et al. Maintenance of long-term clinical benefit with sirolimus-eluting coronary stents: three-year results of the RAVEL trial. Circulation 2005; 111(8):1040–4.

14. Dibra A, Kastrati A, Mehilli J et al; ISAR-DIABETES Study Investigators. Paclitaxel-eluting or sirolimus-eluting stents to prevent restenosis in diabetic patients. N Engl J Med 2005; 353(7):663–70.

15. Windecker S, Remondino A, Eberli FR et al. Sirolimus-eluting and paclitaxel-eluting stents for coronary revascularization. N Engl J Med 2005; 18;353(7):653–62.

16. Moses JW, Stone GW, Nikolsky E et al. Drug-eluting stents in the treatment of intermediate lesions: pooled analysis from four randomized trials. J Am Coll Cardiol 2006; 47(11):2164–71.

17. Rioufol G, Finet G, Ginon I et al. Multiple atherosclerotic plaque rupture in acute coronary syndrome: a three-vessel intravascular ultrasound study. Circulation 2002; 106:804–8.

18. American Heart Association Statistics, 2005.

19. Ross R. Atherosclerosis – an inflammatory disease. N Engl J Med 1999; 340:115–26.

20. Libby P, Ridker PM, Maseri A. Inflammation and atherosclerosis. Circulation 2002; 105:1135–43.

21. Hansson GK. Inflammation, atherosclerosis, and coronary artery disease. N Engl J Med 2005; 352:1685–95.

22. Naghavi M, Libby P, Falk E et al. From vulnerable plaque to vulnerable patient: a call for new definitions and risk assessment strategies: Part I. Circulation 2003; 108(14):1664–72.

23. Drexler H, Zeiher AM. Progression of coronary endothelial dysfunction in man and its potential clinical significance. Basic Res Cardiol 1991; 86(Suppl 2): 223–32.

24. el-Tamimi H, Mansour M, Wargovich TJ et al. Constrictor and dilator responses to intracoronary acetylcholine in adjacent segments of the same coronary artery in patients with coronary artery disease. Endothelial function revisited. Circulation 1994; 89(1):45–51.

25. Reddy KG, Nair RN, Sheehan HM, Hodgson JM. Evidence that selective endothelial dysfunction may occur in the absence of angiographic or ultrasound atherosclerosis in patients with risk factors for atherosclerosis. J Am Coll Cardiol 1994; 23(4):833–43.

26. Sheikine Y, Hansson GK. Chemokines and atherosclerosis. Ann Med 2004; 36(2):98–118.

27. Lucas AD, Greaves DR. Atherosclerosis: role of chemokines and macrophages. Expert Rev Mol Med 2001; 2001:1–18.

28. Stemme S, Hansson GK. Immune mechanisms in atherogenesis. Ann Med 1994; 26(3):141–6.

29. Corti R, Hutter R, Badimon JJ, Fuster V. Evolving concepts in the triad of atherosclerosis, inflammation and thrombosis. J Thromb Thrombolysis 2004; 17(1):35–44.

30. Ito T, Ikeda U. Inflammatory cytokines and cardiovascular disease. Curr Drug Targets Inflamm Allergy 2003; 2(3):257–65.

31. Young JL, Libby P, Schonbeck U. Cytokines in the pathogenesis of atherosclerosis. Thromb Haemost 2002; 88(4):554–67.

32. Hausmann D, Johnson JA, Sudhir K et al. Angiographically silent atherosclerosis detected by intravascular ultrasound in patients with familial hypercholesterolemia and familial combined hyperlipidemia: correlation with high density lipoproteins. J Am Coll Cardiol 1996; 27:1562–70.

33. Schoenhagen P, Nissen SE. Assessing coronary plaque burden and plaque vulnerability: atherosclerosis imaging with IVUS and emerging noninvasive modalities. Am Heart Hosp J 2003; 1(2):164–9.

34. Schoenhagen P, McErlean ES, Nissen SE. The vulnerable coronary plaque. J Cardiovasc Nurs 2000; 15:1–12.

35. Schroeder AP, Falk E. Vulnerable and dangerous coronary plaques. Atherosclerosis 1995; 118(Suppl): S141–9.

36. Vink A, Schoneveld AH, Richard W et al. Plaque burden, arterial remodeling and plaque vulnerability: determined by systemic factors? J Am Coll Cardiol 2001; 38(3):718–23.

37. Virmani R, Burke AP, Farb A, Kolodgie FD. Pathology of the vulnerable plaque. J Am Coll Cardiol 2006; 47(8 Suppl):C13–18.

38. Klein LW. Clinical implications and mechanisms of plaque rupture in the acute coronary syndromes. Am Heart Hosp J 2005; 3(4):249–55.

39. Bekeredjian R, Grayburn PA, Shohet RV. Use of ultrasound contrast agents for gene or drug delivery in cardiovascular medicine. J Am Coll Cardiol 2005; 45(3):329–35.

40. Tsutsui JM, Xie F, Cano M et al. Detection of retained microbubbles in carotid arteries with real-time low mechanical index imaging in the setting of endothelial dysfunction. J Am Coll Cardiol 2004; 44(5): 1036–46.

41. Tsutsui JM, Xie F, Porter RT. The use of microbubbles to target drug delivery. Cardiovasc Ultrasound 2004; 2(1):23.

42. Villanueva FS, Jankowski RJ, Manaugh C, Wagner WR. Albumin microbubble adherence to human coronary endothelium: implications for assessment of endothelial function using myocardial contrast echocardiography. J Am Coll Cardiol 1997; 30: 689–93.

43. Villanueva FS, Wagner WR, Vannan MA, Narula J. Targeted ultrasound imaging using microbubbles. Cardiol Clin 2004; 22(2):283–98.

44. Lindner JR, Ismail S, Spotnitz WD et al. Albumin microbubble persistence during myocardial contrast echocardiography is associated with microvascular endothelial glycocalyx damage. Circulation 1998; 98(20):2187–94.

45. Lindner JR, Dayton PA, Coggins MP et al. Noninvasive imaging of inflammation by ultrasound detection of phagocytosed microbubbles. Circulation 2000; 102(5):531–8.

46. Lindner JR, Coggins MP, Kaul S et al. Microbubble persistence in the microcirculation during ischemia/ reperfusion and inflammation is caused by integrin- and complement-mediated adherence to activated leukocytes. Circulation 2000; 101:668–75.

47. Feinstein SB. The powerful microbubble: from bench to bedside, from intravascular indicator to therapeutic delivery system, and beyond. Am J Physiol Heart Circ Physiol 2004; 287(2):H450–7.

48. Kipshidze NN, Porter TR, Dangas G et al. Systemic targeted delivery of antisense with perflourobutane gas microbubble carrier reduced neointimal formation in the porcine coronary restenosis model. Cardiovasc Radiat Med 2003; 4(3):152–9.

49. Kolodgie FD, John M, Khurana C et al. Sustained reduction of in-stent neointimal growth with the use of a novel systemic nanoparticle paclitaxel. Circulation 2002; 106(10):1195–8.

50. Marks A. Sirolimus for the prevention of in-stent restenosis in a coronary artery. N Engl J Med 2003; 349(14):1307–9.

51. Marx SO, Jayaraman T, Go LO, Marks AR. Rapamycin-FKBP inhibits cell cycle regulators of proliferation in vascular smooth muscle cells. Circ Res 1995; 76:412–17.

52. Gregory CR, Huie P, Billingham ME et al. Rapamycin inhibits arterial intimal thickening caused by both alloimmune and mechanical injury. Transplantation 1993; 55:1409–18.

53. Gallo R, Padurean A, Jayaraman T et al. Inhibition of intimal thickening after balloon angioplasty in porcine coronary arteries by targeting regulators of the cell cycle. Circulation 1999; 99:2164–70.

54. Elloso MM, Azrolan N, Sehgal SN et al. Protective effect of the immunosuppressant sirolimus against aortic atherosclerosis in apo E-deficient mice. Am J Transplant 2003; 3(5):562–9.

55. Basso M, Nambi P, Adelman SJ. Effect of sirolimus on the cholesterol content of aortic arch in ApoE knock-out mice. Transplant Proc 2003; 35:3136–8.

56. Waksman R, Burnett MS, Gulick CP et al. Oral rapamycin inhibits growth of atherosclerotic plaque in apoE knock-out mice. Cardiovasc Radiat Med 2003; 4(1):34–8.

57. Ikonen TS, Gummert JF, Hayase M et al. Sirolimus (rapamycin) halts and reverses progression of allograft vascular disease in non-human primates. Transplantation 2000; 70:969–75.

58. Mancini D, Pinney S, Burkhoff D et al. Use of rapamycin slows progression of cardiac transplantation vasculopathy. Circulation 2003; 108(1):48–53.

59. Eisen H, Kobashigawa J, Starling RC, Valantine H, Mancini D. Improving outcomes in heart transplantation: the potential of proliferation signal inhibitors. Transplant Proc 2005; 37(4 Suppl):4–17S.

60. Keogh A, Richardson M, Ruygrok P et al. Sirolimus in de novo heart transplant recipients reduces acute rejection and prevents coronary artery disease at 2 years: a randomized clinical trial. Circulation 2004; 110(17):2694–700.

61. Kipshidze NN, Porter TR, Dangas G et al. Novel site-specific systemic delivery of Rapamycin with perfluorobutane gas microbubble carrier reduced neointimal formation in a porcine coronary restenosis model. Catheter Cardiovasc Interv 2005; 64(3):389–94.

62. Porter TR, Hiser WL, Kricsfeld D et al. Inhibition of carotid artery neointimal formation with intravenous microbubbles. Ultrasound Med Biol 2001; 27(2): 259–65.

63. Porter TR, Xie F, Knapp D et al. Targeted vascular delivery of antisense molecules using intravenous microbubbles. Cardiovasc Revasc Med 2006; 7(1): 25–33.

64. Grube E, Bullesfeld L. Initial experience with paclitaxel-coated stents. J Interv Cardiol 2002; 15(6): 471–5.

65. Farb A, Heller PF, Shroff S et al. Pathological analysis of local delivery of paclitaxel via a polymer-coated stent. Circulation 2001; 104(4):473–9.

Multislice computed tomography coronary plaque imaging

27

Pim J de Feyter, A Weustink, WB Meijboom, Nico Mollet, and Filippo Cademartiri

INTRODUCTION

The newest generation 64-slice multislice computed tomography (MSCT) allows fast high-resolution imaging of the coronary arteries. MSCT is a tomographic imaging technique and thus provides information about the lumen and wall (plaque) of the coronary arteries. MSCT coronary imaging can be performed in two modes:

- the non-contrast enhanced MSCT mode, which is used for calcium scoring
- the contrast-enhanced MSCT mode, which allows imaging of both non-obstructive and obstructive plaques.[1]

MSCT provides the unique opportunity to non-invasively assess the coronary plaque burden defined as the presence, distribution, and composition of coronary plaques and in addition to evaluate the severity of a luminal stenosis. The clinical and prognostic importance of these findings is currently the topic of many future studies.

CORONARY CALCIFICATION

Since the early 1990s, electron beam computed tomography (EBCT) has been used for the detection and quantification of coronary calcium.[2] Comparative histologic and ultrasound studies have shown that the presence of coronary calcium is almost always associated with the presence of coronary atherosclerosis.[3,4] The amount of coronary calcium is directly related to the extent of the total underlying atherosclerotic plaque burden, although the amount of calcium underestimates the total plaque burden. The absence of coronary calcium does not always exclude the presence of a non-calcified coronary plaque, although the likelihood of such a plaque is very low. In particular, in young patients at high risk, non-calcific plaques may develop and rarely progress to an adverse cardiac event. The prevalence and amount of calcium increase with age in both men and women, but calcifications occur almost 10 years earlier in men, and the calcium score is significantly higher in men (Table 27.1).[5]

Coronary calcium causes high X-ray attenuation and is relatively easily detected by CT. Initially, EBCT was used to detect and quantify coronary calcium and recently spiral CT has also been used for calcium quantification. Agatston et al developed a calcium score based on the product of area and maximal CT density value of the calcium deposits.[2] The Agatston calcium score is now widely used in studies evaluating the predictive value of calcium in asymptomatic individuals.

Earlier large-scale long-term studies have shown that the age- and gender-adjusted calcium score in asymptomatic subjects is highly correlated with the occurrence of adverse cardiovascular events.[6–10]

There has been a debate about the incremental predictive value of the calcium score in addition to the traditional risk factors.

Table 27.1   EBCT calcium score percentiles for 25 251 men and 9995 women within age strata

Calcium score percentiles	Age (years)								
	<40	40–44	45–49	50–54	55–59	60–64	65–69	70–74	>74
Men (N)	3504	4238	4940	4825	3472	2288	1209	540	235
25th percentile	0	0	0	1	4	13	32	64	166
50th percentile	1	1	3	15	48	113	180	310	473
75th percentile	3	9	36	103	215	410	566	892	1071
90th percentile	14	59	154	332	554	994	1299	1774	1982
Women (N)	641	1024	1634	2184	1835	1334	731	438	174
25th percentile	0	0	0	0	0	0	1	3	9
50th percentile	0	0	0	0	1	3	24	52	75
75th percentile	1	1	2	5	23	57	145	210	241
90th percentile	3	4	22	55	121	193	410	631	709

Reprinted from Hoff et al,[5] with permission.
EBCT, electron beam computed tomography.

Several important recent studies have demonstrated that the coronary calcium score is a significant predictor of hard endpoints, all-cause mortality[11] (Table 27.2), or the combination of cardiovascular death and non-fatal myocardial infarction[12] (Table 27.3). This relation was also present in elderly individuals[13] (Table 27.4). In addition, these studies demonstrated that the calcium score offered incremental, predictive value to the predictive value derived from traditional risk factors such as the Framingham score.[11,13]

The role of detection and quantification of coronary calcium in the general population remains a matter of debate. It is now believed that calcium scoring may be useful to reclassify an asymptomatic group of individuals at intermediate risk who have a high calcium score to a high-risk group with subsequent intensive risk factor modification with medical intervention, and those with a negative or low calcium score to a low-risk group in which general lifestyle modification would suffice.[14–16]

Table 27.2   Value of calcium score to predict all-cause mortality in asymptomatic patients

Calcium score	Number of patients	All-cause mortality (%)	Relative risk ratio	Adjusted relative risk
≤10	5.946	1.0 (62)	–	–
11–100	2.044	2.6 (53)	2.47 (1.71; 3.58)	1.64 (1.12; 2.41)
101–400	1.432	3.8 (54)	3.55 (2.46; 5.13)	1.74 (1.16; 2.61)
401–1000	623	6.3 (39)	6.15 (4.11; 9.21)	2.54 (1.62; 3.99)
>1000	332	12.3 (41)	12.3 (8.28; 18.23)	4.03 (2.52; 6.40)

Reprinted from Shaw et al,[11] with permission.
Follow-up = 5 years; mean age = 53 ± 0.1 years (30–85 years); male = 60%; total number of patients = 10.377; 5-year mortality rate = 2.4%.
High rate of self-reported risk factors (72% with two or more risk factors).

Table 27.3 Value of calcium score to predict non-fatal myocordial infarction (MI) and coronary death in asymptomatic adults with coronary risk factors

Calcium score	Events % (MI = 68; death 16)	Hazard ratio (95% CI)
0	4.4 (316)	1.0
1–100	6.5 (321)	1.5 (0.7; 2.9)
101–300	8.8 (171)	2.1 (1.0; 4.3)
>301	15.4 (221)	3.9 (2.1; 7.3)

Follow-up = median 7.0 years; number of patients (NP) = 1029; age = 65.7 (7.8) years; male = 90%.
Reprinted from Greenland,[12] with permission.

CONTRAST-ENHANCED COMPUTED TOMOGRAPHY: CORONARY IMAGING

Current 64-slice MSCT scanners generate high-quality nearly motion-free coronary images at an isotropic spatial resolution of 0.4 mm^3. The tomographic CT coronary images provide information not only about the lumen contour similar to coronary angiography but also about the vessel wall, plaque size, vessel architecture, and composition of plaques similar to intracoronary ultrasound.

MSCT coronary angiography

Contrast-enhanced 64-slice MSCT coronary angiography has a high diagnostic accuracy to detect significant coronary lumen narrowings, as has been reported in four recently published studies.[17–20] The weighted sensitivity, specificity, and negative and positive predictive values were 93%, 96%, 78%, and 99%, respectively (Table 27.5). These data show that current 64-slice MSCT scanners are close to becoming a reliable alternative to invasive diagnostic coronary angiography, and that the time has come for MSCT to slowly enter the phase of clinical acceptance, pending the outcome of MSCT multicenter studies performed in a wide spectrum of patients with suspected or known coronary artery disease.

MSCT coronary plaque imaging

CT imaging of coronary atherosclerotic plaques is even more challenging than visualization of the coronary lumen owing to the smaller dimensions of coronary plaques and the smaller difference between the CT density of non-calcified coronary plaques, adventitial and pericoronary fat tissue.[21]

The diagnostic accuracy of MSCT for identifying non-obstructive coronary plaques with intravascular ultrasound (IVUS) as the standard of reference is reported as between 53% and 95%, depending on the composition of the plaque[22–24] (Table 27.6). Owing to the high density of calcific deposits, the sensitivity of detecting calcific plaques, including the small-sized calcific plaques, is higher. Obviously, with the limited resolution of

Table 27.4 Value of calcium score to predict non-fatal myocardial infarction (MI)/death or total mortality

Calcium score	NP	Non-fatal MI/death NP	RR (95% CI)	Total mortality NP	RR (95% CI)
0–100	905	6	1.0 (reference)	29	1.0 (reference)
101–400	425	10	2.8 (1.0; 7.8)	35	1.9 (1.2; 3.2)
401–1000	269	10	3.9 (1.4; 11.1)	30	2.4 (1.4; 4.2)
>1000	196	14	7.5 (2.8; 20.2)	24	2.7 (1.5; 4.7)

Reprinted from Vliegenthart et al,[13] with permission.
Follow-up = 3.3 ± 0.8 years; mean age = 71.1 ± 5.7 years; male = 43%; total number of patients (NP) = 1795 individuals; RR = relative risk.

Table 27.5   Diagnostic performance of 64-MSCT for detection of significant coronary stenosis (luminal diameter > 50%) segmental analysis

Author	Year	NP	Excluded segments (%)	Sensitivity (%)	Specificity (%)	PPV (%)	NPV (%)
Leschka[17]	2005	67	0	94	95	88	98
Leber[18]	2005	55*	0	76	97	75	97
Raff[19]	2005	70	12	86	95	66	99
Mollet[20]	2005	51	0	99	95	76	99
Total (weighted)		243	4	93	96	78	99

* 4 patients were excluded.
NP, number of patients; PPV, positive predictive value; NPV, negative predictive value.

MSCT, the size of plaques that were not detected by MSCT was obviously smaller. The plaque thickness of detected plaques was 1.5 ± 0.3 mm vs not-detected plaques 0.9 ± 0.3 mm.[22] The plaque volume of detected plaques was 76 ± 10 mm^3 vs 47 ± 11 mm^3 of not-detected plaques.[23] The diagnostic accuracy of detecting non-calcific plaques with the 64-slice MSCT scanner appears to be better compared than with the 16-slice MSCT scanner.

MSCT systematically and significantly underestimated plaque volume compared with intracoronary ultrasound: 24 ± 35 mm^3 and 43 ± 60 mm^3 ($P<0.001$), respectively.[23] The mean plaque cross-sectional area was 8.1 ± 3.8 mm^2 vs 7.3 ± 5.1 mm^2.[22]

Coronary plaques were detected in virtually all symptomatic patients who had undergone invasive diagnostic coronary angiography.[24,25] The frequency of calcific plaques was highest, and was reported as between 56% and 79% (Table 27.7).

The MSCT plaque burden was assessed in 78 patients by determining the number of diseased coronary segments, the distribution of plaques in the coronary tree, the composition of the plaque (calcified, non-calcified, or mixed plaque), and whether a plaque was obstructive or non-obstructive (Figure 27.1).[26] These data show that coronary atherosclerosis is present in the majority of proximal and mid coronary segments, and much less present in the distal coronary segments.

Table 27.6   Diagnostic accuracy of MSCT for detecting plaques

IVUS plaque	MSCT plaque	16-slice MSCT		64-slice MSCT
		Leber[22] sensitivity %	Achenbach[23] sensitivity %	Leber[24] sensitivity %
Any plaque	Any plaque	82 (299/350)	86 (41/50)	84(46/55)
Hypo-/hyperechoic	Non-calcific	78 (149/192)	53 (8/15)	n.a.
Calcific	Calcific	95 (150/158)	92 (33/36)	n.a.
		Specificity %	Specificity %	Specificity %
		92 (484/525)	88 (29/33)	91 (39/43)

Table 27.7 Prevalence of MSCT coronary plaques

	Stable agina[24] (N = 19)	Acute MI[24] (N = 21)	Symptomatic patients[25] (N = 179)
Calcific plaques	79	56	73
Non-calcific plaques	7	24	27
Mixed plaque	13	18	–

It remains to be established whether the MSCT plaque burden imparts an incremental predictive value in addition to the calcium score and traditional risk factors. MSCT high-quality coronary imaging allows assessment of coronary remodeling of diseased coronary segments, which may provide additional information about the propensity of a plaque to rupture. It was shown that MSCT is able to detect both positive remodeling and negative remodeling.[27] This non-invasive information may be helpful to further optimize strategies to treat significant coronary lesions.

A recent study using intracoronary ultrasound as a reference reported that 64-slice CT underestimated the volume of mixed and non-calcified plaques, with overestimation of calcified plaque volume.[28] A non-calcified plaque was correctly identified in 83% of cases, a mixed plaque in 94%, and calcified plaques in 95%.[28]

MSCT IDENTIFICATION OF HIGH-RISK PLAQUES

The identification of a high-risk plaque is currently the subject of intense debate and research. Non-invasive detection of

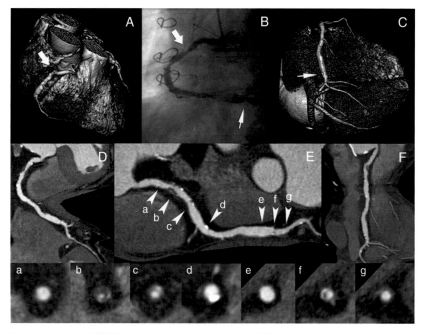

Figure 27.1 Volume-rendered MSCT coronary artery image (A and C) provides a three-dimensional overview of the right coronary artery (RCA), showing a significant lesion in RCA 1 (thick arrow) and a dilated segment RCA 3 with distally an intermediate lesion (thin arrow), which is confirmed with conventional coronary angiography (B). Three orthogonal curved multiplanar reconstructions (D–F) display the RCA throughout the right atrial–ventricular groove. Cross-sectional images clarify the different types of plaque distribution. A normal lumen (a) precedes the non-calcified significant lesion (b) in RCA 1, with distally a mixed non-significant plaque (c), a calcified non-significant plaque (d) in RCA 2, and in the distal segment a dilated vessel (e), a mixed intermediate lesion (f), and a non-significant non-calcified plaque (g) before the crux.

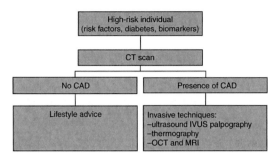

Figure 27.2   Role of MSCT in the detection of coronary plaque. CT, computed tomography; CAD, coronary artery disease; IVUS, intravascular ultrasound; OCT, optical coherence tomography; MRI, magnetic resonance imaging.

a high-risk plaque would be highly desirable and contrast-enhanced MSCT may be helpful in identifying a high-risk plaque. MSCT may play a significant role in the early detection of atherosclerosis (Box 27.1 and Figure 27.2). The calcium score and, potentially, also the total plaque burden may independently (of the traditional risk factors) identify patients at high risk. MSCT allows non-invasive interrogation of the entire coronary tree and thus is able to identify plaques in the high risk proximal and mid coronary segments which are prone to thrombotic occlusions causing acute myocardial infarction.[26] In particular, identification of atherosclerosis in the left main and proximal left anterior

descending coronary artery may be useful because these segments carry an important risk of mortality and morbidity. MSCT may reveal several high-risk plaque characteristics, including non-calcified plaque size (lipid pool?), positive remodeling, localization in high-risk coronary segment, and obstructive nature of plaque.

Most importantly, absence of any detectable coronary atherosclerosis may be associated with an excellent prognosis, whereas presence and extent of coronary atherosclerosis may identify patients who should undergo further intensive investigation with intracoronary techniques to identify a high-risk plaque. Obviously, this approach requires further prospective studies, which are currently being designed.

Box 27.1   Role of MSCT in early detection of coronary atherosclerosis

High-risk patient
Calcium score
Total plaque burden

High-risk coronary tree
Identification of plaques in proximal/mid coronary segments

High-risk coronary plaque
Non-calcified plaque
Large-size plaque
Remodeling
Located in high-risk coronary segments (proximal/mid)
Obstructive plaque

REFERENCES

1. De Feyter PJ, Krestin GP, Cademartiri F, Mollet NRA, Nieman K. Computed Tomography of the Coronary Arteries. London: Taylor & Francis, 2005.
2. Agatston AS, Janowitz WR, Hildner FJ et al. Quantification of coronary artery calcium using ultrafast computed tomography. J Am Coll Cardiol 1990; 15(4):827–32.
3. Rumberger JA, Simons DB, Fitzpatrick LA, Sheedy PF, Schwartz RS. Coronary artery calcium area by electron-beam computed tomography and coronary atherosclerotic plaque area. A histopathologic correlative study. Circulation 1995; 92(8):2157–62.
4. Sangiorgi G, Rumberger JA, Severson A et al. Arterial calcification and not lumen stenosis is highly correlated with atherosclerotic plaque burden in humans: a histologic study of 723 coronary artery segments using nondecalcifying methodology. J Am Coll Cardiol 1998; 31(1):126–33.
5. Hoff JA, Chomka EV, Krainik AJ et al. Age and gender distributions of coronary artery calcium detected by electron beam tomography in 35, 246 adults. Am J Cardiol 2001; 87(12):1335–9.
6. Wong ND, Hsu JC, Detrano RC et al. Coronary artery calcium evaluation by electron beam computed tomography and its relation to new cardiovascular events. Am J Cardiol 2000; 86(5):495–8.
7. Arad Y, Spadaro LA, Goodman K, Newstein D, Guerci AD. Prediction of coronary events with electron beam computed tomography. J Am Coll Cardiol 2000; 36(4):1253–60.
8. Detrano RC, Wong ND, Doherty TM et al. Coronary calcium does not accurately predict near-term future coronary events in high-risk adults. Circulation 1999;

99(20):2633–8. Erratum in Circulation 2000; 101(11): 1355. Circulation 2000; 101(6):697.

9. Raggi P, Callister TQ, Cooil B et al. Identification of patients at increased risk of first unheralded acute myocardial infarction by electron-beam computed tomography. Circulation 2000; 101(8):850–5.

10. Kondos GT, Hoff JA, Sevrukov A et al. Electron-beam tomography coronary artery calcium and cardiac events: a 37-month follow-up of 5635 initially asymptomatic low- to intermediate-risk adults. Circulation 2003; 107(20):2571–6.

11. Shaw LJ, Raggi P, Schisterman E, Berman DS, Callister TQ. Prognostic value of cardiac risk factors and coronary artery calcium screening for all-cause mortality. Radiology 2003; 228(3):826–33.

12. Greenland P, LaBree L, Azen SP, Doherty TM, Detrano RC. Coronary artery calcium score combined with Framingham score for risk prediction in asymptomatic individuals. JAMA 2004; 291(2):210–15.

13. Vliegenthart R, Oudkerk M, Hofman A et al. Coronary calcification improves cardiovascular risk prediction in the elderly. Circulation 2005; 112(4): 572–7.

14. O'Rourke RA, Brundage BH, Froelicher VF et al. American College of Cardiology/American Heart Association Expert Consensus document on electron-beam computed tomography for the diagnosis and prognosis of coronary artery disease. Circulation 2000; 102(1):126–40.

15. Expert Panel on Detection, Evaluation, and Treatment of High Blood Cholesterol in Adults. Executive Summary of the Third Report of the National Cholesterol Education Program (NCEP) Expert Panel on Detection, Evaluation, and Treatment of High Blood Cholesterol in Adults (Adult Treatment Panel III). JAMA 2001; 285:2486–97.

16. Smith SC Jr, Greenland P, Grundy SM. AHA Conference Proceedings. Prevention conference V: Beyond secondary prevention: Identifying the high-risk patient for primary prevention: executive summary. American Heart Association. Circulation 2000; 101(1):111–16.

17. Leschka S, Alkadhi H, Plass A et al. Accuracy of MSCT coronary angiography with 64-slice technology: first experience. Eur Heart J 2005; 26(15):1482–7.

18. Leber AW, Knez A, von Ziegler F et al. Quantification of obstructive and nonobstructive coronary lesions by 64-slice computed tomography: a comparative study with quantitative coronary angiography and intravascular ultrasound. J Am Coll Cardiol 2005; 46(1):147–54.

19. Raff GL, Gallagher MJ, O'Neill WW, Goldstein JA. Diagnostic accuracy of noninvasive coronary angiography using 64-slice spiral computed tomography. J Am Coll Cardiol 2005; 46(3):552–7.

20. Mollet NR, Cademartiri F, van Mieghem CA et al. High-resolution spiral computed tomography coronary angiography in patients referred for diagnostic conventional coronary angiography. Circulation 2005; 112(15):2318–23.

21. Schroeder S, Kopp AF, Baumbach A et al. Noninvasive detection and evaluation of atherosclerotic coronary plaques with multislice computed tomography. J Am Coll Cardiol 2001; 37(5):1430–5.

22. Leber AW, Knez A, Becker A et al. Accuracy of multidetector spiral computed tomography in identifying and differentiating the composition of coronary atherosclerotic plaques: a comparative study with intracoronary ultrasound. J Am Coll Cardiol 2004; 43(7):1241–7.

23. Achenbach S, Moselewski F, Ropers D et al. Detection of calcified and noncalcified coronary atherosclerotic plaque by contrast-enhanced, submillimeter multidetector spiral computed tomography: a segment-based comparison with intravascular ultrasound. Circulation 2004; 109(1):14–17.

24. Leber AW, Knez A, White CW et al. Composition of coronary atherosclerotic plaques in patients with acute myocardial infarction and stable angina pectoris determined by contrast-enhanced multislice computed tomography. Am J Cardiol 2003; 91(6): 714–18.

25. Nikolaou K, Sagmeister S, Knez A et al. Multidetector-row computed tomography of the coronary arteries: predictive value and quantitative assessment of noncalcified vessel-wall changes. Eur Radiol 2003; 13(11):2505–12.

26. Mollet NR, Cademartiri F, Nieman K et al. Noninvasive assessment of coronary plaque burden using multislice computed tomography. Am J Cardiol 2005; 95(10):1165–9.

27. Achenbach S, Ropers D, Hoffmann U et al. Assessment of coronary remodeling in stenotic and nonstenotic coronary atherosclerotic lesions by multidetector spiral computed tomography. J Am Coll Cardiol 2004; 43(5):842–7.

28. Leber AW, Becker A, Knez A et al. Accuracy of 64-slice computed tomography to classify and quantify plaque volumes in the proximal coronary system: a comparative study using intravascular ultrasound. J Am Coll Cardiol 2006; 47(3):672–7.

Magnetic resonance imaging   28

Chun Yuan, William S Kerwin, Vasily L Yarnykh, Jianming Cai, Marina S Ferguson, Baocheng Chu, Tobias Saam, Norihide Takaya, Hunter R Underhill, Fei Liu, Dongxiang Xu, and Thomas S Hatsukami

INTRODUCTION

Much has changed in the field of atherosclerotic plaque imaging since the publication of *'Handbook of the Vulnerable Plaque'*.[1] The accuracy and reproducibility of magnetic resonance imaging (MRI) for assessing atherosclerotic lesion size and composition has been previously reviewed.[2–13] This chapter reviews key recent advances in vulnerable plaque imaging, integration of imaging with hemodynamic and tissue mechanical property studies, and the use of imaging as a biomarker. This review focuses on MR imaging used for the human carotid, aorta, and coronary arteries, and concludes with a discussion of the present and future status of MR plaque imaging.

BACKGROUND

Atherosclerosis is a systemic disease of the vessel wall occurring in the aorta, carotid, coronary, and peripheral arteries. The clinical manifestations of atherosclerosis, which include myocardial, intracranial, visceral, and peripheral ischemia, are a result of thromboembolic events at the site of or downstream from atherosclerotic lesions or from hemodynamic compromise from high-grade stenosis. Autopsy studies of coronary arteries show that plaque rupture, erosion, or calcified nodules are associated with thrombosis.[14–18] Of these, plaque rupture is most implicated, owing to the exposure of thrombogenic subendothelial plaque components to the lumen surface. Histopathologic studies indicate that a vulnerable plaque is characterized by a thinning fibrous cap (FC) overlying a thrombogenic lipid core.[17,19–21] In addition, the size of the lipid/necrotic core, the degree of neovascularization, and the amount of inflammation within the plaque may be important determinants of plaque stability.[21–23]

Imaging atherosclerotic lesions may improve risk stratification and evaluation of patient response to interventions, as well as assist in the identification of novel genetic and molecular determinants of risk. Clinically, the degree of lumen stenosis is used as a measure of atherosclerosis severity. However, it has recently been shown that vessel lumen size measurement may not be the sole indicator of the high-risk plaque. Expansive remodeling will lead to an underestimation of plaque burden when only the lumen size is considered. Plaque tissue components, heavily implicated in plaque vulnerability, may be a more significant indicator of events than lumen size alone. Therefore, angiographic techniques may not adequately detect the vulnerable plaque. The current focus of vascular imaging has been to identify plaque tissue components, measure plaque size (lumen and wall), and when possible, include flow dynamics and mechanical tissue conditions. Furthermore, validated imaging-based biomarkers that can produce quantitative measurements of the properties of atherosclerosis are needed. Of all the non-invasive imaging techniques, MRI shows the most promise for imaging atherosclerosis by providing detailed information about the arterial wall.

RECENT TECHNICAL DEVELOPMENTS

Much of the validation of novel MRI techniques has used examination of excised plaque specimens as the gold standard. This section reviews the need for consensus guidelines and standardized methods to describe the histologic findings, and summarizes new developments in hardware, pulse sequence design, contrast agents, and image analysis tools.

Histologic validation of plaque imaging

Histologic correlation has been the foundation for validating imaging techniques. Recent critical appraisals of the performance, reporting, and interpretation of studies that compare plaque imaging with corresponding histology specimens have produced highly variable results, even for similar imaging techniques. In a systematic review of studies that compare plaque imaging results with those from corresponding histology sections, Lovett et al demonstrate how histologic methods from 73 eligible studies were poorly reported and highly variable; 23% reported reproducibility data for imaging and only 12% reported reproducibility data for histology.[24] Of 29 studies that reported quantitative results of blinded comparisons between plaque imaging and corresponding histology, numerous methodologic deficiencies occurred, making the results highly variable. No study considered the extent in which the lack of reproducibility of histology findings influenced the reported imaging–pathologic correlations. Therefore, pathology correlations in studies of plaque imaging may not be reliable, owing to incomparable and poorly reported histology methods. Lovett et al's review strongly demonstrates the current need to improve the imaging–pathologic correlation methods and opens the door to a consensus-based development of guidelines for such studies.

Developments in hardware

3T magnetic resonance imaging

In a recent study, the benefits of 3 tesla (3T) MRI were explored for evaluation of carotid atherosclerosis. Normal volunteers and subjects with carotid disease were scanned in 1.5T and 3T scanners with a similar protocol providing transverse T1-, T2-, and proton-density (PD)-weighted black-blood images using a fast spin-echo sequence with single (T1-weighted) or multislice (PD-/T2-weighted) double-inversion recovery (DIR) preparation.[25] Wall and lumen signal-to-noise ratio (SNR) and wall/lumen contrast-to-noise ratio (CNR) were compared in 44 artery cross sections. Wall SNR and lumen/wall CNR significantly increased ($P<0.0001$) at 3 T, with a 1.5-fold gain for T1-weighted images and a 1.7/1.8-fold gain for PD-/T2-weighted images. Lumen area, wall area, and mean wall thickness measurements demonstrated good agreement between 1.5 and 3T MRI, with no significant bias ($P = 0.5$), a coefficient of variation (CV) of <10%, and intraclass correlation coefficient (ICC) of >0.95. In summary, this study demonstrated significant improvement in SNR, CNR, and image quality for high-resolution black-blood imaging of carotid arteries at 3T. Morphologic measurements are compatible between 1.5 T and 3 T.

Intravascular magnetic resonance imaging

MRI has proven its ability to assess the composition of the carotid atherosclerotic plaque with good sensitivity and specificity. However, for vessels located deep in the human body, such as the coronary arteries, visualization is limited by poor SNR and spatial resolution, creating marginal results. Intravascular MRI (IVMRI) has shown promise as a technique to improve SNR and spatial resolution of images from deeper vessels. Recently, Larose et al evaluated the capability of in-vivo IVMRI to measure vessel wall size and to discern the composition of human iliac arteries on a 1.5T scanner.[26] Using a 0.030-inch-diameter IVMRI detector coil, the iliac arteries of 25 human subjects were assessed, and MRI results were compared to those of intravascular ultrasound (IVUS). IVMRI readily visualized inner and outer plaque boundaries in all arteries, regardless of the presence of calcification, which precluded accurate assessment with IVUS. There was good interobserver and intraobserver agreement in the interpretation of plaque composition for IVMRI, with kappa ranging from 0.62 to 0.79, compared with only 0.21 for IVUS. The results show that IVMRI can reliably identify plaque composition and size in arteries deep within the body. Although many technical challenges remain, this compelling study points to the feasibility of the use of IVMRI in coronary arteries.

Developments in pulse sequence design

Three-dimensional free-breathing magnetic resonance coronary vessel wall imaging

Until recently, the reproducibility of in-vivo wall thickness measurements of the coronary arteries was limited. Using a refined magnetization preparation scheme, Desai and colleagues demonstrated that the use of black-blood free-breathing three-dimensional (3D) MRI in conjunction with semi-automated analysis software allows for reproducible measurements of right coronary arterial vessel wall thickness.[27] Images were obtained in 18 healthy individuals with no known history of coronary artery disease, and scans were repeated 1 month later in eight subjects. There was a highly significant intraobserver ($r = 0.97$), interobserver ($r = 0.94$), and interscan ($r = 0.90$)

correlation for wall thickness (all $P < 0.001$). ICCs for intraobserver ($r = 0.97$), interobserver ($r = 0.92$), and interscan ($r = 0.86$) analyses were excellent. This technique has great potential in non-invasive longitudinal studies of coronary atherosclerosis.

Simultaneous outer volume and blood suppression by quadruple inversion-recovery

Development of new imaging sequences plays an important role in improvement of the vessel wall imaging. A new multipurpose technique[28] based on the previously described quadruple inversion-recovery (QIR) principle[29] has been recently proposed for imaging the aorta and carotid arteries. This technique combines suppression of signals from the outer volume and inflowing blood by using an SFQIR (small-FOV [field of view] quadruple inversion-recovery) preparative pulse sequence consisting of two double-inversion pulse pairs applied to two orthogonal planes. One of these planes coincides with the imaged slice, while another restricts the FOV in the phase-encoding direction. This allows imaging only the selected small area within the body, while contributions from the outer parts of the object and inflowing blood appear substantially suppressed. An important feature of this method is its ability for multislice acquisition, which considerably improves the time efficiency compared with earlier black-blood sequences such as DIR or QIR. The SFQIR method facilitates the elimination of motion and flow artifacts, reduction of scan time, and improvement in spatial resolution. Because of the considerably reduced scan time and T1-insensitive blood suppression, SFQIR enables a new imaging approach, black-blood dynamic contrast enhancement (DCE),[28] which may improve detection of inflammatory activity and neovascularization in the FC. This capability seems to be rather important for clinical and research applications focused on markers of plaque vulnerability, since the previously described bright-blood DCE method for imaging plaque inflammation[30] fails at the blood–wall interface due to unpredictable signal behavior.

Contrast enhancement and plaque tissue characterization

Gadolinium contrast enhancement

Previous studies using contrast-enhanced MRI (CEMRI) have shown that the FC in atherosclerotic carotid plaques enhances with gadolinium-based contrast agents.[7,10] In a recent publication, Kramer et al demonstrated that CEMRI can reliably distinguish atherosclerotic plaque components in abdominal aortic aneurysms.[31] They found that a higher signal on T2-weighted MRI can identify the FC and thrombus in abdominal aortic aneurysm and that contrast enhancement improves the delineation of the FC.

While the FC may enhance with CEMRI, the lipid-rich necrotic core (LR-NC), lacking both vasculature and matrix, shows no

or only slight enhancement. Cai et al employed this phenomenon to assess whether CEMRI can be used to accurately measure the dimensions of the intact FC and LR-NC (Figure 28.1).[32] In a study of 21 patients, they reported that blinded comparison of MR images and corresponding histology sections showed moderate to good correlation for length ($r = 0.73$, $P < 0.001$) and area ($r = 0.80$, $P < 0.001$) of the intact FC. The mean percentage LR-NC areas (LR-NC area/wall area) measured by CEMRI and histology were 30.1% and 32.7%, respectively, and were strongly correlated across locations ($r = 0.87$, $P < 0.001$). This study affirms that in-vivo high-resolution CEMRI is capable of quantitatively measuring the dimensions of the intact FC and LR-NC. These new parameters can be useful in both the evaluation of plaque vulnerability in providing continuous variables and for characterizing the intact FC and LR-NC in progression and regression studies.

As noted above, differential enhancement of plaque tissues has been observed in advanced carotid atherosclerosis. However, marked enhancement suggests

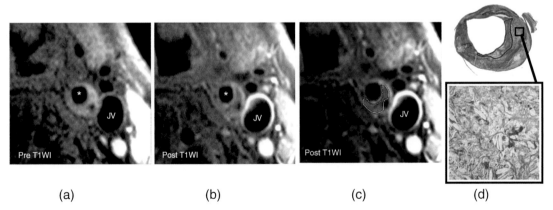

(a)   (b)   (c)   (d)

Figure 28.1   (a) Pre-contrast T1-weighted MR image (T1W1) of the common carotid artery demonstrating a large eccentric plaque in the common carotid artery (* = lumen; JV = jugular vein). (b) Post-contrast T1W1 demonstrates differential enhancement of the fibrous cap and underlying lipid-rich necrotic core. (c) Measurement of the fibrous cap (green) and lipid-rich necrotic core (yellow) areas. (d) Matched histologic cross section of the common carotid artery from the excised specimen with fibrous cap (green) and lipid-rich necrotic core (yellow) outlined. The box demonstrates a high-power view of the lipid-rich necrotic core, demonstrating abundant cholesterol clefts. (Reproduced from Cai et al,[32] with permission.)

the presence of a vascular supply to the plaque (neovasculature) and increased microvessel endothelial permeability that facilitates entry of the contrast agent from the blood plasma. Because neovasculature in-growth into the plaque and increased endothelial permeability are both associated with inflammation,[33–37] plaque enhancement has been argued as an indirect indicator of the degree of vessel wall inflammation. Using a dynamic MRI acquisition protocol in 30 patients scheduled to undergo carotid endarterectomy, the rate of gadolinium uptake in carotid plaques was quantified by measuring time-varying intensities within the plaques to estimate the transfer constant (K^{trans}) into the extracellular space.[38] Measurements of K^{trans} correlated with macrophage content ($r = 0.75$, $P < 0.001$) and neovasculature content ($r = 0.71$, $P < 0.001$). Interestingly, there was a negative correlation between K^{trans} and high-density lipoprotein (HDL) levels ($r = -0.66$, $P < 0.001$). Furthermore, K^{trans} was noted to be significantly higher amongst cigarette smokers compared with non-smokers (mean $= 0.134$ vs 0.074 min^{-1}; $P = 0.01$).

Targeted contrast agents

Molecular MRI has emerged rapidly over the last couple of years.[39] In this technique, selective targeted imaging is performed using contrast agents that bind to specific targets. First attempts in the field of arteriosclerosis used iron oxide particles, which accumulate in macrophages, resulting in a signal void.[40–43] Imaging, then, is best performed with T2*-weighted gradient echo sequences. Other compounds are based on nanoparticles, antibodies, liposomes, or peptides, etc.,[43,44] using targets such as integrins, adhesion molecules, fibrin, or glycoproteins.[43,45–50] Typically, these approaches with paramagnetic compounds result in a local signal amplification and are called 'white-spot imaging'. Sequences need to be heavily T1-weighted in order to observe contrast uptake. Furthermore, adjacent tissue such as the normal vessel wall, fat, and the blood pool need to be signal suppressed.

Targeted contrast agents may soon be able to provide information other than the location of the target. The presence of activated macrophages is an early and consistent marker of the inflammatory nature of atherosclerotic disease. Dextran-coated superparamagnetic iron oxide particles (SPIOs) are avidly endocytosed. These particles have a strong effect on the MR signal and have been proposed as a non-invasive probe for the presence of early non-occlusive atherosclerotic disease. Rogers and Basu recently demonstrated significantly reduced SPIO uptake when pretreated with lovastatin to 61% ($P < 0.001$) and 43% ($P = 0.02$) of control at 1.0 μmol/L and 17.5 μmol/L lovastatin, respectively.[51] Interferon-gamma (IFN-γ, 1000 U/ml) increased SPIO uptake to 163% of control ($P < 0.05$). Interleukin-4 (IL-4, 40 ng/ml) also increased uptake (178% of control, $P < 0.04$). In cells incubated with SPIO in the absence of serum proteins, SPIO uptake fell to 57% of control ($P < 0.001$), concluding that uptake of SPIO by activated macrophages is regulated by endogenous cytokines and serum components as well and exogenous lovastatin. Thus, MRI signal changes after SPIO administration may reflect macrophage phagocytic capacity as well as macrophage presence.

Image analysis tools

Recent developments have clearly demonstrated the ability of MRI in measuring plaque morphology and in identifying plaque tissue composition. It is ideal that image processing techniques can be applied to these images to assist in the tissue identification and quantitation. Image analysis, however, has been challenging. Multiple contrast weighted image acquisition has been the foundation of

MRI plaque characterization, but it creates several limitations arising from acquisition time, motion artifacts, unsuppressed blood flow in black-blood images, and limitations in SNR, CNR, and achievable resolution.

In-vivo supervised classifiers

Hofman et al studied the possibility of using supervised classifiers to quantify the main components of carotid atherosclerotic plaque in vivo on the basis of multicontrast weighted MRI data.[52] Five MR weightings were obtained from 25 symptomatic subjects. Histologic micrographs of endarterectomy specimens from the 25 carotids were used as a standard of reference for training and evaluation. The set of subjects was split into a training set (12 subjects) and an evaluation set (13 subjects). There were four different basic classifiers:

1. Bayes, a standard Bayesian classifier that assumes a multivariate normal distribution for each class.
2. K-nearest neighbor classifier.
3. A feedforward neural network with one hidden layer and four output neurons.
4. Bayes2, a combination of the Bayes classifier with a Parzen classifier that takes into account the spatial context of each pixel.

Two human MRI readers determined the percentages of calcified tissue, fibrous tissue, lipid core, and intraplaque hemorrhage on the subject level for all subjects in the evaluation set. Relatively small amounts of calcium could not be quantified with statistical significance by either the classifiers or the MRI readers. For the other tissues, a simple Bayesian classifier (Bayes) performed better than the other classifiers and the MRI readers. All classifiers performed better than the MRI readers in quantifying the sum of hemorrhage and lipid. This pilot study demonstrated the feasibility of using algorithmic classifiers for quantifying plaque components.

Morphology-enhanced probabilistic plaque segmentation

In another recent publication, Liu et al introduced a novel in-vivo segmentation scheme, referred to as morphology-enhanced probabilistic plaque segmentation (MEPPS), that utilized a method based on a maximum a-posteriori probability Bayesian theory to divide axial, multicontrast weighted images into regions of necrotic core, calcification, loose matrix, and fibrous tissue.[53] The key advantage of this method is that it uses morphologic information, such as local wall thickness, and coupled active contours to limit the impact from noise and artifacts associated with in-vivo imaging. In experiments involving 142 sets of multicontrast images from 26 subjects undergoing carotid endarterectomy, segmented areas of each of these issues per slice agreed with histologically confirmed areas with correlations (r^2) of 0.78, 0.83, and 0.82 for necrotic core, calcification, and fibrous tissue, respectively. In comparison, manual identification of areas blinded to histology yielded correlations of 0.71, 0.76, and 0.78, respectively. These results show that in-vivo automatic segmentation of carotid MRI is feasible and comparable to, or possibly more accurate than, manual reviews of plaque composition.

Use of computer-driven algorithms to validate MRI plaque tissue characterization

Using an ex-vivo classification technique, Clarke et al attempted to systematically validate MRI signals from carotid plaques in 48 carotid endarterectomy specimen cross sections selected from 13 carotid arteries scored with the AHA (American Heart Association) lesion grade determined histopathologically.[54] The specimens were concurrently imaged using a combination of 8 MRI contrast weightings in vitro. A maximum likelihood classification algorithm generated MRI maps of plaque components by using the training data set selected from 12 of the 48 cross sections which constituted only 2.5% of the total plaque cross-sectional area. An AHA lesion grade was assigned correspondingly. Additional analysis compared classification accuracy obtained with a commonly used set of MR contrast weightings (PD, T1, and T2) to accuracy obtained with the combination of PD, T1, and diffusion-weighted (Dw) contrast. For the 8 contrast combination, the sensitivities for fibrous tissue, necrotic core, calcification, and hemorrhage detection were 83%, 67%, 86%, and 77%, respectively. The corresponding specificities were 81%, 78%, 99%, and 97%. Good agreement (79%) between MR and histopathology for AHA classification was achieved. For the PD, T1, and Dw combination, the overall classification accuracy was insignificantly different at 78%, whereas the overall classification accuracy using PD, T1, and T2 contrast weightings was significantly lower at 67%. This systematic study provides further proof that the composition of atherosclerotic plaques determined by high-resolution MRI accurately reflects lesion composition defined by histopathologic examination.

IMAGING USED IN HEMODYNAMIC AND TISSUE MECHANICAL PROPERTY STUDIES

Three-dimensional fluid structure interactions models and quantifying effects of atherosclerotic plaques

The inter-relationship between hemodynamic and mechanical properties of plaque tissue has long been considered as the cause of eventual plaque rupture, and therefore has been an area of active research.[55] The combination of in-vivo imaging and realistic mathematical models provides a unique opportunity to advance our knowledge of this relationship. In a study by Tang et al, MRI-based 3D unsteady models of human atherosclerotic plaques with multicomponent plaque structure and fluid structure interactions (FSI) were used to perform mechanical analysis for human atherosclerotic plaques.[56] The results showed that stress variations on critical sites such as a thin cap can be 300% higher than stress at normal sites. Large areas of calcification altered stress and strain distributions. Plaque cap erosion caused almost no change on maximal stress level at the cap, but led to a 50% increase in maximal strain value. Findings from this study suggested that computational mechanical analysis has the potential to improve the accuracy of plaque vulnerability assessment.

Longitudinal structural determinant of atherosclerotic plaque vulnerability

Although it has been shown that an excessive concentration of stress is related to atherosclerotic plaque rupture, the local determinant of plaque longitudinal stress distribution along the arterial wall remains unclear. Computational analysis of stress distribution using vascular models and 3D IVUS imaging has also proven to be useful in determining atherosclerotic plaque vulnerability. Imoto et al examined the longitudinal structural determinants of plaque vulnerability using a color-coded stress mapping technique for several hypothetical vessel models as well as 3D IVUS images using a finite element analysis.[57] Color maps of equivalent stress distributions within plaques of 3D vessel models as well as longitudinal IVUS plaque images ($n = 15$) were created. They then examined the effects of plaque size, shape, expansive remodeling, calcification, and lipid core on the equivalent stress distribution. The results showed that color mapping of vessel walls reveals a concentration of equivalent stress at the top of the hills and shoulders of homogeneous fibrous plaques. Expansive remodeling and the lipid core augmented the surface equivalent stress, whereas luminal stenosis and superficial calcification attenuated the equivalent stress. The location of excessive stress concentration was modified by the distribution of the lipid core and calcification. The thickness of the FC was inversely related to the equivalent stress within the FC. However, the color mapping of IVUS plaque images showed that the equivalent stress value at the FC varied with changes in plaque shape and superficial calcification, even when the thickness of the FC remained constant. The FCs of the same thickness did not consistently represent the same vulnerability to rupture.

Shear stress and plaque progression and regression in the thoracic aorta

A condition favorable to the development of atherosclerotic lesions is low oscillating shear stress (SS).[58–62] In the descending thoracic aorta, the relationship between plaque distribution and SS has never been characterized. The regression of plaque as the result of lipid-lowering therapy is associated with reverse atherogenic mechanisms. Wentzel et al therefore investigated the role of SS in plaque regression, using MRI.[55] Phase-contrast MRI was performed in the thoracic aorta of eight healthy volunteers to derive typical average SS distribution. Shear stress predicted the location of wall thickness (WT) ($r^2 = 0.29$, $P<0.05$) but did not predict plaque regression. The best predictor of plaque regression was baseline WT. However, the results showed an association between WT and average low SS locations and support the role of local hemodynamics in the development of atherosclerotic lesions in the descending thoracic aorta. SS does not seem to be the major predictor for plaque regression by lipid-lowering interventions, which suggests that other mechanisms are involved in the lipid-reversal mechanism.

IMAGING AS A BIOMARKER FOR PRESENCE OF DISEASE, PROGRESSION, AND ISCHEMIC EVENTS

Correlation of carotid artery mean wall thickness by MRI and intima–media thickness by ultrasound

Whereas B-mode ultrasound has become the gold standard for measuring intima–media thickness (IMT) of the carotid artery, MRI has been proven to non-invasively characterize and quantify carotid plaques. The two modalities used together are a powerful combination for assessing plaque morphology and IMT, which is pivotal for successful treatment. Ideally, only one test would be needed. In the attempt to combine IMT and the characterization of atherosclerotic plaque, Underhill et al compared B-mode ultrasound results with those of cross-sectional, black-blood, T1-weighted MRI to see if MRI alone can determine carotid artery wall thickness.[63] If MRI is viable, future progression studies would benefit from a reduction in cost, simplification of protocol design, and minimization of patient time. The results showed that automated mean wall thickness by MRI is highly correlated with ultrasound measurements of IMT. MRI did, however, overestimate thickness at lower values. This may be due to the inclusion of the adventitia in the MRI measurements. Still, the results suggest that evaluating mean wall thickness with MRI may serve as an alternative to ultrasound. With MRI, it is possible to obtain local detail and systematic atherosclerotic information in one quick examination. Another advantage of using MRI is that it requires no additional imaging requirements. And finally, MRI requires less operator dependence than ultrasound because using MRI for measuring WT relies on well-defined and highly reproducible protocols with similar carotid coverage and image quality across multiple sites and operators.

Quantification of plaque composition by MRI

MRI has been shown to be capable of identifying the presence or absence of major plaque components with good sensitivity and specificity. For progression and regression studies, quantitative measures of the size of these components would be more powerful. Recently, Saam et al evaluated the ability of MRI to quantify major carotid atherosclerotic plaque components in vivo.[64] MR images of carotid plaques from 31 subjects scheduled for carotid endarterectomy and a total of 214 MR imaging locations were matched to corresponding histology sections. For MRI and histology, area measurements of the major plaque components such as LR-NC, calcification, loose matrix, and dense (fibrous) tissue were recorded as percentages of the total wall area. MRI measurements of plaque composition were statistically equivalent to those of histology for the LR-NC (23.7% vs 20.3%; $P = 0.1$), loose matrix (5.1% vs 6.3%; $P = 0.1$), and dense (fibrous) tissue (66.3% vs 64%; $P = 0.4$). Calcification differed significantly when measured as a percentage of wall area (9.4% vs 5%; $P < 0.001$). There was a strong correlation between MRI and histology area measurements (mean per location) for lumen ($r = 0.81$; $P < 0.001$), wall ($r = 0.84$; $P < 0.001$), outer wall ($r = 0.82$; $P < 0.001$), LR-NC ($r = 0.75$; $P < 0.001$), calcification ($r = 0.74$; $P < 0.001$), and loose matrix ($r = 0.70$; $P < 0.001$). There was a moderate correlation between MRI and histology measurements of dense (fibrous) tissue ($r = 0.55$; $P < 0.001$) and a moderate to strong correlation between measurements of hemorrhage ($r = 0.66$; $P < 0.001$). Intrareader reproducibility (ICC; 95% CI) was excellent for area measurements of LR-NC (0.89; 0.75–0.95) and calcification (0.9; 0.77–0.96), and good for hemorrhage (0.74; 0.45–0.89) and for loose matrix (0.79; 0.54–0.91). Inter-reader reproducibility (ICC; 95% CI) was excellent for area measurements of LR-NC (0.92; 0.82–0.97) and calcification (0.95; 0.88–0.98), and good for hemorrhage (0.73; 0.44–0.88) and for loose matrix (0.79; 0.55–0.91). The results demonstrate the potential of multicontrast MRI for the quantitative characterization of the main components of human atherosclerotic plaque in prospective longitudinal studies to examine carotid atherosclerotic plaque progression and regression.

Intraplaque hemorrhage and progression of carotid atherosclerosis

Kolodgie et al suggested that intraplaque hemorrhage may represent a potent atherogenic stimulus by contributing to the deposition of free cholesterol, macrophage infiltration, and the enlargement of the necrotic core.[65] Immunohistochemical staining with the antibody to glycophorin A, a protein specific to erythrocyte membranes, was strongly associated with the size of the necrotic core and degree of macrophage infiltration. They also noted that rabbit lesions with induced intramural hemorrhage had significantly greater lipid content than control lesions without hemorrhage.

Previous MRI studies accurately detected the presence and age of carotid intraplaque hemorrhage.[66,67] Recently, Takaya et al used MRI to test the hypothesis that intraplaque hemorrhage is a predisposing factor in the progression of human atherosclerosis.[68] Twenty-nine subjects (14 cases with intraplaque hemorrhage and 15 controls with comparably sized plaques without intraplaque hemorrhage at baseline) underwent serial carotid MRI examination with a multicontrast weighted protocol (T1, T2, proton density, and 3D time of flight) over a period of 18 months. The volume of wall, lumen, LR-NC, and hemorrhage were measured at baseline and after 18 months. The percent change in wall volume (6.8% vs −0.15%; $P = 0.009$) and LR-NC volume (28.4% vs −5.2%; $P = 0.001$) were significantly greater in plaques with hemorrhage compared to those without hemorrhage at baseline (Figure 28.2). Furthermore, those patients with intra-plaque hemorrhage at baseline were much more likely to have new plaque hemorrhages at 18 months compared with controls (43% vs 0%; $P = 0.006$). In summary, findings from this study strongly suggested that hemorrhage into the carotid atherosclerotic plaque accelerated plaque progression in an 18-month period, and that repeated bleeding into the plaque may produce a stimulus for the progression of atherosclerosis by increasing lipid core and plaque volume and creating new destabilizing factors.

Aortic atherosclerosis and risk factors

Taniguchi et al, using MRI, detected atherosclerotic plaque in the thoracic and abdominal aortas.[69] While the results suggest that thoracic and abdominal aortas may have different susceptibilities to risk factors, plasma inflammatory markers appear to reflect the total extent of aortic atherosclerosis. Although aortic plaques are common in patients with coronary artery disease (CAD), only thoracic plaques were found to be an independent factor for CAD.

Thoracic aorta, carotid intima–media thickness, and the extent of coronary artery disease

The IMT of the common carotid artery and atherosclerosis of the thoracic aorta have been shown to correlate with CAD. In a study that compared the relation between wall changes in the thoracic aorta and the carotid arteries and the angiographic severity and extent of atherosclerotic lesions in coronary arteries in patients with verified CAD, a significant correlation was seen between the extent of coronary artery stenosis and aortic plaque score.[70] Mean carotid IMT was also significantly correlated with coronary artery

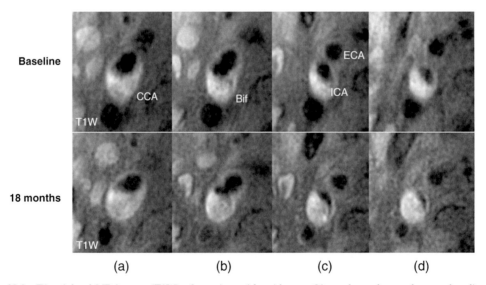

Figure 28.2 T1-weighted MR images (T1W) of a patient with evidence of intraplaque hemorrhage at baseline (top row). The panels from left to right show cross-sectional images of (a) the common carotid artery (CCA), (b) carotid bifurcation (Bif), (c) proximal internal carotid artery (ICA), and (d) the ICA more distally. The lower row shows the matched cross-sectional images on the 18-month follow-up MRI. There is marked decrease in luminal area in the ICA (c and d), and increase in atherosclerotic lesion size in the ICA. (Reproduced from Takaya et al,[68] with permission.)

stenosis extent score. The results showed a clear and significant relationship between wall changes in the thoracic aorta, common carotid IMT, and the angiographic extent of coronary artery stenosis in patients with severe CAD. The findings indicate a potential for B-mode ultrasonography of the carotid arteries and transesophageal echocardiographic aortic examination in the diagnostic and prognostic evaluation of patients with suspected CAD.

MRI and statin-induced cholesterol lowering and plaque regression

A number of recently published studies have demonstrated the utility of MRI for quantifying change in overall plaque burden in response to lipid-lowering therapy. One of the first prospective studies examining the effects of statin therapy was published by Corti et al, where 51 hypercholesterolemic patients were randomized to 20 mg/day ($n = 29$) or 80 mg/day ($n = 22$) of simvastatin.[71] The authors found that aortic vessel wall area decreased by 10% at 12 months and by 15% at 24 months, as assessed by MRI. Carotid vessel wall area decreased by 14% and 18% at 12 and 24 months, respectively. However, no change in lumen size was detected at 6 and 12 months.

In another recently published study, Lima and colleagues reported evidence of significant regression in thoracic aortic atherosclerotic plaques by 6 months after initiation of therapy with simvastatin.[3] Twenty-seven patients were treated with simvastatin 20–80 mg daily. The authors reported a reduction in aortic plaque (AP) volume from 3.3 ± 1.4 cm^3 at baseline to 2.9 ± 1.4 cm^3 at 6 months (12% reduction, $P <0.02$). There was a slight trend toward luminal volume increase (from 12.0 ± 3.9 to 12.2 ± 3.7 cm^3, $P<0.06$). Furthermore, there was a significant correlation between plaque volume regression and changes in LDL-C (low-density lipoprotein cholesterol)

levels (regression coefficient = 7.07, 95% CI 1.3–12.9; $P = 0.02$).

Similar to the findings associated with simvastatin reported above, Yonemura and colleagues demonstrated regression of thoracic aortic plaques amongst patients treated with high-dose atorvastatin therapy.[72] In this study, 40 hypercholesterolemic patients were randomized to receive either 5 mg or 20 mg of atorvastatin. The thoracic and abdominal aorta was imaged with MRI at baseline and 12 months after initiation of treatment. In the high-dose group, vessel wall area (VWA) in the thoracic aorta decreased by 18% ($P<0.001$), whereas VWA increased by 4% in the low-dose group. In the abdominal aorta, there was no evidence of significant regression or progression in VWA (+3%) in the 20 mg group, but significant progression (+12%) in the 5 mg group ($P<0.01$). The degree of plaque regression in the thoracic aorta correlated with reduction in LDL-C ($r= 0.64$). Notably, thoracic aortic regression was also significantly associated with reduction in C-reactive protein (CRP) levels ($r= 0.49$).

Prediction of subsequent ischemic events

In a study involving 154 subjects,[73] baseline MRI findings were compared with clinical outcome for the hypothesis that MRI identification of plaque features, such as intraplaque hemorrhage, thinned/ruptured FC, or large LR-NC, is associated with the development of future ipsilateral carotid-distribution transient ischemic attack (TIA) or stroke. Following the baseline MRI examination, subjects were contacted every 3 months to identify the onset of TIA- or stroke-like symptoms, with a mean follow-up of 38.2 months. There were 12 ipsilateral cerebrovascular events that were felt to be clearly related to the index carotid artery lesion. Cox regression analysis demonstrated a significant association between baseline MRI identification

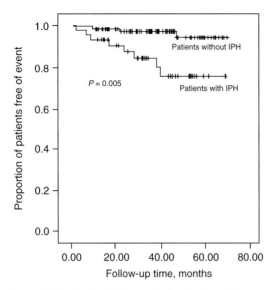

Figure 28.3 Kaplan–Meier survival estimates of the proportion of patients remaining free of ipsilateral transient ischemic attack (TIA) or stroke for subjects with (lower curve) and without (upper curve) intraplaque hemorrhage (IPH). (Reproduced from Takaya et al,[73] with permission.)

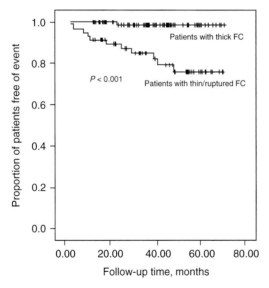

Figure 28.4 Kaplan–Meier survival estimates of the proportion of patients remaining free of ipsilateral transient ischemic attack (TIA) or stroke for subjects with (lower curve) and without (upper curve) thin or ruptured fibrous cap (FC). (Reproduced from Takaya et al,[73] with permission.)

of the following plaque characteristics and subsequent symptoms during follow-up:

- presence of a thin or ruptured FC (hazard ratio [HR] = 17.0; $P < 0.001$)
- intraplaque hemorrhage (HR = 5.2; $P = 0.005$)
- larger mean intraplaque hemorrhage area (HR for 10 mm^2 increase = 2.6; $P = 0.006$)
- larger maximum percent LR-NC (HR for 10% increase = 1.6; $P = 0.004$)
- larger maximum wall thickness (HR for a 1-mm increase = 1.6; $P = 0.008$).

Figures 28.3 and 28.4 demonstrate Kaplan–Meier estimates of stroke and TIA-free survival with and without intraplaque hemorrhage and FC thinning or rupture.

CONCLUSIONS AND FUTURE CHALLENGES

MRI characterization of plaque has been shown to be accurate and reproducible for assessing the structure and key compositional features of carotid and aortic lesions of atherosclerosis. Results from several randomized clinical trials have demonstrated the potential of this non-invasive imaging modality. Furthermore, initial results from single-center studies indicate that MRI is capable of identifying carotid plaque features associated with more rapid progression as well as an increased risk of subsequent TIA or stroke. However, in order to move this technology forward into routine clinical practice, several challenges must be addressed.

First, the promising initial findings from single-center studies must be reproduced on a larger, multicenter scale. This involves the development of a standardized image acquisition protocol that can be applied across the various MRI scanner platforms. Inter-platform reproducibility must be assessed. Specific training in the acquisition of high-resolution MR images of atherosclerosis is needed to insure image quality and reproducible uniform coverage for serial studies. Furthermore, dedicated training in the interpretation of images from this novel technique is required, and further development of analysis tools that improve the efficiency and reproducibility of the review process is needed.

Secondly, improvement in spatial and temporal resolution is needed to extend the MRI technique for better characterization of coronary artery atherosclerosis, and to improve the precision of assessment of fine structures such as the fibrous cap. Reduction in overall scan time will have secondary benefits in terms of improvements in image quality (reduced patient motion), improved patient acceptance, and reduced costs.

Finally, further development of techniques is needed to assess not only the anatomic structure of the atherosclerotic plaque but also its functional state. Promising approaches in this field include novel MRI contrast agents targeted to specific receptors, and combined imaging techniques such as positron emission tomography (PET)-MRI.

In conclusion, the combination of extensive histologic validation and initial results from prospective clinical studies demonstrating associations between MRI plaque findings, progression, and ischemic events demonstrate the great promise of this imaging technique. If confirmed in larger studies, findings from MRI may result in a better understanding of the mechanisms of atherosclerosis progression, discovery of novel risk factors or biomarkers for the disease, and in improved selection of treatment that is tailored to the individual patient.

ACKNOWLEDGMENT

The authors would like to express their gratitude to Andrew Ho and Diana Jensen for their assistance in preparing this chapter.

REFERENCES

1. Waksman R, Serruys PW, eds. Handbook of the Vulnerable Plaque. London: Taylor & Francis; 2004.
2. Kang X, Polissar NL, Han C, Lin E, Yuan C. Analysis of the measurement precision of arterial lumen and wall areas using high-resolution MRI. Magn Reson Med 2000; 44:968–72.
3. Lima JA, Desai MY, Steen H et al. Statin-induced cholesterol lowering and plaque regression after 6 months of magnetic resonance imaging-monitored therapy. Circulation 2004; 110:2336–41.
4. Yuan C, Beach KW, Smith LH, Hatsukami TS. Measurement of atherosclerotic carotid plaque size in vivo using high resolution magnetic resonance imaging. Circulation 1998; 98:2666–71.
5. Toussaint J, Southern JF, Fuster V, Kantor HL. T2-weighted contrast for NMR characterization of human atherosclerosis. Arterioscler Thromb Vasc Biol 1995; 15:1533–42.
6. Shinnar M, Fallon JT, Wehrli S et al. The diagnostic accuracy of ex vivo MRI for human atherosclerotic plaque characterization. Arterioscler Thromb Vasc Biol 1999; 19:2756–61.
7. Yuan C, Kerwin WS, Ferguson MS et al. Contrast-enhanced high resolution MRI for atherosclerotic carotid artery tissue characterization. J Magn Reson Imaging 2002; 15:62–7.
8. Yuan C, Mitsumori LM, Ferguson MS et al. In vivo accuracy of multispectral magnetic resonance imaging for identifying lipid-rich necrotic cores and intraplaque hemorrhage in advanced human carotid plaques. Circulation 2001; 104:2051–6.
9. Hatsukami TS, Ross R, Polissar NL, Yuan C. Visualization of fibrous cap thickness and rupture in human atherosclerotic carotid plaque in vivo with high-resolution magnetic resonance imaging. Circulation 2000; 102:959–64.
10. Wasserman BA, Smith WI, Trout HH3 et al. Carotid artery atherosclerosis: in vivo morphologic characterization with gadolinium-enhanced double-oblique MR imaging initial results. Radiology 2002; 223:566–73.
11. Clarke SE, Hammond RR, Mitchell JR, Rutt BK. Quantitative assessment of carotid plaque composition using multicontrast MRI and registered histology. Magn Reson Med 2003; 50:1199–208.
12. Moody AR, Murphy RE, Morgan PS et al. Characterization of complicated carotid plaque with magnetic resonance direct thrombus imaging in patients with cerebral ischemia. Circulation 2003; 107:3047–52.
13. Murphy RE, Moody AR, Morgan PS et al. Prevalence of complicated carotid atheroma as detected by magnetic resonance direct thrombus imaging in patients with suspected carotid artery stenosis and previous acute cerebral ischemia. Circulation 2003; 107:3053–8.
14. Virmani R, Farb A, Burke AP. Risk factors in the pathogenesis of coronary artery disease. Compr Ther 1998; 24:519–29.

15. Burke AP, Farb A, Malcom GT et al. Coronary risk factors and plaque morphology in men with coronary disease who died suddenly [see comments]. N Engl J Med 1997; 336:1276–82.

16. Farb A, Tang AL, Burke AP et al. Sudden coronary death. Frequency of active coronary lesions, inactive coronary lesions, and myocardial infarction. Circulation 1995; 92:1701–9.

17. Kolodgie FD, Burke AP, Farb A et al. The thin-cap fibroatheroma: a type of vulnerable plaque: The major precursor lesion to acute coronary syndromes. Curr Opin Cardiol 2001; 16:285–92.

18. Burke AP, Kolodgie FD, Farb A et al. Healed plaque ruptures and sudden coronary death: evidence that subclinical rupture has a role in plaque progression. Circulation 2001; 103:934–40.

19. Davies MJ, Thomas AC. Plaque fissuring – the cause of acute myocardial infarction, sudden ischaemic death, and crescendo angina. Br Heart J 1985; 53: 363–73.

20. Davies MJ. Stability and instability: two faces of coronary atherosclerosis. The Paul Dudley White Lecture 1995. Circulation 1996; 94:2013–20.

21. Felton CV, Crrok D, Davies MJ, Oliver MF. Relation of plaque lipid composition and morphology to the stability of human aortic plaques. Arterioscler Thromb Vasc Biol 1997; 17:1337–45.

22. Libby P, Geng YJ, Aikawa M et al. Macrophages and atherosclerotic plaque stability. Curr Opin Lipidol 1996; 7:330–5.

23. Libby P, Galis ZS, Sukhova G, Lee RT. Inflammation and disruption of atherosclerotic plaques. J Vasc Surg 1995; 22:102–3.

24. Lovett JK, Redgrave JN, Rothwell PM. A critical appraisal of the performance, reporting, and interpretation of studies comparing carotid plaque imaging with histology. Stroke 2005; 36:1091–7.

25. Yarnykh VL, Terashima M, Hayes CE et al. Multicontrast black-blood MRI of carotid arteries: comparison between 1.5 and 3 tesla magnetic field strengths. J Magn Reson Imaging 2006; 23:691–8.

26. Larose E, Yeghiazarians Y, Libby P et al. Characterization of human atherosclerotic plaques by intravascular magnetic resonance imaging. Circulation 2005; 112:2324–31.

27. Desai MY, Lai S, Barmet C, Weiss RG, Stuber M. Reproducibility of 3D free-breathing magnetic resonance coronary vessel wall imaging. Eur Heart J 2005; 26:2320–4.

28. Yarnykh VL, Yuan C. Simultaneous outer volume and blood suppression by quadruple inversion-recovery. Magn Reson Med 2006; 55:1083–92.

29. Yarnykh VL, Yuan C. T1-insensitive flow suppression using quadruple inversion-recovery. Magn Reson Med 2002; 48:899–905.

30. Kerwin WS, Yarnykh V, Chu B et al. Incremental contrast-enhanced quadruple inversion recovery MRI for characterizing temporal patterns of enhancement in carotid atherosclerosis. International symposium for magnetic resonance in medicine. Toronto, Canada, 2003.

31. Kramer CM, Cerilli LA, Hagspiel K et al. Magnetic resonance imaging identifies the fibrous cap in atherosclerotic abdominal aortic aneurysm. Circulation 2004; 109:1016–21.

32. Cai J, Hatsukami TS, Ferguson M et al. In vivo quantative measurement of intact fibrous cap and lipid-rich necrotic core size in atherosclerotic carotid plaque: a comparison of high-resolution contrast-enhanced MRI and histology. Circulation 2005; 112:3437–44.

33. O'Brien KD, Allen MD, McDonald TO et al. Vascular cell adhesion molecule-1 is expressed in human coronary atherosclerotic plaques. Implications for the mode of progression of advanced coronary atherosclerosis [see comments]. J Clin Invest 1993; 92:945–51.

34. O'Brien KD, McDonald TO, Chait A, Allen MD, Alpers CE. Neovascular expression of E-selectin, intercellular adhesion molecule-1, and vascular cell adhesion molecule-1 in human atherosclerosis and their relation to intimal leukocyte content. Circulation 1996; 93:672–82.

35. de Boer OJ, van der Wal AC, Teeling P, Becker AE. Leucocyte recruitment in rupture prone regions of lipid-rich plaques: a prominent role for neovascularization? Cardiovasc Res 1999; 41:443–9.

36. Moulton KS, Vakili K, Zurakowski D et al. Inhibition of plaque neovascularization reduces macrophage accumulation and progression of advanced atherosclerosis. Proc Natl Acad Sci USA 2003; 100:4736–41.

37. Celletti FL, Waugh JM, Amabile PG et al. Inhibition of vascular endothelial growth factor-mediated neointima progression with angiostatin or paclitaxel. J Vasc Interv Radiol 2002; 13:703–7.

38. Kerwin WS, O'Brien KD, Ferguson MS et al. Inflammation in carotid atherosclerotic plaque is associated with elevated neovasculature and permeability: a dynamic contrast-enhanced MRI study. Radiology 2006; 241:459–68.

39. Weissleder R, Mahmood U. Molecular imaging. Radiology 2001; 219:316–33.

40. Schmitz SA, Coupland SE, Gust R et al. Superparamagnetic iron oxide-enhanced MRI of atherosclerotic plaques in Watanabe hereditable hyperlipidemic rabbits. Invest Radiol 2000; 35:460–71.

41. Kooi ME, Cappendijk VC, Cleutjens KB et al. Accumulation of ultrasmall superparamagnetic particles of iron oxide in human atherosclerotic plaques can be detected by in vivo magnetic resonance imaging. Circulation 2003; 107:2453–8.

42. Ruehm SG, Corot C, Vogt P, Kolb S, Debatin JF. Magnetic resonance imaging of atherosclerotic plaque with ultrasmall superparamagnetic particles of iron oxide in hyperlipidemic rabbits. Circulation 2001; 103:415–22.

43. Choudhury RP, Fuster V, Fayad ZA. Molecular, cellular and functional imaging of atherothrombosis. Nat Rev Drug Discov 2004; 3:913–25.

44. Wickline SA, Lanza GM. Nanotechnology for molecular imaging and targeted therapy. Circulation 2003; 107:1092–5.

45. Botnar RM, Perez AS, Witte S et al. In vivo molecular imaging of acute and subacute thrombosis using a fibrin-binding magnetic resonance imaging contrast agent. Circulation 2004; 109:2023–9.

46. Sipkins DA, Cheresh DA, Kazemi MR et al. Detection of tumor angiogenesis in vivo by alpha$_v$beta$_3$-targeted magnetic resonance imaging. Nat Med 1998; 4:623–6.

47. Winter PM, Morawski AM, Caruthers SD et al. Molecular imaging of angiogenesis in early-stage atherosclerosis with alpha$_v$beta$_3$-integrin-targeted nanoparticles. Circulation 2003; 108:2270–4.

48. Flacke S, Fischer S, Scott MJ et al. Novel MRI contrast agent for molecular imaging of fibrin: implications for detecting vulnerable plaques. Circulation 2001; 104:1280–5.

49. Yu X, Song SK, Chen J et al. High-resolution MRI characterization of human thrombus using a novel fibrin-targeted paramagnetic nanoparticle contrast agent. Magn Reson Med 2000; 44:867–72.

50. Sirol M, Aguinaldo JG, Graham PB et al. Fibrin-targeted contrast agent for improvement of in vivo acute thrombus detection with magnetic resonance imaging. Atherosclerosis 2005; 182:79–85.

51. Rogers WJ, Basu P. Factors regulating macrophage endocytosis of nanoparticles: implications for targeted magnetic resonance plaque imaging. Atherosclerosis 2005; 178:67–73.

52. Hofman JM, Branderhorst WJ, ten Eikelder HM et al. Quantification of atherosclerotic plaque components using in vivo MRI and supervised classifiers. Magn Reson Med 2006; 55:790–9.

53. Liu F, Xu D, Ferguson MS et al. Automated in vivo segmentation of carotid plaque MRI with morphology-enhanced probability maps. Magn Reson Med 2006; 55:659–68.

54. Clarke SE, Beletsky V, Hammond RR, Hegele RA, Rutt BK. Validation of automatically classified magnetic resonance images for carotid plaque compositional analysis. Stroke 2006; 37:93–7.

55. Wentzel JJ, Corti R, Fayad ZA et al. Does shear stress modulate both plaque progression and regression in the thoracic aorta? Human study using serial magnetic resonance imaging. J Am Coll Cardiol 2005; 45:846–54.

56. Tang D, Yang C, Zheng J et al. Quantifying effects of plaque structure and material properties on stress behaviors in human atherosclerotic plaques using 3D FSI models. J Biomech Eng 2005; 127:1185–94.

57. Imoto K, Hiro T, Fujii T et al. Longitudinal structural determinants of atherosclerotic plaque vulnerability: a computational analysis of stress distribution using vessel models and three-dimensional intravascular ultrasound imaging. J Am Coll Cardiol 2005; 46:1507–15.

58. Zarins CK, Giddens DP, Bharadvaj BK et al. Carotid bifurcation atherosclerosis. Quantitative correlation of plaque localization with flow velocity profiles and wall shear stress. Circ Res 1983; 53:502–14.

59. Ku DN, Giddens DP, Zarins CK, Glagov S. Pulsatile flow and atherosclerosis in the human carotid bifurcation. Positive correlation between plaque location and low oscillating shear stress. Arteriosclerosis 1985; 5:293–302.

60. Irace C, Cortese C, Fiaschi E et al. Wall shear stress is associated with intima–media thickness and carotid atherosclerosis in subjects at low coronary heart disease risk. Stroke 2004; 35:464–8.

61. Gnasso A, Irace C, Carallo C et al. In vivo association between low wall shear stress and plaque in subjects with asymmetrical carotid atherosclerosis. Stroke 1997; 28:993–8.

62. Malek AM, Alper SL, Izumo S. Hemodynamic shear stress and its role in atherosclerosis. JAMA 1999; 282:2035–42.

63. Underhill H, Kerwin WS, Hatsukami TS, Yuan C. Automated measurement of mean wall thickness in the common carotid artery by MRI: a comparison to intima–media thickness by B-mode ultrasound. J Magn Reson Imaging 2006; 24:379–87.

64. Saam T, Ferguson MS, Yarnykh VL et al. Quantitative evaluation of carotid plaque composition by in vivo MRI. Arterioscler Thromb Vasc Biol 2005; 25:234–9.

65. Kolodgie FD, Gold HK, Burke AP et al. Intraplaque hemorrhage and progression of coronary atheroma. N Engl J Med 2003; 349:2316–25.

66. Chu B, Kampschulte A, Ferguson MS et al. Hemorrhage in the atherosclerotic carotid plaque: a high-resolution MRI study. Stroke 2004; 35:1079–84.

67. Kampschulte A, Ferguson MS, Kerwin WS et al. Differentiation of intraplaque vs juxtaluminal hemorrhage/thrombus in advanced human carotid atherosclerotic lesions by in vivo magnetic resonance imaging. Circulation 2004; 110:3239–44.

68. Takaya N, Yuan C, Chu BC et al. Presence of intraplaque hemorrhage stimulates progression of carotid atherosclerotic plaques: a high-resolution MRI study. Circulation 2005; 111:2768–75.

69. Taniguchi H, Momiyama Y, Fayad ZA et al. In vivo magnetic resonance evaluation of associations between aortic atherosclerosis and both risk factors and coronary artery disease in patients referred for coronary angiography. Am Heart J 2004; 148:137–43.

70. Rohani M, Jogestrand T, Ekberg M et al. Interrelation between the extent of atherosclerosis in the thoracic aorta, carotid intima–media thickness and the extent of coronary artery disease. Atherosclerosis 2005; 179:311–16.

71. Corti R, Fuster V, Fayad ZA et al. Effects of aggressive vs conventional lipid-lowering therapy by simvastatin on human atherosclerotic lesions: a prospective, randomized, double-blind trial with high-resolution magnetic resonance imaging. J Am Coll Cardiol 2005; 46:106–12.

72. Yonemura A, Momiyama Y, Fayad ZA et al. Effect of lipid-lowering therapy with atorvastatin on atherosclerotic aortic plaques detected by noninvasive magnetic resonance imaging. J Am Coll Cardiol 2005; 45:733–42.

73. Takaya N, Yuan C, Chu B et al. Association between carotid plaque characteristics and subsequent ischemic cerebrovascular events: a prospective assessment with Magnetic Resonance Imaging - initial results. Stroke 2006; 37:818–23.

SECTION V

Systemic therapy

Influenza vaccination as a strategy to prevent cardiovascular events

29

Mohammad Madjid and S Ward Casscells III

INTRODUCTION

We are born and continue to live during a pandemic of cardiovascular disease (CVD). Coronary heart disease (CHD), a rare disease of the affluent and rich in the late 19th century, rapidly emerged as the main cause of death in the Western world by the mid 20th century and is rising to the number one cause of death in the developing countries as well. Atherosclerosis, the main underlying pathology for coronary artery disease, is a very common finding in adults living in the Western world and can be found even in the young. In fact, multiple autopsy studies have shown that atherosclerotic lesions can be found at very early ages.[1,2] The relation between high plasma concentrations of cholesterol and especially low-density lipoprotein (LDL) cholesterol, smoking, diabetes, and hypertension with atherosclerosis is well established by now. However, new evidence generated during the past two decades has highlighted the critical role of inflammation in atherosclerosis.[3] Atherosclerosis is an inflammatory disease characterized by multifocal lesions and systemic elevations of a number of inflammatory markers such as acute phase proteins, cytokines, and cell adhesion molecules.[4] The natural history of atherosclerosis is one of slow progression over years with a possible abrupt disruption of plaques leading to acute coronary syndromes (ACS). The most common underlying pathophysiologic mechanism of ACS is plaque rupture and subsequent thrombosis at the site of the plaque disruption.[5] A majority of myocardial infarction (MI) cases and sudden cardiac deaths are caused by the rupture of a coronary atherosclerotic plaque.[6] Plaque rupture may be precipitated by external stresses or 'triggers' superimposed on vulnerable coronary plaques.[7] The mechanisms by which certain triggers can induce rupture and instability of the plaques are not completely understood but are believed to involve mechanical tension, chemical changes (low pH), tissue degradation (release of proteolytic enzymes), thinning of the fibrous cap (<65 µm) along with changes in platelet aggregability and blood viscosity.

Several external triggers for acute myocardial infarction (AMI) have been recognized, including strenuous physical activity, emotional stress, cocaine use, sexual activity, extreme air pollution, and catastrophes such as earthquakes or missile attacks.[7] We have been studying the role of influenza as a trigger of AMI.[8] Influenza has a high incidence in adult populations and causes a severe inflammatory response in the body that predisposes the high-risk patients to develop ACS.

INFLUENZA AS A TRIGGER OF ACUTE MYOCARDIAL INFARCTION

Influenza infection causes significant morbidity and mortality in developed and underdeveloped countries. Influenza is currently the fourth major cause of mortality in the USA; however, the actual death toll due to influenza may be even higher than this number.[9] The reported death rate due to influenza is mainly based upon the study of death certificates, which traditionally underestimate death due to influenza. It is estimated that influenza-related morbidity and mortality is approximately three times higher than those calculated based on death certificates. Influenza causes a significant number of AMIs every year; however, cases of fatal AMI due to influenza are generally recorded as CHD-related death and not influenza-related deaths.[9] In fact, we have previously estimated that influenza causes up to 91 000 deaths per year in the USA through triggering of fatal myocardial infarctions alone.[9] This heavy burden is based on the high prevalence of both symptomatic and asymptomatic CHD in the population and a concomitant high incidence of influenza infection each year. The influenza attack rate in a typical year is about 10–20% and, as expected, many of these cases affect patients with CHD.[10] This attack rate (and also the severity of the subsequent acute febrile disease) will be even higher in epidemic and pandemic years. A new influenza pandemic is expected in the near future and may be associated with a remarkably high number of coronary deaths as the main cause of death.[9,11] During most influenza epidemics and pandemics (except for 1918), the mortality rate from cardiovascular causes is about twice that of pneumonia and influenza-related causes.[11] We and others have noticed that influenza can trigger AMI.[8,12–16] Influenza infection can also trigger stroke.[17] The ability of influenza infection to trigger acute cardiovascular events has major clinical and public health implications, as discussed in the following section.

INFLUENZA VACCINE AND CARDIOVASCULAR DISEASES

Considering the triggering role of influenza in causing heart attacks, we hypothesized that influenza vaccination may prevent cardiovascular events in high-risk subjects. In 2000, we reported a case-control study in which we studied 218 patients with CHD. In our study, after adjusting for multiple confounders, we found that receipt of influenza vaccine was associated with a 67% reduction in the risk of recurrent events in CHD patients (odds ratio [OR] = 0.33; 95% CI 0.13–0.82, $P = 0.017$).[18] In another case-control study, Siscovick et al found that influenza vaccine use was associated with a 49% reduction (OR = 0.51; 95% CI 0.33–0.79) in the risk of primary out-of-hospital cardiac arrest.[19]

Lavallée et al, during an influenza epidemic period, studied 270 patients, comprising 90 consecutive elderly patients with brain infarction and 180 population-based controls, and obtained their history of influenza vaccination. After multivariate adjustment, the stroke risk was significantly reduced in the subjects who were vaccinated during the year of the study and in those vaccinated during the last 5 years, with ORs of 0.50 (95% CI 0.26–0.94; $P = 0.033$) and 0.42 (95% CI 0.21–0.81; $P = 0.009$), respectively.[20] Jackson et al studied survivors of a first MI in a well-treated health maintenance organization (HMO) population and found no protective effect from influenza vaccination in reducing recurrent coronary events (adjusted hazard ratio [HR] = 1.18; 95% CI 0.79–1.75).[21]

Kristin Nichol and her colleagues used pooled computerized data from three large managed-care organizations to study a large (>280 000 persons) cohort of community-dwelling elderly (at least 65 years old) and observed that vaccination against influenza was associated with a reduced risk of hospitalization for heart disease (reduction = 19%; $P < 0.001$), cerebrovascular disease (reduction = 16–23%; $P < 0.018$), and reduced all-cause mortality (reduction = 48–50%; $P < 0.001$) during influenza seasons.[22] Gurfinkel and colleagues conducted a pilot randomized clinical trial on 200 MI patients and 101 planned angioplasty/stent patients and found marked mortality reduction in the vaccinated group vs the control group (relative risk [RR] = 0.25; 95% CI 0.07–0.86; P = 0.01).[23] In their study, the triple composite endpoint occurred in 11% of the vaccinated patients vs 23% of the control patients (P = 0.009).[23] The observed reduction in the incidence of cardiovascular death was continued for 1 year after the study (RR = 0.34; 95% CI 0.17–0.71).[24]

Grau et al, in a case-control study, studied 370 consecutive patients with ischemic or hemorrhagic stroke or transient ischemic attack (TIA) and 370 age- and sex-matched population control subjects.[25] Previous influenza vaccination was less common in TIA patients than control subjects (19.2% vs 31.4%; P <0.0001). Influenza vaccination was associated with reduced odds of stroke/TIA even after adjustment for various confounders (OR = 0.46; 95% CI 0.28–0.77).[25] Armstrong et al performed a prospective cohort study on 24 535 patients aged over 75 years from 73 general practices in Great Britain. The difference in all-cause death between vaccinated and unvaccinated people was significant (P = 0.02). In their analysis, influenza-attributable cardiovascular death was lower in vaccinated than unvaccinated subjects (OR = 0.87: 95% CI 0.73–1.02).[26]

The observed reduction in cardiovascular events following influenza vaccine is consistent with supporting studies showing a significant reduction in all-cause morbidity and mortality following influenza vaccination.[27,28] In a meta-analysis of 20 cohort studies, use of influenza vaccine was associated with a 68% reduction in death, and in the case-control studies vaccine was associated with a 30% reduction in deaths from all causes.[29]

MECHANISMS BY WHICH INFLUENZA INFECTION CAN TRIGGER CARDIOVASCULAR EVENTS

Influenza infection can trigger cardiovascular events through several mechanisms as follows.[8, 30–33]

Direct infection of plaques, plaque inflammation, and destabilization

In mouse models, we have shown that influenza virus can directly infect atherosclerotic plaques, reside in the plaques, and increase inflammation at the plaque level.[34] We have also observed that influenza RNA can be detected in aortic tissues taken from a number of patients with aortic aneurysm.[35] In apolipoprotein E (ApoE)-deficient mice, influenza infection is associated with extensive infiltration of inflammatory cells into atherosclerotic plaques along with platelet aggregation.[36] Influenza infection increases levels of circulating tumor necrosis factor-α (TNF-α), which in turn may increase the proliferation and activity of plaque macrophages.[37] Generation of reactive oxygen species after infection may also contribute to the activation of matrix metalloproteinases in the plaques and further destabilization of the plaques.[38,39] In addition, influenza infection increases macrophage trafficking into arterial walls and reverts the anti-inflammatory properties of high-density lipoprotein (HDL) particles (decreased paraoxonase and platelet-activating factor acetyl hydrolase activity).[40,41]

Prothrombotic effects

Influenza infection causes a massive release of proinflammatory and prothrombotic cytokines. This leads to reduction in the clotting time, induction of procoagulant activity in infected endothelial cells, increase in the expression of tissue factor, increased platelet aggregation, decreased plasminogen, and activation of factors X and VII.[18,40–50]

Cardiovascular stress

Influenza is an acute febrile disease that is often associated with tachycardia, release of endogenous catecholamines, psychological distress, dehydration leading to hypotension and hemoconcentration, increased plasma viscosity, hypoxemia and demand ischemia (in severe cases), and endothelial dysfunction.[51] Influenza can also provoke arrhythmias (including atrial fibrillation and flutter) in susceptible patients.[52]

Antigenic cross-reactivity

In our mice experiments, only the atherosclerotic plaques, and not the normal arterial segments, showed excessive inflammation following infection. A possible mimicry of the amino acid sequences involved in cell attachment of viral hemagglutinin with those of ApoB responsible for binding of LDL to high-affinity LDL receptors may exist and contribute to the pathogenesis of vascular complications of influenza.[53] In fact, an ecological study showed an association between the age distribution of death from influenza during the 1918 US Spanish Flu pandemic and the subsequent distribution of CHD death from 1920 to 1985 in survivors from the corresponding birth cohorts.[54] This provocative study suggests that the 1918 influenza pandemic might have had a role in causing the (so-far-unexplained) epidemic of CHD mortality in the 20th century.

EFFECT OF SYSTEMIC INFECTIONS ON CORONARY ARTERY PATHOLOGY

Few data are available on how influenza may directly affect the atherosclerotic plaques in humans. A clue may be found by studying the coronary arteries of atherosclerotic patients dying of influenza or any other systemic infection. We conducted an autopsy study to investigate the effect of sepsis on the coronary arteries of atherosclerotic patients who had an acute systemic infection within 2 weeks prior to their death.[55] In our study, 5 cases (out of 14) and none of the 13 controls (who had atherosclerosis but not a septic disease

before death) had AMI with thrombosis on autopsy. Whereas the luminal stenosis percent did not differ between cases and controls, the macrophage density in plaques was higher (though non-significantly) in cases vs controls.[55] Interestingly, a significantly higher number of macrophages (1577 ± 1872 vs 265 ± 185 per mm^2; $P = 0.047$) and T cells (48.4 ± 45.0 per mm^2 vs 14.1 ± 6.3 per mm^2; $P = 0.002$) were present in the adventitia of coronary arteries of infected patients vs controls. Dendritic cells were more numerous in the plaques (3.2 ± 2.5 vs 0.3 ± 0.5 per mm^2; $P = 0.022$) but not in the adventitia of the septic patients vs control patients.[55]

INFLUENZA VACCINE COVERAGE IN CARDIAC PATIENTS

Despite the proven benefits of influenza vaccine for cardiac patients, the influenza vaccination rate in US CVD patients is low (49% among persons aged 50–64 years and 23% among persons aged 18–49 years).[56] These numbers are far short of the Healthy People 2000 goal of 60% and the Healthy People 2010 goal of 90%.[57] The situation is unsatisfactory in Europe as well. A recent study from Spain reported that only 39.9% and 51.7% of adult patients with CVD received influenza vaccine in 1993 and 2003, respectively.[58] Unfortunately, the benefit of vaccinating cardiovascular patients against influenza is neglected in most cardiology textbooks and cardiology practice guidelines and this may have contributed to cardiologists' failure to adequately vaccinate their patients against influenza.[59] The authors had urged the American Heart Association (AHA) and American College of Cardiology (ACC) to add influenza vaccination to the ACC/AHA guidelines for care of cardiovascular patients since 2003,[8] and fortunately this recommendation was accepted in 2006.[60]

CLINICAL IMPLICATIONS

Influenza is an important trigger for cardiovascular events by increasing plaque and blood vulnerability in high-risk patients. Influenza vaccine is an effective, inexpensive, and safe intervention that is capable of preventing many cardiovascular events and should be vigorously advocated for cardiac patients. During influenza infections, a person's risk of developing a coronary event is very high, and extensive care should be paid to prevent and control such events. Further research is warranted to identify the exact mechanisms by which influenza can affect the vascular system and to develop more efficient methods to prevent the cardiovascular complications of influenza. Use of neuraminidase inhibitors such as oseltamivir may offer additional protection against influenza and randomized outcome clinical trials are needed to assess their potential efficacy in preventing cardiovascular events in high-risk subjects.

ACKNOWLEDGMENT

This work was supported in part by the US DoD grant # W81XWH-04-2-0035.

REFERENCES

1. Pathobiological Determinants of Atherosclerosis in Youth (PDAY) Research Group. Natural history of aortic and coronary atherosclerotic lesions in youth. Findings from the PDAY Study. Arterioscler Thromb 1993; 13(9):1291–8.

2. Enos WF, Holmes RH, Beyer J. Landmark article, July 18, 1953: coronary disease among United States soldiers killed in action in Korea. Preliminary report. JAMA 1986; 256(20):2859–62.

3. Willerson JT, Ridker PM. Inflammation as a cardiovascular risk factor. Circulation 2004; 109(21 Suppl 1): II2–10.

4. Madjid M, Zarrabi A, Litovsky S, Willerson JT, Casscells W. Finding vulnerable atherosclerotic plaques. Is it worth the effort? Arterioscler Thromb Vasc Biol 2004; 24:1775–82.

5. Shah PK. Mechanisms of plaque vulnerability and rupture. J Am Coll Cardiol 2003; 41(4 Suppl S): 15S–22S.

6. Virmani R, Kolodgie FD, Burke AP, Farb A, Schwartz SM. Lessons from sudden coronary death: a comprehensive morphological classification scheme for atherosclerotic lesions. Arterioscler Thromb Vasc Biol 2000; 20(5):1262–75.

7. Muller JE, Abela GS, Nesto RW, Tofler GH. Triggers, acute risk factors and vulnerable plaques: the lexicon of a new frontier. J Am Coll Cardiol 1994; 23(3):809–13.

8. Madjid M, Naghavi M, Litovsky S, Casscells SW. Influenza and cardiovascular disease: a new opportunity for prevention and the need for further studies. Circulation 2003; 108:2730–6.

9. Thompson WW, Shay DK, Weintraub E et al. Mortality associated with influenza and respiratory syncytial virus in the United States. JAMA 2003; 289(2):179–86.

10. Findlay PF, Gibbons YM, Primrose WR, Ellis G, Downie G. Influenza and pneumococcal vaccination: patient perceptions. Postgrad Med J 2000; 76(894):215–17.

11. Madjid M, Casscells SW. Of birds and men: cardiologists' role in influenza pandemics. Lancet 2004; 364(9442):1309.

12. Bainton D, Jones GR, Hole D. Influenza and ischaemic heart disease – a possible trigger for acute myocardial infarction? Int J Epidemiol 1978; 7(3):231–9.

13. Mackenbach JP, Kunst AE, Looman CW. Seasonal variation in mortality in The Netherlands. J Epidemiol Community Health 1992; 46(3):261–5.

14. Meier CR, Jick SS, Derby LE, Vasilakis C, Jick H. Acute respiratory-tract infections and risk of first-time acute myocardial infarction. Lancet 1998; 351(9114):1467–71.

15. Smeeth L, Thomas SL, Hall AJ et al. Risk of myocardial infarction and stroke after acute infection or vaccination. N Engl J Med 2004; 351(25):2611–18.

16. Spodick DH, Flessas AP, Johnson MM. Association of acute respiratory symptoms with onset of acute myocardial infarction: prospective investigation of 150 consecutive patients and matched control patients. Am J Cardiol 1984; 53(4):481–2.

17. Grau AJ, Buggle F, Ziegler C et al. Association between acute cerebrovascular ischemia and chronic and recurrent infection. Stroke 1997; 28(9):1724–9.

18. Naghavi M, Barlas Z, Siadaty S et al. Association of influenza vaccination and reduced risk of recurrent myocardial infarction. Circulation 2000; 102(25): 3039–45.

19. Siscovick DS, Raghunathan TE, Lin D et al. Influenza vaccination and the risk of primary cardiac arrest. Am J Epidemiol 2000; 152(7):674–7.

20. Lavallee P, Perchaud V, Gautier-Bertrand M, Grabli D, Amarenco P. Association between influenza vaccination and reduced risk of brain infarction. Stroke 2002; 33(2):513–18.

21. Jackson LA, Yu O, Heckbert SR et al. Influenza vaccination is not associated with a reduction in the risk of

recurrent coronary events. Am J Epidemiol 2002; 156(7):634–40.

22. Nichol KL, Lind A, Margolis KL et al. The effectiveness of vaccination against influenza in healthy, working adults. N Engl J Med 1995; 333(14):889–93.

23. Gurfinkel EP, de la Fuente RL, Mendiz O, Mautner B. Influenza vaccine pilot study in acute coronary syndromes and planned percutaneous coronary interventions: the FLU Vaccination Acute Coronary Syndromes (FLUVACS) Study. Circulation 2002; 105(18):2143–7.

24. Gurfinkel EP, Leon de la Fuente R, Mendiz O, Mautner B. Flu vaccination in acute coronary syndromes and planned percutaneous coronary interventions (FLUVACS) Study: One-year follow-up. Eur Heart J 2004; 25(1):25–31.

25. Grau AJ, Fischer B, Barth C et al. Influenza vaccination is associated with a reduced risk of stroke. Stroke 2005; 36(7):1501–6.

26. Armstrong BG, Mangtani P, Fletcher A et al. Effect of influenza vaccination on excess deaths occurring during periods of high circulation of influenza: cohort study in elderly people. BMJ 2004; 329(7467):660.

27. Nichol KL, Wuorenma J, von Sternberg T. Benefits of influenza vaccination for low-, intermediate-, and high-risk senior citizens. Arch Intern Med 1998; 158(16):1769–76.

28. Christenson B, Lundbergh P, Hedlund J, Ortqvist A. Effects of a large-scale intervention with influenza and 23-valent pneumococcal vaccines in adults aged 65 years or older: a prospective study. Lancet 2001; 357(9261):1008–11.

29. Gross PA, Hermogenes AW, Sacks HS, Lau J, Levandowski RA. The efficacy of influenza vaccine in elderly persons. A meta-analysis and review of the literature. Ann Intern Med 1995; 123(7):518–27.

30. Madjid M, Aboshady I, Awan I, Litovsky S, Casscells SW. Influenza and cardiovascular disease: is there a causal relationship? Tex Heart Inst J 2004; 31:4–13.

31. Madjid M, Awan I, Ali M, Frazier L, Casscells W. Influenza and atherosclerosis: vaccination for cardiovascular disease prevention. Expert Opin Biol Ther 2005; 5(1):91–6.

32. Madjid M, Litovsky S, Awan I et al. Influenza virus directly infects the atherosclerotic plaques of apo E deficient mice and can be cultured in high titers from the aortic plaques. Eur Heart J 2004; 25(Abs Suppl):99.

33. Madjid M, Litovsky S, Vela D, Casscells SW. Influenza vaccination: an emerging opportunity to prevent cardiovascular disease. Int Congr Ser 2004; 1263: 678–81.

34. Madjid M, Haidari H, Vela D et al. Influenza virus directly infects atherosclerotic plaques of normal and atherosclerotic mice and exacerbates inflammation in the atherosclerotic plaques. Atherosclerosis 2006; 7(3):309.

35. Madjid M, Litovsky S, Sadeghi N et al. Influenza virus in the atherosclerotic plaques of human aortic aneurysms and Apo E deficient mice. Am J Cardiol 2004; 94(Suppl 6A):141E.

36. Naghavi M, Wyde P, Litovsky S et al. Influenza infection exerts prominent inflammatory and thrombotic effects on the atherosclerotic plaques of apolipoprotein E-deficient mice. Circulation 2003; 107(5): 762–8.

37. Epstein SE, Zhou YF, Zhu J. Infection and atherosclerosis: emerging mechanistic paradigms. Circulation 1999; 100(4):e20–8.

38. Rajagopalan S, Meng XP, Ramasamy S, Harrison DG, Galis ZS. Reactive oxygen species produced by macrophage-derived foam cells regulate the activity of vascular matrix metalloproteinases in vitro. Implications for atherosclerotic plaque stability. J Clin Invest 1996; 98(11):2572–9.

39. Kol A, Sukhova GK, Lichtman AH, Libby P. Chlamydial heat shock protein 60 localizes in human atheroma and regulates macrophage tumor necrosis factor-alpha and matrix metalloproteinase expression. Circulation 1998; 98(4):300–7.

40. Van Lenten BJ, Wagner AC, Anantharamaiah GM et al. Influenza infection promotes macrophage traffic into arteries of mice that is prevented by D-4F, an apolipoprotein A-I mimetic peptide. Circulation 2002; 106(9):1127–32.

41. Van Lenten BJ, Wagner AC, Nayak DP et al. High-density lipoprotein loses its anti-inflammatory properties during acute influenza A infection. Circulation 2001; 103(18):2283–8.

42. Jerushalmy Z, Adler A, Rechnic J, Kohn A, de Vries. Effect of myxoviruses on the clotting and clotretracting activities of human blood platelets "in vitro". Pathol Biol (Paris) 1962; 10:41–8.

43. Whitaker AN, Bunce I, Graeme ER. Disseminated intravascular coagulation and acute renal failure in influenza A2 infection. Med J Aust 1974; 2(6): 196–201.

44. Settle H, Glueck HI. Disseminated intravascular coagulation associated with influenza. Ohio State Med J 1975; 71(10):541–3, S47.

45. Terada H, Baldini M, Ebbe S, Madoff MA. Interaction of influenza virus with blood platelets. Blood 1966; 28(2):213–28.

46. Terada H. [Studies on platelets and interaction with particular reference to the interaction of influenza virus with blood platelets]. Nippon Ketsueki Gakkai Zasshi 1969; 32(1):45–51. [in Japanese]

47. Barshtein Iu A, Frolov AF, Persidskii Iu V, Gavrilov SV. [Characteristics of the action of the influenza virus on the microcirculatory vessels in an experiment]. Mikrobiol Zh 1989; 51(4):44–50. [in Russian]

48. Bogomolov BP, Barinov VG, Deviatkin AV et al. [Hemostasis in influenza and acute respiratory viral infections in the middle-aged and elderly]. Ter Arkh 1990; 62(7):98–102. [in Russian]

49. Bouwman JJ, Visseren FL, Bosch MC, Bouter KP, Diepersloot RJ. Procoagulant and inflammatory response of virus-infected monocytes. Eur J Clin Invest 2002; 32(10):759–66.

50. Visseren FL, Bouwman JJ, Bouter KP et al. Procoagulant activity of endothelial cells after infection with respiratory viruses. Thromb Haemost 2000; 84(2):319–24.

51. Marchesi S, Lupattelli G, Lombardini R et al. Acute inflammatory state during influenza infection and endothelial function. Atherosclerosis 2005; 178(2): 345–50.

52. Bourne G, Wedgwood J. Heart-disease and influenza. Lancet 1959; 1(7085):1226–8.

53. Pleskov VM, Bannikov AI, Zaitsev Iu V. [The receptor-mediated endocytosis of influenza viruses and low-density lipoproteins by tissue cells]. Vopr Virusol 1994; 39(3):121–5. [in Russian]

54. Azambuja MI, Duncan BB. Similarities in mortality patterns from influenza in the first half of the 20th century and the rise and fall of ischemic heart disease in the United States: a new hypothesis concerning the coronary heart disease epidemic. Cad Saude Publica 2002; 18(3):557–77.

55. Madjid M, Litovsky S, Vela D et al. Systemic infection leads to infiltration of macrophages in adventitia of human atherosclerotic coronary arteries: clue to triggering effect of acute infections on acute coronary syndromes. Eur Heart J 2003; 24:417.

56. Singleton JA, Wortley P, Lu PJ. Influenza vaccination of persons with cardiovascular disease in the United States. Tex Heart Inst J 2004; 31:22–7.

57. US Department of Health and Human Services. Healthy People 2010: Understanding and Improving Health, 2nd edn. Washington, DC: US Government Printing Office; 2000.

58. Jimenez-Garcia R, Hernandez-Barrera V, Carrasco Garrido P, Del Pozo SV, de Miguel AG. Influenza vaccination among cardiovascular disease sufferers in Spain: related factors and trend, 1993–2003. Vaccine 2006; 24(23):5073–82.

59. Hunt SA, Abraham WT, Chin MH et al. ACC/AHA 2005 Guideline Update for the Diagnosis and Management of Chronic Heart Failure in the Adult: a report of the American College of Cardiology/ American Heart Association Task Force on Practice Guidelines (Writing Committee to Update the 2001 Guidelines for the Evaluation and Management of Heart Failure): developed in collaboration with the American College of Chest Physicians and the International Society for Heart and Lung Transplantation: endorsed by the Heart Rhythm Society. Circulation 2005; 112(12):1825–52.

60. Smith SC Jr, Allen J, Blair SN et al. AHA/ACC guidelines for secondary prevention for patients with coronary and other atherosclerotic vascular disease: 2006 update: endorsed by the National Heart, Lung, and Blood Institute. Circulation 2006; 113(19):2363–72.

Vaccination: bedside

30

Enrique P Gurfinkel and Veronica S Lernoud

INTRODUCTION

Since the Paleolithic and Neolithic Ages, phylogenetic evolution of hominids has faced major challenges that have determined physical and behavioral modifications. However, from a genetic point of view, the genome mutation rate has been estimated as only 0.5% for every 106 years. Unless a different reactive capacity had been achieved, human beings would be vulnerable.[1]

Considering atherosclerosis as a disease affecting modern civilizations at an increasing rate similar to epidemic disorders, hypercholesterolemia could be analyzed within this evolutionary conception. An interesting observation as regards cholesterol levels in mammals and probably hominids through time is the possible role of the diet in the increasing cholesterol levels found in hominids during evolution.

Cholesterol plasma levels are rarely 100 mg/dl in mammals, and these values seem to have been constant through evolution. On the contrary, human beings have struggled through time, reaching higher values of cholesterol, and gradually developing atherosclerosis. Although the relationship between cultural influences and atherosclerosis cannot be denied, there seems to be a more complex mechanism. Actually, many investigators have attempted to develop an atherosclerotic model in animals and astonishingly found that a fatty-rich diet alone could not explain the disease.

The progression of atherosclerosis seems to result from the interaction between external factors and inner determinants. The understanding of these inner determinants has become one of the most novel areas of knowledge to be acquired in the last decade.

In addition, provided human beings are the result of a long and continuous attempt of the immune system to overcome the challenges of exposure to different noxas through evolution, atherosclerosis could be hypothesized as a failure in that chain of adaptive responses.

The adaptive mechanism along mankind's evolution has involved the development of tolerance to common aggressions such as hunger and infections.[1] Cultural modifications in diet and habits are closely related to exposure to varying noxas and antigens through time. However, infectious agents have the capacity to mutate more rapidly than the human genome. For the human immune system to adapt to mutant noxas, recognition of frequent epitopes shared by different antigens has become a survival resource.

Many infectious pathogens (bacteria and viruses) have been isolated from vessel specimens taken of patients suffering from early and advanced stages of atherosclerosis. Consequently, according to the above-mentioned hypothesis, the dynamic concept of the vulnerable plaque (as it has been thoroughly described) should also be considered as an unstable ecosystem within a vulnerable patient in constant evolution.

Comprehension of the linkage between atherosclerosis and the immune system, plus the infectious background and molecular mechanisms involved, has caught the attention of researchers. Numerous trials have attempted to test this relationship between infection and atherosclerosis: some have reached interesting conclusions.

The randomized trial of roxithromycin in non-Q-wave coronary syndromes (ROXIS)[2,3] was a 6-month follow-up trial based on the hypothesis that a significant gap in the rate of clinical events could be obtained with the addition of anti-*Chlamydia* therapy.

Antibiotics act as inhibitors of bacterial replication or induce of a bactericidal effect, but their half-life implies no remnant or prolonged effect following drug discontinuation.[4] By contrast, vaccines have the property of stimulating the immune system and providing an immune memory, which is more in line with the desired effect to combat a disease characterized by its chronic development such as atherosclerosis.

In 2000 Naghavi et al[5] reviewed medical records and found a reduction in the risk of an acute coronary event in the population receiving anti-flu vaccine. Similarly, Lavalle et al[6] described a decrease in the rate of cerebrovascular events among anti-flu vaccinated patients from observational retrospective reports.

Overall, prior trials results have made the invaluable contribution to science of introducing a brand new interpretation of atherosclerosis as a dynamic and molecularly active process closely related to the inflammatory model. They have drawn attention to the role of these pathogens in plaque development and its instability in acute coronary syndromes.

However, any attempt to comprehend the inner mechanisms involved in atherosclerosis and its broad new spectrum of treatment is still on the first step. This step involves selecting the appropriate antigen to be used and the administration technique required in vaccine design.

There are as many microbes linked to atherosclerotic plaques as targets have been chosen for vaccination development (Figures 30.1 and 30.2).

MIMICRY IS BOTH THE CLUE AND THE PITFALL OF VACCINATION EFFICACY IN ATHEROSCLEROSIS

The key to this heterogeneity of molecular and microbial targets seems to be the molecular mimicry of epitopes the immune system is able to recognize. Consequently, cross-reactivity to similar epitopes[7] could explain the reason why no single pathophysiologic model has been able to reproduce atherosclerosis completely until our day (Figure 30.3).

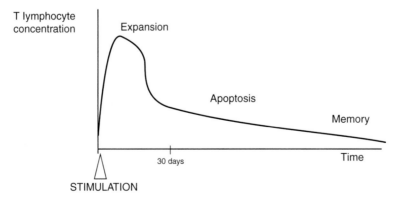

Figure 30.1   Concentration curve of T lymphocytes through time after an antigenic stimulation results in a first stage of cell activation, followed by a stage of apoptosis. The concentration decreases gradually.

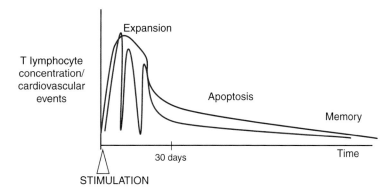

Figure 30.2   The blue line represents T lymphocyte concentration through time. The red line shows cadiovascular events after exposure of the endothelium to antigens. The graphic represents the cumulative amount of cardiovascular events as they correlate with the cellular immune response after a stimulation (superposition of the curve seen in Figure 30.1 and the cumulative event curve).

Regardless of which infectious agent is identified within the plaque, a common denominator is a group of molecules whose function is to stabilize and protect the noxa from the innate immune response. These particles vary in their molecular weights and are called heat shock proteins (HSP), since their concentration increases under stress and inflammatory conditions.[8]

Mimicry between HSP60 from man and from pathogens represents a landmark for the understanding of pathogenesis.

Schematically, a first exposure to a noxa triggers the production of HSP, which enhances a response from the innate immune system in order to protect the dysfunctional infected endothelium. Heat shock proteins activate the proinflammatory genes in endothelial cells, smooth muscle cells, and macrophages, inducing atherogenic effects. Cytokines produced by recluted inflammatory cells (nuclear factor kappa B) intervene, enhancing the adhesion of lymphocytes

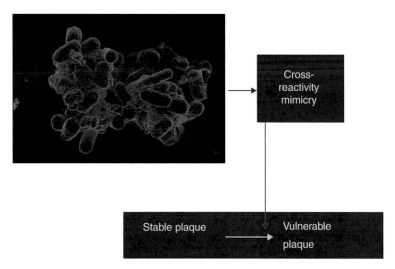

Figure 30.3   Mimicry between influenza virus epitopes (electron microscopy – top left) and endothelial elements results in a cross reaction where immune system interaction leads to alterations within the atherosclerotic plaque: then, a stable plaque would turn into a vulnerable one.

and more macrophages. Antibodies against HSP expressed on cells' surfaces and T lymphocytes exert a cytotoxic effect on affected cells. Once activated, these cells are prone to produce metalloproteinases and tumor necrosis factor-α (TNF-α) that degrade the fibrous lining cap of the atherosclerotic plaque. Subsequently, activated monocytes invade the media intimae. All these steps seem to contribute to inflammation and low-density lipoprotein (LDL) phagocytosis by monocytes.[9] This complex interaction of molecules and cells ultimately predisposes to instability within the plaque (Figure 30.4).

Thus, a stable lesion turns into an unstable one. Once the immune system has had contact with the HSP, the next presentation of these antigens would be followed by a greater immunologic reaction and endothelial dysfunction. The repetitive aggression of oxidized LDL (oxLDL) perpetuates the cycle by recruiting immune cells already competent since their first exposure to HSP. In this model, HSP and oxLDL represent the ultimate responses of the inflammatory chain initiated by infection.[9] They are the newly identified

antigens toward which efforts in designing a vaccine are inclined nowadays.

Recently, the mechanism has been described as a mimicry between HSP60 and oxLDL. This would explain the experiments performed by Dimaguya et al[10] on genetically manipulated mice with targeted deletion of the gene for apolipoprotein E (ApoE-knockout mice) being hypercholesterolemic and on mice lacking LDL receptors when fed with a fatty diet. Not surprisingly, the genetic alteration if not accompanied by the stress influence to the endothelium of a great charge of lipids, would not result in atherosclerotic burden.

One of the most studied agents capable of inducing HSP60 expression and associated to atherosclerosis through many reports worldwide is *Chlamydia pneumoniae*.[9] Saikku[11] noted that patients suffering from myocardial infarction and angina pectoris had a significantly higher percentage of anti-*Chlamydia pneumoniae* IgG (immunoglobulin G) titers compared with asymptomatic controls.

Anti-*Chlamydia pneumoniae* vaccine is considered a possible candidate for

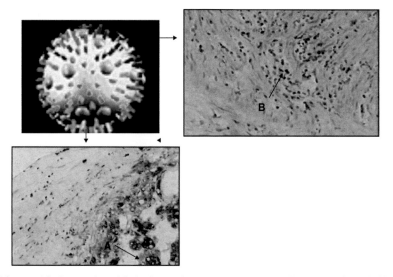

Figure 30.4   Evidence of flu interaction with the innate immune system, promoting macrophage infiltration of the vessel wall and activation of Th1 lymphocytes within the atherosclerotic plaque. (A) Foam cells (macrophages) within vulnerable plaque. (B) Activated T Lymphocytic cells are marked with CD45RO within an inflamed atherosclerotic plaque.

attacking the immunologic arousal from the very beginning. Unfortunately, among the various epitopes constituent of this pathogen, no molecule has been identified that guarantees protective action in humans. A recombinant DNA technique is being used at the basic experimental stage to synthesize a vaccine against bacterial components. Even proteins on the surface of the *Chlamydia* agent known as the 'type III secretion system' are targets of vaccine investigational assays.[9]

Oral and nasal mucosal immunomodulation with HSP in animals has achieved a certain degree of attenuation of atherosclerotic lesions.[8]

Immunomodulation through vaccines against HSP or peptidic epitopes of HSP are promising in shifting the immune reaction from Th1 to Th2 lymphocytes.[12] The immune system responses can be divided into innate and adaptive responses. The innate response represents a burst of inflammatory and toxic response readily active against any antigens. It is started through antigen presentation by macrophages and dendritic cells joined to major histocompatibility complex (MHC) molecules attached to scavenger and Toll-like cell receptors.[13] The adaptive response is specifically targeted towards an antigen, although it needs prior enhancement and recognition to be activated.

The ability to manipulate the immune system through immunomodulation and immunization is a practical clinical bedside therapeutic approach to the vulnerable patient suffering from atherosclerotic disease. Immunization could be passive by means of exposure to hyperimmune sera or recombinant antibodies.[8] On the other hand, active immunization implies antigen manipulation and vaccination in order to induce a protective immune response.[8]

Within the last century, vaccines have almost eliminated the threat of different viral and bacterial agents. Such an achievement is now the goal of scientific research on non-infectious diseases.

A crucial step of immunization is triggering a protective immunologic response, which is represented by the Th2 response. Choosing the right adjuvant ligand to the antigen is the clue for controlling adverse effects of vaccines plus intervening in the extent of the immunologic response obtained (Figure 30.5).

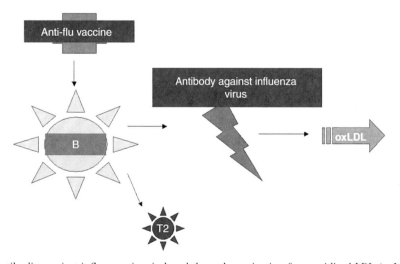

Figure 30.5 Antibodies against influenza virus induced through vaccination favor oxidized LDL (oxLDL) clearance, as they produce antibodies which cross react with oxidized LDL epitopes. In addition, stimulated B lymphocytes enhance a shift in immune response from Th1 to Th2 (T2), which apparently has an atheroprotective effect.

A comprehensive understanding of shifting from Th1 to Th2 requires knowledge of MHC proteins. These proteins are expressed in the membranes of antigen-presenting cells and related to specific recognition by different types of T lymphocytes. MHC class II proteins recognize exogenous antigens and interact with CD4+ T cells; these could also be reckoned as Th1 or Th2. Meanwhile, MHC I proteins remain in the cell's membranes and recognize endogenous antigens. They interact with CD8+ T lymphocytes and correlate to cytotoxic immune reaction.[13]

Certain adjunvants have the property of mimicking the pattern reaction triggered by oxidized LDL, thus becoming particularly useful in vaccination against atherosclerosis. Cytokines and cytokine genes in the form of plasmid DNA have also been tested as adjuvants.[8]

Activation of the immune system could be induced through enhancement of mucosa-associated lymphoid tissue from oral or nasal mucosal membranes.[8] These tissues are rich in dendritic cells and control immune regulatory cytokines. From birth, everything in contact with them is first recognized as an antigen by the organism. Secondly, toleration is achieved through immunomodulation. The same process using a different dose of antigen exposure results in production of high titers of antibodies. Anergy is also developed when antigen-presenting cells induce inactivation of native T cells. As a result, self-antigens are recognized by the immune system and destruction of the organism's own cells is avoided.

Induction of tolerance or antibody production depends on the predominance of a certain type of cytokine in the environment and of the kind of adjuvant ligand associated with the antigen and the presenting cell receptor. Both cytokine and adjuvants are relevant in shifting immune response from Th1 to Th2.[9] Among these determinants, adjuvants such as alum and Freund's have proved to be more appropriate in preferential stimulation of a Th2 response.[8]

Consequently, vaccination could be seen as a two-way opportunity of immunomodulation and therapeutic approach to atherosclerosis: one would be dependent on enhancement of a protective Th2 response, the other would depend on inhibition of the Th1 response.

Animal experiments provide compelling evidence of the important role of Toll-like receptor-mediated innate immune signaling and oxLDL interactions. Furthermore, such interaction between oxLDL and MHC class II proteins with Th CD4+ cells derives from activation of the Th1 response or the Th2 response.[8]

Each pathway implies a different subset of cytokines being produced. The Th1 response secretes interferon-α (IFN-α), the Th2 response secretes interleukins IL-4, IL-5, and IL-10. The former activates cell immune reactions mediated by macrophages, whereas the latter is mediated by humoral immune reactions through activation of B lymphocytes.[14]

Atherosclerotic plaques are characterized by Th1 dominance. Histochemical analyses of vessel lesions detect IG 2a subtype concentrations within them.[12] Although activation involves both lines of Th cells, in atherosclerosis disease there is a tendency toward a predominance of Th1 pathway mechanisms. In recent years, more subsets of Th cells have been identified. Actually, it seems to be T-regulatory cells (T CD4 CD25 subtype) that can trigger a beneficial atheroprotective reaction. At least evidence supporting this hypothesis has been tested in animal models.[8]

Whether this seems to rewrite interpretation of the immunology and atherosclerosis pathogenic paradigm, or merely illustrates the complexity of developing an accurate model of atherosclerosis in humans, remains a question for researchers and physicians.

Meanwhile, attempts to immunize hypercholesterolemic animals with oxLDL have provided interesting results, with 40–70% inhibition of atherosclerosis development.

Oxidized LDL particles, already processed to isolate certain epitopes, have the potential to induce a shift from IgM to IgG antibodies.[12] There is also an association between the increase in specific IgG and the extent of inhibition of atherosclerosis.

Two major subclasses of oxLDL antigens have been identified (specific MDA [malondialdehyde]-modified peptide sequences in ApoB 100 and oxidized phospholipids containing the phosphorylcholine head group), either present as an isolated lipid or covalently bound to an ApoB100 peptide sequence: immunization with the first subclass induces an adaptive T-cell-dependent synthesis of IgG; the second subclass induces an innate-like response with B-cell-dependent IgM synthesis. Both have a relative atheroprotective effect.[12]

There is a limitation to interpreting animal experiments with the above-mentioned vaccines based on oxLDL antigens and their specific fragments as a success for atherosclerosis treatment because most of the experiments have been designed in order to prevent early-vessel lesions at short ages. This represents a clinical limitation, and more research will be needed before wholescale use of such vaccines becomes a standard therapy.

Vaccines targeted against infectious agents and those against HSP60 act within the same ultimate pathway, as already mentioned above. Suppression of plaque inflammatory burst following immunization is documented, with less expression of Th1 cytokines.

A different approach to antiatherosclerotic vaccine is transcription and inclusion of a chimeric polypeptide of tetanus toxic T-cell epitope and a cholesteryl ester transfer protein (CETP) B-cell epitope expressed as inclusion bodies in *Escherichia coli* through genetic manipulation techniques. The preparation was tested on mice for immunization and efficiently evoked an immune response with production of moderate and long-lasting specific antibodies anti CETPC. It seemed to have the potential to inhibit excessive abnormal CETP, thus preventing atherosclerosis.[15,16] Nevertheless, the clinical effect of inhibition of CEPT and adverse events associated with the new vaccine formula need further investigation to be tested in humans.

As we enter the new millennium, the knowledge already accumulated should stimulate laboratories and physicians to apply the evidence to the real patient and find a solution of the therapeutic approach. What we should question nowadays is: Does it seem probable that a vaccine could alter the progression of atherosclerosis?

CONCLUSIVE DECISION MAKING BEDSIDE OF THE VULNERABLE PATIENT

The FLU Vaccination Acute Coronary Syndromes (FLUVACS)[17] trial was designed to explore the immune system and the anti-flu vaccination benefits in acute coronary syndrome patients. It constituted the first randomized, prospective, multicenter, parallel group, and controlled pilot trial directed at proving the immunology and inflammatory hypothesis in atherosclerosis in humans. The analyses implied two different cohorts of patients. A total of 301 patients were enrolled: 151 were assigned to the vaccine group in 2001 and 150 were part of the control group. The inclusion criteria were patients admitted into hospital within the first 72 hours of acute myocardial infarction, either ST- or non-ST-elevation myocardial infarction; there were also 101 patients for planned angioplasty/stenting, referred to as the interventional group. As a result of the intervention, the incidence of cardiovascular death at 1 year was significantly decreased in the vaccinated population in comparison to those who were assumed as the control group.[18] In addition, the hypothesis of an immunomodulation was twice reassured when during the winter of 2002 those not having received the vaccine the previous year were submitted to the treatment group in the context of stable coronary disease.[19] Meanwhile, patients having been vaccinated in the first stage of the trial, were enrolled in the control group. A regression logistic statistical model was used. A major beneficial effect was detected among patients older than 65 years old with non-ST-elevation myocardial infarction, and those having a high-risk score for subsequent adverse events. In the second phase of the study, the combined endpoint of death and myocardial infarction was reduced in the vaccinated group when compared with the control cohort. Less revascularization procedures were required in the vaccination group at 1-year follow-up. The FLU-VACS trial results suggested that the humoral response after vaccination stimulus may reflect migration of committed B lymphocytes.[17]

We developed a subsequent study designed to include apparently healthy subjects who were submitted to anti-flu vaccination and blood sampling at 0, 4, and 12 hours. The same individuals were their own control group as, 1 week later, a placebo was administered and blood sampling was again obtained at the same intervals. Blood samples were tested for measurement of tissue factor pathway inhibitor (TFPI), globulin lysis time, and fibrinogen. At 4 hours from vaccination in the treatment group, a decrease in fibrinogen plasma levels, a prolonged globulin lysis activity, and an increase in TFPI production were documented (Enrique Gurfinkel, pers comm).

A meta-analysis including 20 cohort studies has confirmed a reduction in death rates of 68%.[20] The PRISMA study performed in a population younger than 65 years old with high-risk medical conditions proved the clinical effectiveness of influenza vaccination in this group. Vaccination prevented 78% of deaths (95% CI 39–92%) in PRISMA.[21] As far as science has evolved in the past decade, vaccination seems to be the future goal against the epidemic of atherosclerosis. Even nowadays, commonly used anti-flu vaccines have proved efficient in reducing a hard endpoint as death when applied to coronary patients. Its main effect should be understood as a molecular targeted intervention in order to reduce the inflammatory burst mimicry between infectious agents and endogenous antigens aroused in the human immune system.

A group of experts in various areas – cardiology, neurology, infectology, and internal medicine – gathered at the first Conference on Prevention Strategies for Cardiovascular Diseases through the Application of the Anti-Influenza Vaccine on March 25, 2004. Their recommendations were notified to health authorities by the government.[22,23] Moreover public health decisions have been taken on behalf of these reports. Having assumed atherosclerosis as an inflammatory disease, the World Health Organization (WHO) considered the possible role of anti-flu vaccine as secondary prevention. To achieve most of the beneficial effects observed in all groups of patients, but mainly in those suffering from cardiovascular disease, by means of this inexpensive and profitable resource, vaccination was extended to 50-year-old patients.[24]

Returning to the beginning of our discussion, while desired values of plasmatic cholesterol nowadays are closed to the presumed levels hominids sustained in the Paleolithic Age, statins are the therapeutic resource used. From this perspective, it could be hypothesized that vaccine interaction with the immune system attempts to restore the equilibrium which was altered through exposure to continuous infectious aggression along thousands of years of evolution.

In conclusion, immunomodulation stands as the key to modern therapeutic approaches to the vulnerable patient.

REFERENCES

1. Gurfinkel E. Infection and atherosclerosis. Is this hypothesis still alive? Nat Clin Pract Cardiovasc Med 2006; 3:1.

2. Gurfinkel E, Bozovich G, Daroca A, Beck G, Mautner B. Randomised trial of roxithromycin in non-Q-wave coronary syndromes: ROXIS Pilot Study. Roxis Study Group. Lancet 1997; 350:404–7.

3. Gurfinkel E, Bozovich G, Livellara G et al. Antibiotics for the treatment of non-Q-wave coronary syndromes. The Final Report of the ROXIS Trial. Eur Heart J 1999; 20:121–7.

4. Gurfinkel E, Lernoud V. The role of infection and immunity in atherosclerosis. Expert Rev Cardiovasc Ther 2006; 4(1):131–7.

5. Naghavi M, Barlas Z, Siadaty S et al. Association of influenza vaccination and reduced risk of recurrent myocardial infarction. Circulation 2000; 102:3039–45.

6. Lavalle P, Perchaud V, Gauier/Bertrand M et al. Association between influenza vaccination and reduced risk of brain infarction. Stroke 2002; 33:513–18.

7. Gurevich VS. Influenza, autoimmunity and atherogenesis. Autoimmun Rev 2005; 4:101–5.

8. Nilsson J, Hansson GK, Shah PK. Immunomodulation of atherosclerosis. Implications for vaccine development. Arterioscler Thromb Vasc Biol 2005; 25:18–28.

9. Blasi C. The role of the infectious agents in the pathogenesis and evolution of atherosclerosis. Ann Ital Med Int 2004; 19:249–61.

10. Dimaguya P, Cercek B, Oguchi S et al. Inhibitory effect on arterial injury-induced neointimal formation by adoptive B-cell transfer in rag-1 knockout mice. Arterioscler Thromb Vasc Biol 2002; 22:644–9.

11. Saikku P. Epidemiologic association of Chlamydia pneumoniae and atherosclerosis: the initial serologic observation and more. J Infect Dis 2000; 181 (Suppl 3): S411–13.

12. Fredrikson GN, Andersson L, Soderberg I et al. Atheroprotective immunization with MDA-modified apo B-100 peptide sequences is associated with activation of Th2 specific antibody expression. Autoimmunity 2005; 38(2):171–9.

13. Roitt I, Brostoff J, Male D. Inmunología. Barcelona, Spain: Masson-Salvat Medicina; 1994.

14. Caliguri G, Nicolettei A, Poirier B et al. Protective immunity against atherosclerosis carried by B cells of hypercholesterolemic mice. J Clin Invest 2002; 109:721–4.

15. Gaofu Q, Jie W, Xin Y, Roque RS, Jingjing L. Expressing and purifying an anti-atherosclerosis polypeptide vaccine in Escherichia coli. Protein Expr Purif 2004; 36:198–206.

16. Kermani T, Frishman WH. Nonpharmacologic approaches for the treatment of hyperlipidemia. Cardiol Rev 2005; 13:247–55.

17. Gurfinkel EP, de la Fuente RL, Mendiz O, Mautner B. Influenza vaccine pilot study in acute coronary syndromes and planned percutaneous coronary interventions: the FLU Vaccination Acute Coronary Syndromes (FLUVACS) Study. Circulation 2002; 105:2143–7.

18. Gurfinkel EP, Leon de la Fuente R, Mendiz O, Mautner B. Flu vaccination in acute coronary syndromes and planned percutaneous coronary interventions (FLUVACS) Study. Eur Heart J 2004; 25(1):25–31.

19. Gurfinkel EP, Leon de la Fuente R. Two-year follow-up of the Flu Vaccination Acute Coronary Syndromes (FLUVACS) Registry. Tex Heart Inst J 2004; 31(1):28–32.

20. Werner N, Böhm M. Topic: Cardiovascular disease prevention – risk assessment and management: influenza vaccination in cardiovascular disease. European Society of Cardiology. E-Journal - Vol 8, available at www.escardio.org/knowledge/cardiology–practice/ejournal_vol4/vol4n8.htm/

21. Hak E, Buskens E, van Essen GA et al. Clinical effectiveness of influenza vaccination in persons younger than 65 years with high-risk medical conditions: the PRISMA study. Arch Intern Med 2005; 165:274–80.

22. Resolution from the Argentina Senate 18/March/2004: Health and Sports. Available at www.proyectos.senado.gov.ar/web/owa/web_proce.verexpediente

23. Gurfinkel E, Ameriso S, Belardi J et al. I National Consensus on strategies in primary and secondary prevention of cardiovascular diseases through the application of anti-flu vaccine. Rev Esp Cardiol Suppl 2004; 4:35–41G.

24. Gurfinkel E. The Fluvacs trial in perspective. Rev Esp Cardiol Suppl 2004; 4:25–34G.

Immunomodulation of atherosclerosis

31

Jan Nilsson, Gunilla Nordin Fredrikson, Alexandru Schiopu,
Isabel Gonçalves, Kuang-Yuh Chyu, and Prediman K Shah

INTRODUCTION

Accumulation and oxidation of lipoproteins in the extracellular matrix of the artery wall is a key initiating factor in the development of atherosclerosis.[1,2] It results in activation of an inflammatory response mediated by what is referred to as the innate component of immunity. This part of the immune system provides a rapid and non-specific defense against invading microorganisms but reacts also with modified self-antigens such as oxidized low-density lipoprotein (LDL) and dying cells. The inflammatory response induced by the innate immune system is believed to play a key role in both plaque growth and the development of plaque vulnerability.[3,4] More recently, it has become evident that adaptive immune responses are also critically involved in the disease process. Adaptive immunity is much more complex, specific, and fine-tuned than innate immunity and, as a consequence, may take several days or even weeks to be fully mobilized. It involves a genetic rearrangement process in immunoblasts, leading to generation of a large number of highly antigen-specific T- and B-cell receptors and antibodies. One important function of adaptive immunity is to modulate the inflammatory activity of the innate immune system in order to mount the most appropriate response for each type of challenge. Accordingly, it has

become clear that the immune system represents an interesting target for development of novel therapies for prevention and treatment of cardiovascular disease.[5,6]

INNATE AND ADAPTIVE IMMUNITY IN ATHEROSCLEROSIS

A schematic overview of the innate and adaptive immune systems is given in Figure 31.1. Our understanding of the functional role of the immune system in atherosclerosis is primarily based on mouse studies in which atherosclerosis-susceptible, hypercholesterolemic animals such as ApoE$^{-/-}$ and LDL receptor$^{-/-}$ mice have been cross-bred with mice genetically deficient or transgenically overexpressing specific immune receptors, co-stimulatory factors, and cytokines.

Detection of so-called pathogen-associated molecular patterns (PAMP) by pattern recognition receptors on macrophages and dendritic cells is one of the key elements of the innate immune system. There is a repertoire of pattern recognition receptors binding a wide range of proteins, carbohydrates, lipids, and nucleic acids. Among these pattern recognition receptors are the scavenger receptors and the Toll-like receptors (TLRs).[7] Scavenger receptors mediate removal of modified lipoproteins, apoptotic cells, and some microorganisms, while activation of TLRs

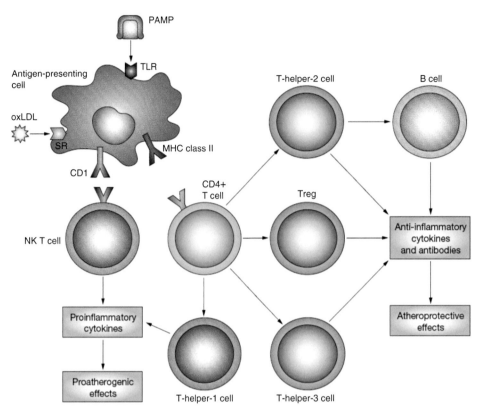

Figure 31.1 A schematic representation of the potential juxtaposed roles of the adaptive immune response to specific antigens. The proatherogenic component results from T-helper-1 cell and natural killer T-cell activation triggered by the presentation of antigens via the major histocompatibility complex class II or CD1 molecules. The atheroprotective component is mediated by the secretion of anti-inflammatory cytokines (such as interleukin-10 and transforming growth factor-β), mediated by T-helper-2, T-helper-3 and regulatory T cells (Treg), and antibody response, mediated by B cells. MHC class I and II, major histocompatibility complex class I and II; NK T cell, natural killer T cell; OxLDL, oxidized low-density lipoprotein; PAMP, pathogen-associated molecular patterns; SR, scavenger receptor; TLR, Toll-like receptor. (Reproduced with permission from Shah et al.[6])

by lipopolysaccharide (LPS) and other microbial antigens induces an inflammatory response. Mice that lack scavenger receptors have been reported to be both more resistant to atherosclerosis development[8,9] as well as more susceptible,[10] making their role in the disease process controversial. A decreased development of atherosclerosis has been observed in animals lacking the membrane-associated TLR signal protein Myd-88,[11,12] as well as in mice lacking the potent proinflammatory cytokine tumor necrosis factor-α (TNF-α).[13] These observations suggest

that hypercholesterolemia is associated with formation of modified self-antigens that interact with pattern recognition receptors causing inflammation and plaque development. They also suggest the possibility that activation of innate pattern recognition receptors by other mechanisms, such as infections, may contribute to the disease process.

Adaptive immune response occurs when a specific antigen, processed and presented by antigen-presenting cells, is recognized by the immune system, leading to proliferation of T and B cells.

Antigens are taken up by dendritic cells and macrophages and presented by major histocompatibility complex (MHC) class II proteins for recognition by specific CD4+ T cells (peptide antigens) or CD1 molecules for natural killer (NK) T cells (lipid-associated antigens). When T cells encounter their specific antigens, an adaptive immune response is activated, including clonal proliferation of the T cell and production of cytokines, and subsequent activation of B cells to produce immunoglobulins.

Hypercholesterolemic mice with severely compromised adaptive immunity, such as severe combined immunodeficiency (SCID) mice, develop markedly less atherosclerosis, suggesting that the net effect of adaptive immune responses to hypercholesterolemia is proatherogenic.[14] This concept is supported by other studies demonstrating that ablation of the CD1[15] and CD4[16] genes in ApoE $^{-/-}$ mice reduce the development of atherosclerosis. A decreased development of atherosclerosis has also been observed in LDL receptor$^{-/-}$ mice lacking B7-1/B7-2[17] and in ApoE$^{-/-}$ mice lacking CD40[18] (all are co-stimulatory molecules expressed by antigen-presenting cells and required for T-cell activation).

Activation of CD4+ T cells by antigen presentation on MHC class II molecules may result in the maturation into several different subtypes of T cells that potentially could have dramatically different effects on the development of atherosclerosis (Figure 31.2). T helper (Th) 1 cells secrete interferon-γ (IFN-γ) and are strongly proinflammatory, Th2 cells produce the anti-inflammatory cytokine interleukin-10 (IL-10) and mediate antibody production, and regulatory T cells (Treg) produce inhibitory signals through immunosuppressive cytokines. Analysis of the cytokine expression in atherosclerotic plaques suggests a dominance of Th1 cells.[19,20] Genetic deletion of components critical for Th1 activity, such as the IFN-γ receptor[21] and T-bet[22] (the transcription factor required for Th1 differentiation), has been found to inhibit atherosclerosis. Interestingly, the opposite effect occurs if components of the alternate pathways, such as IL-10[23,24] and the lymphocyte transforming growth factor-β (TGF-β) receptor,[25] are disrupted. The notion that the alternate pathways are atheroprotective is also supported by the studies of Mallat et al,[26] demonstrating that activation of Treg cells retards the development of atherosclerosis. Accordingly, it appears that the regulation of the CD4+ T-cell differentiation pathway is a critical step in atherosclerosis. It remains to be fully clarified how CD4+ T-cell differentiation is regulated in hypercholesterolemia and atherosclerosis, but if antigen presentation takes place in a proinflammatory environment this generally favors Th1 maturation. Accordingly, it appears likely that antigen presentation that takes place in a plaque with active inflammation would favor maturation of CD4+ T cells into Th1 cells and result in a vicious cycle of further inflammatory stimulation.

INTERACTIONS BETWEEN OXIDIZED LDL AND THE IMMUNE SYSTEM

There is strong evidence that oxidized LDL is the key antigen formed as a consequence of hypercholesterolemia:

1. Oxidized LDL has been identified in atherosclerotic plaques[27] as well as in the circulation of both healthy subjects and patients suffering from cardiovascular disease.[28]
2. T cells specific for oxidized LDL constitute 10–20% of the lymphocyte population in human atherosclerotic plaques[29] and are present also in the circulation.[30]
3. Antibodies specific for oxidized LDL are commonly encountered in man,[31] and animal studies have shown that they are induced by hypercholesterolemia.[32]

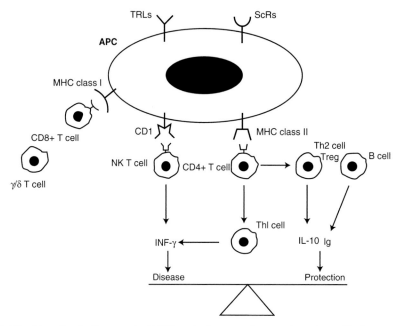

Figure 31.2 Oxidized low-density lipoprotein (LDL) and other proatherogenic antigens bind to scavenger receptors (ScRs) on antigen-presenting cells (APCs). The APCs then present lipid antigens on CD1 receptors and peptide antigens on major histocompatibility complex (MHC) class II molecules. During the development of atherosclerosis, the primary response to this is activation of natural killer (NK) T cells and expression of a Th1 phenotype by CD4+ T cells, resulting in release of interferon-γ (IFN-γ) and progression of disease. This activation pattern is further enhanced by a concurrent activation of Toll-like receptors (TLRs), whereas stimulation of CD8+ T cells by MHC class I molecules as well as activation of γ/γ T cells appear to be of less importance. In contrast, Freund's incomplete adjuvant as well as alum shift activated CD4+ T cells towards development of a Th2 phenotype, leading to expression of anti-inflammatory cytokines, release of immunoglobulins IgG and IgM by B cells and inhibition of disease. Treg regulatory Tcells, IC-10, interleukin-10. (Reproduced with permission from Nilsson J, Circ Res 2005; 96:395–7).[62]

It is important to clarify why oxidized LDL becomes a target for the immune system. As an endogenous structure, LDL is protected by immunologic tolerance. However, the structural change that takes place as LDL is oxidized appears sufficient to break this tolerance. These changes include generation of oxidized phospholipids, breakdown of peptide fragments of ApoB-100 and, perhaps most importantly, aldehyde modification of such fragments.[33] The oxidized phospholipids are recognized by macrophage scavenger receptors that mediate clearance of oxidized LDL from the extracellular space.[34] An innate inflammatory response may be activated by phospholipid metabolites such as phosphatidylcholine and platelet-activating factor (PAF) released from LDL as a result of oxidation or by toxic effects of oxidized LDL on vascular cells.[35] Recent studies have also shown that TLRs are expressed in human and murine atherosclerotic lesions and may be induced by modified lipoproteins.[36–39]

Intracellular processing of oxidized LDL that has been scavenged from the surrounding extracellular matrix subsequently results in presentation of phospholipid and phospholipid–peptide complex antigens by CD1 molecules for NK T cells and peptide antigens by MHC class II molecules for CD4+ T cells (Figure 31.3). As discussed above, in atherosclerosis the predominating response to this antigen presentation appears to be further activation of inflammation and progression of disease.

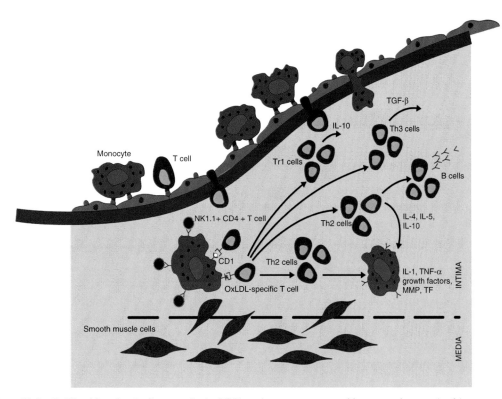

Figure 31.3 Oxidized low-density lipoprotein (oxLDL) antigens are presented by macrophage major histocompatibility complex (MHC) class II proteins for recognition by antigen-specific CD4+ T cells. Activated CD4+ T cells may differentiate into proinflammatory Th1 cells, anti-inflammatory Th2 cells promoting antibody production, Tr1 (T regulatory 1) cells that suppress antigen-induced activation of other CD4+ T cells or transforming growth factor-β (TGF-β)-producing Th3 cells. Presentation of lipid antigens by the macrophage class I-like molecule CD1 results in activation of NK1.1+ CD4+ T cells promoting both Th1 and Th2 responses. The balance between pro- and anti-inflammatory T-cell subsets has a major influence on disease activity and progression. IL, interleukin; MMP, metalloproteinase; TF, tissue factor; TNF-α tumor necrosis factor-α. (Reproduced with permission from Nilsson et al).[5]

MODULATING THE IMMUNE RESPONSE AGAINST OXIDIZED LDL

One approach taken by us and others to clarify the functional importance of immune responses against oxidized LDL has been to actively immunize hypercholesterolemic animals against oxidized LDL. We originally anticipated that this type of immunization would result in a more aggressive immune response against oxidized LDL and an enhanced progression of the disease process. However, unexpectedly, immunization with oxidized LDL was found to confer a partial protection against the development of atherosclerosis.[40,41] The atheroprotective effect of oxidized LDL immunization has later been confirmed in different species and by other research groups.[16,42–46] There are several possible explanations for this outcome:

1. The adjuvants used in the studies (alum and Freund's incomplete adjuvant) favor activation of Th2 responses and may have shifted an endogenous Th1 response against oxidized LDL toward Th2.

2. Antigen presentation following immunization is performed in a non-inflammatory environment (subcutaneous) as opposed to the proinflammatory environment of the atherosclerotic plaque, which again may shift the immune response toward Th2 or induction of tolerance.

3. The results of the knockout experiments discussed above are misleading and also endogenous immune responses against oxidized LDL are in reality atheroprotective.

The third explanation appears the least likely at present in view of the consistency of the experimental findings. The first two explanations are not exclusive and may well both be correct. Immunization with oxidized LDL or peptide antigens from oxidized LDL has been shown to result in an immunoglobulin isotype shift from Th1-specific immunoglobulin IgG2a towards Th2-specific IgG1 in mice,[47] a shift that interestingly also can be observed in response to severe hypercholesterolemia in these animals.[48]

DEVELOPMENT OF IMMUNOMODULATORY THERAPY FOR ATHEROSCLEROSIS – CHALLENGES AND POSSIBILITIES

The observation that immunization with oxidized LDL confers a partial protection against atherosclerosis suggests the fascinating possibility of developing new therapeutic approaches based on selective activation of immune responses against oxidized LDL antigens. However, since oxidized LDL is a complex and poorly characterized particle containing numerous different epitopes that could potentially induce both atheroprotective and atherogenic immune responses, it has become important to obtain a more detailed molecular characterization of the antigens present in oxidized LDL. This information is now starting to become available, making further progress possible

toward development of an immunization-based therapy for atherosclerosis. As discussed above, two major subclasses of oxidized LDL antigens have been identified: oxidized phospholipids containing a phosphorylcholine head group and breakdown peptide fragments of ApoB-100 that become immunogenic because of an altered three-dimensional structure and/or because of aldehyde modification.

The oxidized phospholipid antigens are not exclusively expressed by oxidized LDL but are also found on apoptotic cells and on some microorganisms such as *Streptococcus pneumoniae*.[49] These antigens are recognized by a subclass of IgM referred to as natural antibodies. The natural antibodies can be seen as a humoral equivalent of the cellular pattern recognition receptors. They are usually defined as antibodies that are found in complete absence of exogenous antigenic stimulation and are produced primarily by B-1 cells in the peritoneal cavity and spleen.[50] They provide a first line of defense against invading microorganisms, but react also with self-antigens associated with senescent cells and cellular debris. An additional property of these antibodies that is likely to be important for atherosclerosis is that they inhibit scavenger receptor-mediated uptake of oxidized LDL in macrophages.[51] Binder and co-workers[52] have studied the functional role of antiphospholipid antibodies in atherosclerosis by immunizing LDL receptor knockout mice with *S. pneumoniae*. This treatment was found to result in induction of high levels of oxidized LDL-specific IgM and a modest reduction of atherosclerosis. Stimulation of the immune response against oxidized phospholipids represents one possible approach for development of an immunomodulatory therapy for atherosclerosis. The major challenges associated with this approach are:

- a poor understanding of how the expression of natural antibodies is induced and regulated

- the effect of cross-reactivity with antigens expressed on other structures than oxidized LDL
- the relation to the antiphospholipid antibodies associated with thrombotic disease.

The other major class of antigens in oxidized LDL are the peptide fragments generated as a result of proteolytic degradation and aldehyde modification of ApoB-100, the only protein associated with LDL. These antigens have the advantage of being specific for oxidized LDL because they have a unique amino acid sequence. The antigens presented by MHC class II molecules are generally 13–17 amino acids long, which makes the chance for cross-reactivity with other peptide sequences minimal. A major challenge in this case is that ApoB-100 is such a large protein (4500 amino acids) that it is difficult to know which are the relevant antigen structures. To determine this, we used a library of 302 (20 amino acid-long) polypeptides covering the complete ApoB-100 sequence to construct a corresponding number of malondialdehyde (MDA)- and non-MDA-modified ApoB-100 peptide ELISAs (enzyme-linked immunosorbent assays).[53] We then used these ELISAs to screen human plasma for detection of antibodies recognizing each particular sequence. IgM against more than 100 different MDA-modified ApoB-100 peptide sequences could be detected in pooled plasma from 50 healthy controls, whereas detectable IgG levels were only found against a smaller number of sequences. To investigate the functional role of these immune responses and to determine if they could be responsible for the previously observed atheroprotective effect of oxidized LDL immunization, we immunized ApoE[−/−] mice with the ApoB-100 peptide sequences found to induce antibody expression in man. Immunizations with several of these ApoB-100 peptides were found to reduce atherosclerosis by up to 70%, as well as to decrease macrophage and increase collagen contents of remaining plaques.[47,54] Interestingly, immunization with ApoB-100 peptide sequences that were not homologous between humans and mice did not inhibit atherosclerosis. Immunizations resulted in a marked increase in specific IgG, but had only marginal effects on IgM levels. IgG expression also changed from IgG2a to IgG1, suggesting activation of a Th2 response.[47] The most effective atheroprotective response was found when immunizations were made with the ApoB-100 peptide sequences of amino acids 16–35 (peptide 2), amino acids 631–650 (peptide 45), and amino acids 3136–3155 (peptide 210; Figure 31.4). In these pilot vaccine studies, alum was used as adjuvant and cationized bovine albumin as carrier molecule for the peptides. Present work is focused on determining the most effective composition of a possible future vaccine to be used in human studies, including the most optimal peptide composition and modification, carrier, adjuvant, and route of administration. Following relevant safety and toxicity studies, it is anticipated that clinical phase I studies of a first atherosclerosis vaccine based on ApoB-100 peptides will be carried out sometime in 2008–2009.

ANTIBODY-BASED THERAPY

Generation of specific IgG is a critical mediator of the effect of most vaccines. An increase in specific IgG has also been observed in most (but not all) studies evaluating the effect of immunization with oxidized LDL antigens. To determine the functional role of IgG in mediating the protective effect of immunization with ApoB-100 peptides we used a recombinant library-based technology called n-CoDeR[55] in collaboration with scientists at Bioinvent International (Lund, Sweden) to generate human antibodies against the

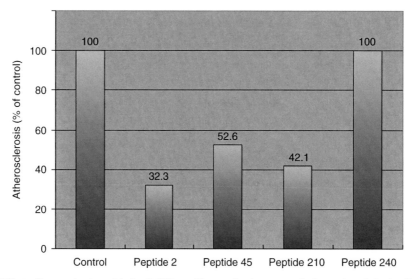

Figure 31.4   Effect of immunization with ApoB-100 peptides on development of atherosclerosis in ApoE$^{-/-}$ mice. Mice were given three weekly immunizations with adjuvant alone (control), peptide 2 (amino acids 16–35), peptide 45 (amino acids 631–650), peptide 210 (amino acids 3136–3155), or peptide 240 (amino acids 3613–3632), starting at 6 weeks of age, and the severity of atherosclerosis in the aorta was determined by oil red-O staining at 25 weeks. Values are expressed as percent of atherosclerosis observed in the controls. Peptide 240 was used as a specificity control because there is no homology between mice and humans for this sequence.

MDA-modified ApoB-100 amino acid sequence 631–650 (peptide 45). This peptide was used to select single chain variable fragments (scFvs) from the library. The resulting scFv, and human full-length IgG1, made utilizing the scFvs bound to oxidized but not to the non-oxidized full-length ApoB-100 and LDL.[56]

The effect of human recombinant anti-MDA-ApoB-100 IgG on atherosclerosis was studied in ApoE$^{-/-}$ mice.[56] A limitation of this model is that the mice will develop an immune response against human IgG that will eventually neutralize the effect of the antibodies. Accordingly, the treatment period was limited to three IgG injections 1 week apart, starting when the mice had reached an age of 21 weeks. The extent of atherosclerosis was measured by en face oil red-O staining of the aorta at 25 weeks. The antibody produced a 50% reduction in atherosclerosis and was also found to reduce inflammation and oxidized LDL deposits in remaining plaques. Similar observations have subsequently been made in other mouse models of atherosclerosis. Another antibody that has atheroprotective effects is a monoclonal antiphosphorylcholine IgM with T15 isotype. A course of 4 weekly treatment of antibody reduced vein graft atherosclerosis in hypercholesterolemic mice.[57] The results are of interest not only because they imply that the effect of active immunization, at least in part, is mediated by antibodies but also because they suggest that it may be possible to develop an antibody-based therapy for atherosclerosis. In contrast to the effect of active immunization that takes up to 2–3 weeks to fully achieve, the effect of antibody treatment should be immediate, making it an attractive option for treatment of vulnerable plaques. In fact, antibodies represent the fastest-growing segment within the biotechnology industry today, and recently several therapeutic antibody-based drugs – e.g. adalimumab (Humira) for treatment of rheumatoid arthritis, rituximab (Rituxan) for treatment of non-Hodgkin's lymphoma, and bevacizumab (Avastin) for treatment of colon carcinoma – have entered the clinic as registered products. The first clinical studies using human recombinant IgG against MDA-ApoB-100 peptides are anticipated to be carried out 2007–2008.

ANTIBODIES AND RISK ASSESSMENT

Another possibility presently being explored is the use of antibodies against oxidized LDL in the imaging of atherosclerotic plaques. Experiments performed by Tsimikas and co-workers in hypercholesterolemic rabbits and LDL-receptor knockout mice demonstrate that intravenously injected ^{125}I-labeled mouse monoclonal antibody specific for MDA-modified LDL (MDA2) has a strong and specific predilection for atherosclerotic lesions but not normal arterial tissue.[58,59] They have subsequently reported that stabilization of existing atherosclerotic lesions by changing the high-fat diet to normal chow resulted in a marked reduction of plaque uptake of ^{125}I-MDA2.[60] These interesting studies suggest the possibility of identifying vulnerable atherosclerotic plaques and monitoring changes in plaque structure by imaging arterial uptake of radio-labeled oxidized LDL antibodies in humans. The recombinant IgG against MDA-modified ApoB-100 peptide sequences described above represent a potential candidate for use in clinical imaging studies of vulnerable plaques, since these antibodies are human and will not give rise to immune responses in man.

An additional, but relatively unexplored, possibility is that the plasma level of autoantibodies against oxidized LDL could serve as a biomarker for disease activity in atherosclerotic plaques. In a study comparing the composition of atherosclerotic plaques from patients undergoing carotid endarterectomy ($n = 114$) with the plasma level of autoantibodies against MDA-ApoB-100 peptide sequences, a significant association was found between high levels of IgG and a more unstable plaque phenotype (more lipid and inflammation and less fibrous tissue), whereas the opposite was found in patients with high IgM levels.[61] It is likely that the higher level of IgG in patients with more vulnerable plaques reflects an increased disease activity. Determination of autoantibody levels has been established as a helpful diagnostic tool in several organ-specific diseases, such as type 1 diabetes, thyroiditis, celiac disease, adrenalitis, pernicious anemia and rheumatic disease. It is likely that this also represents a possible way of monitoring disease activity in cardiovascular disease.

CONCLUSION

Treatment aimed at modulating the immune response against oxidized LDL represents an emerging novel therapy for cardiovascular disease. Results from preclinical studies have been promising and the fact that immune responses against specific oxidized LDL antigens have been associated with cardiovascular disease in clinical studies raises hope that this type of therapy may also be effective in humans. Immunomodulatory treatments, including vaccines and antibodies, are presently being clinically tested in a number of chronic diseases such as cancer, diabetes, Alzheimer's disease, and rheumatoid arthritis. Although the experience from this work has been encouraging, the challenge to establish safety and clinical efficiency should not be underestimated.

REFERENCES

1. Glass CK, Witztum JL. Atherosclerosis: the road ahead. Cell 2001; 104:503–16.

2. Hansson GK. Inflammation, atherosclerosis, and coronary artery disease. N Engl J Med 2005; 352: 1685–95.

3. Binder CJ, Chang MK, Shaw PX et al. Innate and acquired immunity in atherogenesis. Nat Med 2002; 8:1218–26.

4. Hansson GK, Libby P, Schonbeck U, Yan ZQ. Innate and adaptive immunity in the pathogenesis of atherosclerosis. Circ Res 2002; 91:281–91.

5. Nilsson J, Hansson GK, Shah PK. Immunomodulation of atherosclerosis: implications for vaccine development. Arterioscler Thromb Vasc Biol 2005; 25:18–28.

6. Shah PK, Chyu KY, Fredrikson GN, Nilsson J. Immunomodulation of atherosclerosis with a vaccine. Nat Clin Pract Cardiovasc Med 2005; 2:639–46.

7. Gordon S. Pattern recognition receptors: doubling up for the innate immune response. Cell 2002; 111: 927–30.

8. Febbraio M, Podrez EA, Smith JD et al. Targeted disruption of the class B scavenger receptor CD36 protects against atherosclerotic lesion development in mice. J Clin Invest 2000; 105:1049–56.

9. Suzuki H, Kurihara Y, Takeya M et al. A role for macrophage scavenger receptors in atherosclerosis and susceptibility to infection. Nature 1997; 386:292–6.

10. Moore KJ, Kunjathoor VV, Koehn SL et al. Loss of receptor-mediated lipid uptake via scavenger receptor A or CD36 pathways does not ameliorate atherosclerosis in hyperlipidemic mice. J Clin Invest 2005; 115:2192–201.

11. Bjorkbacka H, Kunjathoor VV, Moore KJ et al. Reduced atherosclerosis in MyD88-null mice links elevated serum cholesterol levels to activation of innate immunity signaling pathways. Nat Med 2004; 10:416–21.

12. Michelsen KS, Wong MH, Shah PK et al. Lack of Toll-like receptor 4 or myeloid differentiation factor 88 reduces atherosclerosis and alters plaque phenotype in mice deficient in apolipoprotein E. Proc Natl Acad Sci USA 2004; 101:10679–84.

13. Branen L, Hovgaard L, Nitulescu M et al. Inhibition of tumor necrosis factor-alpha reduces atherosclerosis in apolipoprotein E knockout mice. Arterioscler Thromb Vasc Biol 2004; 24:2137–42.

14. Zhou X, Nicoletti A, Elhage R, Hansson GK. Transfer of CD4(+) T cells aggravates atherosclerosis in immunodeficient apolipoprotein E knockout mice. Circulation 2000; 102:2919–22.

15. Tupin E, Nicoletti A, Elhage R et al. CD1d-dependent activation of NKT cells aggravates atherosclerosis. J Exp Med 2004; 199:417–22.

16. Zhou X, Robertson AK, Rudling M, Parini P, Hansson GK. Lesion development and response to immunization reveal a complex role for CD4 in atherosclerosis. Circ Res 2005; 96:427–34.

17. Buono C, Pang H, Uchida Y et al. B7-1/B7-2 costimulation regulates plaque antigen-specific T-cell responses and atherogenesis in low-density lipoprotein receptor-deficient mice. Circulation 2004; 109: 2009–15.

18. Lutgens E, Cleutjens KB, Heeneman S et al. Both early and delayed anti-CD40L antibody treatment induces a stable plaque phenotype. Proc Natl Acad Sci USA 2000; 97:7464–9.

19. Frostegard J, Ulfgren AK, Nyberg P et al. Cytokine expression in advanced human atherosclerotic plaques: dominance of pro-inflammatory (Th1) and macrophage-stimulating cytokines. Atherosclerosis 1999; 145:33–43.

20. Uyemura K, Demer LL, Castle SC et al. Cross-regulatory roles of interleukin (IL)-12 and IL-10 in atherosclerosis. J Clin Invest 1996; 97:2130–8.

21. Gupta S, Pablo AM, Jiang X et al. IFN-gamma potentiates atherosclerosis in ApoE knock-out mice. J Clin Invest 1997; 99:2752–61.

22. Buono C, Binder CJ, Stavrakis G et al. T-bet deficiency reduces atherosclerosis and alters plaque antigen-specific immune responses. Proc Natl Acad Sci USA 2005; 102:1596–601.

23. Mallat Z, Besnard S, Duriez M et al. Protective role of interleukin-10 in atherosclerosis. Circ Res 1999; 85:e17–24.

24. Pinderski LJ, Fischbein MP, Subbanagounder G et al. Overexpression of interleukin-10 by activated T lymphocytes inhibits atherosclerosis in LDL receptor-deficient mice by altering lymphocyte and macrophage phenotypes. Circ Res 2002; 90: 1064–71.

25. Robertson AK, Rudling M, Zhou X et al. Disruption of TGF-{beta} signaling in T cells accelerates atherosclerosis. J Clin Invest 2003; 112:1342–50.

26. Mallat Z, Gojova A, Brun V et al. Induction of a regulatory T cell type 1 response reduces the development of atherosclerosis in apolipoprotein E-knockout mice. Circulation 2003; 108:1232–7.

27. Palinski W, Rosenfeld ME, Yla-Herttuala S et al. Low density lipoprotein undergoes oxidative modification in vivo. Proc Natl Acad Sci USA 1989; 86:1372–6.

28. Nordin Fredrikson G, Hedblad B, Berglund G, Nilsson J. Plasma oxidized LDL: a predictor for acute myocardial infarction? J Intern Med 2003; 253:425–9.

29. Stemme S, Faber B, Holm J et al. T lymphocytes from human atherosclerotic plaques recognize oxidized low density lipoprotein. Proc Natl Acad Sci USA 1995; 92:3893–7.

30. Frostegård J, Wu R, Giscombe R et al. Induction of T-cell activation by oxidized low density lipoprotein. Arterioscler Thromb 1992; 12:461–7.

31. Nilsson J, Kovanen PT. Will autoantibodies help to determine severity and progression of atherosclerosis? Curr Opin Lipidol 2004; 15:499–503.

32. Palinski W, Tangirala RK, Miller E, Young SG, Witztum JL. Increased autoantibody titers against epitopes of oxidized LDL in LDL receptor-deficient

mice with increased atherosclerosis. Arterioscler Thromb Vasc Biol 1995; 15:1569–76.

33. Palinski W, Witztum JL. Immune responses to oxidative neoepitopes on LDL and phospholipids modulate the development of atherosclerosis. J Intern Med 2000; 247:371–80.

34. Shaw PX, Horkko S, Tsimikas S et al. Human-derived anti-oxidized LDL autoantibody blocks uptake of oxidized LDL by macrophages and localizes to atherosclerotic lesions in vivo. Arterioscler Thromb Vasc Biol 2001; 21:1333–9.

35. Berliner J, Leitinger N, Watson A et al. Oxidized lipids in atherogenesis: formation, destruction and action. Thromb Haemost 1997; 78:195–9.

36. Xu XH, Shah PK, Faure E et al. Toll-like receptor-4 is expressed by macrophages in murine and human lipid-rich atherosclerotic plaques and upregulated by oxidized LDL. Circulation 2001; 104:3103–8.

37. Edfeldt K, Swedenborg J, Hansson GK, Yan ZQ. Expression of toll-like receptors in human atherosclerotic lesions: a possible pathway for plaque activation. Circulation 2002; 105:1158–61.

38. Walton KA, Cole AL, Yeh M et al. Specific phospholipid oxidation products inhibit ligand activation of toll-like receptors 4 and 2. Arterioscler Thromb Vasc Biol 2003; 23:1197–203.

39. Miller YI, Viriyakosol S, Binder CJ et al. Minimally modified LDL binds to CD14, induces macrophage spreading via TLR4/MD-2, and inhibits phagocytosis of apoptotic cells. J Biol Chem 2003; 278: 1561–8.

40. Ameli S, Hultgardh-Nilsson A, Regnstrom J et al. Effect of immunization with homologous LDL and oxidized LDL on early atherosclerosis in hypercholesterolemic rabbits. Arterioscler Thromb Vasc Biol 1996; 16:1074–9.

41. Palinski W, Miller E, Witztum JL. Immunization of low density lipoprotein (LDL) receptor-deficient rabbits with homologous malondialdehyde-modified LDL reduces atherogenesis. Proc Natl Acad Sci USA 1995; 92:821–5.

42. Nilsson J, Calara F, Regnstrom J et al. Immunization with homologous oxidized low density lipoprotein reduces neointimal formation after balloon injury in hypercholesterolemic rabbits. J Am Coll Cardiol 1997; 30:1886–91.

43. Freigang S, Horkko S, Miller E, Witztum JL, Palinski W. Immunization of LDL receptor-deficient mice with homologous malondialdehyde-modified and native LDL reduces progression of atherosclerosis by mechanisms other than induction of high titers of antibodies to oxidative neoepitopes. Arterioscler Thromb Vasc Biol 1998; 18:1972–82.

44. George J, Afek A, Gilburd B et al. Hyperimmunization of apo-E-deficient mice with homologous malondialdehyde low-density lipoprotein suppresses early atherogenesis. Atherosclerosis 1998; 138:147–52.

45. Zhou X, Caligiuri G, Hamsten A, Lefvert AK, Hansson GK. LDL immunization induces T-cell-dependent antibody formation and protection against atherosclerosis. Arterioscler Thromb Vasc Biol 2001; 21: 108–14.

46. Chyu KY, Zhao X, Reyes OS et al. Immunization using an Apo B-100 related epitope reduces atherosclerosis and plaque inflammation in hypercholesterolemic apo E (-/-) mice. Biochem Biophys Res Commun 2005; 338:1982–9.

47. Fredrikson GN, Andersson L, Soderberg I et al. Atheroprotective immunization with MDA-modified apo B-100 peptide sequences is associated with activation of Th2 specific antibody expression. Autoimmunity 2005; 38:171–9.

48. Zhou X, Paulsson G, Stemme S, Hansson GK. Hypercholesterolemia is associated with a T helper (Th) 1/Th2 switch of the autoimmune response in atherosclerotic apo E-knockout mice. J Clin Invest 1998; 101:1717–25.

49. Binder CJ, Shaw PX, Chang MK et al. The role of natural antibodies in atherogenesis. J Lipid Res 2005; 46:1353–63.

50. Boes M. Role of natural and immune IgM antibodies in immune responses. Mol Immunol 2000; 37: 1141–9.

51. Shaw PX, Horkko S, Chang MK et al. Natural antibodies with the T15 idiotype may act in atherosclerosis, apoptotic clearance, and protective immunity. J Clin Invest 2000; 105:1731–40.

52. Binder CJ, Horkko S, Dewan A et al. Pneumococcal vaccination decreases atherosclerotic lesion formation: molecular mimicry between Streptococcus pneumoniae and oxidized LDL. Nat Med 2003; 9:736–43.

53. Fredrikson GN, Hedblad B, Berglund G et al. Identification of immune responses against aldehyde-modified peptide sequences in apo B-100 associated with cardiovascular disease. Arterioscler Thromb Vasc Biol 2003; 23:872–8.

54. Fredrikson GN, Soderberg I, Lindholm M et al. Inhibition of atherosclerosis in apoE-null mice by immunization with apoB-100 peptide sequences. Arterioscler Thromb Vasc Biol 2003; 23:879–84.

55. Soderlind E, Strandberg L, Jirholt P et al. Recombining germline-derived CDR sequences for creating diverse single-framework antibody libraries. Nat Biotechnol 2000; 18:852–6.

56. Schiopu A, Bengtsson J, Soderberg I et al. Recombinant human antibodies against aldehyde-modified apolipoprotein B-100 peptide sequences inhibit atherosclerosis. Circulation 2004; 110:2047–52.

57. Faria-Neto JR, Chyu KY, Li X et al. Passive immunization with monoclonal IgM antibodies against phosphorylcholine reduces accelerated vein graft atherosclerosis in apolipoprotein E-null mice. Atherosclerosis 2005; 189:83–90.

58. Tsimikas S, Palinski W, Halpern SE et al. Radiolabeled MDA2, an oxidation-specific, monoclonal antibody, identifies native atherosclerotic lesions in vivo. J Nucl Cardiol 1999; 6:41–53.

59. Tsimikas S, Shortal BP, Witztum JL, Palinski W. In vivo uptake of radiolabeled MDA2, an oxidation-specific monoclonal antibody, provides an accurate measure of atherosclerotic lesions rich in oxidized LDL and is highly sensitive to their regression. Arterioscler Thromb Vasc Biol 2000; 20:689–97.

60. Torzewski M, Shaw PX, Han KR et al. Reduced in vivo aortic uptake of radiolabeled oxidation-specific antibodies reflects changes in plaque composition consistent with plaque stabilization. Arterioscler Thromb Vasc Biol 2004; 24:2307–12.

61. Goncalves I, Gronholdt ML, Soderberg I et al. Humoral immune response against defined oxidized low-density lipoprotein antigens reflects structure and disease activity of carotid plaques. Arterioscler Thromb Vasc Biol 2005; 25:1250–5.

62. Nilsson J. Regulating protective immunity. Circ Res 2005; 96:395–7.

Multifocal coronary plaque instability: evidence for a systemic inflammatory process

32

James A Goldstein

INTRODUCTION

Coronary plaque rupture resulting in thrombotic occlusion is implicated in the pathogenesis of acute coronary syndromes (ACS).[1–5] Focal flow-limiting coronary stenoses are the targets for revascularization to relieve myocardial ischemia.[6] However, atherosclerosis is a widespread process,[7–9] as most patients harbor diffuse disease. The recognition of the ubiquity of substantial but non-flow-limiting lesions, which may serve as the fodder for subsequent plaque rupture, has resulted in a paradigm shift in thinking about the pathophysiology of coronary artery disease, with the focus no longer solely on the degree of arterial luminal narrowing.[1,6]

Acute coronary syndromes result from rupture of macrophage-rich, inflamed thin-cap fibroatheroma (TCFA) with superimposed thrombus formation.[1,8,9] The angiographic hallmark of ACS is a complex coronary culprit plaque characterized by fissuring, ulceration, haziness, and filling defect, which correlates with pathologic plaque rupture and thrombus.[10–14] Plaque disruption is thought to be a function of the interplay between factors that influence intrinsic plaque vulnerability and extrinsic forces that may precipitate rupture.[1,4,6,10,15–18] Until recently, plaque rupture was thought to reflect local plaque instability attributable to spontaneous or triggered disruption of a lone vulnerable plaque, manifest angiographically or pathologically as a solitary complex unstable lesion. However, the pathophysiologic factors proposed to precipitate plaque instability, whether due to primary weakening of the fibrous cap attributable to inflammation[6,15–18] or the extrinsic influences of intraluminal mechanical forces modulated by sympathetic tone and catecholamines,[19,20] would be expected to exert their effects in a widespread pattern throughout the coronary vasculature. Recent observations now document that many patients with ACS harbor multiple complex unstable plaques by angiography.[21] Multifocal plaque instability is evident not only in coronary vessels but also in peripheral vessels, and peripheral and coronary plaque instability may exist concomitantly.[21,22] These observations support the concept that plaque instability is not merely a local vascular accident, but instead reflects more systemic pathophysiologic processes with the potential to destabilize atherosclerotic plaques throughout the cardiovascular system. This chapter will elucidate clinical and basic science data regarding:

- the prevalence of multifocal plaque instability in the coronary bed of patients with ACS

- evidence of pancoronary inflammation and its relationship to multifocal plaque instability
- links between systemic inflammation, multifocal plaque instability, plaque progression, and clinical outcomes
- evidence for panvascular plaque instability in coronary and extracoronary vascular beds.

PATHOPHYSIOLOGIC ROLE OF INFLAMMATION IN PLAQUE INSTABILITY

Local plaque inflammation and plaque rupture

Pathophysiologic studies have established mechanistic links between inflammation and coronary plaque instability. Local plaque inflammation has emerged as an obligatory feature in events leading to plaque vulnerability and rupture.[4,6,15–18] Macrophages have been implicated in every stage of coronary atherosclerosis, from its initiation to its thrombotic clinical complications.[15–18] Weakening and disruption of its protective fibrous cap appears to be the critical event triggering plaque instability.[2–5,15–18] Autopsy and atherectomy specimens document that, compared with stable lesions in the same patient, unstable plaques manifest active fibrous cap inflammation, particularly activated macrophage infiltration, concentrated at the point of plaque disruption.[15–18,23–25] Macrophages synthesize and secrete matrix metalloproteinases that can degrade and weaken the protective fibrous cap and predispose it to rupture.[26–29] Macrophages also express tissue factor, a potent promoter of coagulation.[30] Immunohistochemical studies of myocardial infarction show other inflammatory cell types at plaque sites, including activated T lymphocytes (which secrete cytokines that regulate plaque destabilization through macrophage activation), smooth muscle cell growth, and extracellular matrix synthesis.[15–18]

Role of systemic inflammation in local vascular plaque instability

There is now abundant evidence that systemic inflammation plays an important pathophysiologic role in coronary plaque instability.[6,15–18] Clinical observations support the concept that systemic processes influence plaque instability, the most important of which appears to be systemic inflammation, which 'fans the flame of plaque vulnerability.'[18] Patients with ACS manifest evidence of a systemic inflammatory reaction, reflected by elevation of C-reactive protein (CRP) and other inflammatory markers, including activation of circulating leukocytes and release of thromboxanes and leukotrienes.[31–36] As gauged by the robust biomarker CRP, inflammation predicts the prognosis of patients with ACS, as well as those with stable angina, and even those without clinically manifest atherosclerosis.[32–35]

Although elevated plasma markers of inflammation might be viewed as a systemic manifestation of local coronary processes, there is a growing chain of evidence to support the notion that an acute inflammatory reaction plays a causative role in atherosclerotic plaque destabilization. The ultimate end-link in the chain is forged by documentation of inflammatory cells, particularly activated macrophages, concentrated at the sites of plaque rupture. There is now abundant serologic and molecular biologic evidence providing the basis for the pathophysiologic link between systemic inflammation and widespread coronary inflammation leading to multifocal plaque instability. Findings of activated leukocytes in the coronary and systemic circulation,[36] together with data demonstrating the release of thromboxanes and leukotrienes during ischemic chest pain, and the presence of elevated serum biomarkers strengthen the connection between systemic and local vascular inflammation.[18] Further upstream in the pathophysiologic chain, it is known that inflammatory mediators not only elevate markers like CRP but also stimulate pathways that weaken the fibrous cap and tip the intraluminal balance toward thrombosis. Importantly, the systemic inflammatory response is associated with generation of markers that provide the basis for postulating mechanisms mediating direct plaque inflammation and destabilization. Patients with ACS manifest elevated serum neopterin, a marker of macrophage activation that is a critical player in plaque inflammation.[37] The detection of elevated serum levels of intercellular adhesion molecule-1 (ICAM-1) and vascular cell adhesion molecule-1 (VCAM-1) provide direct mechanisms by which systemic inflammatory processes mediate local vascular bed inflammation.[36,38–40] ICAM-1, expressed on both resting and activated endothelial cells, promotes adhesion and transendothelial migration of leukocytes from the blood to the arterial intima.[38] VCAM-1, expressed in human coronary atherosclerotic plaques, binds monocytes and T lymphocytes to activated endothelial cells.[36,38–40] Together, these molecular moieties provide the basis for mechanistic links by which inflamed systemic blood may induce local inflammation within the coronary bed.

CORONARY PLAQUE INSTABILITY IS MULTIFOCAL AND PANCORONARY

Given the potential 'pancoronary' impact of these factors adversely influencing plaques, together with the typically diffuse nature of coronary atherosclerosis, it would not be unexpected that plaque instability might develop in a multifocal pattern, resulting in multiple anatomically remote complex unstable plaques, one of which may progress to total occlusion and emerge as the culprit infarct-related lesion. Recent observations from our institution now document that a significant subset of patients with acute myocardial infarction harbor multiple complex coronary plaques, which are associated with adverse clinical outcome.[21,22] In this study of patients with acute transmural myocardial infarction, nearly 40% of patients manifested angiographic evidence of multiple complex coronary plaques (Figure 32.1). Compared to patients with single complex plaques, those with multiple unstable lesions had greater depression of left ventricular function and a less favorable in-hospital course, more often requiring early coronary artery bypass surgery or staged multivessel percutaneous interventions. Importantly, the presence of multiple complex plaques was independently predictive of adverse clinical events over 1 year (Figure 32.2), including an increased incidence of recurrent angina and ACS, higher rates of repeat percutaneous revascularization not only in the initial culprit vessel but also in non-infarct-related lesions previously documented as complex, and a greater likelihood of requiring later coronary artery bypass surgery. These observations led to the concept that plaque instability is not merely a local vascular accident, but probably reflects more systemic pathophysiologic processes with the potential to destabilize atherosclerotic plaques throughout the coronary tree. A wealth of confirmatory data derived from reviews of prior pathologic and angiographic studies, together with more recent investigations employing direct intracoronary imaging techniques and biochemical investigations, now provide abundant evidence that multifocal plaque instability is common in patients with ACS. In fact, multifocal coronary plaque instability may be the rule rather than the exception.

Pathologic evidence of multifocal coronary plaque instability

Multifocal plaque ruptures and multiple coronary thrombi are evident, although

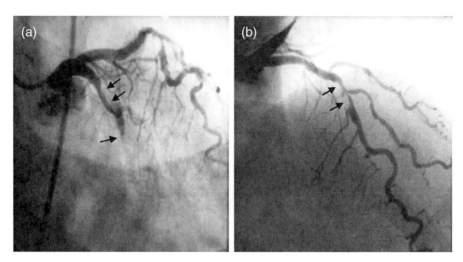

Figure 32.1   Multifocal complex plagues in acute myocardial infarction: angiograms from a patient with acute posterolateral myocardial infarction. (a) Culprit lesion in the circumflex characterized by a long scalloped ulcerated tight stenosis with haziness and ulceration (solid arrows), with a total occlusion just distal (open dark arrow). (b) A cranial view of the left anterior descending coronary artery in the same patient demonstrates a complex ulcerated stenosis with overhanging edges, anatomically remote from the culprit circumflex occlusion. (Reproduced from Goldstein et al,[21] with permission.)

not necessarily commented upon, in autopsy studies of fatal acute ischemic heart disease.[2,3,11,40] One detailed necropsy study of 83 patients dying of acute myocardial infarction documented both extensive multifocal coronary ulceration and multicentric clot formation, with multiple ulcerated plaques in 71% of cases and four or more lesions in 20% of patients.[11] Recent postmortem studies

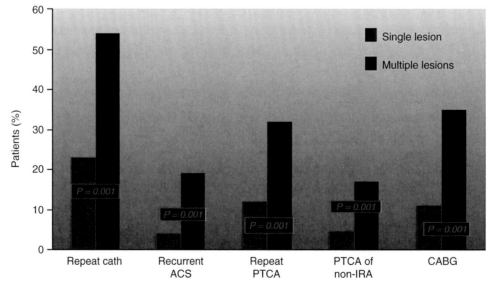

Figure 32.2   Outcomes within 1 year after myocardial infarction in patients with multiple complex plaques or single complex plaques. ACS, acute coronary syndromes; PTCA, percutaneous transluminal coronary angioplasty, CABG, coronaryartery bypass grafting; IRA, infarct-related artery. $P \leq 0.001$ for all comparisons between groups. (Reproduced from Goldstein et al,[21] with permission.)

analyzing plaque inflammatory cell infiltrates in fatal ACS have now documented multiple inflamed plaques.[40]

Angiographic evidence of multifocal plaque instability

Although observations from our laboratory were the first to document the presence of multiple complex coronary plaques and their influence on outcome in patients with acute transmural myocardial infarction,[21,22] multiple complex plaques are evident, though not necessarily commented on, in previous angiographic studies of patients with ACS[37, 41–49] (Table 32.1). The concept of multifocal plaque instability is also supported by angiographic natural history studies documenting rapid progression of culprit and non-culprit complex lesions in patients with ACS.[37, 41–49]

Limitations of angiography in detection of unstable and vulnerable plaques

Although a crucial tool for assessment of patients with coronary artery disease, angiography is well known to underestimate the presence and severity of coronary artery disease in general and has significant limitations in the precise delineation of plaque architecture and biology. Although complex morphology by angiography correlates closely with plaque instability pathologically, and complex plaques are associated with angiographic progression and clinical instability, it is important to emphasize the qualitative nature of angiographic evaluation, for complexity may be in the 'eye of the beholder.'[22] Furthermore, angiographic complexity does not by itself necessarily determine plaque destiny, as some complex plaques may remain stable over time.[50] It is also crucial to emphasize that angiography is an insensitive tool that is only able to detect those plaques that have relatively gross plaque disruption.[22] Observations from intravascular ultrasound (IVUS), angioscopic, and pathologic studies clearly document that the majority of ulcerated plaques are not sufficiently disrupted anatomically to be detected angiographically. Furthermore, it is certain that patients with unstable (and silent) coronary artery disease harbor lipid-rich inflamed 'vulnerable' plaques that have not yet ulcerated and ruptured. Angiography fails to detect the many plaques with subtler but pathologically manifest ulceration and rupture, reflecting only a subset of those coronary lesions that are truly unstable and revealing virtually no insight regarding the many vulnerable but not yet ruptured plaques that serve as the substrate for subsequent coronary events. Therefore, angiographic confirmation of complex plaque undoubtedly represents only the 'tip of the iceberg' of plaque instability and vulnerability.[22]

Table 32.1 Angiographic observations of multiple complex coronary plaques

Author	Type	Observation
Goldstein[21]	AMI	Multiple CP in 40% patients; ↑ coronary events over 1 year
Garcia-Moll[37]	UA	2.6 CP/patient; correlates with activated macrophages (serum neopterin)
Guazzi[42]	MI	Rapid multifocal progression in culprit and non-culprit CP
Theroux[41]	UA	Rapid multifocal progression in culprit and non-culprit CP
Moise[43]	UA	Rapid multifocal progression in culprit and non-culprit CP
Chen[44]	UA	Rapid multifocal progression of CP; ↑ coronary events over 8 months

AMI, acute transmural myocardial infarction; CP, complex plaques; MI, myocardial infarction; UA, unstable angina.

Multifocal plaque instability documented by direct coronary imaging modalities

Observations from direct coronary imaging modalities, including angioscopy, IVUS, and optical coherence tomography, provide morphologic confirmation of multiple unstable plaques in patients with acute coronary syndrome.[51–59] They also emphasize the many subtler plaque ruptures that are not yet angiographically complex and thus lurk beneath the angiographic 'radar screen.' Angioscopic studies document multiple frankly ruptured thrombus-laden plaques as the frequent presence of 'vulnerable yellow' plaques distant from the culprit lesion.[53] IVUS characterization of plaque rupture (ulceration, intimal flap, and aneurysm) correlates strongly with angiographic plaque complexity (Figure 32.3) and provides further confirmatory evidence of multifocal plaque instability in patients with ACS, with additional ruptured plaques remote from the culprit lesion or in non-culprit vessels in up to 80% of cases.[54–56] In contrast, plaque rupture is less commonly seen in those with stable angina.[56–58] TCFAs, which are felt to represent vulnerable but not yet ruptured plaques, are also more frequently observed in a multifocal pattern in patients with ACS compared with stable patients.[59]

CORONARY INFLAMMATION IS WIDESPREAD

Given the pathophysiologic role that systemic inflammation plays in plaque instability, the presence of widespread coronary inflammation and multiple inflamed

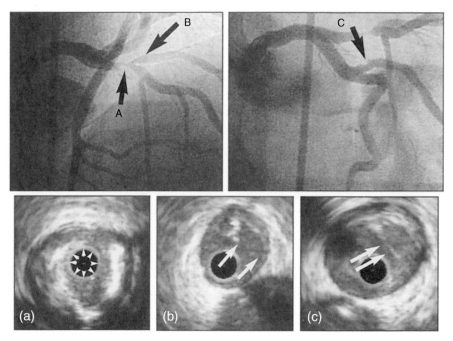

Figure 32.3   Multiple atherosclerotic plaque rupture in acute coronary syndromes (ACS). Angiographic and intravascular ultrasound (IVUS) images of typical multiple unstable coronary lesions. The culprit lesion was subocclusive in the left anterior descending artery (A; arrows underline the arterial lumen); IVUS found two other plaque ruptures in the diagonal artery (B) and in the marginal artery (C), which was the only lesion detected on angiography. The double arrows underline the fibrous capsule rupture edges. (Reproduced from Riouful et al,[53] with permission.)

complex unstable lesions would be expected in patients with ACS. Multifocal and diffuse plaque instability mediated by inflammation is now supported by abundant pathologic and biochemical evidence.[41,60–65] Biochemical evidence that inflammation is not confined to a single plaque but is multifocal and widespread to the entire coronary circulation was first established by documentation of leukocyte activation throughout the coronary circulation in patients with ACS, as indicated by neutrophil myeloperoxidase activity, a marker of inflammation evident in the coronary venous effluent of regions not perfused by the culprit artery (Figure 32.4).[60] Pathoanatomic confirmation of the concept of mutifocal plaque instability is provided by topographic evidence of multifocal inflammatory cell activation in a necropsy study of patients with fatal myocardial infarction, with detailed histopathologic analysis of the

entire coronary tree showing evidence of widespread inflammation not only in the culprit plaques but also in other vessel segments.[61] In that study, both unstable and vulnerable plaques were found to be diffusely infiltrated by inflammatory cells, with an average of nearly 7 vulnerable plaques per patient. Interestingly, although the degree of inflammation in the coronary tree in ACS cases was 3–4-fold that of patients with stable angina, high-grade, though lesser in magnitude, inflammation was present in stable plaques as well.[61] Multifocal inflammatory infiltrate has also been confirmed by optical coherence tomography, which demonstrates significantly greater macrophage density at sites of plaque rupture and increased plaque macrophage density at remote and culprit sites in patients with ACS.[62] Postmortem studies in fatal ACS confirm multicentric coronary inflammation, indicated by activated T lymphocytes

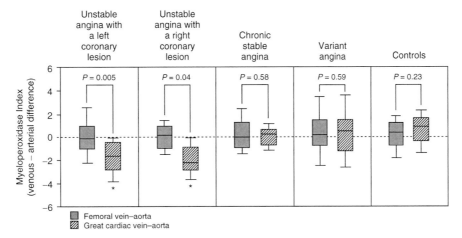

Figure 32.4 Inflammation is pancoronary: widespread coronary inflammation. Venous – arterial differences in myeloperoxidase content across the femoral and coronary vascular beds. Data were presented as medians, with 25th and 75th percentiles (boxes) and 10th and 90th percentiles (I bars). The difference in myeloperoxidase content across the coronary circulation was significantly greater in patients with unstable angina with a left coronary lesion and in patients with unstable angina with a right coronary lesion than in patients with chronic stable angina, patients with variant angina, and control patients. The difference in myeloperoxidase content across the coronary vascular bed was significantly greater than that across the femoral vascular bed in patients with unstable angina with a left coronary lesion and in patients with unstable angina with a right coronary lesion, but not in any of the other three groups. The asterisk indicates $P < 0.05$ for the comparison of the group with unstable angina with a left coronary lesion and unstable angina with a right coronary lesion with the group with chronic stable angina, the group with variant angina, and controls. (Reproduced from Buffon et al,[59] with permission.)

throughout the coronary tree.[41] Inflammation is not confined to epicardial vessels, but also involves small intramural vessels.[63] Further evidence in support of the concept that cardiac inflammation appears to be widespread in patients with ACS is provided by documentation of perivascular and extravascular activation in the ischemic and non-ischemic myocardium of patients with unstable angina,[64] as well as by evidence of interstitial activated T cells expressing HLA-DR in the remote myocardium, observations which suggest that the antigenic stimuli associated with coronary instability are also present in the extravascular compartment.[65] Taken together, these studies challenge the notion that coronary vulnerability responsible for ACS is caused by a single inflamed vulnerable plaque; rather, they suggest diffuse inflammation of the entire coronary tree.

MULTIFOCAL COMPLEX LESIONS, PLAQUE PROGRESSION, AND CLINICAL OUTCOMES

ACS marks patients at higher risk for recurrent instability for weeks to months after resolution of the index clinical event.[1] This increased risk is probably a reflection, at least in part, of pancoronary plaque inflammation, as such patients typically harbor additional foci of coronary vulnerability or frankly complex plaques ripe for rupture and thereby serving as the substrate for subsequent clinical misadventure. Stenosis progression and clinical instability are characteristic of complex coronary lesions. Furthermore, there is a striking association between complex morphology, clinical instability, and prognosis.[21,37,41–49] The concept of multifocal plaque instability is supported by angiographic natural history studies documenting rapid progression of culprit and non-culprit complex lesions in patients with ACS (Table 32.2). Observations from our laboratory were the first to document the presence of multiple complex coronary plaques and their influence on outcome in patients with acute transmural myocardial infarction.[21] Other studies in patients with acute myocardial infarction have demonstrated striking rapid multifocal progression of both infarct-related and non-culprit complex lesions over 1 month.[41] Angiographic natural history studies in patients with

Table 32.2 Multiple complex coronary plaques by direct coronary imaging

Author	Modality	Observation
Asakura[52]	Angioscopy	Multivessel multiple vulnerable plaques in culprit and non-culprit vessels (>3/vessel)
Riouful[53]	IVUS	Plaque rupture distant from culprit in 79% with ACS. Mean 2.08 plaque ruptures/patient
Maehara[54]	IVUS	MPR in 15%, correlates with angiography
Hong[56]	IVUS	MPR in 20% with AMI
Schoenhagen[55]	IVUS	Ulcerated plaque proximal to culprit more common with ACS vs SA (19 vs 4%)
Takano[51]	IVUS	MPR in 24% with AMI
Kotani[57]	IVUS	MPR in 10.5% with AMI
Jang[58]	OCT	Non-culprit TCFA more common in AMI and ACS vs SA

AMI, acute transmural myocardial infarction; ACS, acute coronary syndrome; IVUS, intravascular ultrasound; MPR, multiple plaque rupture; SA, stable angina; OCT, optical coherence tomography; TCFA, thin-cap fibroatheroma.

unstable angina document that complex lesions are at great risk for worsening stenoses, recurrent unstable ischemia, and death.[43–49] Rapid progression is not confined to the initial culprit lesion, but is evident in non-culprit complex lesions as well, consistent with the concept of multifocal plaque instability.[41–47] The angiographic documentation of multiple unstable plaques identifies a subset of patients particularly predisposed to rapid progression of culprit and non-culprit complex lesions, associated with greater risk for recurrent ischemia.[21,32,42]

However, it should be noted that complex angiographic morphology by itself does not determine that a given plaque is necessarily predestined to progression, for some complex lesions may remain stable over time.[50] Although pathologic and IVUS studies have shown that the sequence of plaque rupture and subsequent thrombosis formation is the initiating event for most cases of ACS, rupture of a coronary atheroma appears to be a frequent event that only occasionally leads to luminal obstruction and acute ischemia. Angioscopic follow-up of ruptured plaques shows that non-culprit lesions tend to heal slowly with a progression of angiographic stenosis and suggested that serum CRP might reflect disease activity of the plaque ruptures.[1] Serial IVUS observations in plaque ruptures without significant associated stenosis showed that half of plaques progress, whereas half were healed, and the degree of stenosis tended to diminish over 22 months of medical therapy with statins and antiplatelet therapy.[51] It is not clear why some plaques occlude, whereas many plaque ruptures heal with subsequent fibrosis that may be silent or lead to subsequent chronic luminal narrowing.[66] Presumably, patients with ACS have an underlying biologic milieu predisposing to the development of widespread plaque destabilization and/or thrombus formation.

SYSTEMIC INFLAMMATION, MULTIFOCAL PLAQUE INSTABILITY, AND CLINICAL OUTCOME

Systemic inflammation and multifocal plaque instability

Evidence now buttresses the link between systemic inflammation and the multicentricity of plaque instability. There is a strong correlation between multiple plaque ruptures and the magnitude of systemic inflammation, whether measured by CRP, serum neopterin or other plasma markers indicative of an enhanced systemic inflammatory state (Figure 32.5).[37,57,67–69] Similarly, serum CRP may correlate with the number of TCFAs.[70]

Systemic inflammation is persistent and predicts rapid plaque progression

There is biochemical evidence that systemic inflammation is persistent and linked with recurrent clinical instability. Biochemical evidence of activated systemic inflammatory processes may persist beyond the initial symptomatic ACS episode and correlates with greater risk for recurrent adverse events.[71,72] Elevated CRP measured 1 month after ACS correlates with the number of ruptured plaques by IVUS; not surprisingly, patients with multifocal unstable plaques have worse prognosis.[73] Inflammatory stimulus triggering expression of cellular adhesion molecules is sustained for up to 6 months in patients with acute coronary syndrome.[74,75] Levels of soluble ICAM-1 (sICAM-1), soluble VCAM-1 (sVCAM-1) and soluble E-selection (sE-selectin) are elevated acutely and through 72 hours in patients with ACS (Figure 32.6)[74] and are associated with increased recurrent events. Such processes probably underlie the progression of stable coronary disease to an unstable state, as suggested by the association between serum markers

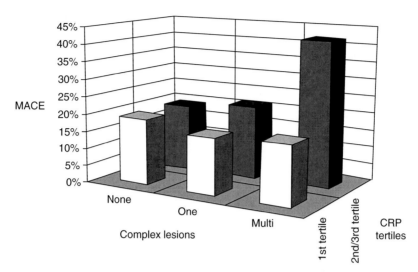

Figure 32.5 Systemic inflammation, multifocal complex plaques, and adverse outcome. Major adverse cardiac events (MACE) (death, non-fatal myocardial infarction, and target vessel revascularization) at 1 year by number of complex coronary lesions and level of systemic inflammation: low = first tertile with C-reactive protein (CRP) level <0.25 mg/dl; high = second and third tertiles with CRP level ≥0.25 mg/dl. (Reproduced from Goldstein et al,[67] with permission.)

of systemic inflammation, macrophage activation, and endothelial cell activation, and the rapid progression of coronary disease in stable angina patients (Figure 32.7).[75]

That these markers remain persistently elevated suggests sustained inflammation reflecting continued accumulation of inflammatory cells at the injured vascular sites. There is also evidence of continued platelet activation after ACS, with levels of

surface E selectin and P selectin remaining elevated for up to 6 months after ACS, consistent with the concept of ongoing activation of platelets and endothelial cells, which may be a consequence of persistent inflammation.[73,76] Sustained enhanced platelet activation induced by persistent inflammation may contribute to the ongoing risk for thrombotically mediated recurrent coronary events. Rapid reduction of recurrent coronary events by

Figure 32.6 Systemic inflammation is persistent after acute coronary syndrome (ACS). Levels of sICAM-1 in ng/ml in UA, NQMI, and control groups at four sampling time points. P values refer to differences in levels of sICAM-1 between the three groups. P< 0.05 for levels of sICAM-1 at 6 months vs levels at 12 months in UA and NQMI groups. sICAM-1, soluble intercellular adhesion molecule-1; NQMI, non-Q-wave myocardial infarction; UA, unstable angina. (Reproduced from Mulvihill et al,[74] with permission.)

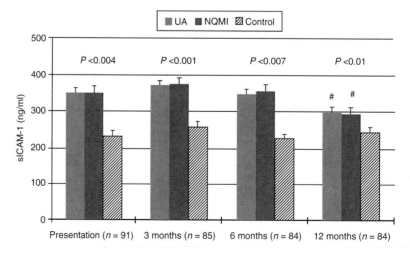

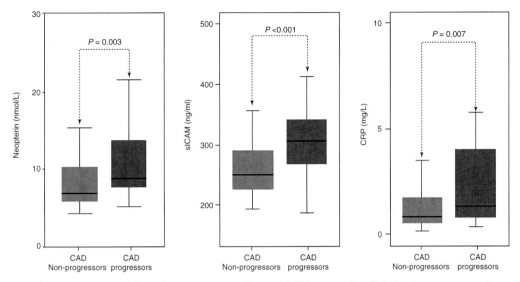

Figure 32.7   Inflammation and rapid coronary artery disease (CAD) progression. Relation between serum C-reactive protein (CRP), neopterin, MMP-2, MMP-9 (Mann–Whitney U Test), sICAM-1, and sVCAM-1 (2-tailed *t*-test) concentrations and rapid CAD progression in 124 patients with CSA (chronic stable angina) awaiting routine coronary angioplasty. (Reproduced from Zouridakis et al,[75] with permission.)

aggressive statin therapy in patients with ACS is consistent with stabilization of vulnerable plaques by anti-inflammatory therapy.[77–80]

Panvascular multifocal plaque instability

Given that atherosclerosis is a systemic vascular process which is rarely if ever confined strictly to the coronary tree, together with findings documenting that coronary plaque instability is not a local vascular accident, but instead more commonly manifests in a multifocal pattern reflecting systemic inflammatory pathophysiologic processes underlying plaque vulnerability and precipitating plaque instability, it should not be surprising that multifocal plaque instability is evident in peripheral vessels, including the carotid artery, thoracic aorta, and femoral arteries,[81–88] and that plaque instability in carotid and coronary beds might occur concomitantly.[82–88]

Clinical implications

In aggregate, these observations support the concept that plaque instability is not merely a local vascular accident, but probably reflects pancoronary pathophysiologic processes with potential to destabilize atherosclerotic plaques throughout diffusely diseased atherosclerotic vascular beds. These findings emphasize that the angiographic documentation of multiple unstable plaques not only influences initial revascularization strategies but also identifies a subset of patients particularly predisposed to rapid plaque progression associated with greater risk for recurrent ischemia. The ultimate goal is to facilitate detection of vulnerable and unstable plaques prior to catastrophic rupture. Unfortunately, we do not yet possess techniques sufficiently accurate to delineate all eroded-ruptured plaques, let alone the many lipid-rich thin-cap potentially 'vulnerable' plaques that have not yet ruptured. Clearly, higher-resolution imaging techniques are necessary to better define coronary plaque architecture with respect to thickness and stability of the protective fibrous cap, presence of inflammation, and extent of the lipid-rich plaque pool. There is also a pressing need for reliable biomarkers that can delineate the local coronary and systemic metabolic and inflammatory processes which underlie plaque destabilization and may better identify the vulnerable patient. Given that plaque instability may be concomitant in coronary and carotid beds, it might be argued that patients with ACS should undergo carotid screening; conversely, those with acute ischemic neurologic syndromes should be monitored closely for progressive and unstable coronary artery disease.

Although local revascularization interventions such as stenting remedy focal disease, to prevent recurrent events a global attack on the metabolic and inflammatory milieu is critical.[6] Just as inflammation underlies the pathophysiology of plaque formation and complications, successful therapeutic strategies appear to exert their beneficial effects through suppression of (combating) inflammation. The cardioprotective benefits of the antiplatelet agent aspirin on recurrent myocardial infarction may be mediated in part by its systemic anti-inflammatory effects. The reduction of recurrent ACS by systemically acting lipid-lowering interventions that reduce CRP[80,81] supports the notion that unstable coronary artery disease is a multifocal process influenced by systemic factors.

REFERENCES

1. Libby P, Theroux P. Pathophysiology of coronary artery disease. Circulation 2005; 111:3481–8.
2. Falk E. Plaque rupture with severe pre-existing stenosis precipitating coronary thrombosis. Characteristics of coronary atherosclerotic plaques underlying fatal occlusive thrombi. Br Heart J 1983; 50:127–34.
3. Davies MJ, Thomas A. Thrombosis and acute coronary artery lesions in sudden cardiac ischemic death. N Engl J Med 1984; 310:1137–40.
4. Falk E, Shah PK, Fuster V. Coronary plaque disruption. Circulation 1995; 92:657–71.
5. Farb A, Burke AP, Tang AL et al. Coronary plaque erosion without rupture into a lipid core. A frequent cause of coronary thrombosis in sudden coronary death. Circulation 1996; 3:1354–63.
6. Libby P. Act local, act global: inflammation and the multiplicity of "vulnerable" coronary plaques. J Am Coll Cardiol 2005; 45:1600–2.
7. Arnett EN, Isner JM, Redwood DR et al. Coronary artery narrowing in coronary heart disease: comparison of cineangiographic and necropsy findings. Ann Intern Med 1979; 91(3):350–6.
8. Tuczu E, Kapadia S, Tutar E et al. High prevalence of coronary atherosclerosis in asymptomatic teenagers and young adults: evidence from intravascular ultrasound. Circulation 2001; 103:2705–10.
9. Mintz GS, Painter JA, Pichard AD et al. Atherosclerosis in angiographically "normal" coronary artery reference segments: an intravascular ultrasound study with clinical correlations. J Am Coll Cardiol 1995; 25:1479–85.
10. Falk E. Unstable angina with fatal outcome: dynamic coronary thrombosis leading to infarction and/or sudden death. Circulation 1985; 71:4:699–708.
11. Frink RJ. Chronic ulcerated plaques: new insights into the pathogenesis of acute coronary disease. J Invasive Cardiol 1994; 6:173–85.
12. Ambrose JA, Winters SL, Stern A et al. Angiographic morphology and the pathogenesis of unstable angina pectoris. J Am Coll Cardiol 1985; 5:609–16.
13. Levin DC, Fallon JT. Significance of the angiographic morphology of localized coronary stenoses: histopathologic correlations. Circulation 1982; 66:316–20.
14. Ambrose JA. Prognostic implications of lesion irregularity on coronary angiography. J Am Coll Cardiol 1991; 18:675–6.
15. Ross. Atherosclerosis: an inflammatory disease. N Engl J Med 1999; 340:115–26.
16. Libby P. Inflammation in atherosclerosis. Nature 2002; 420(6917):868–74.
17. Hansson G. Inflammation, atherosclerosis, and coronary artery disease. N Engl J Med 2005; 352:685–95.
18. Libby P. Inflammation fans the flame of plaque vulnerability. J Am Coll Cardiol 2005; 45:10.
19. Gertz SD, Roberts WC. Hemodynamic shear force in rupture of coronary arterial atherosclerotic plaques. Am J Cardiol 1990; 66:1368–72.
20. Muller JE, Stone PH, Turi ZG. Circadian variation in the frequency of onset of acute myocardial infarction. N Engl J Med 1985; 313:1315–22.
21. Goldstein JA, Demetriou D, Grines CL et al. Multiple complex coronary plaques in patients with acute myocardial infarction. N Engl J Med 2000; 343:915–22.
22. Goldstein JA. Angiographic plaque complexity: the tip of the unstable plaque iceberg. J Am Coll Cardiol 2002; 39:1464–7.
23. Van der Wal AC, Becker AE, Van der Loos CM et al. Site of intimal rupture or erosion of thrombosed

coronary atherosclerotic plaques is characterized by an inflammatory process irrespective of the dominant plaque morphology. Circulation 1994; 89:36–44.

24. Moreno PR, Falk E, Palacios IF et al. Macrophage infiltration in acute coronary syndromes. Implications for plaque rupture. Circulation 1994; 90:775–8.

25. Kovanen PT, Kaartinen M, Paavonen T. Infiltrates of activated mast cells at the site of coronary atheromatous erosion or rupture in myocardial infarction. Circulation 1995; 92:1084–8.

26. Shah PK, Falk E, Badimon JJ et al. Human monocyte-derived macrophages induce collagen breakdown in fibrous caps of atherosclerotic plaques. Potential role of matrix-degrading metalloproteinases and implications for plaque rupture. Circulation 1995; 92(6):1565–9.

27. Galis ZS, Sukhova GK, Lark MW, Libby P. Increased expression of matrix metalloproteinases and matrix degrading activity in vulnerable regions of human atherosclerotic plaques. J Clin Invest 1994; 94:2493–503.

28. Shukhova GK, Schonbeck U, Rabkin E et al. Evidence for increased collagenolysis by interstitial collagenases-1 and –3 in vulnerable human atheromatous plaques. Circulation 1999; 99:2503–9.

29. Zaman A, Helft G, Worthley S, Badimon J. The role of plaque rupture and thrombosis in coronary artery disease. Atherosclerosis 2000; 149:251–6.

30. Thompson SG, Kienast J, Pyke SDM et al. Hemostatic factors and the risk of myocardial infarction or sudden death in patients with angina pectoris. N Engl J Med 1995; 332:635–41.

31. Liuzzo G, Biasucci LM, Gallimore JR et al. The prognostic value of C-reactive protein and serum amyloid A protein in severe unstable angina. N Engl J Med 1994; 331:417–24.

32. Ridker PM, Cushman M, Stampfer MJ et al. Inflammation, aspirin, and the risk of cardiovascular disease in apparently healthy men. N Engl J Med 1997; 336:973–9.

33. Ridker PM, Rifai N, Pfeffer MA et al. Inflammation, pravastatin, and the risk of coronary events after myocardial infarction in patients with average cholesterol levels. Circulation 1998; 98:839–44.

34. Ridker P. Clinical applications of C-reactive protein for cardiovascular disease detection and prevention. Circulation 2003; 107:363–9.

35. Mazzone A, Servi S, Ricevuti G et al. Increased expression of neutrophil and monocyte adhesion molecules in unstable coronary artery disease. Circulation 1993; 88:358–63.

36. Jang Y, Kincoff M, Plow E, Topol E. Cell adhesion molecules in coronary artery disease. J Am Coll Cardiol 1994; 24:1591–601.

37. Garcia-Moll X, Coccolo F, Cole D, Kaski JC. Serum neopterin and complex stenosis morphology in patients with unstable angina. J Am Coll Cardiol 2000; 35:956–62.

38. Boyle J. Association of coronary plaque rupture and atherosclerotic inflammation. J Pathol 1997;181:93–9.

39. Pasterkamp G, Schoneveld AH, van der Wal AC et al. Inflammation of the atherosclerotic cap and shoulder of the plaque is a common and locally observed feature in unruptured plaques of femoral and coronary arteries. Arterioscler Thromb Vasc Biol 1999; 19:54–8.

40. Spagnoli L, Bonanno E, Mauriello A et al. Multicentric inflammation in epicardial coronary arteries of patients dying of acute myocardial infarction. J Am Coll Cardiol 2002; 40:1579–88.

41. Theroux P. Angiographic and clinical progression in unstable angina. Circulation 1995; 91:2295–8.

42. Guazzi M, Bussotti M, Grancini L et al. Evidence of multifocal activity of coronary disease in patients with acute myocardial infarction. Circulation 1997; 96:1145–51.

43. Moise A, Theroux P, Taeymans Y et al. Unstable angina and progression of coronary atherosclerosis. N Engl J Med 1983; 309:685–9.

44. Chen L, Chester MR, Redwood S et al. Angiographic stenosis progression and coronary events in patients with 'stabilized' unstable angina. Circulation 1995; 91:2319–24.

45. Chester MR, Chen L, Kaski JC. The natural history of unheralded complex coronary plaques. J Am Coll Cardiol 1996; 28:604–8.

46. Chen L, Chester MR, Crook R et al. Differential progression of complex culprit stenoses in patients with stable and unstable angina pectoris. J Am Coll Cardiol 1996; 28:597–603.

47. Kaski JC, Chest MR, Chen L, Katritsis D. Rapid angiographic progression of coronary artery disease in patients with angina pectoris. Circulation 1995; 92:2058–65.

48. Freeman MR, Williams AE, Chisholm RJ et al. Intracoronary thrombus and complex morphology in unstable angina. Relation to timing of angiography and in-hospital cardiac events. Circulation 1989; 80:17–23.

49. Davies SW, Marchant B, Lyons JP et al. Irregular coronary lesion morphology after thrombolysis predicts early clinical instability. J Am Coll Cardiol 1991; 18:669–74.

50. Haft JI, Al-Zarka AM. The origin and fate of complex coronary lesions. Am Heart J 1991; 121:1050.

51. Burke AP, Kolodgie FD, Farb A et al. Healed plaque ruptures and sudden coronary death: evidence that subclinical rupture has a role in plaque progression. Circulation 2001; 103:934–40.

51. Takano M, Inami S, Ishibashi F et al. Angioscopic follow-up study of coronary ruptured plaques in nonculprit lesions. J Am Coll Cardiol 2005; 45:652–8.

52. Asakura M, Ueda Y, Yamaguchi O et al. Extensive development of vulnerable plaques as a pan-coronary process in patients with myocardial infarction: an angioscopic study. J Am Coll Cardiol 2001; 37:1284–8.

53. Rioufol G, Finet G, Ginon I et al. Multiple atherosclerotic plaque rupture in acute coronary syndrome: a

three-vessel intravascular ultrasound study. Circulation 2002; 106:804–8.

54. Maehara A, Mintz G, Bui AB et al. Morphologic and angiographic features of coronary plaque rupture detected by intravascular ultrasound. J Am Coll Cardiol 2002; 40:904–10.

55. Schoenhagen P, Stone GW, Nissen SE et al. Coronary plaque morphology and frequency of ulceration distant from culprit lesions in patients with unstable and stable presentation. Atheroscl Thromb Vasc Biol 2003; 23:1895–900.

56. Hong MK, Mintz GS, Lee CW et al. Comparison of coronary plaque rupture between stable angina and acute myocardial infraction: a three vessel intravascular ultrasound study. Circulation 2004; 110:928–33.

57. Kotani J, Mintz G, Castagna M et al. Intravascular ultrasound analysis of infarct-related and non-infarct-related arteries in patients who presented with an acute myocardial infarction. Circulation 2003; 107:2889–93.

58. Jang I, Guillermo J, Tearney J et al. In vivo characterization of coronary atherosclerotic plaques by use of optical coherence tomography. Circulation 2005; 111:1551–5.

59. Buffon A, Biasucci L, Liuzzo G et al. Widespread coronary inflammation in unstable angina. N Engl J Med 2002; 347:5–12.

60. Mauriello A, Sangiorgi G, Fratoni S et al. Diffuse and active inflammation occurs in both vulnerable and stable plaques of the entire coronary tree. J Am Coll Cardiol 2005; 45:1585–93.

61. MacNeill BD, Jang IK, Bouma BE et al. Focal and multi-focal plaque macrophage distributions in patients with acute and stable presentations of coronary artery disease. J Am Coll Cardiol 2004; 44:972–9.

62. Serneri N, Gastone G, Boddi M et al. Immunomediated and ischemia-dependent inflammation of coronary microvessels in unstable angina. Circ Res 2003; 92:1359–66.

63. Lombardo A, Biasucci L, Lanza G et al. Inflammation as a possible link between coronary and carotid plaque instability. Circulation 2004; 109:3158–63.

64. Abbate A, Bonanno E, Mauriello A et al. Widespread myocardial inflammation and infarct-related artery patency. Circulation 2004; 110:46–50.

65. Zairis MN, Papadaki OA, Manousakis SJ et al. C-reactive protein and multiple complex coronary artery plaques in patients with primary unstable angina. Atherosclerosis 2002; 164:355–60.

66. Riouful G, Gilard M, Finet G et al. Evolution of spontaneous atherosclerotic plaque rupture with medical therapy: long-term follow-up with intravascular ultrasound. Circulation 2004; 110:2875–80.

67. Goldstein JA, Chandra HR, O'Neill WW. Relation of number of complex coronary lesions to serum C-reactive protein levels, and major adverse cardiovascular events at one year. Am J Cardiol 2005; 96:56–60.

68. Tanaka, A, Shimada K, Sano T et al. Multiple plaque rupture and C-reactive protein in acute myocardial infarction. J Am Coll Cardiol 2005; 45:1594–9.

69. Burke A, Tracy R, Kolodgie F et al. Elevated C-reactive protein values and atherosclerosis in sudden coronary death: association with different pathologies. Circulation 2002; 105:2019–23.

70. Biasucci LM, Liuzzo G, Grillo RL et al. Elevated levels of C-reactive protein at discharge in patients with unstable angina predict recurrent instability. Circulation 1999; 99:855–90.

71. Biasucci LM, Liuzzo G, Fantuzzi G et al. Increasing levels of interleukin (IL)-1Ra and IL-6 during the first 2 days of hospitalization in unstable angina are associated with increased risk of in-hospital coronary events. Circulation 1999; 99:2079–84.

72. Mulvihill N, Foley BJ, Ghaisas N et al. Early temporal expression of soluble cellular adhesion molecules in patients with unstable angina and subendocardial myocardial infarction. Am J Cardiol 1999; 83:1265–7.

73. Ault K, Cannon C, Mitchell J et al. Platelet activation in patients after an acute coronary syndrome: results from the TIMI-12 trial. J Am Coll Cardiol 1999; 33:634–9.

74. Mulvihill NT, Foley JB, Murphy R, Crean P, Walsh M. Evidence of prolonged inflammation in unstable angina and non-Q wave myocardial infarction. J Am Coll Cardiol 2000; 36:1210–16.

75. Zouridakis E, Avanzas P, Arroyo-Espliguero R, Fredericks S, Kaski JC. Markers of inflammation and rapid coronary artery disease progression in patients with stable angina pectoris. Circulation 2004; 110:1747–53.

76. Cannon CP, Weintraub WS, Demopoulos LA et al. Comparison of early invasive conservative strategies in patients with unstable coronary syndromes treated with the glycoprotein IIb/IIIa inhibitor tirofiban. N Engl J Med 2004; 344:1879–87.

77. Schwartz GG, Olsson AG, Ezekowitz MD et al. Effects of atorvastatin on early recurrent ischemic events in acute coronary syndromes: The MIRACL study: a randomized controlled trial. J Am Coll Cardiol 2001; 285(13):1711–18.

78. Nissen S, Tuzcu M, Schoenhagen P et al. Statin therapy, LDL cholesterol, C-reactive protein, and coronary artery disease: N Engl J Med 2005; 352:29–38.

79. Ridker PM, Cannon CP, Morrow D et al. (PROVE IT-TIMI 22) Investigators. C-reactive protein levels and outcomes after statin therapy. N Engl J Med 2005; 352:20–8.

80. Kinlay S, Schwartz G, Olsson A et al. High-dose atorvastatin enhances the decline in inflammatory markers in patients with acute coronary syndromes in the MIRACL study. Circulation 2003; 108:1560–6.

81. Amarenco P, Duyckaerts C, Tzourio C et al. The prevalence of ulcerated plaques in the aortic arch in patients with stroke. N Engl J Med 1992; 326:221–5.

82. Rothwell PM, Villagra R, Gibson R, Donders RC, Warlow CP. Evidence of a chronic systemic cause of instability of atherosclerotic plaques. Lancet 2000; 355:19–24.

83. Cohen A, Tzourio C, Bertrand B et al. Aortic plaque morphology and vascular events: a follow-up study in patients with ischemic stroke. Circulation 1997; 96:3838–41.

84. Saito D, Shiraki T, Oka T et al. Morphologic correlation between atherosclerotic lesions of the carotid and coronary arteries in patients with angina pectoris. Circulation 1999; 63:522–6.

85. Honda O, Sugiyama S, Kugiyama K et al. Echolucent carotid plaques predict future coronary events in patients with coronary artery disease. J Am Coll Cardiol 2004; 43:1177–84.

86. Kato M, Dote K, Habara S et al. Clinical implications of carotid artery remodeling in acute coronary syndrome: ultrasonographic assessment of positive remodeling. J Am Coll Cardiol 2003; 42:1026–32.

87. Vink A, Schoneveld AH, Richard W et al. Plaque burden, arterial remodeling and plaque vulnerability: determined by systemic factors? J Am Coll Cardiol 2001; 38:718.

88. Lombardo A, Biasucci L, Lanza G et al. Inflammation as a possible link between coronary and carotid plaque instability. Circulation 2004; 109:3158–63.

Stem cell therapy in heart disease

Emerson C Perin, Guilherme V Silva, and James T Willerson

INTRODUCTION

Despite efforts such as revascularization to halt the progression to ischemic heart failure, ventricular remodeling is still a growing danger. Efforts to treat severely compromised hearts refractory to medical therapy have included heart transplantation and mechanical ventricular assistance.[1] Until now, cardiologists believed that beyond revascularization and medical therapy, the process of ischemic heart failure was irreversible because the heart lacked the capacity to renew itself.

However, new insights into the mechanisms of cardiac repair have provided evidence that the adult heart can repair itself and that vasculogenesis (new vessel formation from a precursor cell) may not occur solely during embryonic development.[2–5] These insights, in turn, have sparked strong interest in the field of stem cell therapy. Prompted by evidence that adult bone marrow harbors a reservoir of enormously plastic cells,[6] animal experiments have generated evidence supporting the use of stem cells for repairing cardiac tissue in diverse clinical scenarios.[7] Moreover, the groundbreaking work by Anversa et al[8] with the discovery of cardiac stem cells has disproved the theory that the heart is a postmitotic organ. Solid evidence has emerged from that work substantiating the heart's self-healing capacity.

The idea of using stem cells for cardiac repair by replacing or healing myocardium has been met both with enthusiasm and disbelief. Many controversies exist, and basic mechanistic questions have yet to be answered. Although some of the body's natural healing response is being elucidated, the main pathways of heart self-regeneration remain unclear. However, stem cell therapy for cardiac diseases is becoming a clinical reality. Several strategies have been tested with promising initial results. This chapter, aimed at the clinical cardiologist who will ultimately deliver this investigational therapy to patients, outlines the basic concepts of stem cell therapy and reviews the clinical data available from phase 1 and 2 trials.

STEM CELL IDENTIFICATION

Each adult stem cell subtype can be identified by cell surface receptors that selectively bind to particular signaling molecules. Differences in structure and binding affinity allow for a remarkable multiplicity of receptors. Normally, cells utilize these receptors and the molecules that bind to them to communicate with other cells and perform the proper function of the tissue to which they belong (e.g. contraction, secretion, synaptic transmission). Each type of adult stem cell has a certain receptor or combination of receptors (i.e. marker) that distinguishes it from other stem cell types.

Stem cell markers are often given letter and number codes based on the molecules that bind to them. A cell presenting the stem cell antigen-1 receptor is identified as Sca-1$^+$. Cells exhibiting Sca-1 but not the CD34 antigen or lineage-specific antigen (Lin) are identified as CD34$^-$Sca-1$^+$Lin$^-$. This particular combination of surface receptors identifies mesenchymal stem cells (MSCs).

Newer strategies for stem cell identification have been developed based on knowledge of metabolic cell characteristics. A primitive and multipotential subpopulation of bone marrow mononuclear cells has been identified on the basis of the intracellular presence of aldehyde dehydrogenase (ALDH). Those cells can be 'marked' on the basis of the presence of ALDH and are called aldehyde dehydrogenase-bright cells (ALDH^{br} cells), allowing for their separation from a bone marrow aspiration mononuclear subpopulation under fluorescence-activated cell sorter (FACS) analysis.

STEM CELLS AND CARDIAC REPAIR

Stem cells are self-replicating cells capable of generating, sustaining, and replacing terminally differentiated cells.[9,10] Stem cells can be subdivided into two large groups: embryonic and adult. Embryonic stem cells are present in the earliest stage of embryonic development – the blastocyst. Embryonic stem cells are pluripotent (i.e. capable of generating any terminally differentiated cell in the human body).[11] All the body's organs arise, through a series of divisions and differentiations, from the original embryonic stem cells that form the blastocyst.

Adult stem cells are intrinsic to specific tissues of the postnatal organism and are committed to differentiate into those tissues.[12] Adult stem cells yield mature differentiated cells capable of performing the specialized function(s) of that tissue in helping to maintain organ homeostasis. Each type of differentiated cell has its own phenotype (i.e. observable characteristics), including shape or morphology; interactions with surrounding cells and extracellular matrix; expression of particular cell surface proteins (receptors); and behavior. Adult tissue-specific stem cells are present in other self-renewable organs such as the liver, pancreas, skeletal muscle, and skin.[12] The heart, which until very recently was considered a terminally differentiated, postmitotic organ with a finite store of myocytes established at birth, might now be added to this list. It has recently been observed that hematopoietic stem cells (HSCs) can transdifferentiate into cardiomyocytes[13,14] and that stem cells may reside in the heart.[15] These resident cardiac stem cells are thought to occupy niches in the atria and apex and have been observed in the border zones of myocardial infarcts.[16,17] Such observations have, in turn, drastically changed our understanding of the cardiac repair process. Now it appears that resident cardiac stem cells and possibly bone marrow-derived stem cells may be able to repair the damaged heart. Once adequate signaling is established with cytokines and growth factors, bone marrow cells are mobilized.[18] Strengthening this concept is evidence from animal studies showing that acute myocardial infarction (AMI) repair involves bone marrow cells[19] and by evidence of chimerism in transplanted hearts.[20]

Further evidence for a dynamic cardiac renewal process in the adult heart comes from the recent identification of a novel population of early tissue-committed stem cells that may be part of a group of circulating progenitor cells involved in cardiac repair.[21] The particularities and interactions of resident and circulating stem cells in this setting continue to be delineated.

Stem cells and atherosclerosis

Studies by several research groups have shown that cells derived from bone marrow accelerate the re-endothelialization process.[22] Further evidence has emerged asserting that the presence of risk factors and the aging process can lead to bone marrow failure and the depletion of progenitor cells needed for vascular repair.[23–25] This may also be true in inflammatory states such as diabetes mellitus and coronary artery disease. Fadini et al[26] have demonstrated decreased endothelial progenitor cell (EPC) levels in patients with diabetes. They hypothesize that the extreme depletion of circulating EPCs in diabetic patients may be involved in the pathogenesis of peripheral vascular complications.[26] Walter et al[27] have demonstrated that the reduced neovascularization capacity of EPCs in patients with coronary artery disease (CAD) derives from an impaired CXCR4 signaling pathway. CXCR4 is a cytokine receptor essential for the migration and homing of hematopoietic stem cells.

Dong et al[28] have summarized the role of bone marrow in vascular repair. In the presence of competent bone marrow, the inflammatory signals (cytokines, etc.) generated by vascular injury result in the recruitment of bone marrow progenitor cells that are capable of arterial repair, thus providing a negative feedback loop that, in turn, shuts down the production of inflammatory mediators leading to homeostasis. By contrast, in the presence of a senescent bone marrow, the inflammatory signals do not result in mobilization of progenitor cells capable of healing. Instead, these factors may lead to the development of atherosclerosis and further injury by amplification of the inflammatory signaling. Inflammation in itself has been shown to create vascular injury that perpetuates the disease state.

STEM CELL TYPES

Adult bone marrow-derived stem cells

Adult bone marrow-derived stem cells are the cell type most widely utilized in cardiac stem cell therapy. A very heterogeneous subset, termed autologous bone marrow-derived mononuclear cells (ABMMNCs), is composed of small amounts of stromal or MSCs, hematopoietic progenitor cells (HPCs), EPCs, and more committed cell lineages such as natural killer lymphocytes, T lymphocytes, B lymphocytes, and others.

Bone marrow stem cells are aspirated from the patient's iliac crest under local anesthesia. The mononuclear subfraction of the aspirate is isolated by means of Ficoll density centrifugation, filtered through a 100 μm nylon mesh to remove cell aggregates or bone spicules, and washed several times in phospate-buffered saline solution before being used immediately for therapy or expanded in an endothelial cell-specific culture medium. Endothelial progenitor cells can be harvested from peripheral blood.

So far, the most important bone marrow subtypes utilized for cardiac repair have been MSCs, EPCs, or, alternatively, the whole ABMMNC fraction.

Mesenchymal stem cells

Adult MSCs are cells from any adult tissue that can be expanded in culture, can renew themselves, and can differentiate into several specific mesenchymal cell lineages. These cells are present in different niches throughout the body, such as bone marrow and adipose tissue.[29] Adult MSCs are extremely plastic, with the potential to terminally differentiate in vitro and in vivo into mesenchymal phenotypes such as bone,[30,31] cartilage,[32] tendon,[33,34] muscle,[13,35] adipose tissue,[36,37] and hematopoiesis-supporting stroma.[32]

Mesenchymal stem cells are CD45⁻ CD34⁻ bone marrow cells that can be readily grown in culture. They are evidently rare in the bone marrow (<0.01% of nucleated cells, by some estimates) and thus 10 times less abundant than HSCs. To obtain necessary numbers for therapy, MSCs need to be cultured at least 20 days, which would directly affect any clinical strategy for treating AMI that involves autologous MSCs.

Adult bone marrow MSCs, which are easy to manipulate genetically and weakly immunogenic, represent another potential source of allogeneic stem cells.[38] Allogeneic MSCs actually inhibit T cells in culture,[39] and several in-vivo studies have achieved good engraftment of allogeneic MSCs without rejection.[38]

Our group at the Texas Heart Institute was the first to study mesenchymal cell injections in a large-animal model of chronic myocardial ischemia.[40] In brief, we used ameroid constrictors to induce ischemia in 12 dogs. One month later, we directly injected the myocardium of each dog with 100 million MSCs or saline as a control. Subsequent two-dimensional echocardiography showed improved systolic function both at rest and during stress in the treated dogs (Figure 33.1). Histopathologic studies showed that the MSCs had transdifferentiated into endothelial and smooth muscle cells (Figures 33.2 and 33.3) and improved vascularization (Figure 33.4).

Genetically modified MSCs have been preliminarily tested as an alternative therapeutic strategy. Genetically modified MSCs should, in theory, overcome one of the main drawbacks of cell therapy: short-term survival of stem cells. Furthermore, these cells could potentially be used as 'couriers' to deliver genes or as a factory by encoding genes that would secrete key substances to enhance angiogenesis (e.g. vascular endothelial growth factor [VEGF]).

Endothelial progenitor cells

Endothelial progenitor cells can be isolated from the mononuclear fraction of the bone marrow or peripheral blood, as well as from fetal liver or umbilical cord blood.[41–45] Heterologous, homologous, and autologous EPCs have been shown to engraft at sites of active neovascularization in widely ranging animal models of ischemia.[43]

Endothelial progenitor cells can differentiate into endothelial cells, smooth muscle cells, or cardiomyocytes, both in vitro and in vivo. Different research groups have identified EPCs by using various methodologies.[2,46–50]

'Immature' or 'primitive' EPCs have a profile similar to that of HSCs; both cell types are thought to result from a common precursor, the hemangioblast.[51] Within the bone marrow, immature EPCs and HSCs share common cell surface markers: CD34, CD133, and VEGF receptor 2 (VEGFR-2, also known as KDR/FLK-1). Similarly, in the peripheral circulation, the more primitive cell population – with its capacity for differentiating into EPCs – expresses CD34, VEGFR-2, and CD133. In the peripheral circulation, the more committed EPCs lose CD133 but retain CD34 and VEGFR-2 expression. Some circulating EPCs and, to a greater extent, more differentiated EPCs, start expressing the endothelial lineage-specific marker vascular endothelial (VE) cadherin or E-selectin. However, when immature EPCs follow the hematopoietic path, the surface markers of CD133 and VEGFR-2 are extinguished because stem/progenitor cell markers are not expressed on differentiated hematopoietic cells.

Our characterization of EPCs and identification of those subtypes most useful for cardiac cell therapy has advanced rapidly but is still incomplete.[43] Nonetheless, as the positive results of initial preclinical and clinical studies have shown, EPCs show great therapeutic promise.

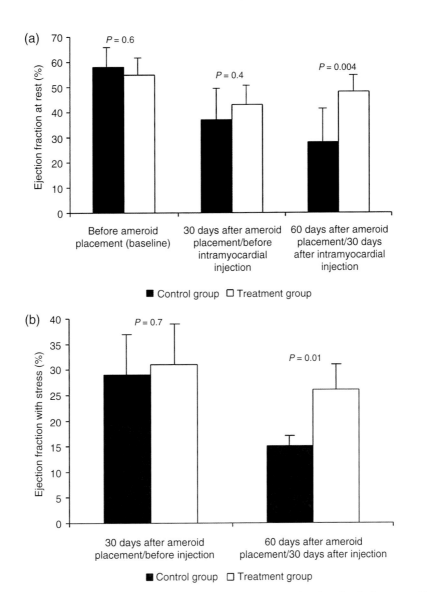

Figure 33.1   (a) Left ventricular ejection fraction at rest. Assessments were made at baseline before ameroid placement (left), 30 days later at time of cell or saline injection (middle), and 60 days after ameroid placement (right). (b) Left ventricular ejection fraction with stress. Assessments were made before and 30 days after intramyocardial injection. (Reproduced from Silva et al,[40] with permission.)

Other bone marrow stem cells

Recently, Kucia et al[52] published the first evidence that postnatal bone marrow harbors a non-hematopoietic cell population that expresses markers for cardiac differentiation. This finding corroborates the early work of Deb et al,[53] who isolated Y-chromosome-positive cardiac myocytes from female recipients of male bone marrow. The percentage of cardiomyocytes that harbored the Y chromosome was quite small (only 0.23%), but there was no evidence of either pseudonuclei or cell fusion.

Two new bone marrow cardiac precursors have been identified: ABMMNCs

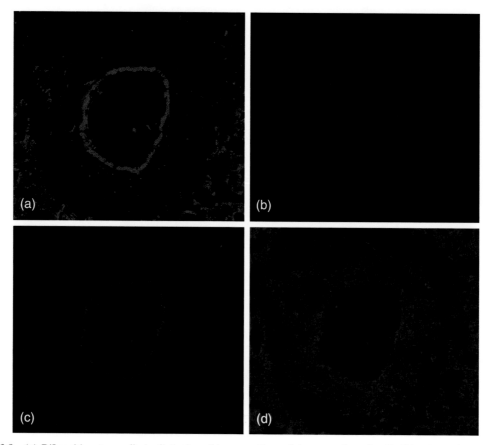

Figure 33.2   (a) DiI-positive stem cells (red) in the mid myocardium of the anterolateral wall. (b) α-Smooth muscle actin staining with FITC (green) showing cross section of vessel wall. (c) Stained areas showing co-localization (yellow) of stem cells and smooth muscle cells, suggesting transformation of stem cells into smooth muscle cells. The vessel shown is in the myocardial interstitium. Arrows point to vessel media. (Reproduced from Silva et al,[40] with permission.)

expressing cardiac markers within a population of non-hematopoietic CXCR4+/Sca-1+/Lin−/CD45− ABMMNCs in mice and within a population of non-hematopoietic CXCR4+/CD34+/AC133+/CD45− ABMMNCs in humans. These non-hematopoietic ABMMNCs expressing cardiac precursors are mobilized into the peripheral blood after a myocardial infarction (MI) and home in on the infarcted myocardium in an SDF-1-CXCR4-, HGF-c-Met-, and LIF-LIF-R-dependent manner.[52]

Skeletal myoblasts

Skeletal myoblasts are adult, tissue-specific stem cells[54] located between the basal lamina and the sarcolemma on the periphery of the mature skeletal muscle fiber.[55] Also known as muscle satellite cells, these small, mononuclear cells are activated by biochemical signals to divide and differentiate into fusion-competent cells after muscle injury.

The use of skeletal myoblasts for cardiac repair originated from earlier attempts where fetal cardiomyocytes were used. When injected into the border zone of an AMI, fetal cardiomyocytes can engraft and survive.[56] Despite initial encouraging results in animal models, however, clinical use of fetal cardiomyocytes has not been pursued because of ethical issues and the limited availability of these cells.

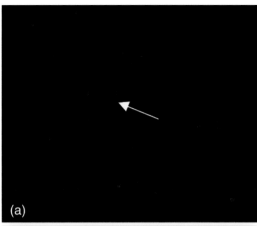

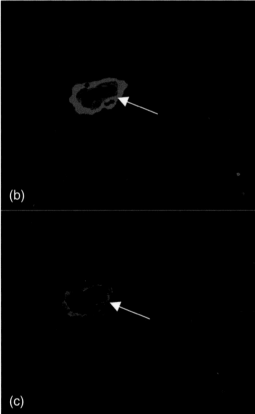

Figure 33.3 (a) Factor VIII staining with FITC (green) showing a thin vessel wall. (b) DiI-positive mesenchymal stem cells (red) in a vessel of the anterolateral wall. (c) Co-localization (yellow) of MSCs and endothelial cells, indicating transformation of MSCs into endothelial cells. (d) DAPI stain showing labeled endothelial nuclei. (Reproduced from Silva et al,[40] with permission.)

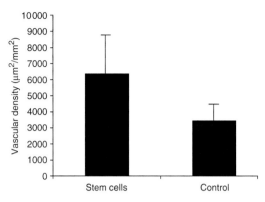

Figure 33.4 Vascular density was statistically greater in the anterolateral walls of animals that received the stem cells. (Reproduced from Silva et al,[40] with permission.)

Skeletal myoblasts can survive prolonged periods of hypoxia.[57] Like fetal cardiomyocytes, skeletal myoblasts can also survive and engraft when injected into the border zone of an AMI.

Embryonic stem cells

As gradually revealed over the past two decades, embryonic stem cells (ESCs) are derived from the cell mass of blastocysts in mice and humans. Murine ESC lines have been shown in vitro to differentiate into cells (hematopoietic progenitors, adipocytes, hepatocytes, smooth muscle cells, endothelial cells, neurons, and others) associated with each of the three layers.[58,59] More importantly, they have been shown to differentiate into cardiomyocytes[60] in response to appropriate stimuli and specific signaling factors. Hepatocyte growth factor, epidermal growth factor, basic fibroblast growth factor, platelet-derived growth factor, retinoic acid, vitamin C, and overexpression of γ-aminobutyric acid transporter all enhance this differentiation process in vitro. However, the ideal combination of these factors for enhancing ESC differentiation into cardiomyocytes remains unknown.

Because ESCs are pluripotent and can proliferate indefinitely, they may have an important potential role in cardiac regeneration. However, initial preclinical work (unpublished data) has evidenced tumorigenesis after intramyocardial injection of this cell type.

Although ethical issues involving the use of human ESCs have slowed research in several countries, including the USA, enthusiasm about their future clinical utilization remains high.

Resident cardiac stem cells

Myocyte replication is the failing heart's attempt to compensate for a limited capacity for hypertrophy. When Urbanek et al[17] used Ki-67 (a nuclear protein expressed during cell division) to assess the mitotic activity of myocytes, they observed significantly greater mitotic activity at infarct border zones than in distant myocardium or undiseased control hearts. The evidence that cardiac myocytes divide shortly after an MI led investigators to search for the origin of the dividing myocytes.[61] This culminated in the description of resident cardiac stem cells (CSCs).[15–17,62]

The developing and adult heart has a cell pool that has been described as the CSC side-population pool. These cells share the ability to efflux the Hoechst 33342 dye as the bone marrow side-population. Those cells are CD31+, raising suspicion that they are of bone-marrow origin rather than of true cardiac origin. Recently, an Sca-1, CD31− cardiac side-population was identified; its cells have a high regenerative potential and are able to terminally differentiate into myocytes. Anversa et al[61] have proposed a hierarchy of CSC growth and differentiation (Figure 33.5).

The current understanding of the CSCs' biology points to a homeostatic equilibrium of cell apoptosis and cell formation in normal hearts on the basis of the CSC compartment. Once disease ensues, such as chronic myopathic disease, this equilibrium is disrupted, favoring apoptosis. It is unclear why the CSC pool also has limited regeneration capacity in the setting of acute myocardial injury. Future understanding of the biology of CSCs might provide better regenerative strategies after AMI and in the setting of chronic heart failure.

Alternative sources of stem cells

Fat-derived stem cells

Despite successful preclinical and clinical utilization of bone marrow cells and skeletal myoblasts, the search continues for an ethical, easily accessible, high-yield source of stem cells. Mesenchymal stem cells have been isolated from adipose tissue, placental tissue, and umbilical cord blood. A number of studies have shown adipose-derived mesenchymal stem cells (AMSCs) to be pluripotent and capable of differentiating into multiple cell lineages along the myogenic, osteogenic, neurogenic, and hematopoietic pathways.[63–65] Research to characterize AMSCs better and to evaluate their safety and efficacy in preclinical studies is ongoing.

Placental-derived stem cells

By means of dissection and proteinase digestion, large numbers of viable mononuclear cells can be harvested from the human placenta at term, and a mesenchymal cell population with characteristic expression of CD9, CD29, and CD73 can be obtained in culture. The in-vitro growth behavior of such placenta-derived mesenchymal cells is similar to that of human bone marrow mesenchymal progenitor cells.[66] Transdifferentiation experiments have shown a potential for differentiation along osteogenic, chondrogenic, adipogenic, and myogenic lines.[66] The human placenta at term might be an easily accessible, ample source of multipotent mesenchymal progenitor cells and is also under preclinical investigation.

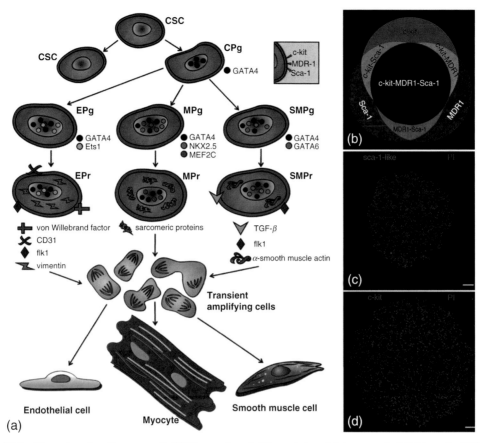

Figure 33.5   Hierarchy of cardiac stem cell (CSC) growth and differentiation. (a) Asymmetrical division of a CSC into a daughter CSC and a daughter cardiac progenitor (CPg). CPg gives rise to myocyte progenitor (MPg) and precursor (MPr), endothelial cell (EC) progenitor (EPg) and precursor (EPr), and smooth muscle cell (SMC) progenitor (SMPg) and precursor (SMPr). Precursors become transient amplifying cells, which divide and differentiate into mature myocytes, ECs, and SMCs. CSCs are lineage-negative cells that express only the stem cell-related antigens c-kit, MDR1, or Sca-1. Progenitors express stem cell antigens and transcription factors of cardiac cells but do not exhibit specific cytoplasmic proteins. Precursors possess stem cell antigens, transcription factors, and membrane and cytoplasmic proteins typical of myocytes, ECs, and SMCs. Amplifying cells have nuclear, cytoplasmic, and membrane proteins of cardiac cell lineages but are negative for stem cell antigens. TGF-β indicates transforming growth factor-β receptor. (b) Colocalization of c-kit, MDR1, and Sca-1 in CSCs. Areas corresponding to cells positive for one antigen only were enlarged three times. (c, d) Clones derived from a single Sca-1-like-positive cell (c, yellow) and a single c-kit-positive cell (d, green). Scale bars = 100 μm. (Reproduced from Anversa et al,[8] with permission.)

Cord blood-derived stem cells

Cord blood has long been used as a source of MSCs for bone marrow transplantation. The stem cell compartment is more abundant and less mature in cord blood than in bone marrow. Moreover, MSCs in cord blood have a higher proliferative potential because of their extended life span and longer telomeres.[67] Not only can cord-blood MSCs be harvested without morbidity to the donor but also they display a robust in-vitro capacity for directable or spontaneous differentiation into mesodermal, endodermal, and ectodermal cell fates. Cord-blood MSCs are CD45⁻ and HLA-II⁻ and can be expanded without losing their pluripotency. Therefore, cord blood is also undergoing preclinical evaluation as a possible easily accessible source of multipotent cells.

STEM CELL DELIVERY METHODS

The current understanding of stem cell biology and kinetics gives us important clues about how we should deliver them. The efficacy of therapeutic stem cells will obviously depend largely on successful delivery. Stem cells have been delivered indirectly through peripheral and coronary veins and coronary arteries. Alternatively, they have been delivered directly by intramyocardial injections via surgical, transendocardial, or transvenous approaches. Another potential delivery strategy is the mobilization of stem cells from the bone marrow by means of cytokine therapy with or without peripheral harvesting.

Stem cell mobilization

In humans, progenitor cells from the bone marrow mobilize after an AMI. This response suggests a 'natural' attempt at cardiac repair.[3] In theory, therapeutic mobilization of bone marrow progenitor cells after an AMI would amplify the existing healing response. Because of its simplicity, mobilization of stem cells is therefore an attractive delivery strategy,[68,69] not only obviating the need for invasive harvesting or delivery procedures but also taking advantage of the clinical procedures already established for the use of progenitor cell-mobilizing granulocyte colony-stimulating factor (G-CSF) in treating hematologic disorders.

Intravenous infusion

Peripheral (intravenous) infusion of stem cells as performed in bone marrow transplantation would be a very convenient – not to mention simple, widely available, and inexpensive – way of delivering therapeutic stem cells to myocardial targets. A study in a mouse model has confirmed that bone marrow cells infused into the peripheral circulation do indeed home in on peri-infarct areas.[70] However, the number of cells that reach the affected area is very small, and this technique would be most applicable after an AMI, because the technique would rely on physiologic homing signals alone.

The major drawback to using an intravenous route of cell delivery would be the possibility that the therapeutic cells would become trapped in the microvasculature of the lungs, liver, and lymphoid tissues. This theoretical limitation of systemic transvenous delivery of stem cells has been confirmed experimentally. In a study by Toma et al,[71] human MSCs were injected into the left ventricular cavity of experimental mice; 4 days later, an estimated 0.44% of the injected cells remained in the myocardium, and the rest had localized to the spleen, liver, and lungs. Other studies using the systemic delivery approach have produced similar results, with very low local cell retention rates of less than 5%.[72,73] Thus, the transvenous delivery route appears unlikely to achieve the local cell concentration needed to produce a significant therapeutic benefit.

Retrograde coronary venous delivery

Two methodologies have been described for delivering therapeutic agents via the coronary venous system. Low-pressure delivery aims to increase the time that the agent is in contact with the vessels without disrupting the venous endothelium.[74–76] High-pressure delivery aims to create a biologic reservoir of product by disrupting the tight endothelial junctions of the venocapillary vasculature and mechanically driving cells across them into the myocardial interstitium.[77–79] Another, newer technique involves a new catheter that has proximal and distal balloons that occlude coronary flow and therefore theoretically allow greater contact between therapeutic cells and the coronary venous system.

Clinical experience with retrograde venous infusion is limited, and several key issues, such as optimal delivery pressure, volume, and infusion time, remain to be resolved.[80,81]

Intracoronary infusion

Intracoronary infusion has been the most popular method of delivering stem cells in the clinical setting, especially after AMI. Intracoronary stem cell delivery 4–9 days after AMI is relatively safe.[82–88] The technique is similar to that for coronary angioplasty, which involves over-the-wire positioning of an angioplasty balloon in a coronary artery. Coronary blood flow is transiently stopped for 2–4 minutes while stem cells are infused under pressure. This maximizes their contact with the microcirculation of the infarct-related artery, thereby optimizing their homing time. Again, this delivery technique would be suitable only in the setting of acute ischemia when adhesion molecules and cytokine signaling are temporarily up-regulated.

Results of recent studies have challenged the safety and effectiveness of intracoronary delivery. There is growing evidence of very low retention of stem cells in target regions and of increased restenosis rates associated with this delivery method.

Intramyocardial injection

Intramyocardial injection has been performed in the clinical setting of chronic myocardial ischemia. It is the preferred delivery route in patients with chronic total occlusion of coronary arteries and in patients with chronic conditions (e.g. congestive heart failure) that involve weaker homing signals. In theory, intramyocardial injection should be the most suitable route for delivering larger cells such as skeletal myoblasts and MSCs, which are prone to microvascular 'plugging.' Intramyocardial injection can be performed via transepicardial, transendocardial, or transcoronary venous routes.

Transepicardial injection

Transepicardial injection of stem cells has been performed during open surgical revascularization procedures to deliver the cells to infarct border zones or areas of infarcted or scarred myocardium. Because a sternotomy is required, this approach is highly invasive and associated with surgical complications. However, in the setting of a planned open heart procedure, the ancillary delivery of cell therapy in this fashion can be easily justified. Interestingly, not all areas of the myocardium (e.g. the interventricular septum) can be reached via a direct external approach.

The main advantages of direct surgical injection are its proven safety in several preclinical and human trials[19,40,89–94] and ease of use. However, it is also costly and offers a very unsophisticated targeting opportunity. The surgeon uses visual assessment only to inject the border of the infarcted area or scar tissue. In addition, the safety of direct surgical injection in patients with recent AMI has not been tested in large clinical trials.

Transendocardial injection

Transendocardial injection is performed via a percutaneous femoral approach. An injection-needle catheter is advanced in retrograde fashion across the aortic valve and positioned against the endocardial surface. Stem cells are then injected directly into targeted areas of the left ventricular wall. Three catheter systems are currently available for transendocardial cell delivery: the Stiletto™ (Boston Scientific, Natick, MA), the BioCardia helical infusion (BioCardia South, San Francisco, CA), and the Myostar™ (Biosense Webster, Diamond Bar, CA).

The Stiletto is used under fluoroscopic (usually biplanar) guidance. Drawbacks of the approach are the bidimensional orientation and lack of precision associated with fluoroscopy. Another drawback is the inability to characterize the underlying or target myocardium.

The BioCardia delivery system uses a catheter whose deflectable tip includes a helical needle for infusion. Initial preclinical experience with this system has provided preliminary evidence of its safety and feasibility.[95] More extensive preclinical experience with this catheter is needed before future human trials can begin.

The Myostar injection catheter takes advantage of non-fluoroscopic magnetic guidance.[96] Injections are targeted with the help of a three-dimensional left ventricular 'shell,' or NOGA electromechanical map (EMM) (Biosense Webster, Markham, ON, Canada), representing the endocardial surface of the left ventricle. The shell is constructed by acquiring a series of electrocardiogram-gated points at multiple locations on the endocardial surface. Ultralow magnetic fields (10^{-} to 10^{-6} T) generated by a triangular magnetic pad positioned beneath the patient intersect with a sensor just proximal to the deflectable tip of a 7F mapping catheter, which helps determine the real-time location and orientation of the catheter tip inside the left ventricle. The NOGA system algorithmically calculates and analyzes the movement of the catheter tip or the location of an endocardial point throughout systole and diastole. That movement is then compared with the movement of neighboring points in an area of interest. The resulting value, called linear local shortening (LLS), is expressed as a percentage that represents the degree of mechanical function of the left ventricular region at that endocardial point. Data are obtained only when the catheter tip is in stable contact with the endocardium. This contact is determined automatically.

The mapping catheter also incorporates electrodes that measure endocardial electrical signals (unipolar or bipolar voltage).[96] Voltage values are assigned to each point acquired during left ventricular mapping, and an electrical map is constructed concurrently with the mechanical map. Each data point has an LLS value and a voltage value. When the map is complete, all the data points are integrated by the NOGA workstation into a three-dimensional, color-coded map of the endocardial surface, as well as 9- and 12-segment bull's-eye views that show average LLS and voltage values in each myocardial segment. These maps can be spatially manipulated in real time on a Silicon Graphics workstation (Silicon Graphics, Inc., Mountain View, CA). The three-dimensional representations acquired during the cardiac cycle can also be used to calculate left ventricular volume and ejection fraction.

The three-dimensional EMM serves both therapeutic and diagnostic purposes. On the one hand, it allows the catheter to be maneuvered through the left ventricle and oriented for transendocardial injections. On the other hand, it allows ischemic areas (i.e. those with low LLS and preserved unipolar voltage [UniV]) to be distinguished from infarcted areas (i.e. those with low LLS and low UniV).[97] Moreover, the Myostar catheter (Figure 33.6) allows myocardial viability to be assessed at each specific injection site where the catheter touches the endocardial surface. The operator is thus able to target therapy to viable tissue (where neoangiogenesis may be possible) or non-viable tissue (where the target of cell therapy may be a scarred area).[98–103] Because of the patchy nature of human ischemic heart disease, the ability to characterize the underlying myocardial tissue is important when delivering stem cells.

Comparisons of delivery methods

The biodistribution of intravenously injected allogeneic MSCs has been recently described.[104] Oxine-labeled MSCs were injected intravenously 72 hours after occlusion/reperfusion in 7 dogs. Initially, cells

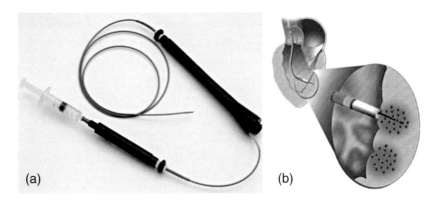

Figure 33.6   (a) Myostar catheter with attached syringe. (b) Artist's illustration showing the catheter traversing the aortic valve and transendocardial extension of the needle with cell delivery (inset). (Reproduced from Perin et al,[124] with permission.)

were trapped in the lungs; within 24 hours after injection, they had been redistributed into the liver and spleen. Focal uptake and persistence of the stem cells was observed in a mid anterior wall location corresponding to the infarcted target area.

Few studies have compared the different modes of cell delivery. Hou et al[105] have described the fate of peripheral blood mononuclear cells (PBMNCs) 1 hour after direct surgical injection, intracoronary infusion, and retrograde venous infusion in an acute swine ischemia/reperfusion model. Overall, PBMNCs concentrated significantly more in the pulmonary vasculature and parenchyma than in the myocardium. Direct surgical injection resulted in significantly less pulmonary retention (26%) than did either intracoronary infusion (47%) or retrograde venous infusion (43%). Cells were scarcely present in the liver and spleen. Myocardial homing, even in a setting of intense homing signaling, was limited in all three approaches, although direct intramyocardial injection (11.3%) achieved better homing and engraftment than did either intracoronary infusion (2.6%) or retrograde venous infusion (3.2%).

Together, these data suggest that none of these three delivery strategies are more than modestly efficient at delivering cells to targeted regions. This limitation is of special concern in the case of intracoronary

delivery, which is the stem cell delivery method most widely used after AMI. This has several important clinical implications for the future of cardiac stem cell therapy:

- higher doses might be needed to achieve desired therapeutic effects
- new (e.g. combined) delivery strategies need to be considered
- myocardial homing and signaling must be better understood
- recipients of systemically delivered cells must be followed up carefully and closely.

CLINICAL TRIALS OF CARDIAC STEM CELL THERAPY

Stem cell therapy for acute myocardial infarction

Most of the clinical experience gained with stem cells has involved therapy for AMI, particularly intracoronary infusion of bone marrow cells, since skeletal myoblasts are too large for this purpose. Table 33.1 summarizes the experience to date. In all of these trials, revascularization was performed promptly after the index MI, and left ventricular systolic compromise was minor (in the BOOST trial, the baseline left ventricular ejection fraction [LVEF] was 50%[88]).

In the Transplantation of Progenitor Cells and Regeneration Enhancement in

Table 33.1 Cell therapy trials in patients with acute myocardial infarction

Study	[n]	Cell type	Dose	Delivery	Time after AMI	Outcomes Improved	Outcomes No change
Strauer et al[87]	10 treated, 10 controls*	MNC	$2.8 \pm 2.2 \times 10^7$	IC	5–9 days	Regional wall motion;† infarct size; ↓ perfusion†	Global LVEF; LVEDV†
TOPCARE-AMI[82,83,86]	29 MNC, 30 CPC, 11 controls*	MNC	$2.1 \pm 0.8 \times 10^8$	IC	5 ± 2 days	Regional wall motion;† global LVEF;† infarct size;†↓ coronary flow†	LVEDV†
		CPC	$1.6 \pm 1.2 \times 10^7$				
Fernandez-Aviles et al[85]	20 treated, 13 controls*	MNC	$7.8 \pm 4.1 \times 10^7$	IC	14 ± 6 days	Regional wall motion;† global LVEF†	LVEDV†
Kuethe et al[119]	5 treated	MNC	$3.9 \pm 2.3 \times 10^7$	IC	6 days	Regional wall motion;† global LVEF†	Regional wall motion;† global LVEF†
BOOST[88]	30 treated, 30 controls	NC	$2.5 \pm 0.9 \times 10^9$	IC	6 ± 1 day	Regional wall motion; global LVEF	LVEDV; infarct size
Chen et al[84]	34 treated, 35 controls	MSC	$4.8–6.0 \times 10^{10}$	IC	18 days	Regional wall motion; global LVEF; infarct size↓; LVEDV↓	
Vanderheyden et al[120]	12 treated, 10 controls*	CD133+	$6.6 \pm 1.4 \times 10^6$	IC	14 ± 6 days	Regional wall motion;† global LVEF; perfusion†	Regional wall motion;† global LVEF†

MNC, bone marrow-derived mononuclear cells; CPC, circulating blood-derived progenitor cells; NC, bone marrow-derived nucleated cells; MSC, bone marrow-derived mesenchymal stem cells; CD133+, bone marrow-derived CD133+ cells; IC, intracoronary; AMI, acute myocardial infarction; LVEF, left ventricular ejection fraction; LVEDV, left ventricular end-diastolic volume.
*Non-randomized control groups.
†Effects reported only within cell therapy groups. Study by Vanderheyden et al[120] has been presented in abstract form only. Values are means ± SD.
Adapted from Wollert KC, Drexler H. Clinical applications of stem cells for the heart. Circ Res 2005; 96(2):151–63.

Acute Myocardial Infarction (TOPCARE-AMI) trial, patients were randomized to receive either bone marrow-derived mononuclear cells or EPCs via intracoronary infusion.[106] Compared with the non-randomized control patients, treated patients had a significantly improved global LVEF, as assessed by left ventricular angiography, regardless of cell type used. In a subgroup of this study population, LVEF was significantly increased, as assessed by cardiac magnetic resonance imaging (MRI), and infarct size was reduced, as assessed by late-enhancement MRI.[107] Interestingly, the infused cells' ability to migrate was the most important predictor of infarct remodeling. Coronary flow reserve also increased, which is suggestive of neovascularization.

The 1-year results of TOPCARE-AMI reinforce the notion that stem cells protect against ventricular remodeling. Despite the limited number of patients, contrast-enhanced MRI revealed a significantly increased LVEF ($P < 0.001$), significantly reduced infarct size ($P < 0.001$), and the absence of reactive hypertrophy, suggesting that the infarcted ventricles had been functionally regenerated. Scientific criticism of this trial has focused on the cell delivery method, which included transient coronary occlusion and flow cessation, and its potential for ischemic preconditioning. Such preconditioning has been shown to improve outcomes during AMI and may have contributed to the functional improvement noted in this trial. Moreover, the occurrence of in-stent thrombosis in one patient 3 days after undergoing cell therapy has raised safety concerns.

In a study by Bartunek et al,[108] 35 patients were infused with AC133+ bone marrow cells after AMI. The mean dose was 12.6 million cells, and the mean infusion was 11.4 days after the index event. At 4-month follow-up, treated patients had an improved mean LVEF but higher rates of stent restenosis, stent reocclusion, and de-novo coronary artery lesions than did the controls.

The intracoronary route has also been used to deliver autologous MSCs. Chen et al[109] recently reported the first randomized clinical trial of these cells in 69 patients who underwent a primary percutaneous coronary intervention within 12 hours after an AMI. Either an MSC or saline infusion was injected into the target coronary artery. At 3-month follow-up, left ventricular perfusion and the LVEF had significantly improved in the treatment group.

In the randomized BOOST trial,[88] patients received either bone marrow-derived ABMMNCs or no treatment at all (no placebo). Stem cell therapy resulted in an increased LVEF and a reduced end-systolic volume, as assessed by MRI. This improvement was attributed principally to increased contractility of the peri-infarct zones. Unlike earlier non-randomized trials, the BOOST trial did not show a significant reduction in infarct size.

The 18-month follow-up of patients in the BOOST trial was recently published.[110] The initial improvement in LVEF in the cell-treated group was not sustained when compared to the control group. However, the speed in which there was LVEF recovery over the 18 months was significantly higher in the cell-treated group.

A study by Janssens et al[111] sheds further insight into the intracoronary delivery of ABMMNCs after AMI. In a series of 67 patients, ABMMNCs were infused 24 hours after mechanical reperfusion. The primary endpoint of LVEF at 4-month follow-up was similar between the cell-treated and placebo groups. However, the cell-treated group had smaller infarct sizes and better recovery in regional systolic function.

Taken together, the phase I intracoronary delivery trials have taught us that the magnitude of improvement after intracoronary infusion of stem cells is modest and possibly mediated through prevention of remodeling. Overall, the small (less than 5%) cell engraftment after intracoronary delivery could potentially explain its modest therapeutic benefits. More specifically, in Janssens et al's study, the importance of cell delivery timing is once more evident. Early infusion of stem cells may result in even lower engraftment rates or higher rates of cell death given the adverse environment into which the cells are delivered. Alternatively, the modest therapeutic benefit could be due to patient selection. All of the intracoronary studies were performed in patients with small areas of infarction and a preserved LVEF. As mentioned earlier, animal models of cell delivery have repeatedly shown the superior engraftment of cells via intramyocardial delivery.

The feasibility and efficacy of G-CSF therapy and subsequent intracoronary infusion of collected peripheral blood stem cells were prospectively investigated in the Myocardial Regeneration and Angiogenesis in Myocardial Infarction with G-CSF and Intracoronary Stem Cell Infusion (MAGIC) randomized clinical trial,[112] which showed improved cardiac function and promotion of angiogenesis in MI patients. However, the trial raised important safety questions. Intracoronary infusion of G-CSF-stimulated peripheral blood stem cells apparently aggravated restenosis after coronary stenting, leading to early termination of the trial. Meanwhile, no temporal association between increased restenosis rate and stenting near the time of intracoronary cell administration has been noted in other studies that have not used G-CSF stimulation.

Stem cell mobilization

A different therapeutic strategy using G-CSF involved mobilization of CD34$^+$ cells from the bone marrow to the peripheral blood.[18] Thirty patients in the superacute phase of MI underwent primary percutaneous revascularization. Eighty-five minutes after revascularization, 15 patients were randomized to begin receiving G-CSF stimulation for up to 6 days. At 1-year follow-up, the G-CSF-treated patients had significantly improved LVEF and stable end-diastolic diameters.

The safety of G-CSF stimulation in patients with CAD has been questioned in two recent studies. Hill et al[113] report the results of administration of 10 μg/kg/day of G-CSF for 5 days in patients with chronic CAD ($n = 16$). There was no clinical benefit as assessed by exercise stress testing and dobutamine cardiac MRI. Additionally, 2 patients in the G-CSF group developed serious adverse events related to the therapy (1 non-ST elevation MI; 1 MI causing death). Zbinden et al[114] also tested the efficacy of the same G-CSF dose in patients with chronic CAD ($n = 7$). The invasive endpoint collateral flow index was significantly better in the G-CSF-treated patients than in the placebo group. However, 2 patients in the G-CSF-treated group developed acute coronary syndrome during treatment.

In a study by Zohlnhofer et al,[115] 56 AMI patients were assigned to receive G-CSF treatment after successful percutaneous coronary intervention. Those patients were compared with 58 patients assigned to receive a placebo. The G-CSF treatment did not influence infarct size, left ventricular function, or coronary restenosis, and G-CSF was not associated with adverse outcomes.

Collectively, the G-CSF trials point to an ineffective therapy after AMI, and in the chronic setting that could be potentially dangerous, due to systemic inflammatory effects that probably lead to acute coronary syndromes.

Stem cells for chronic ischemic heart disease

Outside the AMI setting, stem cells have been used to treat patients with ischemic heart disease with or without systolic functional compromise and patients unsuitable for myocardial revascularization (Table 33.2). Autologous bone

Table 33.2 Cell therapy trials in patients with ischemic cardiomyopathy

Study	[n]	LVEF	Cell type	Dose	Time after MI	Delivery	Outcomes[‡]
Menasche et al[91]	10 treated	24 ± 4%	Myoblasts	8.7 ± 1.9 × 10^8	3–228 months	Transepicardial (during CABG)*	Regional wall motion↑; global LVEF↑
Herreros et al[90]	11 treated	36 ± 8%	Myoblasts	1.9 ± 1.2 × 10^8	3–168 months	Transepicardial (during CABG)[†]	Regional wall motion↑; global LVEF↑; viability in infarct area↑
Siminiak et al[92]	10 treated	25–40%	Myoblasts	0.04–5.0 × 10^7	4–108 months	Transepicardial (during CABG)[†]	Regional wall motion↑; global LVEF↑
Chachques et al[121]	20 treated	28 ± 3%	Myoblasts	3.0 ± 0.2 × 10^8	Not reported	Transepicardial (during CABG)*	Regional wall motion↑; global LVEF↑; viability in infarct area↑
Smits et al[122]	5 treated	36 ± 11%	Myoblasts	2.0 ± 1.1 × 10^8	24–132 months	Transendocardial (guided by EMM)	Regional wall motion↑; global LVEF↑
Stamm et al[93,94]	12 treated	36 ± 11%	CD133+	1.0–2.8 × 10^6	3–12 weeks	Transepicardial (during CABG)*	Global LVEF↑; LVEDV↓; perfusion↑
Assmus et al[123]	51 MNC, 35 CPC, 16 controls	40 ± 11%	MNC	1.7 ± 0.8 × 10^8	3–144 months	IC	Global LVEF↑ (only in MNC group)
			CPC	2.3 ± 1.2 × 10^7			

LVEF, left ventricular ejection fraction; CD133+, bone marrow-derived CD133+ cells; MNC, bone marrow-derived mononuclear cells; CPC, circulating blood-derived progenitor cells; MI, myocardial infarction; CABG, coronary artery bypass grafting; EMM, electromechanical mapping; IC, intracoronary; LVEDV, left ventricular end-diastolic volume.
*CABG of non-injected territories only.
[†]CABG of injected and non-injected territories.
[‡]Effects only within cell therapy groups. Study by Assmus et al[123] has been presented in abstract form only. Values are means ± SD.
Adapted from Wollert KC, Drexler H. Clinical applications of stem cells for the heart. Circ Res 2005; 96(2):151–63.

marrow stem cell therapy has been used to treat patients with chronic myocardial ischemia, including ischemic heart failure with or without systolic functional compromise, and patients ineligible for myocardial revascularization (Table 33.3). The preliminary clinical evidence supports the efficacy of this new therapy, and, at this point, all evidence appears to substantiate its safety.

Tse et al[116] have reported that transendocardial injection of ABMMNCs in 8 patients with severe ischemic heart disease led to preserved left ventricular function. At 3-month follow-up, heart failure symptoms and myocardial perfusion had improved, especially in the ischemic region, as shown by cardiac MRI.

Fuchs et al[99] studied the clinical feasibility of transendocardial delivery of filtered unfractionated autologous bone marrow-derived (not mononuclear) cells in 10 patients with severe, symptomatic, chronic myocardial ischemia not amenable to conventional revascularization. Twelve targeted injections (0.2 ml each) were administered into ischemic, non-infarcted myocardium identified previously by single-photon emission computed tomography (SPECT) perfusion imaging. No serious adverse effects (i.e. arrhythmia, infection, myocardial inflammation, or increased scar formation) were noted. Moreover, even though treadmill exercise duration results did not change significantly (391 ± 155 vs 485 ± 198 seconds; $P = 0.11$), there was improvement in Canadian Cardiovascular Society angina scores (3.1 ± 0.3 vs 2.0 ± 0.94; $P = 0.001$) and in stress scores in segments within the injected regions (2.1 ± 0.8 vs 1.6 ± 0.8; $P < 0.001$).

Our group performed the first clinical trial of transendocardial injection of ABMMNCs to treat heart failure patients.[117] This study, performed in collaboration with physicians and scientists at the Hospital Pro-Cardiaco in Rio de Janeiro, Brazil, used EMM-guided transendocardial delivery of stem cells. The results of 2- and 4-month non-invasive and invasive follow-up evaluations[117] and of 6- and 12-month follow-up evaluation[118] have already been published.

A total of 21 patients were enrolled. The first 14 constituted the treatment group, and the last 7 patients the control group. Baseline evaluations included complete clinical and laboratory tests, exercise stress (ramp treadmill) studies, two-dimensional Doppler echocardiography, SPECT perfusion scanning, and 24-hour Holter monitoring. ABMMNCs were harvested, isolated, washed, and resuspended in saline for injection via NOGA catheter (15 injections of 0.2 ml, totalling 30×10^6 cells per patient) in viable myocardium (unipolar voltage ≥ 6.9 mV). All patients underwent non-invasive follow-up tests at 2 months, and the treatment group also underwent invasive studies at 4 months, using standard protocols and the same procedures as at baseline. The demographic and exercise test variables did not differ significantly between the treatment and control groups. There were no procedural complications. At 2 months, there was a significant reduction in the total reversible defect in the treatment group and between the treatment and control groups ($P = 0.02$) on quantitative SPECT analysis. At 4 months, the LVEF improved from a baseline of 20% to 29% ($P = 0.003$) and the end-systolic volume decreased ($P = 0.03$) in the treated patients. Electromechanical mapping revealed significant mechanical improvement in the injected segments ($P < 0.0005$). In our opinion, this established the safety of transendocardial injection of ABMMNCs and warranted further investigation of this therapy's efficacy endpoints. This trial was important because for the first time myocardial perfusion and cardiac function were observed to improve in a group of severely impaired patients treated solely with stem cells. The significant improvement seen at 2 and 4 months was maintained at 6 and

Table 33.3 Cell therapy trials in patients with myocardial ischemia and no revascularization option

Study	[n]	LVEF	Cell type	Dose	Delivery	Outcomes	
						Subjective	Objective
Hamano et al[89]	5 treated		MNC	$0.3–2.2 \times 10^9$	Transepicardial (during CABG)		Perfusion↑[†]
Tse et al[116]	8 treated	58 ± 11%	MNC	From 40 ml BM	Transendocardial (guided by EMM)	Angina↓[†]	Perfusion↑;[†] regional wall motion↑[†]
Fuchs et al[99]	10 treated	47 ± 10%	NC	$7.8 \pm 6.6 \times 10^7$	Transendocardial (guided by EMM)	Angina↓[†]	Perfusion↑[†]
Perin et al[117,124]	14 treated, 7 controls*	30 ± 6%	MNC	$3.0 \pm 0.4 \times 10^7$	Transendocardial (guided by EMM)	Angina↓; NYHA class↓	Perfusion↑; regional wall motion↑;[†] global LVEF↑

LVEF, left ventricular ejection fraction; MNC, bone marrow-derived mononuclear cells; NC, bone marrow-derived nucleated cells; BM, bone marrow; CABG, coronary artery bypass grafting; EMM, electromechanical mapping; NYHA, New York Heart Association.
*Non-randomized control group.
[†]Effects reported only within cell therapy groups. Values are means ± SD.
Adapted from Wollert KC, Drexler H. Clinical applications of stem cells for the heart. Circ Res 2005; 96(2):151–63.

Table 33.4 Comparison of clinical values for the treatment and control groups at baseline, 2 months, 6 months, and 12 months

	Baseline		2 months		6 months		12 months		P*
	Treatment	Control	Treatment	Control	Treatment	Control	Treatment	Control	
SPECT:									
Total reversible defect, %	14.8 ± 14.5	20 ± 25.4	4.45 ± 11.5	37 ± 38.4	8.8 ± 9	32.7 ± 37	11.3 ± 12.8	34.3 ± 30.8	0.01
Total fixed defect (50%), %	42.6 ± 10.3	38 ± 12	39.8 ± 6.9	39.1 ± 11.2	38 ± 6.7	36.4 ± 12	38.2 ± 8.5	35.2 ± 9.3	0.3
Ramp treadmill:									
VO$_2$ max, ml/kg/min	17.3 ± 8	17.5 ± 6.7	23.2 ± 8	18.3 ± 9.6	24.15 ± 7	17.3 ± 6	25.1 ± 8.7	18.2 ± 6.7	0.03
METS	5.0 ± 2.3	5.0 ± 1.91	6.6 ± 2.3	5.2 ± 2.7	7.19 ± 2.4	4.92 ± 1.7	7.2 ± 2.5	5.1 ± 1.9	0.02
LVEF	30 ± 6	37 ± 14	37 ± 6	27 ± 6	30 ± 10	28 ± 4	35.1 ± 6.9	34 ± 3	0.9
Functional class:									
NYHA	2.2 ± 0.9	2.7 ± 0.8	1.5 ± 0.5	2.4 ± 1.0	1.3 ± 0.6	2.4 ± 0.5	1.4 ± 0.7	2.7 ± 0.5	0.01
CCSAS	2.6 ± 0.8	2.9 ± 1.0	1.8 ± 0.6	2.5 ± 0.8	1.4 ± 0.5	2 ± 0.1	1.2 ± 0.4	2.7 ± 0.5	0.002
PVC, n	2507 ± 6243	672 ± 1085	901 ± 1236	2034 ± 4528	3902 ± 8267	1041 ± 1971	–	–	0.4
dQRS, ms	136 ± 15	145 ± 61	145.9 ± 25	130 ± 27	144.8 ± 25	140 ± 61	–	–	0.62
LAS 40, ms	50 ± 24	70 ± 76	54 ± 33	48 ± 20	25 ± 25	66 ± 79	–	–	0.47
RMS 40, µV	22.2 ± 22	23.3 ± 23	23.3 ± 19	24.6 ± 28	25 ± 25	30 ± 27	–	–	0.7

SPECT, single-photon emission computed tomography; METS, metabolic equivalents; LVEF, left ventricular ejection fraction; PVC, premature ventricular contraction; LAS 40, duration of terminal low-amplitude signal less than 40 mV; RMS 40, root-mean-square voltage in the terminal 40 ms of the QRS complex; dQRS, filtered QRS duration; NYHA, New York Heart Association; CCSAS, Canadian Cardiovascular Society Angina Score.

*P for comparisons between treatment and control groups by ANOVA.

Adapted from Perin EC et al.[117]

12 months, even as exercise capacity improved slightly (Table 33.4). Monocyte, B-cell, hematopoietic progenitor cell, and early hematopoietic progenitor cell subpopulations correlated with improvement in reversible perfusion defects at 6 months (Table 33.5).

We recently described the postmortem study of one of our patients who received ABMMNCs.[118] Eleven months after performing the treatment, we observed no abnormal or disorganized tissue growth, no abnormal vascular growth, and no enhanced inflammatory reactions. Histologic and immunohistochemical findings from infarcted areas of the anterolateral ventricular wall (areas that had received bone marrow cell injections) were reported. The histologic findings from the anterolateral wall region were subsequently compared with findings from within the interventricular septum (which had normal perfusion in the central region and no cell therapy) and findings from the previously infarcted inferoposterior

Table 33.5 Correlation of bone marrow mononuclear cell subpopulations and reduction in total reversible perfusion defects

Cell population and phenotype	r	P
Hematopoietic progenitor cells (CD45^{lo}CD34$^+$)	0.6	0.04
Early hematopoietic progenitor cells (CD45^{lo}CD34$^+$HLA-DR$^-$)	0.6	0.04
CD4$^+$ T cells (CD45$^+$CD3$^+$CD4$^+$)	0.5	0.1
CD8$^+$ T cells (CD45$^+$CD3$^+$CD8$^+$)	0.5	0.07
B cells (CD45$^+$CD19$^+$)	0.7	0.02
Monocytes (CD45$^+$CD14$^+$)	0.8	0.03
NK cells (CD45$^+$CD56$^+$)	0.1	0.9
B-cell progenitors (CD34$^+$CD19$^+$)	0.5	0.3
CFU-F	0.7	0.06

r, Pearson correlation coefficient; CFU-F, fibroblast colony-forming unit; NK, natural killer.
Adapted from Perin EC et al.[117]

ventricular wall (which had extensive scarring and no cell therapy).

The observed effects of cell therapy were quite intriguing:

1. The cell-treated infarcted areas of this patient's heart had a higher capillary density than did the non-treated, infarcted areas.
2. Smooth muscle α-actin-positive pericytes and mural cells proliferated exclusively in the cell-treated area.
3. These pericytes and mural cells expressed specific cardiomyocyte proteins.

The angiogenesis literature makes clear that pericytes are essential for long-lasting physiologic angiogenesis. In our postmortem study, the cell-injected wall had marked areas of pericyte and mural cells hyperplasia. The observed hypertrophic pericytes, though still located in the vascular wall, expressed specific myocardial proteins and were found in locations distant from the vessel walls, suggesting detachment. Migratory pericytes and mural cells were found in adjacent tissue (in the vicinity of cardiomyocytes) either isolated or in small clumps. Closer to cardiomyocytes, the expression of myocardial proteins was enhanced, yielding brighter immunostaining throughout the whole cytoplasm. Within the posterior wall, none of this was seen, and small blood vessels were rare. Although it would be premature to arrive at any definitive conclusions about ABMMNC efficacy on the basis of one postmortem study, the above findings in the cell-treated wall are consistent with neoangiogenesis. If confirmed in future human studies, these findings would corroborate most of the preclinical studies in chronic myocardial ischemia models.

Clinical trials of skeletal myoblasts have focused on the treatment of patients with ischemic cardiomyopathy and systolic dysfunction. Overall, these trials have resulted in improved segmental contractility and global LVEF. The preferred delivery route has been surgical intramyo-cardial injection, and one feasibility trial of transendocardial injection has been reported in the literature so far.

Conclusions

Stem cell therapy for cardiac diseases is slowly becoming a reality. Solid preclinic evidence of efficacy has accumulated over the years, and translational research is ongoing. Despite many unresolved issues related to treatment dose, timing, and delivery, the clinical potential of stem cell therapy for cardiovascular disease is enormous. The expectations of both patients and clinicians for this new therapeutic modality, however, are high and will require continued cooperation and close collaboration between basic and clinical researchers.

The discovery of the full potential of this novel therapy will ultimately lead to a more complete understanding of the healing process of the heart.

REFERENCES

1. Radovancevic B, Vrtovec B, Frazier OH. Left ventricular assist devices: an alternative to medical therapy for end-stage heart failure. Curr Opin Cardiol 2003; 18:210–14.

2. Asahara T, Murohara T, Sullivan A et al. Isolation of putative progenitor endothelial cells for angiogenesis. Science 1997; 275:964–7.

3. Shintani S, Murohara T, Ikeda H et al. Mobilization of endothelial progenitor cells in patients with acute myocardial infarction. Circulation 2001; 103:2776–9.

4. Rumpold H, Wolf D, Koeck R et al. Endothelial progenitor cells: a source for therapeutic vasculogenesis? J Cell Mol Med 2004; 8:509–18.

5. Asahara T, Masuda H, Takahashi T et al. Bone marrow origin of endothelial progenitor cells responsible for postnatal vasculogenesis in physiological and pathological neovascularization. Circ Res 1999; 85:221–8.

6. Krause DS. Plasticity of marrow-derived stem cells. Gene Ther 2002; 9:754–8.

7. Perin EC, Geng YJ, Willerson JT. Adult stem cell therapy in perspective. Circulation 2003; 107:935–8.

8. Anversa P, Kadstura J, Leri A et al. Life and death of cardiac stem cells: a paradigm shift in cardiac biology. Circulation 2006; 113:1451–63.

9. Blau HM, Brazelton TR, Weimann JM. The evolving concept of a stem cell: entity or function? Cell 2001; 105:829–41.

10. Weissman IL. Stem cells: units of development, units of regeneration, and units in evolution. Cell 2000; 100:157–68.

11. Thomson JA, Itskovitz-Eldor J, Shapiro SS et al. Embryonic stem cell lines derived from human blastocysts. Science 1998; 282:1145–7.

12. Korbling M, Estrov Z. Adult stem cells for tissue repair – a new therapeutic concept? N Engl J Med 2003; 349:570–82.

13. Ferrari G, Cusella-De Angelis G, Coletta M et al. Muscle regeneration by bone marrow-derived myogenic progenitors. Science 1998; 279:1528–30.

14. Graf T. Differentiation plasticity of hematopoietic cells. Blood 2002; 99:3089–101.

15. Beltrami AP, Barlucchi L, Torella D et al. Adult cardiac stem cells are multipotent and support myocardial regeneration. Cell 2003; 114:763–76.

16. Oh H, Bradfute SB, Gallardo TD et al. Cardiac progenitor cells from adult myocardium: homing, differentiation, and fusion after infarction. Proc Natl Acad Sci USA 2003; 100:12313–18.

17. Urbanek K, Quaini F, Tasca G et al. Intense myocyte formation from cardiac stem cells in human cardiac hypertrophy. Proc Natl Acad Sci USA 2003; 100:10440–5.

18. Iwami Y, Masuda H, Asahara T. Endothelial progenitor cells: past, state of the art, and future. J Cell Mol Med 2004; 8:488–97.

19. Orlic D, Kajstura J, Chimenti S et al. Bone marrow cells regenerate infarcted myocardium. Nature 2001; 410:701–5.

20. Quaini F, Urbanek K, Beltrami AP et al. Chimerism of the transplanted heart. N Engl J Med 2002; 346:5–15.

21. Kucia M, Ratajczak J, Ratajczak MZ. Bone marrow as a source of circulating CXCR4+ tissue-committed stem cells. Biol Cell 2005; 97:133–46.

22. Raffi S, Lyden D. Therapeutic stem and progenitor cell transplantation for organ vascularization and regeneration. Nat Med 2003; 9:702–12.

23. Vasa M, Fichtlscherer S, Aicher A et al. Number and migratory activity of circulating endothelial progenitor cells inversely correlate with risk factors for coronary artery disease. Circ Res 2001; 89:E1–7.

24. Werner N, Kosiol S, Schiegl T et al. Circulating endothelial progenitor cells and cardiovascular outcomes. N Engl J Med 2005; 353:999–1007.

25. Schmidt-Lucke C, Rössig L, Fichtlscherer S et al. Reduced number of circulating endothelial progenitor cells predicts future cardiovascular events. Proof of concept for the clinical importance of endogenous vascular repair. Circulation 2005; 111:2981–7.

26. Fadini GP, Miorin M, Facco M et al. Circulating endothelial progenitor cells are reduced in peripheral vascular complications of type 2 diabetes mellitus. J Am Coll Cardiol 2005; 45:1449–57.

27. Walter DH, Haendeler J, Reinhold J et al. Impaired CXCR4 signaling contributes to the reduced neovascularization capacity of endothelial progenitor cells

from patients with coronary artery disease. Circ Res 2005; 97:1142–51.

28. Dong C, Crawford LE, Goldschmidt-Clermont PJ. Endothelial progenitor obsolescence and atherosclerotic inflammation. J Am Coll Cardiol 2005; 45: 1458–60.

29. Baksh D, Song L, Tuan RS. Adult mesenchymal stem cells: characterization, differentiation, and application in cell and gene therapy. J Cell Mol Med 2004; 8:301–16.

30. Bruder SP, Jaiswal N, Haynesworth SE. Growth kinetics, self-renewal, and the osteogenic potential of purified human mesenchymal stem cells during extensive subcultivation and following cryopreservation. J Cell Biochem 1997; 64:278–94.

31. Bruder SP, Kurth AA, Shea M et al. Bone regeneration by implantation of purified, culture-expanded human mesenchymal stem cells. J Orthop Res 1998; 16:155–62.

32. Kadiyala S, Young RG, Thiede MA et al. Culture expanded canine mesenchymal stem cells possess osteochondrogenic potential in vivo and in vitro. Cell Transplant 1997; 6:125–34.

33. Awad HA, Butler DL, Boivin GP et al. Autologous mesenchymal stem cell-mediated repair of tendon. Tissue Eng 1999; 5:267–77.

34. Young RG, Butler DL, Weber W et al. Use of mesenchymal stem cells in a collagen matrix for Achilles tendon repair. J Orthop Res 1998; 16:406–13.

35. Galmiche MC, Koteliansky VE, Briere J et al. Stromal cells from human long-term marrow cultures are mesenchymal cells that differentiate following a vascular smooth muscle differentiation pathway. Blood 1993; 82:66–76.

36. Dennis JE, Merriam A, Awadallah A et al. A quadripotential mesenchymal progenitor cell isolated from the marrow of an adult mouse. J Bone Miner Res 1999; 14:700–9.

37. Prockop DJ. Marrow stromal cells as stem cells for nonhematopoietic tissues. Science 1997; 276:71–4.

38. Pittenger MF, Martin BJ. Mesenchymal stem cells and their potential as cardiac therapeutics. Circ Res 2004; 95:9–20.

39. Tse WT, Pendleton JD, Beyer WM et al. Suppression of allogeneic T-cell proliferation by human marrow stromal cells: implications in transplantation. Transplantation 2003; 75:389–97.

40. Silva GV, Litovsky S, Assad JA et al. Mesenchymal stem cells differentiate into an endothelial phenotype, enhance vascular density, and improve heart function in a canine chronic ischemia model. Circulation 2005; 111:150–6.

41. Murohara T, Ikeda H, Duan J et al. Transplanted cord blood-derived endothelial precursor cells augment postnatal neovascularization. J Clin Invest 2000; 105:1527–36.

42. Quirici N, Soligo D, Caneva L et al. Differentiation and expansion of endothelial cells from human bone marrow CD133(+) cells. Br J Haematol 2001; 115:186–94.

43. Hristov M, Erl W, Weber PC. Endothelial progenitor cells: mobilization, differentiation, and homing. Arterioscler Thromb Vasc Biol 2003; 23:1185–9.

44. Harraz M, Jiao C, Hanlon HD et al. CD34- blood-derived human endothelial cell progenitors. Stem Cells 2001; 19:304–12.

45. Nieda M, Nicol A, Denning-Kendall P et al. Endothelial cell precursors are normal components of human umbilical cord blood. Br J Haematol 1997; 98:775–7.

46. Gehling UM, Ergun S, Schumacher U et al. In vitro differentiation of endothelial cells from AC133-positive progenitor cells. Blood 2000; 95:3106–12.

47. Gunsilius E, Petzer AL, Duba HC et al. Circulating endothelial cells after transplantation. Lancet 2001; 357:1449–50.

48. Hatzopoulos AK, Folkman J, Vasile E et al. Isolation and characterization of endothelial progenitor cells from mouse embryos. Development 1998; 125: 1457–68.

49. Lin Y, Weisdorf DJ, Solovey A et al. Origins of circulating endothelial cells and endothelial outgrowth from blood. J Clin Invest 2000; 105:71–7.

50. Peichev M, Naiyer AJ, Pereira D et al. Expression of VEGFR-2 and AC133 by circulating human CD34(+) cells identifies a population of functional endothelial precursors. Blood 2000; 95:952–8.

51. Shi Q, Rafii S, Wu MH et al. Evidence for circulating bone marrow-derived endothelial cells. Blood 1998; 92:362–7.

52. Kucia M, Dawn B, Hunt G et al. Cells expressing early cardiac markers reside in the bone marrow and are mobilized into the peripheral blood after myocardial infarction. Circ Res 2004; 95:1191–9.

53. Deb A, Wang S, Skelding KA et al. Bone marrow-derived cardiomyocytes are present in adult human heart: a study of gender-mismatched bone marrow transplantation patients. Circulation 2003; 107:1247–9.

54. Dowell JD, Rubart M, Pasumarthi KB et al. Myocyte and myogenic stem cell transplantation in the heart. Cardiovasc Res 2003; 58:336–50.

55. Menasche P. Cellular transplantation: hurdles remaining before widespread clinical use. Curr Opin Cardiol 2004; 19:154–61.

56. Leor J, Patterson M, Quinones MJ et al. Transplantation of fetal myocardial tissue into the infarcted myocardium of rat. A potential method for repair of infarcted myocardium? Circulation 1996; 94:II332–6.

57. Tambara K, Sakakibara Y, Sakaguchi G et al. Transplanted skeletal myoblasts can fully replace the infarcted myocardium when they survive in the host in large numbers. Circulation 2003; 108 (Suppl 1): II259–63.

58. Cowan CA, Klimanskaya I, McMahon J et al. Derivation of embryonic stem-cell lines from human blastocysts. N Engl J Med 2004; 350:1353–6.

59. Itskovitz-Eldor J, Schuldiner M, Karsenti D et al. Differentiation of human embryonic stem cells into

embryoid bodies compromising the three embryonic germ layers. Mol Med 2000; 6:88–95.

60. Sachinidis A, Fleischmann BK, Kolossov E et al. Cardiac specific differentiation of mouse embryonic stem cells. Cardiovasc Res 2003; 58:278–91.

61. Anversa P, Sussman MA, Bolli R. Molecular genetic advances in cardiovascular medicine: focus on the myocyte. Circulation 2004; 109:2832–8.

62. Messina E, De Angelis L, Frati G et al. Isolation and expansion of adult cardiac stem cells from human and murine heart. Circ Res 2004; 95:911–21.

63. Dragoo JL, Choi JY, Lieberman JR et al. Bone induction by BMP-2 transduced stem cells derived from human fat. J Orthop Res 2003; 21:622–9.

64. Safford KM, Hicok KC, Safford SD et al. Neurogenic differentiation of murine and human adipose-derived stromal cells. Biochem Biophys Res Commun 2002; 294:371–9.

65. Zuk PA, Zhu M, Ashjian P et al. Human adipose tissue is a source of multipotent stem cells. Mol Biol Cell 2002; 13:4279–95.

66. Wulf GG, Viereck V, Hemmerlein B et al. Mesengenic progenitor cells derived from human placenta. Tissue Eng 2004; 10:1136–47.

67. Erices A, Conget P, Minguell JJ. Mesenchymal progenitor cells in human umbilical cord blood. Br J Haematol 2000; 109:235–42.

68. Lew WY. Mobilizing cells to the injured myocardium: a novel rescue strategy or an unwelcome intrusion? J Am Coll Cardiol 2004; 44:1521–2.

69. Maekawa Y, Anzai T, Yoshikawa T et al. Effect of granulocyte-macrophage colony-stimulating factor inducer on left ventricular remodeling after acute myocardial infarction. J Am Coll Cardiol 2004; 44:1510–20.

70. Saito T, Kuang JQ, Bittira B, Al-khadi A, Chiu RC. Xenotransplant cardiac chimera: immune tolerance of adult stem cells. Ann Thorac Surg 2002; 74:19–24; discussion.

71. Toma C, Pittenger MF, Cahill KS et al. Human mesenchymal stem cells differentiate to a cardiomyocyte phenotype in the adult murine heart. Circulation 2002; 105:93–8.

72. Aicher A, Brenner W, Zuhayra M et al. Assessment of the tissue distribution of transplanted human endothelial progenitor cells by radioactive labeling. Circulation 2003; 107:2134–9.

73. Barbash IM, Chouraqui P, Baron J et al. Systemic delivery of bone marrow-derived mesenchymal stem cells to the infarcted myocardium: feasibility, cell migration, and body distribution. Circulation 2003; 108:863–8.

74. Boekstegers P, von Degenfeld G, Giehrl W et al. Myocardial gene transfer by selective pressure-regulated retroinfusion of coronary veins. Gene Ther 2000; 7:232–40.

75. Murad-Netto S, Moura R, Romeo LJ et al. Stem cell therapy with retrograde coronary perfusion in acute myocardial infarction. A new technique. Arq Bras Cardiol 2004; 83:352–4; 349–51.

76. von Degenfeld G, Raake P, Kupatt C et al. Selective pressure-regulated retroinfusion of fibroblast growth factor-2 into the coronary vein enhances regional myocardial blood flow and function in pigs with chronic myocardial ischemia. J Am Coll Cardiol 2003; 42:1120–8.

77. Herity NA, Lo ST, Oei F et al. Selective regional myocardial infiltration by the percutaneous coronary venous route: a novel technique for local drug delivery. Catheter Cardiovasc Interv 2000; 51:358–63.

78. Hou D, Maclaughlin F, Thiesse M et al. Widespread regional myocardial transfection by plasmid encoding Del-1 following retrograde coronary venous delivery. Catheter Cardiovasc Interv 2003; 58:207–11.

79. Raake P, von Degenfeld G, Hinkel R et al. Myocardial gene transfer by selective pressure-regulated retroinfusion of coronary veins: comparison with surgical and percutaneous intramyocardial gene delivery. J Am Coll Cardiol 2004; 44:1124–9.

80. Thompson CA, Nasseri BA, Makower J et al. Percutaneous transvenous cellular cardiomyoplasty. A novel nonsurgical approach for myocardial cell transplantation. J Am Coll Cardiol 2003; 41:1964–71.

81. Siminiak T, Fiszer D, Jerzykowska O et al. Percutaneous trans-coronary-venous transplantation of autologous skeletal myoblasts in the treatment of post-infarction myocardial contractility impairment: the POZNAN trial. Eur Heart J 2005; 26:1188–95.

82. Assmus B, Schachinger V, Teupe C et al. Transplantation of Progenitor Cells and Regeneration Enhancement in Acute Myocardial Infarction (TOPCARE-AMI). Circulation 2002; 106:3009–17.

83. Britten MB, Abolmaali ND, Assmus B et al. Infarct remodeling after intracoronary progenitor cell treatment in patients with acute myocardial infarction (TOPCARE-AMI): mechanistic insights from serial contrast-enhanced magnetic resonance imaging. Circulation 2003; 108:2212–8.

84. Chen SL, Fang WW, Ye F et al. Effect on left ventricular function of intracoronary transplantation of autologous bone marrow mesenchymal stem cell in patients with acute myocardial infarction. Am J Cardiol 2004; 94:92–5.

85. Fernandez-Aviles F, San Roman JA, Garcia-Frade J et al. Experimental and clinical regenerative capability of human bone marrow cells after myocardial infarction. Circ Res 2004; 95:742–8.

86. Schachinger V, Assmus B, Britten MB et al. Transplantation of progenitor cells and regeneration enhancement in acute myocardial infarction: final one-year results of the TOPCARE-AMI Trial. J Am Coll Cardiol 2004; 44:1690–9.

87. Strauer BE, Brehm M, Zeus T et al. Repair of infarcted myocardium by autologous intracoronary mononuclear bone marrow cell transplantation in humans. Circulation 2002; 106:1913–18.

88. Wollert KC, Meyer GP, Lotz J et al. Intracoronary autologous bone-marrow cell transfer after myocardial infarction: the BOOST randomised controlled clinical trial. Lancet 2004; 364:141–8.

89. Hamano K, Nishida M, Hirata K et al. Local implantation of autologous bone marrow cells for therapeutic

angiogenesis in patients with ischemic heart disease: clinical trial and preliminary results. Jpn Circ J 2001; 65:845–7.

90. Herreros J, Prosper F, Perez A et al. Autologous intramyocardial injection of cultured skeletal muscle-derived stem cells in patients with non-acute myocardial infarction. Eur Heart J 2003; 24:2012–20.

91. Menasche P, Hagege AA, Vilquin JT et al. Autologous skeletal myoblast transplantation for severe postinfarction left ventricular dysfunction. J Am Coll Cardiol 2003; 41:1078–83.

92. Siminiak T, Kalawski R, Fiszer D et al. Autologous skeletal myoblast transplantation for the treatment of postinfarction myocardial injury: phase I clinical study with 12 months of follow-up. Am Heart J 2004; 148:531–7.

93. Stamm C, Kleine HD, Westphal B et al. CABG and bone marrow stem cell transplantation after myocardial infarction. Thorac Cardiovasc Surg 2004; 52:152–8.

94. Stamm C, Westphal B, Kleine HD et al. Autologous bone-marrow stem-cell transplantation for myocardial regeneration. Lancet 2003; 361:45–6.

95. Amado LC, Saliaris AP, Schuleri KH et al. Cardiac repair with intramyocardial injection of allogeneic mesenchymal stem cells after myocardial infarction. Proc Natl Acad Sci USA 2005; 102:11474–9.

96. Sarmento-Leite R, Silva GV, Dohman HF et al. Comparison of left ventricular electromechanical mapping and left ventricular angiography: defining practical standards for analysis of NOGA maps. Tex Heart Inst J 2003; 30:19–26.

97. Perin EC, Silva GV, Sarmento-Leite R et al. Assessing myocardial viability and infarct transmurality with left ventricular electromechanical mapping in patients with stable coronary artery disease: validation by delayed-enhancement magnetic resonance imaging. Circulation 2002; 106:957–61.

98. Fuchs S, Baffour R, Zhou YF et al. Transendocardial delivery of autologous bone marrow enhances collateral perfusion and regional function in pigs with chronic experimental myocardial ischemia. J Am Coll Cardiol 2001; 37:1726–32.

99. Fuchs S, Satler LF, Kornowski R et al. Catheter-based autologous bone marrow myocardial injection in no-option patients with advanced coronary artery disease: a feasibility study. J Am Coll Cardiol 2003; 41:1721–4.

100. Kamihata H, Matsubara H, Nishiue T et al. Improvement of collateral perfusion and regional function by implantation of peripheral blood mononuclear cells into ischemic hibernating myocardium. Arterioscler Thromb Vasc Biol 2002; 22:1804–10.

101. Kawamoto A, Tkebuchava T, Yamaguchi J et al. Intramyocardial transplantation of autologous endothelial progenitor cells for therapeutic neovascularization of myocardial ischemia. Circulation 2003; 107:461–8.

102. Kornowski R, Fuchs S, Tio FO et al. Evaluation of the acute and chronic safety of the biosense injection catheter system in porcine hearts. Catheter Cardiovasc Interv 1999; 48:447–53; discussion 54–5.

103. Kornowski R, Leon MB, Fuchs S et al. Electromagnetic guidance for catheter-based transendocardial injection: a platform for intramyocardial angiogenesis therapy. Results in normal and ischemic porcine models. J Am Coll Cardiol 2000; 35:1031–9.

104. Kraitchman DL, Tatsumi M, Gilson WD et al. Dynamic imaging of allogeneic mesenchymal stem cells trafficking to myocardial infarction. Circulation 2005; 112:1451–61.

105. Hou D, Youssef EA, Brinton TJ et al. Radiolabeled cell distribution after intramyocardial, intracoronary, and interstitial retrograde coronary venous delivery: implications for current clinical trials. Circulation 2005; 112:I150–6.

106. Assmus B, Schachinger V, Teupe C. Transplantation of progenitor cells and regeneration enhancement in acute myocardial infarction (TOPCARE-AMI). Circulation 2002; 106:3009–17.

107. Britten MB, Abolmaali ND, Assmus B et al. Infarct remodeling after intracoronary progenitor cell treatment in patients with acute myocardial infarction (TOPCARE-AMI): mechanistic insights from serial contrast-enhanced magnetic resonance imaging. Circulation 2003; 108:2212–18.

108. Bartunek J, Vanderheyden M, Vandekerckhove B et al. Intracoronary injection of CD133-positive enriched bone marrow progenitor cells promotes cardiac recovery after recent myocardial infarction: feasibility and safety. Circulation 2005; 112:I178–83.

109. Chen SL, Fang WW, Ye F et al. Effect on left ventricular function of intracoronary transplantation of autologous bone marrow mesenchymal stem cell in patients with acute myocardial infarction. Am J Cardiol 2004; 94:92–5.

110. Meyer GP, Wollert KC, Lotz J et al. Eighteen months' follow-up data from the randomized, controlled BOOST (BOne marrOw transfer to enhance ST-elevation infarct regeneration) trial. Circulation 2006; 113:1287–94.

111. Janssens S, Dubois C, Bogaert J et al. Autologous bone marrow-derived stem-cell transfer in patients with ST-segment elevation myocardial infarction: double-blind, randomised controlled trial. Lancet 2006; 367:113–21.

112. Kang HJ, Kim HS, Zhang SY et al. Effects of intracoronary infusion of peripheral blood stem-cells mobilised with granulocyte-colony stimulating factor on left ventricular systolic function and restenosis after coronary stenting in myocardial infarction: the MAGIC cell randomised clinical trial. Lancet 2004; 363:751–6.

113. Hill JM, Syed MA, Arai AE. Outcomes and risks of granulocyte colony-stimulating factor in patients with coronary artery disease. J Am Coll Cardiol 2005; 46:1643–8.

114. Zbinden S, Zbinden R, Meier P, Windecker S, Seiler C. Safety and efficacy of subcutaneous-only granulocyte-macrophage colony-stimulating factor for collateral growth promotion in patients with coronary artery disease. J Am Coll Cardiol 2005; 46:1636–42.

115. Zohlnhofer D, Ott I, Mehilli J et al; REVIVAL-2 Investigators. Stem cell mobilization by granulocyte colony-stimulating factor in patients with acute myocardial infarction: a randomized controlled trial. JAMA 2006; 295:1003–10.

116. Tse HF, Kwong YL, Chan JK et al. Angiogenesis in ischaemic myocardium by intramyocardial autologous bone marrow mononuclear cell implantation. Lancet 2003; 361:47–9.

117. Perin EC, Dohmann HF, Borojevic R et al. Improved exercise capacity and ischemia 6 and 12 months after transendocardial injection of autologous bone marrow mononuclear cells for ischemic cardiomyopathy. Circulation 2004; 110:II213–18.

118. Dohmann HF, Perin EC, Takiya CM et al. Transendocardial autologous bone marrow mononuclear cell injection in ischemic heart failure: postmortem anatomicopathologic and immunohistochemical findings. Circulation 2005; 112:521–6.

119. Kuethe F, Richartz BM, Sayer HG et al. Lack of regeneration of myocardium by autologous intracoronary mononuclear bone marrow cell transplantation in humans with large anterior myocardial infarctions. Int J Cardiol 2004; 97:123–7.

120. Vanderheyden M, Mansour S, Vandekerckhove B et al. Selected intracoronary CD133+ bone marrow cells promote cardiac regeneration after acute myocardial infarction. Circulation 2004; 110 (Suppl III):324–5.

121. Chachques JC, Herreros J, Trainini J et al. Autologous human serum for cell culture avoids the implantation of cardioverter-defibrillators in cellular cardiomyoplasty. Int J Cardiol 2004; 95 (Suppl 1):S29–33.

122. Smits PC, van Geuns RJ, Poldermans D et al. Catheter-based intramyocardial injection of autologous skeletal myoblasts as a primary treatment of ischemic heart failure: clinical experience with six-month follow-up. J Am Coll Cardiol 2003; 42:2063–9.

123. Assmus B, Honold J, Lehmann R et al. Transcoronary transplantation of progenitor cells and recovery of left ventricular function in patients with chronic ischemic heart disease: results of a randomized, controlled trial. Circulation 2004; 110(Suppl III):238.

124. Perin EC, Dohmann HF, Borojevic R et al. Transendocardial, autologous bone marrow cell transplantation for severe, chronic ischemic heart failure. Circulation 2003; 107:2294–302.

125. Wollert KC, Drexler H. Clinical applications of stem cells for the heart. Circ Res 2005; 96(2): 151–63.

SECTION VI

Local therapy

Photodynamic therapy

34

Ron Waksman

INTRODUCTION

Photodynamic therapy (PDT) involves photosensitizing (light-sensitive) drugs, light, and tissue oxygen to treat a wide range of medical conditions primarily in the oncology field. Photosensitizing agents, many of which are porphyrins or chemicals of similar structure, are administered locally or parenterally and selectively absorbed or retained within the tissues targeted for therapy. This differential selectivity or retention promotes selective damage when the target tissue is exposed to light of an appropriate wavelength; the surrounding normal tissue, containing little or no drug, absorbs little light and is thus spared injury.[1,2] PDT clinical research has historically focused primarily and successfully on cancer treatment;[3-6] however, it has shown promise as a breakthrough treatment in ophthalmic, urologic, autoimmune, and cardiovascular diseases. Any disease associated with rapidly growing tissue, including the formation of abnormal blood vessels, can potentially be treated with this technology. For the cardiovascular system, selectivity renders PDT particularly appealing in treating restenosis and atherosclerotic illnesses such as coronary artery disease, in which other catheter-based approaches are relatively non-selective and carry a substantial risk of damage to the normal arterial wall.[7] Recently there have been preclinical and clinical studies targeted to examine the utility of PDT for vascular applications. This chapter summarizes the mechanisms of action, PDT systems, and the results of these preclinical and clinical studies.

MECHANISMS OF ACTION

Photodynamic therapy is a non-thermal, photochemical process that involves the administration of a photosensitizer followed by light activation, which corresponds to the sensitizer's profile. Based on the differential accumulation of a photosensitizer in the target tissue, PDT uses light absorption to produce photochemical reactions through the production of free radical moieties without the generation of heat. These free radical moieties are produced either by the photosensitizer itself or by energy transfer to ambient molecular oxygen, causing cytotoxic effects on tissue and cells. The tissue is subsequently photoilluminated at the wavelength that favors maximal absorption by the photosensitized drug. Light is usually in the form of red light derived from a laser; however, it can originate from collimated or diffuse illuminators as well (e.g. high-power lamps and light-emitting diode [LED] panels).[8] For intravascular application, light is delivered to the treatment site directly with either balloon catheter-based illumination systems[9,10] or optical fibers with cylindrically emitting diffusing fibers.

The photobiologic response (direct, rapid cell apoptosis and delayed necrosis from neovascular damage) becomes maximal within several days.[1,11-13] Throughout this process, the drug serves as a catalyst for energy transfer, whereas light absorption leads to the formation of cytotoxic-reactive oxygen species such as singlet oxygen, a highly reactive, oxidizing agent with very short diffusion distances (≤ 0.1 μm).

Cell death is thus confined to those illuminated areas in which there is an adequate presence of the sensitized drug.[14] PDT demonstrated in numerous trials and in different animal models the potential of eradication of medial smooth muscle proliferation following endothelial denudation in the rat and rabbit model. A strong correlation exists between the depletion of potential neointimal precursor cells at acute time points and inhibition of intimal hyperplasia over the long term after PDT.[15,16] This observation suggests that the main mechanisms are by apoptosis and DNA fragmentation.

PHOTOSENSITIZERS AND PHOTODYNAMIC THERAPY SYSTEMS

While laser balloon systems have been purported to have therapeutic vascular effects,[17,18] the goal of illumination for PDT is to have no intrinsic biologic activity due to thermal effects from the light source. Early PDT agents were activated at wavelengths of 630–670 nm. At those wavelengths, blood and tissue substantially attenuated the delivery of light to target cells.[19] Tissue optics suggested that higher wavelengths were desired for penetration and photosensitizer activation, with a maximal absorption in the range of 700–800 or 950–1100 nm.[20]

Hematoporphyrin derivative was the first of a number of photosensitizers with demonstrable, selective accumulation within atherosclerotic plaque,[21] which displays in-vitro preferential uptake by human plaque. Administration of the photosensitizing agent 5-aminolevulinic acid has been accomplished by topical, systemic, and local internal routes in a variety of malignant and dysplastic conditions.[14,22] However, its administration can elicit hemodynamic changes (depression of systemic and pulmonary pressures and pulmonary resistance) that could limit its ultimate utility in cardiovascular applications.[23]

Biotechnology has developed a new generation of selective photosensitizers and catheter-based technological advances in light delivery, which have allowed the introduction of PDT into the vasculature. Two of these systems are Antrin phototherapy and PhotoPoint PDT.

Antrin phototherapy is a combination of endovascular illumination and motexafin lutetium (MLu, Antrin), an expanded porphyrin (texaphyrin) that accumulates in plaque. Texaphyrins can disrupt the intracellular oxidation–reduction balance and alter bioenergetic processes within target cells. When activated by various energy forms (e.g. ionizing radiation, chemotherapy, or light), they may also be able to reduce or eliminate diseased tissue targets. Interest in the texaphyrin family of molecules as therapeutic agents for cardiovascular disease is based on tissue selectivity, cellular localization, and light activation properties. This phototherapy has been shown to reduce plaque in animal models and generates cytotoxic singlet oxygen that has been shown to induce apoptosis in macrophages and smooth muscle cells.[8] Antrin is excited by red light that penetrates tissue and blood, is synthetic and water soluble, localizes in atheroma, and has a short plasma half-life.[24]

A specialized diode laser, which produces a consistent 730 nm red light, has been developed for use with MLu in the catheterization laboratory. This approximates the size of a standard desk top PC with a touch screen control system that allows easy testing of the light fiber and calibration before endovascular illumination. The optical fiber is 0.018 inch in diameter, can be delivered through angioplasty balloon catheters and standard transfer catheters, and has been delivered to allow illumination at sites where standard interventional technologies can be delivered.[8]

PhotoPoint PDT is a combination endovascular therapy designed to systemically deliver a photosensitizer drug

(MV0611) that is capable of being taken up by macrophages and other plaque inflammatory cells. MV0611, gallium chloride mesoporphyrin dimethyl ester (Miravant Pharmaceuticals Inc., Santa Barbara, CA), was discovered through rational drug screening for use in cardiovascular applications. The interaction between MV0611 and intravascular light generates reactive oxygen species, causing targeted medial smooth muscle cell apoptosis and depletion of neointimal precursor cells in rat carotid and porcine coronary arteries.[7,25,26]

PHOTODYNAMIC THERAPY FOR RESTENOSIS PREVENTION

Smooth muscle cell migration and proliferation are the main mechanisms for restenosis following intervention. PDT has shown its ability to eradicate smooth muscle cells following injury in animal models. Also, PDT is known to increase collagen cross linkage in the extracellular matrix, creating a barrier to smooth muscle cell attachment, proliferation, and migration.[27] Restenosis, the major limitation of the long-term success of percutaneous coronary interventions, is probably best treated with brachytherapy, which uses ionizing radiation. PDT, however, which in contrast to brachytherapy uses non-ionizing radiation, has emerged as another possible strategy.[28]

Using the novel photosensitizer molecule, MV0611, Waksman et al examined the effects of intracoronary PhotoPoint PDT in a porcine stented model of restenosis. MV0611 was given systemically followed by intravascular laser light, which was selectively delivered to porcine coronary arteries using a light diffuser centered with a balloon catheter. Bare metal stents were then implanted at the treatment site in the PDT ($n = 5$) or control ($n = 4$) arteries. Thirty days later, vessels were analyzed by histopathology and histomorphometry and showed that PDT reduced percent area stenosis compared with controls ($39 \pm 3\%$ vs $55 \pm 4\%$, $P < 0.01$). Luminal area was increased with PDT and a maximal re-endothelialization score was observed by gross histology in all PDT and control stents. No cases of aneurysm formation or thrombosis presented. Here, intracoronary PDT inhibited vascular neointima formation without impairing endothelial regeneration in the 30-day porcine model of in-stent restenosis.[29]

Further studies with the use of the same system on a balloon overstretch injury model in the pig demonstrated significant inhibition of neointima formation, with vascular remodeling and absence of fibrin deposition or thrombus formation. Other studies on the use of PDT on arteriovenous grafts demonstrated depletion of neointimal precursor cells in the vessel wall. These observations support the notion that PDT can be selectively targeted to smooth muscle cells and fibroblasts, and can attenuate the restenosis process following intervention.

CLINICAL TRIALS FOR RESTENOSIS PREVENTION

In a phase I trial of PDT with Antrin, Rockson et al demonstrated that photoangioplasty with Antrin is well tolerated and safe in the endovascular treatment of atherosclerosis. This was an open-label, single-dose, escalating drug and light-dose study that was originally not designed to examine clinical efficacy; however, several secondary endpoints suggested a favorable therapeutic effect. Clinical evaluation, serial quantitative angiography, and intravascular ultrasonography were performed on a study population, which consisted of patients with symptomatic claudication and objectively documented peripheral arterial insufficiency ($n = 47$; 51 procedures). The standardized classification of clinical outcomes of the 47 patients at follow-up showed improvement in 29 (62%), no change in 17 (36%), and moderate worsening in 1 (2%).[30]

Bisaccia et al used photopheresis for the first time to prevent restenosis. A total of 78 patients with single-vessel coronary artery disease were enrolled; 41 in the control group and 37 in the photopheresis group. Clinical restenosis occurred in significantly less photopheresis patients than control patients (8% vs 27%; $P = 0.04$), with a relative risk of 0.30 (95% CI, 0.09–1.00).[31]

In an original study including seven patients with symptomatic restenosis of the superficial femoral artery within 6 months of angioplasty (one patient with two lesions in the same artery), Mansfield et al determined that at 48 (mean) months after PDT, no patients developed critical limb ischemia or ulceration and there were no arterial complications.[32] Only one of eight lesions treated by angioplasty with adjuvant PDT developed symptomatic restenosis at the treated site over a 4-year interval. Although the study was uncontrolled and had a small number of patients, the authors reported that adjunctive PDT seems to hold considerable promise as a new strategy to prevent restenosis after angioplasty.[32]

Kereiakes et al, in a phase I peripheral artery disease study, showed that Antrin phototherapy at 28 days follow-up produced a quantitative angiography that demonstrated a 50% improvement in luminal diameter, with no adverse vascular responses, and no deleterious effects on treated arterial segments. Investigators concluded that a potential role for MLu phototherapy in the treatment of atherosclerosis is supported by angiography, intravascular ultrasound, ankle brachial index, and clinical outcome measures. Kereiakes et al also performed a coronary arterial disease phase I study using Antrin phototherapy. At 30 days, death, stroke, emergent coronary artery bypass graft, and stent thrombosis were all 0%, with target vessel revascularization at 1.3%. Quantitative results at 6 months revealed that binary restenosis was 33.8% ($n = 71$), late lumen loss was 1.02 mm (in the stent segment), and there were no clinically significant differences between the stent, balloon injury, illumination, and analysis segments. There was a very low incidence of geographic miss (8%), no evidence of significant edge stenosis, and the maximum well-tolerated drug dose and a range of tolerated light doses were identified.[24]

PHOTODYNAMIC THERAPY AND ATHEROSCLEROTIC PLAQUE

Acute coronary syndromes arising from plaque rupture are one of the leading causes of cardiovascular-related mortality.[33–36] In sudden coronary death and acute myocardial infarction, lesions resembling plaque rupture (thin-cap fibroatheroma, vulnerable plaque) have been reported in other arterial sites remote from the culprit plaque.[37,38] Chronic inflammation caused by macrophage infiltration, foam cell formation, size of necrotic core, fibrous cap, and degradation of collagen are intrinsic to the natural history of symptomatic and asymptomatic atherosclerotic disease. However, these vulnerable, unstable plaques are considered 'rupture-prone' because of the higher (10–15%) incidence of repeat acute myocardial infarction in patients previously presenting with acute myocardial infarction.[36,39] This evidence suggests that the genesis and etiology of plaque disease are complex and diverse. Human plaques vary morphologically in length, volume, and location, and are composed of heterogeneous cellular components. However, plaque inflammation and degree of stenosis,[33,39] independently or collectively, play a critical role in promoting plaque instability. Therefore, a versatile therapeutic paradigm, that can be localized either to a region of the plaque that is rupture-prone or to a length of artery with significant plaque burden, to simultaneously reduce plaque inflammation and acutely promote plaque healing and stabilization without remodeling, is required.

PDT is being utilized as a treatment modality for proliferative neoplasms[40–42] and age-related macular degeneration.[43] Recently, endovascular PDT has emerged as a promising therapy for the treatment of restenosis following injury[32,44] and in short-term studies has shown efficacy in limiting atherosclerotic plaque inflammation in animal models.[7,45]

Atherosclerosis, a vascular inflammatory disease, involves the pathologic development of fatty plaques in a heterogeneous cell matrix.[46] The atherosclerotic plaque target requires radial light delivery, with penetration to a specific target depth, to gain the desired vascular effect. Interest in PDT for treating atherosclerosis has increased in recent years because of the advent of new drugs with fewer side effects and more powerful, less-expensive devices. PDT application can be integrated into traditional vascular procedures with or without stent implantation.[8]

Chen et al explored the effect of altering the intracellular redox state on PDT-induced cell death by depleting intracellular glutathione stores with the use of butathione sulfoximine (BSO), a specific inhibitor of γ-glutamyl cysteine synthetase. Alone, BSO had no effect on macrophage viability; however, treatment of the cells with the antioxidant N-acetyl cysteine (NAC) significantly reduced cell death induced by PDT. In contrast to PDT, macrophage apoptosis induced by exogenous C2-ceramide was largely unaffected by treatment with BSO or NAC. Investigators concluded that, taken, together, these observations suggested that apoptosis initiated by PDT is redox sensitive and that distinct signaling cascades may be operative in PDT compared with certain non-PDT pathways.[47]

Chen et al also examined the mechanism of cell death induced by PDT with MLu by using annexin V staining of macrophages and smooth muscle cells. Here, PDT increased the number of apoptotic macrophages 4.2 ± 1.2-fold (mean ± SD, $n = 4$) and the number of apoptotic smooth muscle cells 4.0 ± 1.9-fold ($n = 3$). The percentage of necrotic cells did not increase from baseline after PDT.[47]

In a vein-graft model, Yamaguchi et al[48] found that PDT could effectively reduce intimal hyperplasia. Inferior vena cava-grafted rats were injected with MLu (10 mg/kg) 4 or 12 weeks after grafting. Light therapy was performed 24 hours after MLu injection. PDT at 4 weeks after surgery significantly reduced the intima–media ratio, whereas treatment at 12 weeks did not reduce the intima–media ratio. Activated macrophages were observed 4 weeks after grafting; however, a significant reduction occurred in these cells by 12 weeks. Thus, it appeared that the mechanism by which PDT works may be related to the targeting of activated macrophages in these models of vascular disease.[8]

Targeting entire plaque cell populations, in their study, Waksman et al also examined the effects of the photosensitizing drug MV0611. New Zealand White rabbits received MV0611 (2 mg/kg intravenously), followed by light delivery using a Miravant catheter-based diode laser (15 J/cm²) 4 hours post-injection. PDT induced a significant reduction (92 ± 6%) in the population of nuclei of all cell types in plaques relative to controls ($P < 0.01$). Results indicated that PDT with MV0611 induces significant depletion of plaque cell populations.[46]

Waksman's findings indicate that optimized PhotoPoint PDT simultaneously causes plaque stabilization while promoting vessel healing and repair. At 7 days post-treatment, PDT caused a decrease in plaque macrophage cell content throughout the entire 2 cm PDT-treated vessel segment.

This effect was sustained at 28 days post-treatment, regardless of elevated cholesterol, an acute stimulus for inflammation. By 28 days post-PDT, plaque matrix was almost entirely repopulated by densely populated α-actin positive smooth muscle cells, predictive of plaque stabilization and healing.[49,50] Cell proliferation analysis by Ki67 showed only 1% of the smooth muscle cells were in G2 or S phases of the cell cycle, suggesting that at 28 days post-PDT, the majority of plaque cells are non-proliferating, with limited potential for plaque growth or restenosis at this time. Moreover, the endothelium, which was previously denuded, appeared intact at 28 days post-PDT. Collectively, the cellular changes induced by MV0611-PDT led to significantly reduced neointimal growth with complete vascular healing.

A pivotal component of PDT in promoting plaque stabilization is sustained macrophage removal. Cytokines released by macrophages promote further atherogenesis[51,52] and continuous macrophage infiltration and degradation over time cause the accumulation of lipoproteins and aggregation of free cholesterol that contribute to necrotic lipid core formation,[53] leading to plaque instability.[54] Moreover, release of macrophage metalloproteinases and other proteolytic enzymes is considered, in part, to weaken the fibrous cap and promote plaque rupture.[55,56] The finding that macrophage reinfiltration was prevented by MV0611-PDT treatment at 28 days is surprising given that plasma cholesterol levels, a potent stimulus for macrophage activation, remained elevated until the time of sacrifice. These data suggest that factors other than cholesterol contribute to plaque macrophage infiltration and that stabilizing effects of PDT on plaque matrix may selectively inhibit macrophage migration. In-vitro collagen gel studies, for the purpose of understanding PDT mechanisms of cell migration in restenosis, have shown that the effects of PDT at the molecular level are complex. On the one hand, PDT may cross-link collagen,[57] providing a temporary barrier to invading smooth muscle cells.[27] Yet, at the same time, PDT has been shown to promote accelerated endothelialization.[58] Whereas it is possible that the reconstituted endothelium may be functionally altered to delay macrophage adhesion and migration, the precise mechanisms of action that prevent the influx of macrophages into the intimal layer are unclear.

A critical component of plaque healing and repair is that following treatment with MV0611-PDT, the intimal matrix was repopulated by smooth muscle cells by 28 days with an absence of macrophages. Although similar changes in plaque cell composition (favorable to plaque stabilization) have been reported in rabbits maintained either on a 16-month hypolipidemic diet or 12 months of chronic pravastatin therapy,[59,60] the rapid change in plaque composition induced by PDT is striking. Moreover, whereas statins have shown long-term clinical efficacy for reducing atherosclerosis in humans,[61] they are unsuitable for acute management of plaques that are rupture prone.[62] In contrast, the acute plaque stabilizing effects of MV0611-PDT may prove to be of therapeutic benefit since a complete change in plaque cell composition was rapidly achieved by 28 days. Temporal studies to understand the source(s) of newly populated smooth muscle cells are ongoing.

At 28 days post-treatment, MV0611-PDT-treated arteries were significantly less occluded than untreated contralateral control arteries. The effects of PDT in reducing neointimal growth while simultaneously stabilizing multiple plaques of varying degrees of stenosis, without inducing effects on remodeling, remain unsurpassed by existing intravascular therapies. Given that these effects were observed throughout the entire 2 cm treated length of artery, these data suggest that PDT may prove effective for the treatment of regional atherosclerosis in humans. Moreover, systemic photosensitizer administration may allow for multiple-vessel segment treatments within a single intervention, and may prove more cost-effective, for example, than the deployment of multiple stents. Also, from a safety perspective, catheter removal post-PDT treatment may avoid some of the pathologic phenomena that are typically associated with stents, such as hypersensitivity, late-stage thrombosis, delayed healing, malapposition, restenosis, adventitial fibrosis, and impaired re-endothelialization.[63,64] Moreover, a well-tolerated biologic response with appropriate vessel healing may compare favorably with drug-eluting stents that could be challenged in their capacity to locally deliver the combination of drugs required to reduce inflammation yet promote healing and repair mechanisms.

REGIONAL PHOTODYNAMIC THERAPY WITH LS11 FOR VULNERABLE PLAQUE

Another interesting approach is with the photoreactive agent LS11, an amphiphilic molecule (water soluble) approved in Japan for use in phase II cancer and retinal trials. It is activated by LED for 5–10 minutes after infusion, and there is no need for laser activation. The molecule has shown its capabilities for selective accumulation in the atherosclerotic plaque; its mechanism of action is by disassociation of the cholesterol ester bond and depletion of cholesterol from the plaque.[65] In addition, there is degradation of macrophages and expulsion of foam cells from the subintima. Another interesting feature of this molecule is its ability to enhance intraplaque neovessel closure while sparing adventitial vasa vasorum. These phenomena were the basis for treatment of macular degeneration with this agent. Therefore, the concept of this molecule is to treat proximal coronary

segments to close intraplaque neovessels, reduce the risk of intraplaque hemorrhage, or recruitment of inflammatory cells (macrophages and T lymphocytes) or erythrocyte-derived cholesterol deposition, matrix depletion, fibrous cap thinning, and promote plaque stabilization and potentially plaque regression.

CONCLUSION

Photodynamic technology for vascular applications holds promise and expectation to play a role for both the prevention of restenosis, as a modality to attenuate atherosclerotic plaques, and perhaps to passivate vulnerable plaques. Nevertheless, the challenge is in finding the optimal dose for both the drug (photosensitizer) and the light (the energy source) to achieve these targets safely without affecting the integrity of the vessel or exposing the patients to additional risk. If proven in clinical trials, we will find catheter-based photodynamic therapy playing a pivotal role in interventional cardiology.

REFERENCES

1. Henderson B, Dougherty T. How does photodynamic therapy work? Photochem Photobiol 1992; 55:145–57.
2. Dougherty T. Photosensitizers: therapy and detection of malignant tumors. Photochem Photobiol 1987; 45: 879–89.
3. Dougherty TJ, Gomer CJ, Henderson BW et al. Photodynamic therapy. J Natl Cancer Inst 1998; 90:889–905.
4. Pass Hi. Photodynamic therapy in oncology: mechanisms and clinical use. J Natl Cancer Inst 1993; 85:443–56.
5. Prewitt TW, Pass HI. Photodynamic therapy for thoracic cancer: biology and applications. Sem Thorac Cardiovasc Surg 1993; 5:229–37.
6. Woodburn KW, Fan Q, Kessel D et al. Phototherapy of cancer and atheromatous plaque with texaphyrins. J Clin Laser Med Surg 1996; 14:343–8.
7. Rockson SG, Lorenz DP, Cheong W-F et al. Photoangioplasty: an emerging clinical cardiovascular role for photodynamic therapy. Circulation 2000; 102:591–6.
8. Chou TM, Woodburn KW, Cheong W-F et al. Photodynamic therapy: applications in atherosclerotic vascular disease with motexafin lutetium. Catheter Cardiov Interv 2002; 57:387–94.

9. Spears JR. Percutaneous laser treatment of atherosclerosis: an overview of emerging techniques. Cardiovasc Intervent Radiol 1986; 9:303–12.

10. Jenkins MP, Buonaccorsi GA, Mansfield R et al. Reduction in the response to coronary and iliac artery injury with photodynamic therapy using 5-aminolaevulinic acid. Cardiovasc Res 2000; 45:478–85.

11. Kessel D, Luo Y, Deng Y et al. The role of subcellular localization in initiation of apoptosis by photodynamic therapy. Photochem Photobiol 1997; 65:422–6.

12. Sluiter W, de Vree W, Pietersma A et al. Prevention of late lumen loss after coronary angioplasty by photodynamic therapy: role of activated neutrophils. Mol Cell Biochem 1996; 157:233–8.

13. Reed M, Miller F, Wieman T et al. The effect of photodynamic therapy on the microcirculation. J Surg Res 1988; 45:452–9.

14. Nyamekye I, Anglin S, McEwan J et al. Photodynamic therapy of normal and balloon-injured rat carotid arteries using 5-amino-levulinic acid. Circulation 1995; 91:417–25.

15. Grove RI, Leitch I, Rychnovsky S et al. Current status of photodynamic therapy for the prevention of restenosis. In: Waksman, R, ed. Vascular Brachytherapy, 3rd edn. New York: Futura 2002:339–45.

16. Barton JM, Nielsen HV, Rychnovsky S et al. PhotoPoint™ PDT inhibits intimal hyperplasia in arteriovenous grafts. Presented at CRT 2003, January 26–29. Washington, DC.

17. Spears JR, James LM, Leonard BM et al. Plaque-media rewelding with reversible tissue optical property changes during receptive cw Nd:YAG laser exposure. Lasers Surg Med 1988; 8:477–85.

18. Cheong WF, Spears JR, Welch AJ. Laser balloon angioplasty. Crit Rev Biomed Eng 1991; 19:113–46.

19. Vincent GM, Fox J, Charlton G et al. Presence of blood significantly decreases transmission of 630 nm laser light. Lasers Surg Med 1991; 11:399–403.

20. Doiron DR, Keller GS. Porphyrin photodynamic therapy: principles and clinical applications. Curr Prob Dermatol 1986; 15:85–93.

21. Spears J, Serur J, Shropshire D et al. Fluorescence of experimental atheromatous plaques with hematoporphyrin derivative. J Clin Invest 1983; 71:395–9.

22. Kennedy J, Marcus S, Pottier R. Photodynamic therapy (PDT) and photodiagnosis (PD) using endogenous photosensitization induced by 5-aminolevulinic acid (ALA): mechanisms and clinical results. J Clin Laser Med Surg 1996; 14:289–304.

23. Herman M, Webber J, Fromm D et al. Hemodynamic effects of 5-aminolevulinic acid in humans. J Photochem Photobiol B 1998; 43:61–5.

24. Kereiakes DJ. Photodynamic therapy: clinical. Presented at CRT 2003, January 26–29. Washington, DC.

25. Wilson A, Leitch IM, Diaz E et al. Endovascular photodynamic therapy with the new photosenitizer MV0611 reduces neo-intimal cell content in a rodent arterial injury model. Circulation 2001; 104(Suppl II): 663.

26. Yazdi H, Kim H-S, Seabron R et al. Cellular effects of intracoronary photodynamic therapy with the new photosensitizer MV0611 in normal and balloon-injured porcine coronary arteries. Acute and long term effects. Circulation 2001;104 (Suppl II): 388.

27. Overhaus M, Heckenkamp J, Kossodo S et al. Photodynamic therapy generates a matrix barrier to invasive vascular cell migration. Circ Res 2000; 86:334–40.

28. Mansfield R, Bown S, McEwan J. Photodynamic therapy: shedding light on restenosis. Heart 2001; 86:612–18.

29. Waksman R, Leitch I, Roessler J et al. Intracoronary photodynamic therapy reduces neointimal growth without suppressing re-endothelialisation in a porcine model. Heart 2006; 92:1138–44.

30. Rockson SG, Kramer P, Razavi M et al. Photoangioplasty for human peripheral atherosclerosis: results of a phase I trial of photodynamic therapy with motexafin lutetium (Antrin). Circulation 2000; 102:2322–4.

31. Bisaccia E, Palangio M, Gonzalez J et al. Photopheresis. Therapeutic potential in preventing restenosis after percutaneous transluminal coronary angioplasty. Am J Cardiovasc Drugs 2003; 3:43–51.

32. Mansfield RJR, Jenkins MP, Pai ML et al. Long-term safety and efficacy of superficial femoral artery angioplasty with adjuvant photodynamic therapy to prevent restenosis. B J Surg 2002; 89:1538–9.

33. Farb A, Burke AP, Tang AL et al. Coronary plaque erosion without rupture into a lipid core: a frequent cause of coronary thrombosis in sudden coronary death. Circulation 1996; 93:1354–63.

34. Virmani R, Kolodgie F, Burke A et al. Lessons from sudden coronary death: a comprehensive morphological classification scheme for atherosclerotic lesions. Arterioscler Thromb Vasc Biol 2000; 20:1262–75.

35. Kolodgie F, Burke A, Farb A et al. The thin-cap fibroatheroma: a type of vulnerable plaque: the major precursor lesion to acute coronary syndromes. Curr Opin Cardiol 2001; 16:285–92.

36. Naghavi M, Libby P, Falk E et al. From vulnerable plaque to vulnerable patient: a call for new definitions and risk assessment strategies: part I. Circulation 2003; 108:1664–72.

37. Rioufol G, Finet G, Ginon I et al. Multiple atherosclerotic plaque rupture in acute coronary syndrome. Circulation 2002; 106:804–8.

38. Haft J. Multiple atherosclerotic rupture in acute coronary syndrome. Circulation 2003; 107:e65–6.

39. Burke A, Farb A, Malcom G et al. Coronary risk factors and plaque morphology in men with coronary disease who died suddenly. N Engl J Med 1997; 336:1276–82.

40. Gomer C, Rucker N, Ferrario A, Wong S. Properties and applications of photodynamic therapy. Radiat Res 1989; 120:1–18.

41. Henderson B, Waldow S, Mang T et al. Tumor destruction and kinetics of tumor cell death in two experimental mouse tumors following photodynamic therapy. Cancer Res 1985; 45:572–6.

42. Prout GJ, Lin C, Benson RJ et al. Photodynamic therapy with hematoporphyrin derivative in the treatment of superficial transitional-cell carcinoma of the bladder. N Engl J Med 1987; 317:1251–5.

43. Thomas E, Snyder W. Photodynamic therapy with tin ethylpurpurin. In: Gragoudas ES, Miller JW, Zografos L, eds. Photodynamic Therapy for Ocular Diseases: Lippincott, Williams & Williams; 2004:231–46.

44. Kim H-S, Waksman R, Yazdi HA et al. Intracoronary photodynamic therapy with the new photosensitizer MV0611 inhibits neointimal formation in porcine coronary arteries after balloon injury. Circulation 2001; 104:624.

45. Hayase M, Woodburn KW, Perlroth J et al. Photoangioplasty with local motexafin lutetium delivery reduces macrophages in a rabbit post-balloon injury model. Cardiovasc Res 2001; 49:449–55.

46. Waksman R, Yazdi H, Seabron R et al. Cellular effects of photodynamic therapy on rabbit atherosclerotic plaques. Presented at Transcatheter Cardiovascular Therapeutics (TCT), 2002. [abstract]

47. Chen Z, Woodburn KW, Shi C et al. Photodynamic therapy with motexafin lutetium induces redox-sensitive apoptosis of vascular cells. Arterioscler Thromb Vasc Biol 2001; 21:759–64.

48. Yamaguchi A, Woodburn KW, Hayase M, Robbins RC. Reduction of vein graft disease using photodynamic therapy with texafin lutetium in a rodent isograft model. Circulation 2000; 102:III275–80.

49. Kockx M, De Meyer G, Buyssens N et al. Cell composition, replication, and apoptosis in atherosclerotic plaques after 6 months of cholesterol withdrawal. Circ Res 1998; 83:378–87.

50. Burke A, Kolodgie F, Farb A et al. Healed plaque ruptures and sudden coronary death: evidence that subclinical rupture has a role in plaque progression. Circulation 2001; 103:934–40.

51. Galis Z, Sukhova G, Lark M et al. Increased expression of matrix metalloproteinases and matrix degrading activity in vulnerable regions of human atherosclerotic plaques. J Clin Invest 1994; 94:2493–503.

52. Aikawa M, Rabkin E, Okada Y et al. Lipid lowering by diet reduces matrix metalloproteinase activity and increases collagen content of rabbit atheroma. Circulation 1998; 97:2433–44.

53. Guyton J, Klemp K. Development of the lipid-rich core in human atherosclerosis. Arterioscler Thromb Vasc Biol 1996; 16:4–11.

54. Bloch K. Cholesterol: evolution of structure and function. In: Vance DE, Vance J, eds. Biochemistry of Lipids, Lipoproteins and Membranes. Amsterdam, Netherlands: Elsevier; 1991:363–81.

55. Galis Z, Khatri J. Matrix metalloproteinases in vascular remodeling and atherogenesis: the good, the bad, and the ugly. Circ Res 2002; 90:251–62.

56. Libby P, Lee R. Matrix matters. Circulation 2000; 102:1874–84.

57. Waterman P, Overhaus M, Heckencamp J et al. Mechanisms of reduced vascular cell migration after photodynamic therapy. Photochem Photobiol 2001; 75:46–50.

58. Adili F, Scholz T, Hille M et al. Photodynamic therapy mediated induction of accelerated re-endothelialisation following injury to the arterial wall: implications for the prevention of postinterventional restenosis. Eur J Vasc Endovasc Surg 2002; 24:166–75.

59. Aikawa M, Rabkin E, Voglic S et al. Lipid lowering promotes accumulation of mature smooth muscle cells expressing smooth muscle myosin heavy chain isoforms in rabbit atheroma. Circ Res 1998; 83:1015–26.

60. Fukumoto Y, Libby P, Rabkin E et al. Statins alter smooth muscle cell accumulation and collagen content in established atheroma of Watanabe heritable hyperlipidemic rabbits. Circulation 2001; 103:993–9.

61. Maron DJ, Fazio S, Linton MF. Current perspectives on statins. Circulation 2000; 101:207–13.

62. Ambrose J, Martinez E. A new paradigm for plaque stabilization. Circulation 2002; 105:2000–4.

63. Farb A, Burke AP, Kolodgie FD et al. Pathological mechanisms of fatal late coronary stent thrombosis in humans. Circulation 2003; 108:1701–6.

64. Virmani R, Guagliumi G, Farb A et al. Localized hypersensitivity and late coronary thrombosis secondary to a siroliumus-eluting stent: should we be cautious? Circulation 2004; 109:701–5.

65. Hayashi J, Saito T, Aizawa K. Change in chemical composition of lipids accumulated in atheromas of rabbits following photodynamic therapy. Lasers Surg Med 1997; 21:287–93.

Stenting the vulnerable plaque   35

Probal Roy and Ron Waksman

INTRODUCTION

Coronary artery disease (CAD) consistently remains the leading cause of death in the USA.[1] Despite great advances in medical and revascularization therapies, CAD continues to exert enormous morbidity, mortality, and cost. Erosion or rupture of the vulnerable plaque is pivotal in the pathophysiology of acute coronary syndromes.[2] Insights into the pathology and detection of the vulnerable plaque have been described elsewhere.[3] Currently, medical therapy is the mainstay of treatment for the vulnerable plaque. The heavy burden of CAD that persists despite available therapy highlights the need for an alternative strategy, perhaps local or regional therapy. Among the local therapies proposed are balloon angioplasty, stents, local delivery of drugs, cryoplasty, sonotherapy, radiation, and photodynamic therapy. The focus of this chapter is the potential role of stents in vulnerable plaque management, including the rationale for stenting non-obstructive lesions, mechanical plaque stabilization, the benefits and risks of stenting, desirable stent designs, and proposed clinical trials to assess the utility of such therapy.

RATIONALE FOR STENTING THE VULNERABLE PLAQUE

Acute coronary syndromes arise from plaque erosion or rupture, which results in thrombus formation and acute vessel occlusion.[4] Atherosclerotic plaques that were subjected to mechanical intervention usually scarred, some restenosed, but rarely ruptured. Falk et al established that the majority of plaque ruptures resulting in myocardial infarction arise from lesions that were non-obstructive prior to the event[5] (Figure 35.1). While obstructive lesions (diameter stenosis >70%) mainly undergo revascularization for symptom relief, non-obstructive lesions are usually left untreated. These lesions have the potential to progress and become obstructive or rupture and result in myocardial infarction or unstable angina. The question is whether prophylactic treatment of these non-obstructive lesions will reduce late progression or plaque rupture. The logic behind such an approach is that the segment that was subjected to mechanical intervention will heal with scar formation and this scar will

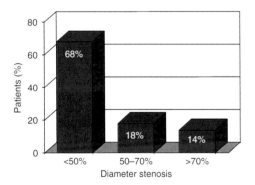

Figure 35.1 Severity of coronary artery stenosis before acute myocardial infarction. This graph illustrates that the majority of acute myocardial infarcts arise from plaque rupture of non-obstructive lesions. (Reproduced from Falk et al,[5] with permission.)

guard the segment from rupture or progression.[6] To reduce morbidity, mortality, and costs associated with acute coronary syndromes, it becomes apparent that greater attention needs to be given to the prevention of non-obstructive plaque rupture. The challenge is to understand which lesions are at risk and which should be treated or left alone.

Increasingly, acute coronary syndromes are being recognized as the result of a systemic inflammatory response diffusely affecting the entire coronary tree.[7–9] Aspirin, β-blockers, angiotensin-converting enzyme inhibitors, and HMG-CoA (3-hydroxy-3-methylglutaryl coenzyme A) reductase inhibitors are the mainstays of therapy for CAD; they all have biologic plausibility and proven clinical efficacy.[10] Systemic therapies for the prevention of vulnerable plaque are partially effective but not bulletproof. The event rate in the PROVE IT-TIMI 22 (Pravastatin or Atorvastatin Evaluation and Infection Therapy – Thrombolysis in Myocardial Infarction 22) trial of 22.4% at 24 months, despite maximal medical therapy with high-dose atorvastatin and antiplatelet therapy, highlights the need for a complementary strategy.[11]

Although the concept of systemic inflammation is attractive, a few issues need to be raised. Inherent to the natural history of the vulnerable plaque is its unpredictable nature. The majority of plaque ruptures heal spontaneously and are clinically inconsequential.[6] Generally, the vast majority of acute coronary syndromes are attributed to a solitary 'culprit' plaque rupture despite the presence of other ruptured plaques.

The detection of the vulnerable plaque and vulnerable patient remains challenging but crucial when considering focal therapy. Invasive detection of potential vulnerable plaque is challenging and has not been proven with the non-invasive or invasive imaging modalities available. Another approach, therefore, is

to detect regions of risk for myocardial infarction and to apply the therapy primarily to plaques at these regions. Wang et al reported the spatial distribution of acute myocardial infarction in the coronary tree and suggested that this may guide physicians as to which segments of the coronary tree focal therapy should be applied regardless of the imaging of these plaques. The investigators tested the hypothesis that thrombotic occlusion in acute myocardial infarction occurs in a non-uniform distribution throughout the coronary tree. The sites of occlusion in 208 consecutive patients presenting with acute myocardial infarction were mapped. Thrombotic occlusions were clustered to the proximal third of the major epicardial vessels. For each 10 mm increment from the ostium, the probability of occlusion decreased by 13–30%. Ninety percent of left anterior descending artery occlusions were located in the first 40 mm of the vessel (Figure 35.2). The authors concluded that the non-uniform distribution of thrombotic occlusion identifies high-risk zones which could be targeted for detection and therapeutic purposes.[12] The prevention of plaque rupture in the proximal segments of the epicardial vessels is expected to be associated with prognostic benefit, given the substantial amount of myocardium subtended.

The rationale for stenting the vulnerable plaque is primarily to seal potential sites of plaque rupture and hence prevent sudden death and non-fatal myocardial infarction. We anticipate that this will result in significant healthcare cost savings in terms of hospital admissions, medications, revascularization procedures, devices, and rehabilitation. The prevalence of the disease, failure of medical therapy, the focal nature of clinically significant plaque rupture, and identification of high-risk segments are sound rationale to pursue a focal management strategy for the vulnerable plaque. With the introduction of drug-eluting stents (DES), which have demonstrated a

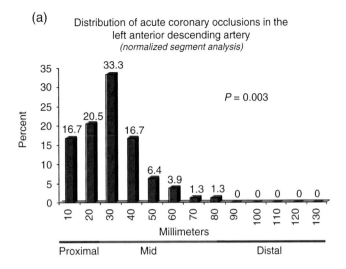

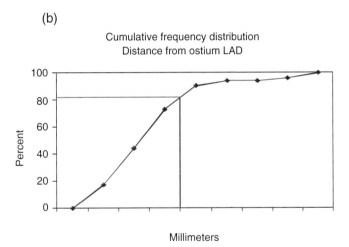

Figure 35.2 (a) Spatial distribution of thrombotic occlusion in patients presenting with acute myocardial infarction. (b) The non-uniform distribution to the proximal left anterior descending artery (LAD) was reproduced in the other epicardial vessels. (Reproduced from Wang et al,[12] with permission.)

low risk of restenosis and thrombosis, prophylactic stenting of high-risk segments to prevent plaque rupture is a provocative strategy and should be further explored.

MECHANICAL STABILIZATION OF VULNERABLE PLAQUE

Over a decade ago, the concept of mechanical plaque sealing by coronary angioplasty was introduced by Meier et al.[6]

Balloon dilatation induces the splitting of plaque, which subsequently results in tissue reaction. The initially observed smooth muscle-rich intima transforms into a collagen-rich layer and thus results in mechanical stabilization.[13] These architectural changes induced by balloon angioplasty, which result in scarring of the treated segment, prevent the segment from supporting atherosclerotic plaque in the future. The inherent risks of acute closure and restenosis with balloon dilatation made widespread adoption of this approach unattractive for the prevention of the vulnerable plaque.

Implantation of a bare metal stent (BMS) in a diseased segment results in mechanical compression of the soft tissue matrix, replacement of the previous thin cap with a thick fibrous cap, minimization of the lipid core, and replacement of the thin plaque shoulders by neointima[14] (Figure 35.3). These changes again result in the segment being unable to give rise to atherosclerotic plaque and subsequent plaque rupture. The potential benefit of preventing a plaque rupture against the risk of restenosis made translating this strategy into clinical practice problematic. The emergence of the DES, which has substantially reduced restenosis rates, may make the stenting of non-obstructive vulnerable plaque justifiable. The benefits will need to be considered in light of the small, but not insignificant, risk of late stent thrombosis in the DES era.

EXPERIENCE IN STENTING NON-OBSTRUCTIVE PLAQUE

Experience in stenting non-obstructive lesions is not extensive, with very limited published data. Mercado et al published outcomes of patients with mild coronary stenoses (diameter stenosis <50%) with either balloon angioplasty or stenting. They reported a combined 1-year mortality and non-fatal myocardial infarction rate of 4.8% and 3.1% in the balloon angioplasty and stenting groups, respectively. These rates did not differ significantly from those for obstructive lesions. Nevertheless, the high revascularization rate prohibited the authors from advocating the use of balloon angioplasty or BMS for the treatment of non-obstructive lesions.[15]

As mentioned earlier, the substantial reduction in restenosis rates with the emergence of the DES has resulted in renewed interest in stenting vulnerable plaques. Hoye et al published a small series of 20 patients (23 lesions) who were treated with sirolimus-eluting stents for non-obstructive lesions. They reported survival free from major adverse events of 95% beyond 1 year. The impressive finding was that no patient required revascularization.[16] Although the number of subjects in this study was small, it supported the notion that DES were safe in the treatment of vulnerable plaques and reduced restenosis rates, which meant this was a feasible strategy.

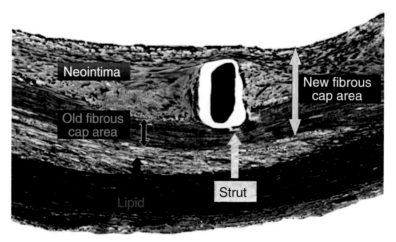

Figure 35.3 Histologic changes seen with mechanical stabilization of atherosclerotic plaque with a bare metal stent. (Reproduced from Echiverri and Moreno,[14] with permission.)

A pooled analysis of four randomized clinical trials (SIRIUS, TAXUS IV, FUTURE I, and FUTURE II) published recently has provided further insight into the use of DES in non-obstructive lesions. Of a total of 2478 randomized patients, 167 with intermediate lesions were inadvertently treated with either DES or BMS. Major adverse cardiac events at 1 year were 5.6% vs 25.4% (P = 0.0003) for DES and BMS, respectively, with this difference driven by target vessel revascularization rates (3.4% vs 20.3%, P = 0.0004). The finding that no patient developed stent thrombosis was encouraging. The authors concluded that DES are safe in the treatment of intermediate lesions and that their efficacy may allow a shift toward an invasive strategy.[17]

The current data relate to the treatment of non-obstructive lesions. It must be noted that none of the above investigations attempted to further delineate these plaques as vulnerable or not. Nevertheless, DES use is both safe and efficacious in the treatment of non-obstructive plaque. Certain issues arise from the potential use of DES for the sealing of vulnerable plaque. First, the risk of myocardial infarction for a given patient must be assessed and weighed against the risks of stent thrombosis and restenosis. The risk for myocardial infarction is variable and difficult to predict, but must be significantly greater than the potential risks for DES placement for this to be a justifiable strategy. From the CASS registry, the risk of myocardial infarction for a stenosis <50% over a 3-year period was estimated to be 2%. The corresponding figure was 7% for a 50–70% severe stenosis.[18] The risk of clinical restenosis at 12 months from the large DES randomized trials is <5%.[19,20] Stent thrombosis, a potentially fatal condition, has been found to occur in <1% of cases at long-term follow-up.[21] It is the balance of these risks that will drive the argument to stent non-obstructive vulnerable plaque or not.

A strategy of targeting vulnerable plaque in the proximal epicardial vessel may result in a long stented segment that carries higher rates of stent thrombosis and restenosis.[21,22] Stenting long segments may also result in the loss of side branches and higher rates of post-procedural creatinine kinase (CK) elevation.[23] Another issue arising from DES use for the treatment of non-obstructive lesions is cost. Bosch et al reported a cost-effective analysis of a hypothetical approach of using DES for the treatment of vulnerable plaque. In their analysis they suggest that this strategy is more cost-effective than current practice.[24] The results of this hypothetical model could be verified by a cost-effective analysis of a prospective randomized trial.

PROPOSED CLINICAL TRIALS

Currently there are no randomized clinical trials supporting the use of DES for the treatment of the vulnerable non-obstructive plaque. The *P*rospective *R*andomized *E*valuation of Sirolimus-Eluting *V*elocity Stent in Patients with *A*cute Coronary Syndrome and *I*ntermediate *L*esions (PREVAIL) study was designed to address the safety and efficacy of the sirolimus-eluting stent in lesions of intermediate significance after a 'culprit' lesion has been treated successfully. Here, the high-risk patient is randomized to either medical therapy or percutaneous coronary intervention to an intermediate lesion using a sirolimus-eluting stent. Outcomes of death, myocardial infarction, target vessel revascularization, and lesion progression will be assessed at 12 months[25] (Figure 35.4). This is the first planned, randomized trial seeking to establish the benefit of mechanical stabilization of the non-obstructive vulnerable plaque. The results of this trial and others have the potential to initiate a paradigm shift in vulnerable plaque management.

Figure 35.4   Prospective Randomized Evaluation of Sirolimus-Eluting Velocity Stent in Patients with Acute Coronary Syndrome and Intermediate Lesions (PREVAIL) study patient algorithm. ACS, acute coronary syndromes; TRS, timi risk score; CRP, C-reactive protein; PCI, percutaneous coronary intervention; DES, drug-eluting stents; MI, myocardial infarction; TVR, target vessel revascularization; (Reproduced with permission from Cardiovascular Institute Philadelphia, Philadelphia, PA, Cardiovascular Research Foundation, New York.[25])

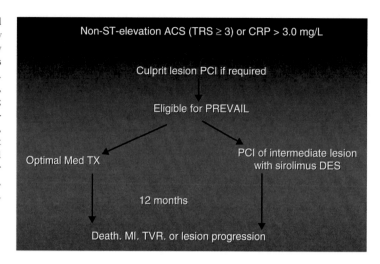

FEATURES OF DEDICATED STENTS FOR THE PREVENTION OR MANAGEMENT OF VULNERABLE PLAQUE

Of all the modalities under consideration for vulnerable plaque management, the DES is the most likely to gain widespread clinical acceptance. Despite the availability of this technology, evidence from randomized clinical trials is required to demonstrate that the risk of DES placement is outweighed by the potential risk of plaque rupture and infarction. When considering alternative stent designs, it is necessary to review the desirable characteristics of the stent for plaque passivation. The major consideration regarding stent design for the treatment of vulnerable plaques is minimization of vessel wall injury and, hence, the reduction of potential restenosis or stent thrombosis risk. Desirable technical features of the stent for vulnerable plaque passivation are as follows:

- hybrid multimodular stent design
- highly conformable stent
- relatively low radial force
- wall thickness <100 μm
- strut thickness <75 μm
- strut alignment parallel to blood flow
- strut with blunted edges

- balanced strut density
- bio-inert material composition
- passive coating.

The permanent nature of metallic stents carries with it disadvantages. Late stent thrombosis is a major concern in the DES era and the prevention of this catastrophic event requires prolonged antiplatelet therapy. Permanent metallic stents incite both neointimal proliferation and chronic inflammation, which ultimately lead to restenosis. The bioabsorbable stent potentially can eliminate these long-term issues.[26] Although initial experiences in human coronary arteries is promising, we await results of randomized clinical trials.[27] The bioabsorbable stent may be particularly advantageous in vulnerable plaque management where it is imperative to reduce risks of stent insertion to make it a viable strategy. The delivery of drugs (sirolimus) and genes on the bioabsorbable stent platform are also being investigated.[26]

CONCLUSIONS

Stenting the non-obstructive vulnerable plaque remains a contentious issue in interventional cardiology. Although the implantation of DES has been shown to be safe in intermediate lesions, there is currently no evidence that stenting vulnerable plaque to prevent myocardial infarction carries prognostic benefit. Nevertheless, the rationale to pursue this strategy is strong. The results of clinical trials and the emergence of improved therapeutic options are required to allow physicians to adopt a stenting strategy for vulnerable plaque which may then complement current systemic treatments.

REFERENCES

1. National Health and Nutrition Examination Survey III, NHANES III, 1988–94 http://www.cdc.gov/nchs/about/major/nhances/nh3data.htm.
2. Corti R, Farkouh ME, Badimon JJ. The vulnerable plaque and acute coronary syndromes. Am J Med 2002; 113:668–80.
3. Muller JE, Tawakol A, Kathiresan S, Narula J. New opportunities for identification and reduction of coronary risk: treatment of vulnerable patients, arteries, and plaques. J Am Coll Cardiol 2006; 47(8 Suppl):C2–C6.
4. Fuster V, Lewis A. Connor Memorial Lecture: mechanisms leading to myocardial infarction: insights from studies of vascular biology. Circulation 1994; 90:2126–46.
5. Falk E, Shah PK, Fuster V. Coronary plaque disruption. Circulation 1995; 92:657–71.
6. Meier B, Ramamurthy S. Plaque sealing by coronary angioplasty. Cathet Cardiovasc Diagn 1995; 36:295–2977.
7. Goldstein JA, Demetriou D, Grines CL et al. Multiple complex coronary plaques in patients with acute myocardial infarction. N Engl J Med 2000; 343:915–22.
8. Buffon A, Biasucci LM, Liuzzo G et al. Widespread coronary inflammation in unstable angina. N Engl J Med 2002; 347:5–12.
9. Rioufol G, Finet G, Ginon I et al. Multiple atherosclerotic plaque rupture in acute coronary syndrome: a three-vessel intravascular ultrasound study. Circulation 2002; 106:804–8.
10. Ambrose JA, D'Agate DJ. Classification of systemic therapies for potential stabilization of the vulnerable plaque to prevent acute myocardial infarction. Am J Cardiol 2005; 5:379–82.
11. Scirica BM, Morrow DA, Cannon CP et al; PROVE IT-TIMI 22 Investigators. Intensive statin therapy and the risk of hospitalization for heart failure after an acute coronary syndrome in the PROVE IT-TIMI 22 study. J Am Coll Cardiol 2006; 47:2326–31.
12. Wang JC, Normand SL, Mauri L, Kuntz RE. Coronary artery spatial distribution of acute myocardial infarction occlusions. Circulation 2004; 110:278–84.
13. Inoue K, Nakamura N, Kako T et al. Serial changes of coronary arteries after percutaneous transluminal coronary angioplasty: histopathological and immunohistochemical study. Am J Cardiol 1994; 24:279–91.
14. Echiverri D, Moreno P. Mechanical stabilization of vulnerable plaque with BMS. ACC 2003; 52nd Annual Scientific Session.
15. Mercado N, Maier W, Boersma E et al. Clinical and angiographic outcome of patients with mild coronary lesions treated with balloon angioplasty or coronary stenting. Implications for mechanical plaque sealing. Eur Heart J 2003; 24:541–51.
16. Hoye A, Lemos PA, Arampatzis CA et al. Effectiveness of sirolimus-eluting stent implantation for coronary narrowings <50% in diameter. Am J Cardiol 2004; 94:112–14.
17. Moses JW, Stone GW, Nikolsky E et al. Drug-eluting stents in the treatment of intermediate lesions: pooled analysis from four randomized trials. J Am Coll Cardiol 2006; 47:2164–71.
18. Ellis S, Alderman E, Cain K et al. Prediction of risk of anterior myocardial infarction by lesion severity and measurement method of stenoses in the left anterior descending coronary distribution: a CASS Registry Study. J Am Coll Cardiol 1988; 11:908–16.
19. Holmes DR Jr, Leon MB, Moses JW et al. Analysis of 1-year clinical outcomes in the SIRIUS trial: a randomized trial of a sirolimus-eluting stent versus a standard stent in patients at high risk for coronary restenosis. Circulation 2004; 109:634–40.
20. Stone GW, Ellis SG, Cox DA et al; TAXUS-IV Investigators. One-year clinical results with the slow-release, polymer-based, paclitaxel-eluting TAXUS stent: the TAXUS-IV trial. Circulation 2004; 109:1942–7.
21. Park DW, Park SW, Park KH et al. Frequency of and risk factors for stent thrombosis after drug-eluting stent implantation during long-term follow up. Am J Cardiol 2006; 98:352–6.
22. Moses JW, Leon MB, Popma JJ et al. SIRIUS Investigators. Sirolimus-eluting stents versus standard stents in patients with stenosis in a native coronary artery. N Engl J Med 2003; 349:1315–23.
23. Chu WW, Kuchulakanti PK, Torguson R et al. Impact of overlapping drug-eluting stents in patients undergoing percutaneous coronary intervention. Catheter Cardiovasc Interv 2006; 67:595–9.
24. Bosch JL, Beinfeld MT, Muller JE, Brady T, Gazelle GS. A cost-effectiveness analysis of a hypothetical catheter-based strategy for the detection and treatment of vulnerable coronary plaques with drug-eluting stents. J Interv Cardiol 2005; 18:339–49.
25. Cardiovascular Institute Philadelphia, Philadelphia, PA, Cardiovascular Research Foundation, New York. Prospective Randomized Evaluation of Sirolimus-Eluting Velocity Stent in Patients with Acute Coronary Syndrome and Intermediate Lesions. CRT 2005 (unpublished).
26. Waksman R. Vulnerable plaque intervention. Local and regional therapy. CRT 2006 (unpublished).
27. Tamai H, Igaki K, Kyo E et al. Initial and 6-month results of biodegradable poly-l-lactic acid coronary stents in humans. Circulation 2000; 102:399–404.

SECTION VII

Clinical management

PREVAIL* study

Heidar Arjomand, Roxana Mehran, George Dangas, and Sheldon Goldberg

36

INTRODUCTION

Atherosclerotic coronary artery disease (CAD) is the leading cause of morbidity and mortality in industrialized countries.[1] Clinical manifestations of CAD include sudden cardiac death and acute coronary syndromes (ACS) of unstable angina, non-ST-elevation myocardial infarction (MI), and ST-elevation MI. Most acute ischemic events are caused by rupture or superficial erosion of coronary plaques at sites with only mild to moderate luminal stenosis.[2] Coronary plaques which are prone to rupture, the so-called *vulnerable plaques*, tend to have a thin fibrous cap and a large lipid core. Recent data indicate that patients with ACS manifest multiple ruptured/vulnerable plaques in addition to the culprit lesion causing the index ischemic event.[3–6] These additional ruptured plaques may be associated with a poor long-term prognosis. The significance of this issue is evidenced by the fact that patients with ACS account for approximately 1.4 million hospitalizations each year in the USA, and more than 2 million admissions worldwide.[1]

CLINICAL EVENTS RELATED TO THE NON-TARGET LESION

Recent landmark randomized trials demonstrated that drug-eluting stents significantly reduce the rates of restenosis and target lesion revascularization (TLR). However, the reduction of late events unrelated to restenosis remains a clear target for future study and intervention.[7–9]

In a long-term (7–11 years) follow-up study of 405 patients undergoing coronary stenting, Kimura et al demonstrated that stented lesions were stable, and late cardiac events occurred predominantly due to progressive disease at non-target sites.[10]

Based on the obligatory, FDA (Food and Drug Administration)-required, long-term clinical follow-up, Cutlip et al evaluated 5-year outcome of 1228 patients treated with second-generation coronary stents. They showed that during the first year after stent implantation, the clinical events (mainly MI and repeat TLR) were related to the index procedure resulting from restenosis.[11] However, during the following 4 years, events related to the target lesions occurred less frequently, and non-target lesion events dominated (Figure 36.1). Notably, the presence of diabetes and multivessel disease were strong predictors of events related to both restenotic and de-novo lesions. Of particular interest, >50% of patients with restenosis also sustained a clinical event unrelated to the restenotic lesion.[11]

CORONARY PLAQUE MORPHOLOGY: COMPLEX VERSUS SIMPLE PLAQUE; RUPTURED VERSUS STABLE

Coronary lesions/plaques have been classified as simple or complex based on their angiographic features.[12,13] A significant

---

*Prospective *R*andomized *E*valuation of Sirolimus-Eluting *V*elocity Stent in Patients with *A*cute Coronary Syndrome and *I*ntermediate *L*esions.

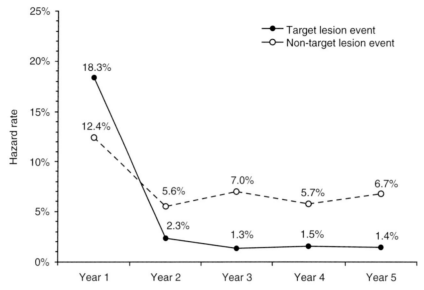

Figure 36.1 Hazard rates per year for target lesion events – death, myocardial infarction (MI), acute coronary syndromes (ACS), congestive heart failure (CHF) or target lesion revascularization clearly attributed to target lesion – and non-target lesion events – death, MI, ACS, CHF, or repeat revascularization not clearly attributed to the target lesion – derived from life table survival analysis. (Reproduced with permission from Cutlip et al.[11])

number of ACS patients have multiple complex coronary plaques that are associated with adverse clinical outcomes. In an angiographic study by Goldstein et al, 40% of patients with acute MI had multiple complex plaques.[12] As compared to patients with a single complex plaque, patients with multiple complex coronary plaques more commonly required urgent coronary bypass surgery (27% vs 5.2%, $P < 0.001$). These patients also had worse 1-year outcomes, with an increased incidence of recurrent ACS and repeat percutaneous or surgical revascularization (Figure 36.2)

Figure 36.2 Outcomes within 1 year after myocardial infarction in patients with multiple complex plaques or single complex plaques ($P < 0.001$ for all comparison between the two groups). PTCA, percutaneous transluminal coronary angioplasty; CABG, coronary artery bypass grafting. (Reproduced with permission from Goldstein et al.[12])

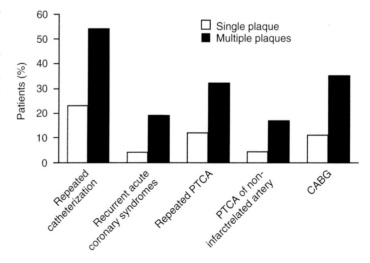

and a trend toward increased 1-year mortality (17% vs 12.4%, $P = 0.32$). Multivariate analysis showed that the presence of multiple complex plaques was an independent predictor of adverse outcomes.[12]

Among the currently available diagnostic modalities, intravascular ultrasound (IVUS) remains the gold standard for assessment of coronary plaque morphology.[13–15] In a study of 24 patients with ACS, Rioufol et al performed IVUS examination of all three major coronary arteries. In total, 50 plaque ruptures (mean = 2.08 per patient; range 0–6) were identified.[15] Of these 24 patients, 79% had at least one ruptured plaque distinct from the culprit lesion (Figure 36.3). More importantly, the ruptured plaques were found in a different artery in 71% of the patients. Interestingly, only 37.5% of plaque ruptures were on the culprit lesions, most likely due to the overlying thrombus covering and masking the underlying ulcerations or ruptures. These data indicate that patients with ACS harbor multiple ruptured plaques in addition to the culprit lesion causing the index ischemic event. In contrast to the poor prognosis associated with the angiographically identified multiple complex plaques,[12] IVUS-identified multiple ruptured plaques were not associated with a poor prognosis at 10-month follow-up.[15] However, this study was limited by the lack of a control group and small number of patients.

CONCEPT OF INTERMEDIATE CORONARY LESION

There is significant evidence indicating that the majority of cases of sudden cardiac death and MI result from the rupture or superficial erosion of coronary plaques at sites with only mild to moderate luminal stenosis.[2–4] There are also compelling data that plaque composition and *vulnerability*, rather than stenosis severity, are the most important determinants of the development of thrombus-mediated acute coronary syndromes.[5,6]

Lesions resulting in 30–70% diameter stenosis (visual assessment) are usually considered as intermediate in severity.[16–21] There is a continuing dispute as to whether an intervention on such intermediate lesions is justified.

If the anginal syndrome is obvious and/or there is evidence of ischemia on non-invasive testing, revascularization is usually performed.[22] If the results of non-invasive testing are inconclusive or contradictory, adjunctive diagnostic modalities to guide management are used.[16,23–25] This includes the assessment of the hemodynamic significance of the lesion using pressure-derived myocardial fractional flow reserve (FFR) or the evaluation of the vessel lumen by using IVUS.[16,23–25] In several studies, deferring of coronary intervention for intermediate stenosis with normal physiology (FFR ≥ 0.75) was consistently associated with considerable (8.7–11%) rates of clinical events at 6-month to 2-year follow-up.[17,26,27]

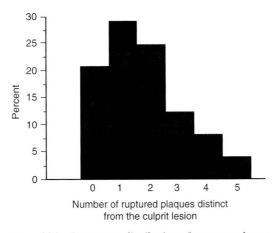

Figure 36.3 Percentage distribution of coronary plaque ruptures other than the culprit lesion. In 79% of cases, at least one such plaque rupture was found. (Reproduced with permission from Rioufol et al.[15])

CLINICAL EVENTS AFTER NOT PERFORMING PERCUTANEOUS CORONARY INTERVENTION FOR INTERMEDIATE LESIONS

In a study of patients with multivessel disease, Berger et al showed that percutaneous coronary intervention (PCI) of hemodynamically non-significant stenoses can be safely deferred.[28] This study analyzed the outcome of 102 patients with multivessel CAD in whom at least one vessel was treated by PCI and at least one other vessel was deferred on the basis of an FFR measurement >0.75 during the same session. At a mean follow-up of 29 ± 18 months, no death occurred. Major adverse cardiac events or MACE (death, MI, and repeat revascularization) occurred in 9% of patients at 12 months and 13% of patients at 36 months. These events were related to 22 (9.2%) arteries. Among them, only 8 (6.3%) events were related to one of the initially deferred vessels, whereas 14 (12.3%) MACE were related to one of the initially treated coronary arteries (Table 36.1).[28]

Moreover, data derived from the IVUS analysis on intermediate lesions indicated that medically treated patients with minimal luminal area ≥ 4.0 mm^2 by IVUS had only an 8% rate of cardiac events after 13 months.[21]

RELATIONSHIP OF INTERMEDIATE LESIONS WITH RECURRENT CLINICAL EVENTS AND C-REACTIVE PROTEIN LEVELS

Available data indicate that C-reactive protein (CRP) is a strong independent predictor of future cardiac events, both in patients with stable CAD and those with unstable ischemic syndromes.[29-31]

In a study of patients with intermediate lesions, Meuwissen et al suggested that an approach combining physiologic information and local and/or systemic inflammatory markers might be valuable in decision making regarding revascularization in these patients.[19] This study evaluated 71 patients with intermediate lesions (diameter stenosis 30–70% by visual estimation) and deferred revascularization based on FFR of ≥ 0.75. At a mean follow-up of 318 days, there was an 8% rate of MACE (all TLR). In the majority of patients, MACE occurred relatively early (within 6 months) and was strongly associated with a higher level of preprocedure CRP. All but one event occurred in the group with CRP levels >5.0 mg/L, resulting in rates of MACE 27.8% in these patients. Another interesting observation was the significant lesion progression with QCA (quantitative coronary angiography) diameter stenosis, increasing from 46.1% at baseline to 62.0% at follow-up in patients with MACE.[19]

Table 36.1   Rates of events related to vessels with deferred intervention vs vessels treated with PCI in patients with multivessel disease

Parameter	Patients with CAD (n =102)	
	Arteries treated with PCI (n = 102)	Arteries with deferred PCI (n = 127)
Baseline FFR, mean ± SD	0.57 ± 0.13	0.86 ± 0.06
Baseline diameter stenosis, mean ± SD, %	68 ± 14	47 ± 12
Follow-up:		
Death	0	0
MACE	12.3%	6.3%

Based on data from Berger et al.[28]
CAD, coronary artery disease; PCI, percutaneous coronary intervention; FFR, fractional flow reserve; MACE, major adverse cardiac events.

IMPACT OF DRUG-ELUTING STENTS ON CLINICAL EVENTS RELATED TO INTERMEDIATE LESIONS

Drug-eluting stents have revolutionized the treatment of patients with angiographically severe coronary lesions.[7,8] Preliminary data indicate that drug-eluting stents may change the current treatment paradigm of intermediate lesions. Based on data from the prospective RESEARCH Registry of patients treated with sirolimus-eluting stents, Hoye et al evaluated the outcome of 20 consecutive patients with 23 angiographically mild (<50% by QCA), de-novo lesions.[32] In this small series, survival free of major adverse events was 95% at a mean follow-up of 399 days with no cases of TLR and no subacute/delayed stent thrombosis.[32]

Larger series representing pooled analysis of four prospective randomized controlled trials (SIRIUS, TAXUS IV, FUTURE I, and FUTURE II)[7–9] showed that the treatment of intermediate lesions (baseline QCA as <50% diameter stenosis) with drug-eluting stents was safe with very low rates of in-hospital and 30-day complications (1.1% both).[33] In comparison to bare metal stents, drug-eluting stents resulted in a significant reduction in restenosis (1.8% vs 34%) and, consequently, dramatically lower rates of TLR (1.2% vs 20.3%), target vessel revascularization (TVR) (3.4% vs 20.3%), and MACE (5.6% vs 25.4%) at 1-year follow-up (Figure 36.4).[33]

These favorable outcomes in patients with intermediate coronary lesions make drug-eluting stents a potentially safe treatment modality for intermediate coronary lesions, which may decrease the propensity to plaque progression and rupture.

RISK STRATIFICATION OF PATIENTS WITH CORONARY ARTERY DISEASE

Thrombolysis In Myocardial Infarction (TIMI) risk score

Recent data have shown the usefulness of risk-stratification models in the management of patients with non-ST-elevation ACS.[34,35] One such model is the Thrombolysis In Myocardial Infarction (TIMI) risk score, which includes several readily available clinical variables (Box 36.1).[34] In the TACTICS-TIMI-18 trial, the primary endpoint of death, non-fatal MI, or rehospitalization for an ACS at 6 months, was significantly lower with use of the early invasive strategy (15.9% vs 19.4% with use of the conservative strategy, odds ratio [OR] = 0.78; 95% CI 0.62–0.97; $P = 0.025$).[35] In this trial, the

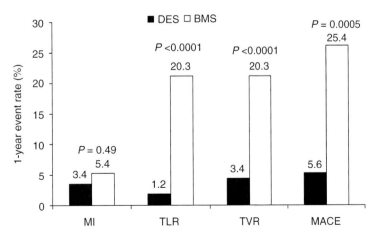

Figure 36.4 Rates of major adverse cardiac events MACE in patients with intermediate lesions treated with drug-eluting stents (DES) vs. bare-metal stents (BMS) in SIRIUS, TAXUS-IV, FUTURE-1 and FUTURE-2 randomized trials. (based on data from Reference 33, Mosses JW, et al. J Am Coll Cardio 2006; 47:216-217)

Box 36.1 TIMI risk score, initially derived and validated based on the data from the ESSENCE and TIMI-11B trials

TIMI risk score
1. Age ≥ 65
2. ≥ 3 risk factors
3. ≥ two episodes of chest pain within 24 hours
4. Prior aspirin use
5. Known CAD (coronary lesion ≥ 50%)
6. ST-segment deviation
7. Elevation of cardiac markers

Based on data from Antman.[34]
TIMI, Thrombolysis in Myocardial Infarction; CAD, coronary artery disease.

usefulness of the TIMI risk score in risk stratification and treatment of ACS patients was again confirmed; only patients with intermediate and high TIMI risk scores actually benefited from an early invasive treatment strategy (Figure 36.5). In patients with intermediate to high TIMI risk score, 16–20% of patients experienced an ischemic event (death, non-fatal MI, or rehospitalization for ACS) at 6 months despite being treated with invasive strategy of early revascularization.[35] Thus, the TIMI risk score seems to be a useful tool in initial risk stratification and subsequent management of patients with non-ST-elevation ACS.

Inflammatory markers and the risk of repeat coronary events

Atherosclerosis was originally considered a bland lipid storage disease. The process, now better known as atherothrombosis, actually involves an ongoing inflammatory response.[2] Recent advances have established a fundamental role of inflammation in mediating all stages of this disease, from initiation through progression and, ultimately, the thrombotic complications of atherothrombosis.

To date, elevated levels of several inflammatory mediators among apparently healthy men and women have proven to

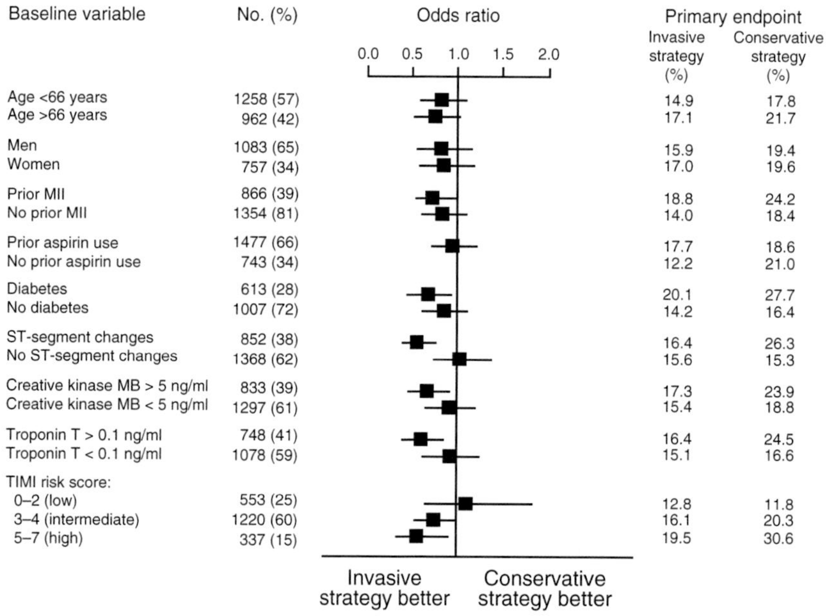

Baseline variable	No. (%)	Odds ratio	Primary endpoint Invasive strategy (%)	Primary endpoint Conservative strategy (%)
Age <66 years	1258 (57)		14.9	17.8
Age >66 years	962 (42)		17.1	21.7
Men	1083 (65)		15.9	19.4
Women	757 (34)		17.0	19.6
Prior MII	866 (39)		18.8	24.2
No prior MII	1354 (81)		14.0	18.4
Prior aspirin use	1477 (66)		17.7	18.6
No prior aspirin use	743 (34)		12.2	21.0
Diabetes	613 (28)		20.1	27.7
No diabetes	1007 (72)		14.2	16.4
ST-segment changes	852 (38)		16.4	26.3
No ST-segment changes	1368 (62)		15.6	15.3
Creative kinase MB > 5 ng/ml	833 (39)		17.3	23.9
Creative kinase MB < 5 ng/ml	1297 (61)		15.4	18.8
Troponin T > 0.1 ng/ml	748 (41)		16.4	24.5
Troponin T < 0.1 ng/ml	1078 (59)		15.1	16.6
TIMI risk score:				
0–2 (low)	553 (25)		12.8	11.8
3–4 (intermediate)	1220 (60)		16.1	20.3
5–7 (high)	337 (15)		19.5	30.6

Odds ratio scale: 0.0 0.5 1.0 1.5 2.0

Invasive strategy better ← | → Conservative strategy better

Figure 36.5 Rates of the primary endpoint of death, non-fatal myocardial infarction (MI), or rehospitalization for an acute coronary syndrome at 6 months in TACTICS-TIMI-18 trial, according to baseline characteristics. (Reproduced with permission from Cannon et al.[35])

have predictive value for future vascular events. In particular, prospective epidemiologic studies have found increased vascular risk in association with increased basal levels of cytokines such as interleukin-6 (IL-6) and tumor necrosis factor-α (TNF-α), cell adhesion molecules such as soluble intercellular adhesion molecule-1 (sICAM-1), P-selectin, and E-selectin, and downstream acutephase reactants such as CRP, fibrinogen, and serum amyloid A.[29,36–39]

Of these markers, the most promising inflammatory biomarker appears to be CRP, a classical acute-phase reactant.[29–31,39] Several population-based studies have demonstrated that baseline CRP levels predict future cardiovascular events (Figure 36.6).[29]

Available data indicate that CRP testing may thus have a major adjunctive role in the global assessment of cardiovascular risk. In both stable and unstable angina, elevated CRP levels predict future events independent of coronary angiography. The association between CRP levels and future cardiovascular events has also been found to be independent of age, smoking, cholesterol levels, diabetes, and other major cardiac risk factors. A CRP level of <1.0 mg/L is considered to denote a low risk, 1.0–3.0 mg/L is an intermediate risk, and >3.0 mg/L is a high risk of future cardiac events (Figure 36.7).[40]

The suggested usefulness of combining physiologic information and local and/or systemic inflammatory markers in decision making regarding revascularization in patients with intermediate stenoses was already discussed.[19] In the study by Meuwissen et al, when angioplasty for intermediate lesions (diameter stenosis 30–70%) was deferred based on FFR ≥0.75, there was an 8% rate of MACE (all TLR) at a mean follow-up of 318 days. Remarkably, in the majority of patients, MACE occurred relatively early (within 6 months) after the diagnostic angiography

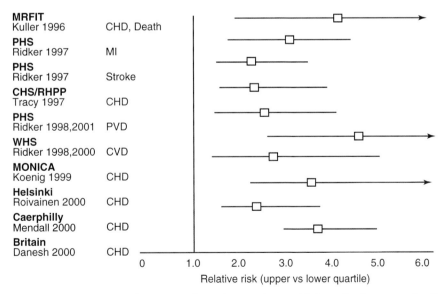

Figure 36.6 Prospective studies of high-sensitivity C-reactive protein as a risk factor for future vascular disease. CHD, coronary heart disease; MRFIT, Multiple Risk Factor Intervention Trial; PHS, Physicians' Health Study; CHS/RHPP, Cardiovascular Health Study and the Rural Health Promotion Project; WHS, Women's Health Study; PVD, pulmonary vascular disease; CVD, cardiovascular disease; and MONICA, Monitoring Trends and Determinants in Cardiovascular Disease. (Reproduced with permission from Ridker.[29])

Figure 36.7 Cumulative rate of myocardial infarction or coronary heart disease death. (a) Data for men; (b) data for women. Unadjusted hazard ratios (and 95% CIs) for each group compared with reference group (CRP <1 mg/L) are shown. Solid line indicates CRP <1 mg/L; dotted line, CRP 1–3 mg/L; and dashed line, CRP >3 mg/L. (Reproduced with permission from Cushman et al.[40])

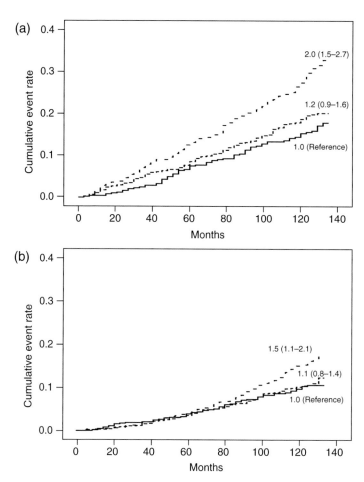

Diabetes mellitus, metabolic syndrome, and coronary artery disease progression

Prospective data indicate that diabetes mellitus is associated with a substantial increase in all-cause and CAD mortality. The presence of both diabetes and CAD identifies a particularly high-risk group. In a prospective cohort study of 91 285 US male physicians aged 40–84 years, the relative risk (RR) of CAD death was 3.3 (95% CI 2.6–4.1) among men with diabetes and without CAD, but RR = 5.6 (95% CI 4.9–6.3) among men with CAD and without diabetes, and RR = 12.0 (95% CI 9.9–14.6) among men with both diabetes and CAD.[41]

Clinical outcome after PCI is significantly worse in diabetic patients than in patients without diabetes. In a consecutive series of patients with successful stent placement, comprising 715 patients with diabetes and 2839 patients without diabetes, the primary clinical endpoint, event-free survival at 1 year, was significantly lower in diabetic than in non-diabetic

and was strongly associated with higher level of preprocedure CRP; and all but one event occurred in the group with significantly elevated CRP levels, resulting in rates of MACE of 27.8% in these patients.[19]

patients (73.1% vs 78.5%, $P <0.001$). The incidence of both restenosis (37.5% vs 28.3%, $P<0.001$) and stent vessel occlusion (5.3% vs 3.4%, $P = 0.04$) was significantly higher in diabetic patients.[42] Diabetes was identified as an independent risk factor for adverse clinical events and restenosis in multivariate analyses.[42] In a study on 99 diabetic patients with multivessel CAD treated with PCI during 2000–2001, 1-year event-free survival was 67%.[43] Importantly, disease progression contributed to 57% of repeat revascularization procedures.[43]

In a study of 2000 patients, Kugelmass et al reported that diabetic patients, compared with non-diabetic patients, tended to have more TLR (13.6% vs 8.9%; $P = 0.07$) and more TVR (17.6% vs 12.7%; $P = 0.06$). In addition, diabetic patients were 1.6 times more likely to have a second PCI procedure in another vessel ($P = 0.013$), 2.4 times more likely to undergo bypass surgery ($P = 0.003$), 1.9 times more likely to undergo an additional revascularization procedure ($P <0.001$), and 1.8 times more likely to experience any major adverse cardiac events ($P <0.001$) than non-diabetic patients during 1-year follow-up.[44]

The metabolic syndrome, characterized by a constellation of fasting hyperglycemia, hypertriglyceridemia, low high-density lipoprotein (HDL) cholesterol, hypertension, and/or abdominal obesity, was found to worsen prognosis of patients with CAD. The recent Women's Ischemia Syndrome Evaluation (WISE) study evaluated relationships between angiographic CAD, the metabolic syndrome, and cardiovascular events among 755 women referred for coronary angiography.[45] In this study, compared with women with normal metabolic status, women with the metabolic syndrome had a significantly lower 4-year survival rate (94.3% vs 97.8%, $P = 0.03$) and event-free survival from MACE (death, non-fatal myocardial infarction, stroke, or congestive heart failure; 87.8% vs 93.5%, $P = 0.003$).[45]

RATIONALE FOR PREVAIL STUDY DESIGN

In the current era, despite optimal systemic therapy with antiplatelet agents, anti-ischemic medications, and plaque-modifying agents such as statins, the risk of recurrent ischemic events remains high.[29–31,35] Based on data from both randomized controlled trials and population-based studies, patients with non-ST-elevation ACS and TIMI risk score of ≥3 and patients with CRP >3.0 mg/L are at high risk for future cardiovascular events.[31,35,40] Available data indicate that non-culprit intermediate lesions may be responsible for the majority of cardiac events in such patients. As such, these non-culprit intermediate lesions constitute potential targets for secondary prevention and reduction of future cardiac events in high-risk patients.

It is well-known that PCI of severe coronary lesions relieves angina in patients with stable coronary disease. However, PCI of the lesions that are of intermediate severity by angiographic assessment, but have characteristics of vulnerable lesions, is expected to prevent death and MI in high-risk patients with ACS. The *purpose* of the PREVAIL study is to evaluate the safety and therapeutic efficacy of optimal medical therapy plus PCI of intermediate, and presumably vulnerable, lesions with sirolimus drug-eluting stents, compared with optimal medical treatment alone, on angiographic lesion progression in high-risk patients. Once the safety and initial efficacy of such a strategy is established, future PREVAIL studies will ideally focus on evaluation of PCI of intermediate, and presumably vulnerable, lesions in reducing death, MI, and TVR (Figure 36.8).

The PREVAIL study will include high-risk ACS patients with non-culprit intermediate de-novo coronary lesions (Box 36.2). Enrollment in the PREVAIL study is conditional on the successful performance of

Figure 36.8 Proposed flow chart for PREVAIL study. ACS = acute coronary syndrome; TIMI = Thrombolysis In Myocardial Infarction; QCA = quantitative coronary angiography; IVUS = intravascular ultrasound; SES = sirolimus-eluting stent; w/DES = with drug-eluting stents.

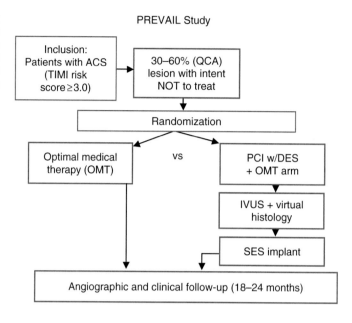

culprit single-vessel PCI. However, if angiography shows non-obstructive disease, patients can be eligible for PREVAIL without any PCI of the presumed culprit lesion. Patients with acute ST-elevation-MI, prior coronary artery bypass grafting (CABG), and renal insufficiency will be excluded (Box 36.3).

As shown in Figure 36.8, patients with ACS and high-risk features (TIMI risk score ≥3) are considered for enrollment in the PREVAIL study. Informed consent is obtained prior to the diagnostic coronary angiography. When eligible, patients will undergo PCI of the culprit lesion with sirolimus-eluting stents. Then, patients

---

Box 36.2 Inclusion criteria for PREVAIL study

Clinical inclusion criteria
Patients undergoing PCI for:
- Non-ST elevation ACS with TIMI risk score ≥3 (stratified by elevated CRP ≥3.0 mg/L and diabetes mellitus or metabolic syndrome)

Angiographic inclusion criteria (Intermediate lesion)
- Lesion of intermediate severity (angiographic diameter stenosis in the range of 25–50% by QCA, which corresponds to 40–70% by visual estimation)
- Complex lesion morphology defined by Ambrose criteria[13]
- Vessel size >2.5 mm and <3.5 mm
- Not more than three intermediate lesions in one epicardial vessel territory (main vessel and side-branches)

PCI, percutaneous coronary intervention; ACS, acute coronary syndromes; CRP, C-reactive protein; TIMI, Thrombolysis in Myocardial Infarction; QCA, quantitative coronary angiography.

Box 36.3 Exclusion criteria for PREVAIL study

- Acute ST-elevation myocardial infarction within 72 hours
- Cardiogenic shock
- Prior coronary artery bypass grafting
- Renal insufficiency (creatinine >2.0 mg/dl)
- Left main coronary artery disease with stenosis >50%
- Left ventricular ejection fraction <30%
- Warfarin therapy
- Treatment with drug-eluting stent (DES) in the preceding 3 months
- In-stent restenotic lesion at time of enrollment after implantation of DES
- Aorto-ostial location of the intermediate lesion
- Intermediate lesion is located at bifurcation with a side branch reference vessel diameter >2.5 mm that necessitates the treatment of both branches

will be evaluated for the presence of intermediate lesions (30–60% by QCA) which would otherwise not be treated by stenting. At this point, patients with intermediate lesions will be randomized to either the 'combined' treatment group or 'medical' treatment group. The combined treatment group includes PCI of intermediate lesions with sirolimus-eluting stent plus optimal medical therapy. The medical treatment group includes optimal medical therapy alone. At least a subgroup of patients undergoing PCI of intermediate lesions will undergo baseline and follow-up IVUS evaluation. The PREVAIL study will include angiographic (and IVUS in the specific subgroup) follow-up at 18 months and clinical follow-up at 24 months. The primary endpoint of the initial PREVAIL study is angiographic lesion progression, while the future PREVAIL studies will include clinical events (death, MI, repeat revascularization) as primary endpoints.

The PREVAIL study will also include ancillary biochemical and imaging substudies to evaluate the impact of inflammatory markers and the newer imaging modalities in predicting clinical events related to both culprit lesions and non-culprit intermediate lesions.

SUMMARY

Most acute ischemic events are caused by rupture or superficial erosion of coronary plaques with mild to moderate stenosis. Patients with ACS manifest multiple ruptured coronary plaques which may be responsible for recurrent ischemic events such as death and MI. Current treatment of patients with ACS includes PCI of the culprit lesion causing the index ischemic event. There is significant controversy regarding optimal treatment of intermediate, and potentially vulnerable, lesions in high-risk ACS patients. In addition to optimal adjunctive medical therapy, the PREVAIL study will evaluate the effect of PCI,

with sirolimus-eluting stents, of such intermediate, and potentially vulnerable, lesions on angiographic lesion progression. Then, the PREVAIL study will aim to evaluate the efficacy of PCI, with sirolimus-eluting stents, of intermediate, and potentially vulnerable, lesions in reducing recurrent ischemic events such as death, MI, and repeat revascularization in high-risk ACS patients.

REFERENCES

1. Smith SC Jr, Blair SN, Bonow RO et al. AHA/ACC Guidelines for Preventing Heart Attack and Death in Patients With Atherosclerotic Cardiovascular Disease: 2001 update. A statement for healthcare professionals from the American Heart Association and the American College of Cardiology. J Am Coll Cardiol 2001; 38:1581–3.
2. Fuster V, Moreno PM, Fayad ZA et al. Atherothrombosis and high-risk plaque: Part I: Evolving concepts. J Am Coll Cardiol 2005; 46:937–54.
3. Braunwald E, Antman EM, Beasley JW et al; American College of Cardiology; American Heart Association. Committee on the Management of Patients With Unstable Angina. ACC/AHA 2002 guideline update for the management of patients with unstable angina and non-ST-segment elevation myocardial infarction – summary article: a report of the American College of Cardiology/American Heart Association task force on practice guidelines (Committee on the Management of Patients With Unstable Angina). J Am Coll Cardiol 2002; 40:1366–74.
4. Farb A, Burke AP, Tang AL et al. Coronary plaque erosion without rupture into a lipid core. A frequent cause of coronary thrombosis in sudden coronary death. Circulation 1996; 93:1354–63.
5. Falk E, Shah PK, Fuster V. Coronary plaque disruption. Circulation 1995; 92:657–71.
6. Loree HM, Kamm RD, Stringfellow RG et al. Effects of fibrous cap thickness on peak circumferential stress in model atherosclerotic vessels. Circ Res 1992; 71:850–8.
7. Moses JW, Leon MB, Popma JJ et al, For the SIRIUS Investigators. Sirolimus-eluting stents versus standard stents in patients with stenosis in a native coronary artery. N Engl J Med 2003; 349:1315–23.
8. Stone GW, Ellis SG, Cox DA et al; TAXUS-IV Investigators. A polymer-based, paclitaxel-eluting stent in patients with coronary artery disease. N Engl J Med 2004; 350:221–31.
9. Grube E, Sonoda S, Ikeno F et al. Six- and twelve-month results from first human experience using everolimus-eluting stents with bioabsorbable polymer. Circulation 2004; 109:2168–71.
10. Kimura T, Abe K, Shizuta S et al. Long-term clinical and angiographic follow-up after coronary stent

placement in native coronary arteries. Circulation 2002; 105:2986–91.

11. Cutlip DE, Chhabra AG, Baim DS et al. Beyond restenosis: five-year clinical outcomes from second-generation coronary stent trials. Circulation 2004; 110:1226–30.

12. Goldstein JA, Demetriou D, Grines CL et al. Multiple complex coronary plaques in patients with acute myocardial infarction. N Engl J Med 2000; 343: 915–22.

13. Pasterkamp G, Falk E, Woutman H et al. Techniques characterizing the coronary atherosclerotic plaque: influence on clinical decision making? J Am Coll Cardiol 2000; 36:13–21.

14. Yamagishi M, Terashima M, Awano K et al. Morphology of vulnerable coronary plaque: insights from follow-up of patients examined by intravascular ultrasound before an acute coronary syndrome. J Am Coll Cardiol 2000; 35:106–11.

15. Rioufol G, Finet G, Ginon I et al. Multiple atherosclerotic plaque rupture in acute coronary syndrome: a three-vessel intravascular ultrasound study. Circulation 2002; 106:804–8.

16. Pijls NH, De Bruyne B, Peels K et al. Measurement of fractional flow reserve to assess the functional severity of coronary-artery stenoses. N Engl J Med 1996; 334:1703–8.

17. Chamuleau SA, Meuwissen M, Koch KT et al. Usefulness of fractional flow reserve for risk stratification of patients with multivessel coronary artery disease and an intermediate stenosis. Am J Cardiol 2002; 89:377–80.

18. Miller DD, Donohue TJ, Younis LT et al. Correlation of pharmacological ^{99m}Tc-sestamibi myocardial perfusion imaging with poststenotic coronary flow reserve in patients with angiographically intermediate coronary artery stenoses. Circulation 1994; 89:2150–60.

19. Meuwissen M, de Winter RJ, Chamuleau SA et al. Value of C-reactive protein in patients with stable angina pectoris, coronary narrowing (30% to 70%), and normal fractional flow reserve. Am J Cardiol 2003; 92:702–5.

20. Bech GJ, De Bruyne B, Bonnier HJ et al. Long-term follow-up after deferral of percutaneous transluminal coronary angioplasty of intermediate stenosis on the basis of coronary pressure measurement. J Am Coll Cardiol 1998; 31:841–7.

21. Abizaid AS, Mintz GS, Mehran R et al. Long-term follow-up after percutaneous transluminal coronary angioplasty was not performed based on intravascular ultrasound findings: importance of lumen dimensions. Circulation 1999; 100:256–61.

22. Smith SC Jr, Dove JT, Jacobs AK et al; American College of Cardiology/American Heart Association task force on practice guidelines (Committee to revise the 1993 guidelines for percutaneous transluminal coronary angioplasty); Society for Cardiac Angiography and Interventions. ACC/AHA guidelines for percutaneous coronary intervention (revision of the 1993 PTCA guidelines) – executive summary: a report of the American College of Cardiology/American Heart Association task force on practice guidelines (Committee to revise the 1993 guidelines for percutaneous transluminal coronary angioplasty) endorsed by the Society for Cardiac Angiography and Interventions. Circulation 2001; 103:3019–41.

23. Fearon WF, Takagi A, Jeremias A et al. Use of fractional myocardial flow reserve to assess the functional significance of intermediate coronary stenoses. Am J Cardiol 2000; 86:1013–14, A10.

24. De Bruyne B, Paulus WJ, Pijls NH. Rationale and application of coronary transstenotic pressure gradient measurements. Cathet Cardiovasc Diagn 1994; 33:250–61.

25. Briguori C, Anzuini A, Airoldi F et al. Intravascular ultrasound criteria for the assessment of the functional significance of intermediate coronary artery stenoses and comparison with fractional flow reserve. Am J Cardiol 2001; 87:136–41.

26. Bech GJ, De Bruyne B, Pijls NH et al. Fractional flow reserve to determine the appropriateness of angioplasty in moderate coronary stenosis: a randomized trial. Circulation 2001; 103:2928–34.

27. Rieber J, Schiele TM, Koenig A et al. Long-term safety of therapy stratification in patients with intermediate coronary lesions based on intracoronary pressure measurements. Am J Cardiol 2002; 90:1160–4.

28. Berger A, Botman KJ, MacCarthy PA et al. Long-term clinical outcome after fractional flow reserve-guided percutaneous coronary intervention in patients with multivessel disease. J Am Coll Cardiol 2005; 46:438–42.

29. Ridker PM. High-sensitivity C-reactive protein: potential adjunct for global risk assessment in the primary prevention of cardiovascular disease. Circulation 2001; 103:1813–18.

30. Mueller C, Buettner HJ, Hodgson JM et al. Inflammation and long-term mortality after non-ST elevation acute coronary syndrome treated with a very early invasive strategy in 1042 consecutive patients. Circulation 2002; 105:1412–15.

31. Ridker PM, Cannon CP, Morrow D et al; PROVE IT-TIMI 22 Investigators. C-reactive protein levels and outcomes after statin therapy. N Engl J Med 2005; 352:20–8.

32. Hoye A, Lemos PA, Arampatzis CA et al. Effectiveness of sirolimus-eluting stent implantation for coronary narrowings <50% in diameter. Am J Cardiol 2004; 94:112–14.

33. Moses JW, Nikolsky E, Mintz GS et al. Drug-eluting stents in the treatment of intermediate lesions: pooled analysis from four randomized trials. American Heart Association Scientific Sessions, 2005, Dallas, TX. Oral presentation.

34. Antman EM, Cohen M, Bernink PJ et al. The TIMI risk score for unstable angina/non-ST elevation MI: a method for prognostication and therapeutic decision making. JAMA 2000; 284:835–42.

35. Cannon CP, Weintraub WS, Demopoulos LA et al; TACTICS-TIMI-18 Investigators. Comparison of early invasive and conservative strategies in patients with unstable coronary syndromes treated with the glycoprotein IIb/IIIa inhibitor tirofiban. N Engl J Med 2001; 344:1879–87.

36. Kannel WB, Wolf PA, Castelli WP et al. Fibrinogen and risk of cardiovascular disease. The Framingham Study. JAMA 1987; 258:1183–6.

37. Ma J, Hennekens CH, Ridker PM et al. A prospective study of fibrinogen and risk of myocardial infarction in the Physicians' Health Study. J Am Coll Cardiol 1999; 33:1347–52.

38. O'Malley T, Ludlam CA, Riemermsa RA et al. Early increase in levels of soluble inter-cellular adhesion molecule-1 (sICAM-1); potential risk factor for the acute coronary syndromes. Eur Heart J 2001; 14:1226–34.

39. Anderson R, Dart AM, Starr J et al. Plasma C-reactive protein, but not protein S, VCAM-1, von Willebrand factor or P-selectin, is associated with endothelium dysfunction in coronary artery disease. Atherosclerosis 2004; 172:345–51.

40. Cushman M, Arnold AM, Psaty BM et al. C-reactive protein and the 10-year incidence of coronary heart disease in older men and women: the cardiovascular health study. Circulation 2005; 112:25–31.

41. Lotufo PA, Gaziano JM, Chae CU et al. Diabetes and all-cause and coronary heart disease mortality among US male physicians. Arch Intern Med 2001; 161:242–7.

42. Elezi S, Kastrati A, Pache J et al. Diabetes mellitus and the clinical and angiographic outcome after coronary stent placement. J Am Coll Cardiol 1998; 32:1866–73.

43. Loutfi M, Mulvihill NT, Boccalatte M et al. Impact of restenosis and disease progression on clinical outcome after multivessel stenting in diabetic patients. Catheter Cardiovasc Interv 2003; 58:451–4.

44. Kugelmass AD, Cohen DJ, Houser F et al. The influence of diabetes mellitus on the practice and outcomes of percutaneous coronary intervention in the community: a report from the HCA database. J Invasive Cardiol 2003; 10:568–74.

45. Marroquin OC, Kip KE, Kelley DE et al; Women's Ischemia Syndrome Evaluation Investigators. Metabolic syndrome modifies the cardiovascular risk associated with angiographic coronary artery disease in women: a report from the Women's Ischemia Syndrome Evaluation. Circulation 2004; 109:714–21.

Regulatory issues of the Food and Drug Administration*

37

Felipe Aguel, Andrew Farb, and Elias Mallis

INTRODUCTION

The mission of the US Food and Drug Administration (FDA) is to promote and protect public health. Among the numerous ways the FDA seeks to accomplish this mission is through regulatory supervision of medical drugs, devices, and biologics that are clinically evaluated and granted market entry into the USA. While the FDA's regulatory history of medical drugs is well established over the course of 100 years, triggered by the passage of the Federal Food and Drugs Act of 1906, the FDA's history of regulation of medical devices is much shorter, and was initiated with the passage of the Medical Device Amendments on May 28, 1976.

In its first few years of existence, the FDA's Center for Devices and Radiological Health (CDRH), which regulates medical devices, classified medical devices that were known to be in use at that time into one of three classes (I, II, or III) based on the risks associated with their use. Class III was reserved for the highest-risk devices, and Class I was reserved for the lowest-risk devices. Accordingly, the level of evidence needed for novel devices to gain market entry was predicated upon this classification. A Class III medical device may require

*The views and opinions presented in this article are those of the authors and do not necessarily reflect those of the US Food and Drug Administration, the US Department of Health and Human Services, or the Public Health Service.

a combination of bench, animal, and clinical data to support market approval, whereas a Class I medical device might rely solely on descriptive information.

Over the past 30 years, the world of medicine has rapidly evolved with new technologic advances, including an explosion of complex medical devices that have advanced medical care beyond what were imagined or predicted when CDRH was established. However, the FDA's basic tenet and approach to novel technologies and devices established in the 1976 Amendments has not changed; specifically, a risk–benefit analysis is applied to evaluate the safety and effectiveness of a new device that is being considered for market entry. Thus, the FDA assesses whether the benefit provided by the use of the new device outweighs the safety risk imposed by its use.

Over the past few years, the scientific research and medical community has shown significantly increased interest in the diagnosis and treatment of vulnerable atherosclerotic plaque, with an emphasis on advancing technologies that will ultimately assist patients who are at risk for acute coronary ischemic syndromes.

This chapter describes the FDA's current approach to the evaluation of novel diagnostic and therapeutic advances in the field of vulnerable plaque. To complement this broad guidance, the FDA recognizes that specific guidance to the regulatory community may be needed on a more detailed, technical basis. One significant mechanism for this important communication to take place is with the Pre-Investigational Device Exemption (Pre-IDE) Program. This forum may serve as a valuable and timely platform for the regulatory community to seek FDA counsel on issues pertaining to the overall regulatory paradigm, as well as bench, in-vitro, animal, and clinical evaluation of the novel device.[1]

DATA USED TO DEMONSTRATE SAFETY AND EFFECTIVENESS OF ARTERIAL DIAGNOSTIC CATHETERS

Safety and effectiveness data are typically reviewed at two primary milestones during the regulatory life cycle of a device: data and other related information are first reviewed at the time an investigational device exemption (IDE) is submitted by a sponsor who seeks approval to commence a clinical trial of a novel device; secondly, data are subsequently reviewed within the context of a market application. For the IDE review, the FDA determines whether a sponsor has demonstrated a sufficient level of probable safety and reasonable expectation of device effectiveness to allow for a study to be initiated (and approved). During review of the market application, the FDA will either review a premarket notification (or 510(k)) or a Premarket Approval (PMA) application to determine whether a device will be granted market entry. The bar for market entry under a 510(k) application (or 510(k) clearance) is demonstration of substantial equivalence between the new device and a device previously cleared under a 510(k) application. The bar for market entry under a PMA is demonstration of reasonable assurance of safety and effectiveness. In an IDE application, all available bench and animal data as well as any clinical data collected previously, either as part of another approved IDE or as part of a study conducted outside the United States (OUS), are evaluated. As part of the market application, the data

included in the IDE, any additional non-clinical data collected but not assessed during the IDE review, and the clinical data collected under the approved IDE should be provided.

The type and amount of data needed to support either an IDE or a market application for arterial diagnostic catheters (ADCs) are largely dependent on the intended use and proposed marketing claims. A tool indication is one where a measurement of a physiologic, physical, or another parameter is provided to the user, usually the physician or healthcare professional, with no association of what the parameter means or predicts clinically. In this context, it is up to the user to decide how to apply the information obtained from the tool device. A diagnostic indication is one where such information is used to provide a diagnosis of or predictive information related to a disease condition or where the information provided has established clinical utility that is widely accepted. Examples of tool claims potentially relevant to the investigation of vulnerable plaque include measurements of temperature, elasticity, material content, and specific anatomic features of an arterial segment or atherosclerotic lesion. Examples of diagnostic claims include classification of an atherosclerotic lesion as a vulnerable plaque or as a thin-cap fibroatheroma (TCFA), and a computer-aided diagnosis that recommends further intervention.

The FDA's ADC guidance document, 'Coronary and Peripheral Arterial Diagnostic Catheters',[2] stipulates that a risk analysis should be the impetus behind the testing conducted to demonstrate the safety of a device. The recommended risk analysis approach is described in detail in the internationally recognized consensus standard 'Medical devices – Application of risk management to medical devices'.[3] Thus, the bench and animal testing needed to demonstrate the probable safety of a device prior to initiation of a clinical study will be device-specific. When determining the necessary bench testing, one needs to consider the device design and operating principle, as well as the patient population in which the device will be indicated. The safety of ADCs should be demonstrated using a combination of bench, animal, and US or appropriate OUS clinical data.

The FDA believes that the most robust and least burdensome way to demonstrate the effectiveness of ADCs is to compare the accuracy of the novel device to a clinically accepted gold standard. However, the FDA recognizes that a gold standard may not exist or may not be ethically feasible to attain clinically (e.g. when histology is the only available gold standard) in many cases. Therefore, it is expected that the demonstration of effectiveness of an ADC may rely heavily on bench and animal data. In such cases, bench and animal experiments should be scientifically and statistically robust and simulate worst-case clinical conditions as best possible (e.g. use of device motion and circulating blood). Clinical data should be used to corroborate that the non-clinical effectiveness data are clinically applicable in a patient population for whom the device will be indicated. A natural history study may be necessary to provide evidence in support of the claim. The use of natural history studies is described later in this chapter.

Figure 37.1 depicts a generalized overview of the bench, animal, and clinical data that may be used to support the safety and effectiveness of ADCs. A natural progression from bench testing to animal testing and, after IDE approval, to clinical studies is indicated by the arrow on the left of Figure 37.1. This figure does not describe formal regulatory requirements, but instead represents just one possible regulatory strategy a sponsor may use to get an ADC to the market. The entries in Figure 37.1 are described in more detail below, and references to appropriate guidance documents and standards are provided.

Bench testing

The FDA expects that bench testing used to support the decision to initiate a clinical study under an IDE should (1) demonstrate probable safety for use in humans and (2) create a reasonable expectation of effectiveness. Below is a description of bench testing that is expected to be common to most ADCs. Because it would be impossible to include all possible variations in device design and operating principle, the list is not meant to be all-inclusive, but rather a likely starting point to provide a thorough risk analysis.

Mechanical safety

The mechanical testing performed should be consistent with any applicable standards and guidance documents.[4,5] These tests include:

- catheter stiffness
- tip stiffness
- tip attachment strength
- torsional strength
- joint strength
- fatigue tolerance
- catheter leakage (if applicable)
- balloon inflation, burst strength, and leakage (if applicable)
- others, as per risk analysis.

Particular attention should be paid to the site where the catheter will be used. For example, if the catheter employs a balloon, and that balloon can be used near atherosclerotic lesions that may include a TCFA, the possibility of plaque rupture or dislodgement induced by the balloon should be considered in addition to the standard mechanical bench tests.

Electrical safety and electromagnetic compatibility

It is recommended that electrical safety testing be conducted as per the recognized consensus standard IEC 60601-1[6] and that

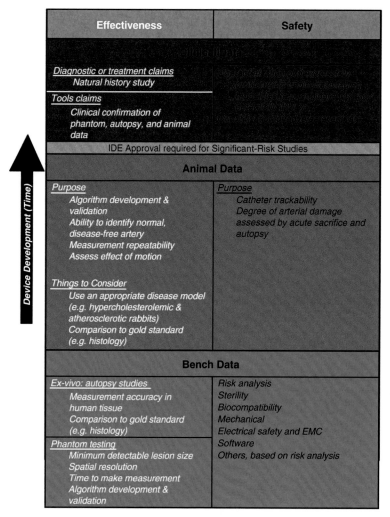

Figure 37.1   Schematic of safety and effectiveness data that can be used to support an arterial diagnostic catheter's safety and effectiveness. On the left column are data to support device effectiveness; on the right column are data to demonstrate device safety. The veritcal axis represents time. The backgound color of items in the figure depict bench, animal, and clinical testing. The yellow band represents the submission of an IDE application seeking approval from FDA to begin a clinical study.

electromagnetic compatibility testing be conducted as per the recognized consensus standard IEC 60601-1-2.[7] Note that the IEC 60601-1-2 standard does not cover wireless communications. A novel device which employs wireless communications for any purpose may be subject to additional testing specific to the wireless communications technology used in the device.

Biocompatibility

The FDA recommends that biocompatibility testing be conducted in accordance with the internationally recognized consensus standard 'ISO 10993-1: Biological evaluation of medical devices'.[8] For ADCs intended for use for less than 24 hours, biocompatibility testing should be conducted as specified in ISO 10993-1 for external communicating devices in limited duration contact with circulating blood. This testing includes cytotoxicity, sensitization, irritation or intracutaneous reactivity, systemic toxicity, and hemo-compatibility (i.e. hemolysis, platelet and complement activation, and thrombo-genicity).

Packaging, shelf life, and sterilization

Packaging, shelf life,[9] and sterilization[10–12] validation reports should be submitted to appropriately demonstrate the sterility of the device prior to use. Testing should be conducted following shelf-life validation as well as full-sterilization cycles. If tests are conducted on unvalidated samples, a justification should be given for why shelf-life testing (e.g. accelerated aging) and sterilization are irrelevant to the test(s) conducted. The sterilization information submitted should include:

- a description of the sterilization method used
- a description of the packaging, including sterile barrier(s)
- the method used to validate the sterilization cycle
- sterility assurance level (SAL) specification
- pyrogenicity information
- if the sterilization method is ethylene oxide, a listing of the ethylene oxide sterilization residuals[13] (i.e. residual ethylene oxide and ethylene chlorohydrin).

Other safety testing

Additional safety testing may be necessary, depending on the technology and operating principles of the device. For example, ADCs that employ a laser light source should have appropriate laser safety testing. ADCs that directly contact the arterial wall should be assessed for the contact force and why such contact force does not represent a potential hazard to the patient. In all cases, the bench testing should be driven by the risk analysis of the novel device.

Software

Depending on the nature of the device design, operating principle, and intended use, the software employed within ADCs raises a moderate or a major level of concern, as defined in the FDA Software Guidance.[14] The appropriate software documentation needed to support the application is described in this guidance. Further, if the ADC utilizes off-the-shelf software (e.g. Microsoft Windows operating system), documentation specified in the Off-the-Shelf Software guidance document[15] would be needed.

Phantom effectiveness testing

The first step a sponsor may take to demonstrate the effectiveness and accuracy of a novel device is to perform adequate testing on phantoms. Phantom testing may be used to demonstrate proof of principle, as well as spatial measurement resolution. Phantoms should be designed to simulate, as best as possible, the clinical conditions in which the novel device will be used; for example, the phantom should be sized and shaped appropriately. The test should include circulating blood at body temperature, physiologic flow rates, and if possible, simulated motion. A justification should be provided for phantom characteristics that do not mimic in-vivo conditions.

Animal testing

For tool claims, it is expected that evidence will rely heavily on animal data to demonstrate device accuracy compared with a gold standard such as histology. It is therefore imperative that the most appropriate animal model be used, taking into consideration the disease state, clinical conditions, and intended use of the device. For vulnerable plaque tools, a disease model such as atherosclerotic rabbits should be considered. For histologic methods used to assess device accuracy, care is needed to precisely register the device measurement site with the histology site. Importantly, an animal model is an effective way to assess measurement reproducibility via repeated measurements and the device's ability to identify a 'normal' or disease-free artery.

Assessment of device effectiveness using autopsy specimens

Examination of human arterial autopsy specimens is an ex-vivo method of measuring device performance. In these studies, device measurement or diagnosis is compared with histologic analysis. It is important to use fresh human arteries, for the histology to be performed by a qualified pathologist, and to derive a predictive value or correlation between histologic and device measurements. Animal testing and ex-vivo human autopsy studies are discussed further below.

VULNERABLE PLAQUE TARGETS FOR DETECTION

Ruptured atherosclerotic plaques are responsible for 60–70% of fatal coronary thrombi, and numerous pathologic studies have demonstrated that the TCFA is the precursor lesion (i.e. the pathologic correlate of most vulnerable plaques) of plaque rupture.[16,17] In brief, these lesions are characterized by a thin fibrous cap, a large lipid core, and chronic inflammation. While the pathogenesis of the development of TCFAs and the transformation of stable plaques to vulnerable plaques remains incompletely understood, coronary artery morphologic studies from coronary death victims provide the foundation for the development of vulnerable plaque diagnostic devices. The fibrous cap of atherosclerotic plaques contains smooth muscle cells (SMCs) and a collagen-rich extracellular matrix. Fibrous caps in unstable plaques responsible for sudden coronary death have fewer SMCs than stable plaques. Furthermore, reduced fibrous cap thickness is a feature of TCFAs, and with a cap thickness of less than 65 μm, the cap is considered 'rupture-prone.' Cap thickness is inversely proportional to the concentration of activated plaque inflammatory cell infiltration. Plaque instability is augmented by inflammatory cell products such as matrix metalloproteinases, which are capable of degrading collagen. Other correlates of plaque vulnerability include the absolute size of the lipid core and the percent of the total plaque size occupied by the lipid core; a larger lipid pool indicates a greater propensity for plaque rupture. More recently, plaque hemorrhage, angiogenesis, and arterial remodeling have been associated with progressive arterial stenosis and plaque vulnerability.

The pathology of TCFAs offers multiple potential targets for device assessment of plaque instability. Among the various structural atherosclerotic plaque elements, a device might be designed to measure fibrous cap thickness, concentration of activated inflammatory cells in the fibrous cap, fibrous cap SMC and type 1 collagen content, lipid core area (absolute size and size as a percent of total plaque size), positive arterial remodeling, plaque neovascularization, and increased vascularity of the adventitia. Probes for non-structural factors associated with plaque vulnerability may be developed to evaluate local concentrations of proinflammatory cytokines, matrix metalloproteinases, adhesion molecules, myeloperoxidase, C-reactive protein, and evidence of cellular apoptosis. Initial studies suggest that physical properties such as increased plaque temperature (a marker of inflammation) and focally increased intraplaque strain indicate enhanced plaque vulnerability. Given the complexity of TCFAs and the correlations among the various structural, molecular, and physical elements, it could be expected that second- and third-generation vulnerable plaque detection devices will assess multiple plaque features to increase their diagnostic severity and specificity.

FEASIBILITY AND NATURAL HISTORY STUDIES IN THE DEVELOPMENT OF VULNERABLE PLAQUE DETECTION DEVICES

Demonstration of acceptable device safety is paramount in preclinical animal studies and initial human feasibility studies related to novel vulnerable plaque device development. In animal studies, it can be expected that placement of devices within the coronary arteries may acutely produce focal superficial arterial injury (e.g. endothelial disruption, sparse acute inflammation, and minute thrombus deposition), but diagnostic devices should not be associated with significant vascular damage (e.g. medial dissection, perforation, or luminal thrombosis). Similarly, it is expected that longer-term animal studies will show healing of the superficial arterial damage (characterized by mild neointimal thickening), but the use of these diagnostic devices should not produce new moderate or severe stenotic lesions. While it is understood that a detailed histologic evaluation is unavailable in initial human testing of intracoronary vulnerable plaque detection devices, evidence of device safety should be assessed via traditional coronary imaging modalities (angiography and potentially IVUS) and clinical markers of myocardial ischemia and infarction.

In preclinical development, TCFA detection devices may utilize algorithms to detect plaque features of interest based on histologic studies of ex-vivo human coronary arteries. These challenging pathologic studies require:

- accurate pathologic definitions that are relevant to the device's tool or diagnostic claims
- precise registration of histologic sections with device acquisition data
- acceptable sensitivity and specificity for lesion detection.

It is recommended that these algorithms should be tested against independent sets of teaching and learning libraries of lesions. Depending on device claims (tool vs diagnostic), an assessment based on ex-vivo human coronary arteries may be quantitative (e.g. identification of a lipid core that occupies greater than a certain percentage of the total plaque area) or qualitative

(e.g. identification of an acceptably defined TCFA). Disease animal models, such as atherosclerotic rabbits, may be particularly useful in the assessment of lesion characteristics that support tool or diagnostic claims (e.g. devices that assess the presence of plaque lipid).

Animal studies and human feasibility testing should also provide an initial assessment of device efficacy and potential clinical utility. Important information on device handling (imaging through a blood pool, imaging during cardiac motion, and device trackability) within the coronary vasculature can be obtained from animal coronary studies and initial clinical trials. Lesion algorithms can be tested for their correlation with ex-vivo pathologic studies, and reproducibility of serial measurements can be assessed. Identification of vulnerable plaques in patients is likely to result in treatment decisions that may lead to aggressive medical therapy or invasive interventions. Therefore, while most attention is appropriately focused on lesion identification, vulnerable plaque detection devices should also demonstrate an acceptable level of negative predictive accuracy. To this end, preclinical animal and ex-vivo human coronary studies can be instrumental in demonstrating the device can accurately identify the absence of vulnerable lesion characteristics (i.e. demonstrating normal arterial architecture or an absence of vulnerable plaque features).

After the completion of initial feasibility studies, natural history studies are recommended to fully assess the safety and efficacy of novel vulnerable plaque detection devices. As noted above, there is no unifying morphologic definition of a vulnerable plaque, which increases the difficulty in the assessment of vulnerable plaques. There are obvious limitations of extrapolating findings from ex-vivo studies performed on the benchtop, including registration of histology with device-derived data, sampling errors, tissue processing, and fixation artifacts, and tissue shrinkage secondary dehydration. Natural history studies are therefore needed to assess whether plaque features assessed by vulnerable plaque detection devices are clinically relevant. For example, natural history studies might address questions such as:

- Is it worth the time, effort, and cost to measure lipid content, cap thickness, or plaque inflammation?
- Does a particular lesion feature have prognostic value for future events?
- Does a vulnerable plaque detection device provide value added to other traditional lesion features or other, perhaps less-invasive, clinical markers?

Natural history studies may take two forms: (1) studies which evaluate whether specifically identified vulnerable plaques transform into culprit lesions associated with clinical events and (2) studies which evaluate whether the presence of vulnerable plaque is associated with clinical events without necessarily demonstrating that the identified vulnerable lesion evolved into the culprit lesion. The challenges associated with the execution of natural history studies should be recognized. Regarding the first type of study presented above, it would be difficult to determine if a clinical event (acute coronary ischemic syndrome) occurred at the site of a previously identified vulnerable plaque; doing so would require the return of the patient for repeat imaging. This type of vulnerable plaque 'local lesion' proof of principle study is made more problematic by

- the relatively small number of events, leading to large sample sizes
- inability to predict the timing of events
- need for return visits to the institution where the initial imaging of vulnerable plaques was performed
- markedly low autopsy rates.

If only subjects with events are re-imaged, the status of lesions in patients without events will remain unknown. Finally, data interpretation may be confounded by a myriad of clinical covariates and treatments. In contrast to a vulnerable plaque 'local lesion' proof of principle, one could consider a 'global' proof of principle of the utility of vulnerable plaque detection (as presented in the second type of natural history study presented above). The ultimate question in the assessment of these lesions is whether the presence of vulnerable plaques identifies patients at significantly increased risk of clinical events without necessarily confirming the vulnerable plaque as the culprit lesion on follow-up imaging studies.

TRIALS OF SYSTEMIC AND LOCAL THERAPIES FOR VULNERABLE PLAQUES

Natural history studies of vulnerable plaque detection devices provide a basis for future randomized studies of systemic or local therapies that are specifically directed at vulnerable plaques. Potential study design schemes for systemic or local vulnerable plaque therapies are given below.

Example 1: systemic therapy for vulnerable plaques

In this example, patients at high risk for events (e.g. those who have had a recent acute coronary syndrome) would be recruited. Vulnerable plaque imaging would be performed, and the patient would be randomized to either systemic therapy or placebo (or aggressive medical therapy vs less-aggressive medical therapy). The endpoint for this study would be the occurrence of coronary events, and subjects could be offered an option for late imaging to evaluate morphologic changes in plaques as a potential secondary endpoint. Subsequent imaging could address whether a vulnerable lesion(s) appears less 'vulnerable' (based on what their device measures) after systemic treatment.

Example 2: systemic therapy for vulnerable plaques (variation)

A variation on the above design would involve a similar patient population (those at a high risk for events), but would initially randomize subjects into two groups: those with vulnerable plaque imaging and those without vulnerable plaque imaging. Both groups would then be further randomized to aggressive or less-aggressive medical treatment in a 2 × 2 design. Events serve as the main endpoint, and this design allows one to address the question of whether vulnerable plaque detection itself is clinically useful.

Example 3: local therapy for vulnerable plaques

It has been postulated that vulnerable but non-flow-limiting lesions could be 'stabilized' via local treatment. Such a treatment strategy might take subjects at high risk for events, identify vulnerable lesions, and then randomize them to local therapy vs no local therapy; subsequent clinical events would be an endpoint. The risks associated with local lesion treatment (such as destabilizing existing vulnerable plaques or producing new stenotic lesions) must be considered in any local therapy study design. Late imaging to evaluate changes in the morphology of vulnerable plaques would be an optional secondary endpoint to determine if local therapy renders lesions less vulnerable. Studies of local therapy of vulnerable plaque rely on the assumptions that the vulnerable plaque device demonstrates acceptable diagnostic sensitivity and specificity, vulnerable plaque detection is clinically relevant, and treatment directed to vulnerable plaque is clinically beneficial.

CONCLUSIONS

The field of vulnerable plaque is significant as it has a far-reaching potential impact on the early diagnosis and treatment of patients at risk for acute coronary syndrome and other clinical events. The FDA's role in the advancement of this field is equally far reaching, as it is charged with the evaluation of novel drugs, devices, and biologics which may be sought for market entry. Specific to novel devices, the FDA expects to evaluate these technologies within the context of the various regulatory applications (e.g. IDE, 510(k), and/or PMA) and will employ a risk-based approach to ultimately determine whether the novel device has demonstrated a reasonable assurance of safety and effectiveness. The FDA envisions the paradigm for ADCs to be determined by whether the device is a tool or diagnostic. In addition, the FDA envisions a significant role for natural history studies and for trial designs for evaluation of systemic and local therapies for vulnerable plaque. Ultimately, with each of these approaches, the FDA will collaborate with the scientific research and medical community in order to formulate an approach to ensure the appropriate and safe delivery of diagnostic and therapeutic medical devices to the public. Use of the Pre-IDE review process is encouraged so that the scientific, regulatory pathway, and other technical issues related to the novel device, may be identified and addressed in order to facilitate a streamlined regulatory review process.

REFERENCES

1. Blue Book Memorandum D95-1, Goals and Initiatives for the Pre-IDE Program. Accessed December 2006 on http://www.fda.gov/cdrh/d951.html
2. Coronary and Peripheral Arterial Diagnostic Catheters. Accessed December 2006 on http://www.fda.gov/cdrh/ode/guidance/1228.pdf
3. ISO 14971:2000, Medical devices – Application of risk management to medical devices.
4. Guidance on Premarket Notification [510(k)] Submission for Short-term and Long-term intravascular catheters, section II.D.b. Accessed December 2006 on http://www.fda.gov/cdrh/ode/824.pdf
5. ISO 10555-1, Sterile, single-use intravascular catheters – Part 1: General requirements.

6. IEC 60601-1-1:2000, Medical electrical equipment –
    Part 1: General requirements for safety; safety require-
    ments for medical electrical systems.

7. IEC 60601-1-2, 2nd Edition, 2001, Medical electrical
    equipment – Part 1–2: General requirements for safety;
    electromagnetic compatibility – requirements and tests.

8. ISO 10993-1:2003(E), Biological evaluation of medical
    devices.

9. Shelf Life of Medical Devices. Accessed December
    2006 on http://www.fda.gov/cdrh/ode/415.pdf

10. ISO 11134:1993, Sterilization of health care products –
    Requirements for validation and routine control-
    industrial moist heat sterilization.

11. ISO 11135:1994, Medical devices – validation and rou-
    tine control of ethylene oxide sterilization.

12. ISO 11737-1:1995, Sterilization of medical devices –
    microbiological methods – Part 1: Estimation of the
    population of microorganisms on product.

13. ISO 10993-7:1995 (R) 2001, Biological evaluation of
    medical devices – Part 7: Ethylene oxide sterilization
    residuals.

14. Guidance for the Content of Premarket Submission
    for Software Contained in Medical Devices. Accessed
    December 2006 on http://www.fda.gov/cdrh/ode/
    guidance/337.pdf

15. Off-The-Shelf Software Use in Medical Devices.
    Accessed December 2006 on http://www.fda.gov/
    cdrh/ode/guidance/585.pdf

16. Farb A, Burke AP, Tang AL et al. Coronary plaque
    erosion without rupture into a lipid core: A frequent
    cause of coronary thrombosis in sudden coronary
    death. Circulation 1996; 93:1354–63.

17. Virmani R, Kolodgie FD, Burke AP, Farb A, Schwartz
    SM. Lessons from sudden coronary death: a compre-
    hensive morphological classification scheme for ath-
    erosclerotic lesions. Arterioscler Thromb Vasc Biol
    2000; 20:1262–75.

Investing in vulnerable plaque   38

*Jan David Wald**

INTRODUCTION

Vulnerable plaque (VP) is at an important juncture in its maturation. Research in the field has been active for a number of years, and investigators are making good progress. Still there are a great many technical and other questions to answer. Other chapters in this book address the current state of VP technology. We focus on a more mundane topic: what criteria might be used to make investments in vulnerable plaque? Because we live in a world where funding for research and development must be constantly sought after, perhaps it is time to ask what it will take to migrate the discoveries made to date and have them realized as manufactured products. This will take hard currency to accomplish, so we will try to address in this chapter what it might take to realize this goal.

Funding agencies (government agencies, private sources, institutional investors), like every business, want to see a return on their investment. The kind of return required, proof-of-concept, prototype demonstration, financial return, differs depending on the source of funding involved. But it is required nonetheless. In this chapter, we focus on financial return, and try to address the question: What will make investors invest in vulnerable plaque technology and product opportunities?

*This chapter was written by Jan D Wald PhD, Health Care Analyst with AG Edwards & Sons, Inc., Member SIPC. Opinions are subject to change without notice; additional information is available on request.

Let us begin by seeing what is actually happening in the financing marketplace to assess the investor psyche. The figures below show the size of the US market for venture and private financing for healthcare vs other sectors.

WHERE ARE HEALTHCARE DOLLARS GOING NOW: WHAT IS VP'S SHARE?

Healthcare competes with other market sectors for capital resources. We have segmented the US financing markets into broad categories: Healthcare, Information Technology, Consumer Products, and Other. We have also segmented the US Healthcare market into Biopharma, Services, Medical Devices, Information Services, and Other. We have chosen to look at these markets in terms of financing rounds, in order to assess the degree of interest in the major categories. We have also chosen to examine the markets in terms of funding, to see the distribution of US dollars ($) over time and in terms of median amounts raised, to help understand the dynamics of the marketplace.

We should say at the start that there appears to be continued interest in funding healthcare ventures, even though (in absolute dollars) funding is down considerably. As can be seen from Figures 38.1 and 38.2, the number of financing rounds for key sectors has decreased sharply, from 6310 in 2000 to 2226 in 2004. That number is likely to be down in 2005 as well. For the first three quarters of 2005,

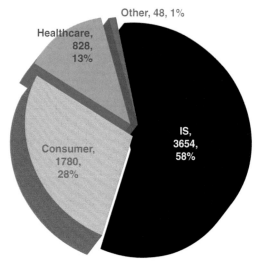

Figure 38.1   US financing rounds by industry: 2000. IS, Information Services. (Reproduced from Ernst & Young,[1] with permission.)

look at total funding, in 2000 approximately $94.5 billion was raised, while in 2004 $21.5 billion was raised. It appears that 2005 will be flat to slightly down compared with 2004. In 2000 Healthcare received 10% of funding, while in 2004 it received approximately 32%, so even though in absolute dollars funding was down, Healthcare did receive a larger share of the pie (Figures 38.3 and 38.4). Once again, Consumer Products took the biggest hit, but Information Services also lost a bit of ground. Healthcare appears to be doing well, considering a smaller amount is being raised now than compared with earlier this decade, especially since it seems, on average, more dollars are going to fewer companies. This can be seen as well looking at Figures 38.5 and 38.6. The median amount raised in 2000 per company was $7.0 million for Healthcare and this grew to $7.5 million in 2004. So far in 2005, it looks as if the median amount raised is $8.0 million. The other major markets have actually decreased per company: Information Services, from $10.0 million in 2000 to $7.0 million in 2004, and Consumer from $9.0 million to

there have only been 1605 financing rounds. The largest decrease in rounds has been in the Consumer Products market (28% to 12%), while healthcare has moved from 13% of rounds to 24% of them. If we

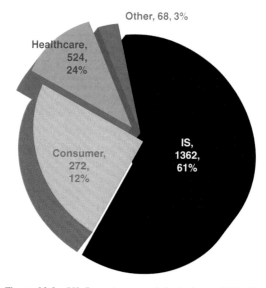

Figure 38.2   US financing rounds by industry: 2004. IS, Information Services. (Reproduced from Ernst & Young,[1] with permission.)

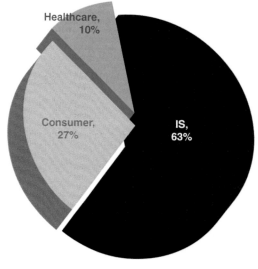

Figure 38.3   US funding by industry: 2000. IS, Information Services. (Reproduced from Ernst & Young,[1] with permission.)

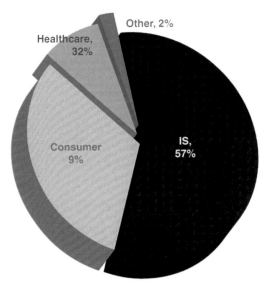

Figure 38.4   US funding by industry: 2004. IS, Information Services. (Reproduced from Ernst & Young,[1] with permission.)

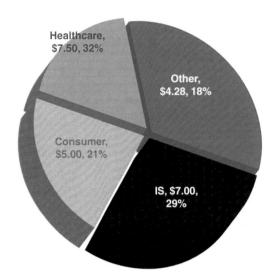

Figure 38.6   Median invested in US industry segments: 2004. IS, Information Services. (Reproduced from Ernst & Young,[1] with permission.)

$5 million. There does appear to be continued interest in funding Healthcare startups, but investors are becoming more selective.

If we look at Healthcare funding, this has dropped dramatically as well: from $9.5 billion down to $6.9 billion in 2004. Year to date, 2005 points toward a flat if not slightly down environment compared with 2004. Biopharma still remains the largest and fastest growing segment in Healthcare (Figures 38.7 and 38.8). On a percentage

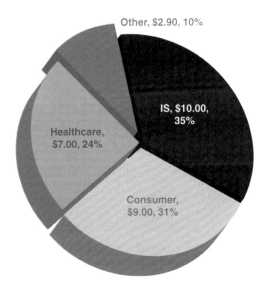

Figure 38.5   Median invested in US industry segments: 2000. IS, Information Services. (Reproduced from Ernst & Young,[1] with permission.)

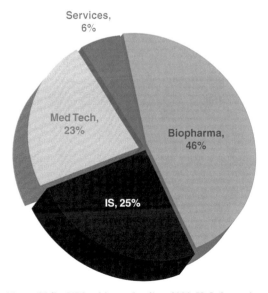

Figure 38.7   US healthcare funding: 2000. IS, Information Services. (Reproduced from Ernst & Young,[1] with permission.)

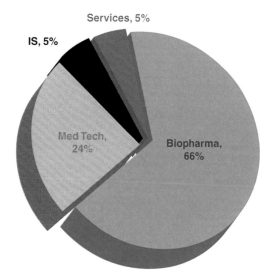

Figure 38.8   US healthcare funding: 2004. IS, Information Services. (Reproduced from Ernst & Young,[1] with permission.)

basis Medical Technology has held its own, however, and Information Services funding has declined sharply, while Services has fallen but has had a less precipitous decline than Information Services. Looking at the median investments in US Healthcare, we see that Biopharma has experienced the second largest increase, Services the largest, and Medical Devices the smallest increase. Information Services has declined by just under 40%. Healthcare dollars appear to be being spent on Biopharma and Medical Devices in aggregate. Larger dollar amounts appear to be going to each Information Services program, but there are many less of them being funded.

What this means for the vulnerable plaque community is that healthcare funding today appears to be fairly equivalent to 2000, but investors are being more selective than they once were. A higher percentage of dollars are being spent on healthcare projects, but the absolute dollars being devoted to healthcare has declined dramatically. The salad days where start-ups just needed a business plan and a smile are over, but from what

we see in the numbers, good ideas and programs are likely to be given consideration and can be funded.

WHAT DO INVESTORS LOOK FOR?

Investors are, by nature, risk adverse, even those investors that fund early-stage ventures. It is, and always has been, the risk–reward ratio that entices investors: early stage 60:1 to late stage 15:1. But all investors look at almost the same criteria when deciding to fund projects. They tend to look for:

- large markets
- acceptable risks
- winner technology/approach
- reasonable timelines
- physician acceptance
- a solid and credible management team, usually with device experience.

Large markets are desirable because even though the product being developed may satisfy a medical need, it may not be profitable enough to pursue. If the market for a drug is $300 million per year, that market size may not be enough to justify its development. Orphan drugs find themselves in this very situation. Large markets, such as drug-eluting stents or congestive heart failure devices, are easy to justify as fundable. We have seen small companies benefit from this market dynamic. The risk must also be acceptable to investors no matter what stage, early or late, they are investing in. Risk is hard to quantify, but can be assessed by looking at the technical concept itself, the competitive landscape to see who and what else might be there, and the regulatory and reimbursement environment, since issues in either of these can have dire consequences for when a product might be marketable. If there are many competing technologies or approaches, investors will also demand some indication as to why one might be better than another, or, at the very least, that there is room for more than one. The timelines themselves must also be reasonable. Investors are thought to look a quarter ahead, but we can attest that investors' time horizons can be 5–10 years out, though most investors only look out about 2 years. One of the most important parameters is physician acceptance. Acceptance can influence a revenue ramp for the product, which can impact when the product or the company reaches profitability. Finally, management quality is also key to funding. While this seems almost a tautology, it is something that should not be underestimated. Device experience is not necessary, but can help a great deal. Strong, existing, industry relationships management should help to open doors for partnerships from a research and development (R&D), regulatory, and sales channel development standpoint and also attract a solid supporting team, board members, and scientific advisors – all of which are important to investors.

It makes sense to ask how vulnerable plaque will fare when these parameters are used to assess its investment potential.

ARE THE MARKETS LARGE ENOUGH?

Cardiovascular disease remains the number one killer in the USA. In 2002, according to the *2005 Heart and Stroke Statistical Update* from the American Heart Association (AHA),[2] 38% of deaths in the USA were due to cardiovascular disease. The cost of treating heart disease in 2005 was $393.5 billion. Also, in 1999, $26.3 billion in payments were made to Medicare beneficiaries for cardiovascular disease-related hospital expenses, an average of $7883 per discharge. Treatment for Medicare patients totaled $10.7 billion in 1999. Each admission for a myocardial infarction (MI) costs $10 336 on average, $11 270 for atherosclerosis, and $3472 for

other heart ailments. In 2002, it is estimated that 1 200 000 Americans, 2 200 000 worldwide, will have a new or recurrent cardiovascular heart disease (about 700 000 will be new), about 865 000 will have new or recurrent MIs, about 565 000 (1 130 000 worldwide) will be first attacks, and 300 000 (600 000 worldwide) will be recurrent attacks. Approximately 25% of men and 38% of women who experience a coronary attack in a given year will die from it. Survivors have a 1.5–15.0 times greater chance of illness and death than the general population. Within 6 years after a recognized MI, 18% of men and 35% of women will have another attack, 7% of men and 6% of women will experience sudden death, about 22% of men and 46% of women will be disabled with heart failure, and 8% of men and 11% of women will have a stroke. About 400 000 (800 000 worldwide) new cases of stable angina appear in the USA per year and about 150 000 (300 000 worldwide) cases of unstable angina[3] will occur in a given year.[4]

We are about to present a market model that attempts to size the VP investment opportunity. Because of space limitations, we are only going to present a best-case scenario. We would be surprised if this case were to be realized, so it might be advisable to discount our numbers used here between 30% and 50% out of conservatism. We do believe, however, that the numbers represent a reasonable view of the market's upside potential.

We have identified two paths to diagnosis and treatment: one from the interventionalists' community and the other from screenings that could occur during routine office visits or cardiologist work-ups. It is very likely that interventionalists will identify VP patients first, and this is where the first patient pool, we believe, will come from. But we also think, eventually, patients will be referred from screenings, like those we see currently for cholesterol.

This is likely because these patients are probably symptomatic.

Secondly, the VP investment opportunity will only be realized if the clinician see its diagnosis as a component of patient care. The acceptance of these physicians is critical for investors, and if subsequent education and training is not forthcoming, investors will either not invest or lose interest.

Thirdly, more than natural history and device/drug approval trials will be necessary. We believe that outcome improvements must also be demonstrated.

Finally, the acceptance and use of the diagnostics will depend on their sensitivity and specificity. Highly sensitive, but nonspecific tests may not be investable ideas. Highly specific, but insensitive tests may be useful, but in limited circumstances.

All of these factors influence market size, but they also impact the investment horizon – more on this topic in a later section.

Peer-reviewed studies and existing market research suggest a large opportunity. We must take account of the opportunity for detecting and treating vulnerable plaques, unstable non-obstructive plaques, in order to size the market properly. Burke et al[5] suggest that between 70% and 85% of all acute coronary interventions (ACI) occur because of the rupture of these vulnerable plaques. Therefore, diagnosing and treating these plaques will more than likely lead to significant opportunities for companies pursuing this market. Figure 38.9 shows the number of procedures, diagnostic and therapeutic, that were performed worldwide in 2001. Assuming a 3% growth rate per year, we have calculated the 2008/2010 vulnerable plaque market opportunity for diagnostic and therapeutic devices (also shown in Figure 38.9).

Our reasoning is as follows. New procedures, i.e. over the 3% core growth rate, will be driven from two sources: referral patterns established by vascular companies, such as Guidant, Johnson & Johnson, Medtronic, and Boston Scientific, to drive new stent (or alternative therapy) sales, and VP indications established from clinical trials by VP diagnostic and therapeutic companies themselves as they prove their technology and drive the business accordingly. At first, we believe that vascular companies will drive patients toward increasing diagnostic screening. Patients need to be identified if these companies plan to sell more therapeutic devices. We would expect the companies to see the therapeutic opportunity translate into more stent sales. This is not a new strategy for these companies. Figure 38.10 depicts a likely referral process. It begins with general screening and becomes more

Figure 38.9 Worldwide angioplasty diagnostic and therapy procedures. Market size: current number of procedures and centers. PTCA, percutaneous transluminal coronary angioplasty; DX, diagnostic. (Courtesy of AG Edwards, Inc.)

MARKET	PTCA/ STENT	DX PROCEDURES	TOTAL ANNUAL PROCEDURE VOLUMES	NUMBER OF CENTERS
USA	1,203,800	2,291,900	3,495,700	1,500
EUROPE	1,112,350	1,437,473	2,549,823	930
JAPAN	175,692	702,768	878,460	1,100
TOTAL	2,491,842	4,432,141	6,282,009	3,530

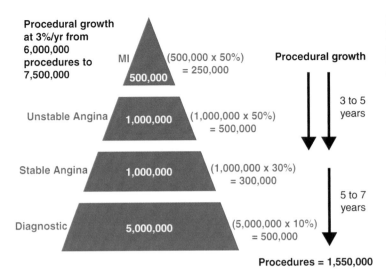

Figure 38.10 Vulnerable plaque procedural growth in the USA. Available procedures in 2008/2009. MI, myocardial infarction. (Courtesy of AG Edwards, Inc.)

selective, and, potentially, invasive as the patient passes through the steps. We have assumed approximately 18 000 000 in the USA (using 2001 data) will be screened, using high cholesterol screening as our baseline, and that a third of them will move to more specific blood screenings (we used other screening percentages, e.g. colonoscopy screening pass-throughs as the standard). From those patients we have assumed 20% of them will move on to either non-invasive or invasive screening, coming to about 1 000 000 patients in the USA and 2 000 000 worldwide that are indicated for some type of therapy.

Figure 38.11 depicts the scenario we envision will evolve. Companies will first diagnose and treat ACI patients and then move on to unstable angina, stable angina, and general diagnostics. We have asked practitioners in the field to tell us how many of the patients in each of those groups are likely to undergo a diagnostic or therapeutic procedure, and we have reflected this in Figure 38.11. Physicians reported 50% of patients with ACI and unstable angina, 30% of patients with stable angina, and 10% of patients in the general diagnostic category. The time frame for indications coming to market is

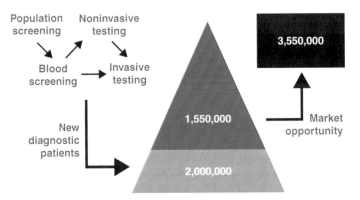

Figure 38.11 Combined US market procedural opportunities. Vulnerable plaque market opportunity: 2008/2010 procedures. (Courtesy of AG Edwards, Inc.)

also identified: 3–5 years for ACI and unstable angina and 5–7 years for stable angina and diagnostics. With these assumptions, there are likely to be as many as 1.6 million procedures performed by 2008/2010.

Figure 38.11 looks at the combined market opportunity growing procedures from both sources. Doing so, new procedures could total 3 550 000. Figure 38.12 shows the potential size of the 2008/2010 market: a $3.2 billion diagnostic market and a $5.3 billion therapeutic market. Diagnostic market size depends on assuming a $900 cost for the single-use catheter involved in the procedure. The therapeutic market assumes one-half of the patients diagnosed will be treated and that, in those treated, 1.5 stents will be used per procedure, with an average price over the years of $1,950 per stent.

There appears to be a considerable diagnostic and therapeutic market for vulnerable plaque, answering the question posed as the title of this section. Again, we should remind readers that we have offered a best case, but one that does point to an attractive market opportunity. The question still remains as to whether or not a viable product can be developed and funded.

DIAGNOSTIC APPLICATION

3,550,000 (Diagnostic procedures)

X $900 (Catheter system cost)
_____
$3.2 billion

A tantalizing thought

THERAPEUTIC APPLICATION

1,800,000 (1/2 of patients will be treated)

X $2925 (1.5 stents implanted/procedure
           — $1950/stent)
_____
$5.3 billion

Figure 38.12 Worldwide total diagnostic and therapeutic market opportunity in dollars.

ARE THE TIMELINES REASONABLE?

Investment timelines depend on the investor's horizon. Using an approach adopted by the US Government (Figure 38.13) for

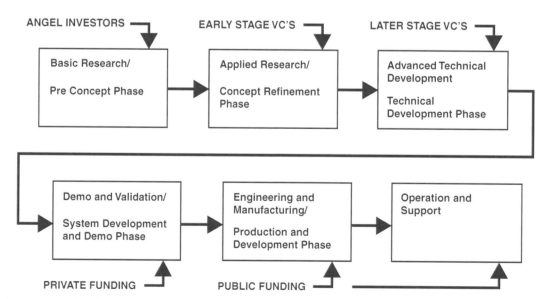

Figure 38.13 Development stages for product development and funding sources for them. VC, venture capitalist. (Courtesy of AG Edwards, Inc.)

program acquisition, we can see the various time points at which investors are likely to fund programs. We can also see from Figure 38.13 that what the various stages of development there are and how funding might relate to the different stages. Investors that 'get in' early will want a higher return on their investment, as they are accepting greater risk (≥60%). One might ask where we would place VP programs at this time. Our best guess is between applied research, where the goal is to demonstrate technical feasibiity, and advanced technology development, where the goal is engineering and manufacturability (i.e. can the product actually be engineered so that it is manufacturable for a reasonable cost). At this point, investors are most likely looking for a 30–50% return on their investment.

Figure 38.14 shows a notional timeline for first product introductions. We assume that products are being developed today, and these will be used in the natural history trials that will take place for the next 2–3 years. The natural history trials are going to be the pacing item, we believe, for when products will be marketable. At this point we have assumed the normal Food and Drug Administration (FDA) submission timeline: 2 years for the clinical trials and 1 year for the review. We should emphasize that this timeline is notional. As there is no sense yet as to what the endpoints and follow-up requirements the FDA or other regulatory authorities might want, it is hard to predict what the timeline might be. Figure 38.14 is a start, though.

Once the VP products are approved, there is really no way to predict yet what the adoption rate might be. This will be influenced by referrals and how real the need is perceived to be by practitioners. Using minimally invasive surgery (MIS) as an example, it took 6–7 years before the diagnostic/therapy took hold. We would expect the time needed to be less, but how much really depends on the benefit

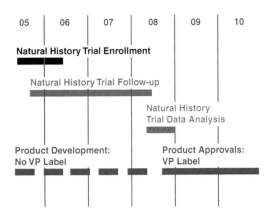

Figure 38.14 A nominal timeline for product development and approval. Natural history trial timelines: from enrollment to vulnerable plaque (VP) labeling. (Courtesy of AG Edwards, Inc.)

perceived and the practicality of the means for diagnosis.

IS THE RISK ACCEPTABLE?

Financial risk is defined as the standard deviation from the return investors can expect from an investment. The narrower the band, the less risk there is thought to be; the wider the band, the more risky the investment. There is also the assumption that the expected return must be larger to counter the riskier investments. We have spoken about this earlier.

Vulnerable plaque, at this juncture, is an early-stage investment. How should investors think about it? Different risk factors can be used to assess a company's risk. We break risk down into technical (technology and clinical), market (need and acceptance), reimbursement, and regulatory. If a company can manage these risks, we believe, it will be successful. We are going to focus on the first two risks, as the latter will become more important as the companies move closer to advanced development. Even at this stage of development, companies should not ignore them – they may come back later to bite them with a vengeance.

The technology risks really dominate at this time. First of all, is VP a systemic disease, a focal disease, or a systemic disease that needs to be treated focally? There is no consensus yet, though we have detected a move toward the conclusion that focal treatments will be part of the physician's toolbox. Another question that remains is whether systemic or local diagnostic tools will be needed. Will biomarkers be enough to determine whether there are vulnerable plaques or not, or will non-invasive or invasive diagnostic approaches be needed to determine vulnerability? One can also ask whether non-invasive magnetic resonance imaging (MRI), computed tomography (CT) scans, etc., be adequate for the task, or will invasive approaches based on near-infrared (NIR), intravascular ultrasound (IVUS), optical coherence tomography (OCT), laser, or other energy sources be needed? There are no definitive answers to these questions to date.

Investors want some assurance that they are going down a promising path. We have summarized in Figure 38.15 our assessment as to the progress companies are making on eliminating technical risk. In summary, we have not seen a great deal of progress, from the investors' perspective, though we do believe that real technical progress is being made. One of the reasons why we cannot point to appreciable progress is because of the lack of meaningful clinical data. We should be helped by the natural history trials Guidant and Bristol-Myers Squibb, among others, have begun. From these trials, we should get an indication whether VP lesions can be detected prior to rupture. There will still be a lot of work to do. There are detection methods being used in these studies, IVUS and thermography, but these approaches will have to go through regulatory approvals prior to their being marketed. More important,

	2003	2004	2005
VP as clinical area of interest	↗	→	→
Clinical Data	↗	→	→
Technology (Detection)	↗	→	→
• Non-invasive Med Tech	→	↘	↘
• Invasive Med Tech	→	↘	↘
Technology (Therapy)	↗	↗	→
• Traditional (Stents)	↗	↗	→
• Technology (Novel)	→	→	→
• Pharmaceuticals	→	→	→
Identifiable Candidates	→	→	↘
• Detection	→	↘	↘
• Therapy	↑	↑	→
Investing Horizon	↘	↘	↘
• Venture	→	→	→
• Private	↘	↘	↘
• Public	↓	↓	↓

Figure 38.15   An investor's assessment of progress and fundability. VP, vulnerable plaque. (Courtesy of AG Edwards, Inc.)

these tools will have to demonstrate that they are at least equivalent and, more likely, better than standard medical treatment. That may not be all that easy or the outcome all that certain. We are not suggesting that the path toward VP approval is different than other diagnostic or therapeutic programs that are breaking new ground. But from an investment perspective, any clarity would add to the investability of a program or product.

Therapy is another issue, though we do not believe that being able to deliver therapy is that much of a concern for investors. Coronary stents will most likely be used at first, with specially designed stents being developed later. There are also other alternative therapies, nanotechnology, and other localized delivery mechanisms that can be developed and used. For now, we believe investors are satisfied that there is a therapy that can treat vulnerable plaques if they can be detected.

As for marketing risk, we do believe that the need has been identified: 70–80% of all heart attacks may be caused by vulnerable plaques. The benefit in terms of lives saved and healthcare costs, if VP can be detected and treated, is well understood. Acceptance is another issue, and we will discuss that in more detail in the next section.

WHAT WILL THE ACCEPTANCE CURVES LOOK LIKE?

Trying to predict acceptance rates is tough. We do have some good examples of what can happen. As we mentioned before, MIS took 6–7 years to become the standard of care, though investors had predicted a much quicker response. Drug-eluting stents, on the other hand, were expected to be immediately accepted, and they were. A recent surprise was the speed at which cardiac resynchronization devices were accepted. Referral patterns were unclear; it was a new technology, and yet

the response was almost immediate. One might ask where VP acceptance will fall within this continuum.

Acceptance is likely to depend early on the specificity and sensitivity of the diagnostics available. We do believe interventional cardiologists will drive the initial adoption rate. The patients will already be in the Cath Lab, but we are uncertain as to how many will perform the additional procedure to determine if there are vulnerable plaques. A good deal of education and training might be necessary.

Acceptance will also depend on clinical trial data. We can expect to learn about the disease progression from natural history trials. We may also learn about which markers are predictors of VP and how promising the detection methods deployed in these trials are. What will not be assessed is the safety and efficacy of these approaches. We will, however, be able to get some read on the viability of stenting as it is likely that if these patients are treated for vulnerable plaques, it will be with stents. If one looks at the amount and kind of data used to evaluate the benefits of drug-eluting stents, there may be considerable time and effort spent before these devices are marketed. We do believe that any diagnostic or therapy is going to have to demonstrate a benefit, and that may be more than just equivalence with current practices. These studies are likely to be large and time consuming. Investors will want to know there is a reasonable chance of success before funding these activities.

Because of the complexity of the issues involved with identifying and treating VP, we do believe that investors will want to be able to predict a physician acceptance rate, and one that will see revenues climb quickly if the studies' outcomes are positive. This means that investors and companies should be taking a very close look at the regulatory strategy any company is pursuing. Time to market is also certainly an important criterion, but one must also ask which products will come to market.

Will there be enough data to support the labeling the company receives from the regulatory authorities? Will the labeling be all inclusive, or will only a small subset of patients be able to benefit and larger patient pools will have to grow as more studies are completed that widen the indication? How many of these studies will be needed? If one uses drug-eluting stents as an example, Boston Scientific has performed or is performing six clinical trials and at least four large registries. In cardiac rhythm management (CRM), there have been a number of studies that have enlarged the patient pool: AVID, MADIT, MUSTT, MADIT II, COMPANION, and SCD-HeFT.

We would suggest that acceptance will probably come in two waves: first from the interventional cardiologist, and then from more general screening. We would expect the first wave to be relatively quick. We could use the rate of IVUS penetration as a starting point to understand what the uptake rate might be. If noninvasive techniques are used, the penetration rate might be quicker. For the second wave, general screening, we would assume that timelines associated with cholesterol screening or hypertension screening might serve as good benchmarks.

We would assume it will take 2–3 years to penetrate the interventional cardiologist patient pool to about 60%. We believe it might take 6–10 years to penetrate the screening market to cut in half the remaining unpenetrated market. Still, as we suggested in an earlier section, the market is large enough that even with these penetration rates, companies in the VP space can be profitable. Investors will have to determine if their investment horizon fits with penetration rates such as we have outlined.

SUMMARY

Vulnerable plaque is at an investment crossroads. Natural history trials are beginning that should help investors to determine the viability of the market opportunity. New approaches will be tried in these trials and others will be developed concurrently. Investors will have to sort out which technologies provide the best opportunity for them, and right now, we would have to say that data will tell the tale, and there is not a great deal of data available. Early-stage investors are the most likely to see the VP opportunity at this time, but that will probably change as these programs mature. Progress is being made, investments are being made, and more are likely to come as the technology matures and clinical data become available.

REFERENCES

1. Ernst & Young. 3Q05 Ernst & Young/VentureOne Venture Capital Report.
2. American Heart Association. 2005 Heart Disease and Stroke Statistics. Dallas, TX; American Heart Association, 2005.
3. American Heart Association. 2005 Heart Disease and Stroke Statistics (At a Glance). Dallas, TX; American Heart Association, 2005.
4. American Heart Association. 2005 Heart Disease and Stroke Statistics. Dallas, TX; American Heart Association, 2002 update.
5. Burke AP, Kolodgie FD, Farb A et al. Healed plaque ruptures and sudden coronary death evidence that subclinical rupture has a role in plaque progression. Circulation 2001; 103:934–40.

Index

Note: Page references in italics refer to Figures; those in **bold** refer to Tables

acquired immune system *31, 32*
actinomycin D 314
acute coronary syndrome (ACS)
    endothelial markers of 121-38
    incidence of thin-cap atheroma in 23
    lesions leading to 16-18
    pathophysiology *142*
    plaque disruption in 43
    protective effect of HDL 41
    role of platelets 39, 40-1, 43
    yellow plaque in 6
acute myocardial infarction (AMI) 172
    influenza as trigger of 353-4
    MMPs in 57
    non-ST-elevation myocardial infarction (NSTEMI) 316
    ST-elevation myocardial infarction (STEM1) 170-1, 316
    thin-cap atheroma in 23
    thrombosis and 40
adalimumab 379
adhesion molecules 32, 303
    see also intercellular adhesion molecule (ICAM-1)
adipose-derived mesenchymal stem cells (AMSCs) 406
AFCAPS/TexCAPS study 144
Agatston calcium score 327, **328**
albumin/dextran perfluorobutane gas microbubble carriers
    (PGMCs) 317-19
aldehyde dehydrogenase (ALDH) 400
anger as trigger of acute cardiovascular disease 88-9
anger management training 93
angina, stable
    lipoprotein-associated phospholipase A_2 and 160
    ROS in 70
angina, unstable 8
    lipoprotein-associated phospholipase A_2 and 160
    ROS in 70
    thrombotic occlusion in 47
angiography 169-77, 180
    geometry of plaque 176
    limitations in detecting vulnerable plaque 176-7
    multifocal coronary plaque 387
    percent diameter stenosis 171-4
    plaque location 170-1
    plaque morphology 174-6
angioplasty 7
angioscopy 5-6, 9, 175
angiotensin II 70-1
angiotensin-converting enzyme (ACE) inhibitor 7, 438
    in acute risk prevention 93, 94
    HOPE trial 81
    lipoprotein-associated phospholipase A_2 and 160
animal models 103-13
    complex atherosclerosis 105-11
    desirable features 103-4, **104**

animal models *(Continued)*
    plaque rupture and 105, 251
    porcine model 43, 110-11, *110, 111-12,* 112-13, *113*
    rabbit models 108-10
    vulnerable endpoints in 104-5, **104**
    see also mouse models
annexin 305-7
anti-CD40L monoclonal antibody 46
antidepressants 93
anti-HSP65 antibody 78
antioxidant mechanisms 69
antioxidant responsive elements (AREs) 235
antiplatelet agents 81
antisense therapy for c-myc AVI-4126 323
antithrombin III 35
Antrin phototherapy 428
anxiety as trigger of acute cardiovascular disease 89
ApoB100/LDLR- transgenic mice 107
ApoE-/- mice 32, 34, 35, 44, 296
    MMPs in 58-60
apolipoprotein E (ApoE) deficiency 236
apoptosis, role of 21-2
apparent diffusion coefficient (ADC) 256
ARIC (Atherosclerosis Risk in Communities) study
    76, 91, 148, 154-7, 162
arterial diagnostic catheter safety 462-6
    animal testing 465
    bench testing 463-5
    biocompatibility 464
    effectiveness wing autopsy specimens 466
    electrical safety and electromagnetic compatibility 463-4
    mechanical safety 463
    packaging, shelf life and sterilization 465
    phantom effectiveness testing 465
    software 465
ascorbic acid 69
aspirin 81, 87, 93, 94, 438
Asymptomatic Carotid Surgery Trial (ACST) (MRC) 80
atherogenesis, platelets in 44-5
atherosclerosis 40-1
    activate platelets in *2*
    angiotensin in 70-1
    development 41-5, *41, 42*
    fibrous cap disruption in 35
    genetics 78
    plaque classification 13, **14**
    plaque composition 13-16
    platelets in 45
    stem cells and 401
    thrombosis and 40-1
Atherosclerosis Risk in Communities (ARIC)
    study 76, 91, 148, 154-7, 162
atherothrombosis 40, 41-5

atorvastatin 180
autologous bone marrow derived mononuclear cells
        (ABMMNCs) 401, 403-4, 413-16

B lymphocytes 30, 32
bare metal stent (BMS) 440-1
B-cell receptors (BCRs) 32
BEAST technique 202
bereavement as trigger of acute cardiovascular disease 89
beta2GPI 33
beta-amyloid precursor protein 44
beta-blockers 6, 87, 93-4, 96, 438
bevacixumab 379
BioCardia helical infusion catheter 409, 410
biomarkers 70-9, 121, 141-50
    see also endothelial biomarkers
Blind Deconvolution 224
bone marrow-derived stem cells, adult 401
bone morphogenic protein-4 (BMP-4) 234
BOOST trial 411, 413
bootstrap error-adjusted single-sample theory (BEAST)
        technique 202
butathione sulfoximine (BSO) 431

C-natriuretic protein (CNP) 234
cadherin 402
calcification 15
    Agatston calcium score 327, **328**
    multislice computed tomography (MSCT) 327-8
calcified nodules 16, *16*, 18
calcium channel blockers in acute risk prevention 94
CAPTURE trial 146, 147, 148
carbon nanotubes 290
CARDIA study 160
CARESS trial 81
Carotid and Vertebral Artery Transluminal Angioplasty
        Study (CAVATAS) trial 80
carotid duplex ultrasound (CDUS) 79-80
carotid endarterectomy (CEA) 77, 80
Carotid Reascularization Endarterectomy versus Stent Trial
        (CREST) 81
Carotid Revascularization Using Endarterectomy or Stenting
        Systems (CaRESS) 81
carotid vulnerable plaque 75-82
    definition 75-6
    pathology and pathophysiology 76-7
cascade polymers 290
catalase 69
cathepsins 34-5
    B 34
    H 34
    L 34
    S 34, 35
    D 34
    F 34
    K 34, 35
CAVATAS trial 80
CD3+ macrophages 78
CD9 406
CD11b/CD18 (Mac-1) 45
CD25 33
CD28 32
CD29 406
CD31+ 70
CD34 402
CD34+ 70
CD39 39
CD40 30, 34, 56, 57, 248
CD40+ 70
CD40–CD40L system 32, 126

CD40L 17, 30, 34, 35, 46, 56
    soluble (CD40L) 46
CD68+ macrophages 77, 78
CD73 406
CD80/86 32
CD133 402
chemokine (C-C motif) receptor-2 (CCR2) 30
chemokines 30, 32
Chlamydia pneumoniae 364-5
cholesterol clefts 15
cholesteryl ester transfer protein (CETP) 367
chymase 238
cigarette smoking 39
classification (AHA) of atherosclerotic lesions 8
clopidogrel 81
Clopidogrel and Aspirin for Reduction of Emboli in
        Symptomatic Carotid Stenosis (CARESS) trial 81
coagulation 35-6
collagen 18, 76
compound B-mode ultrasound 79
computed tomography (CT) 160, 177, 252
    contrast-enhanced 329-31
'contact facilitated drug delivery' 298
contact thermography 270
contrast enhancement MRI (CEMRI) 338-9
    gadolinium contrast enhancement 338-9
    image analysis tools 339-41
    superparamagnetic iron oxide particles (SPIOs) 339
    targeted contrast agents 339
conventional B-mode ultrasound 79-80
copper–zinc SOD 69
cord blood-derived stem cells 407
coronary artery disease (CAD), endothelial
        biomarkers in 125
Coronary Artery Surgery Study (CASS) 171
contrast-enhanced CT coronary imaging 329-31
COX-1 234
C-reactive protein (CRP) 282, 384
    as biomarker 143-5
    cardiac risk and 78
    clinical instability and 135
    pathophysiologic effects *144*
    plaque vulnerability and 30, 33, 46-7
crown ether (CE) fibrin-targeted nanoparticles 297
cryotherapy 7
CX3CR1 30
CXCR3 30
CXCR4 401
cyclo-oxygenase 2 17
CYPHER coronary stent 321
cystatin C 34, 35
cysteine proteases 76
cytokines 30, 32

Dahl salt-sensitive hypertensive rats 107
definition of plaque vulnerability 3, 4-7
    functional 4
    histologic 4-5
    prospective 5-7
dendrimers 290
dendritic cells 30
Determinants of Onset of Myocardial Infarction Study
        (ONSET) 88, 89
diabetes 39, 43
    coronary artery disease progression and 454-5
    intracoronary thermography in 282
    stem cells and 401
diagnostic criteria 76
diaminobutane (DAB) dendrimers 290
diffuse reflectance near-infrared spectroscopy 6

diltiazem 94
disrupted (thrombosed) plaques 7
doxorubicin 290
doxycycline 82
    MMP expression and 60-1
drug-eluting stents (DES) 438-40, 440-1

echogenic liposomes (ELIPS) 293
electromagnetic spectrum *200*
electron beam tomography (EBT) 23
embryonic stem cells 405-6
endothelial biomarkers 121-38
    balance of endothelial products with diametrical roles 135
    best-marker concept 125
    CAD pathophysiology and 135
    combinatorial 134, **137**, 138
    context analysis 126
    current 123, 127-35
    endothelial activation, site of 135
    feasibility of detectable levels demonstrated 127-34
    functional significance and 125-6
    LOX-1 (lectin-like oxidized LDL) 126
    mechanisms of release and half-lives 136-8
    multifaceted endothelial involvement and 125
    normal endothelial functions and 112-15
    panel of biomarkers 134
    plaque type-specific 136
    prioritization strategies 127
    proinjury endothelial dysfunctions 134
    projected functional impact of endothelial activation 136
    rationale and concepts 121-7
    as stand-alone tests 127
    stepwise framework of analysis of development 136
    uniformity of parameters used or comparative analysis
        designs 136
endothelial cells (ECs) 44
endothelial dysfunction 121, **123-4**
    biomarkers of **128-33**
    progression to plaque 141-3
endothelial dysfunction score 138
endothelial functions **123-4**
endothelial microparticles (EMPs) 125
endothelial nitric oxide synthase (eNOS) 143, 234
endothelial progenitor cells 402
endothelial thrombomodulin/protein C pathway 70
endothelin-1 (ET-1) 41, 135, 143, 234
endovascular therapy 80-1
ENRICHD trial 93
environmental stress as trigger of acute cardiovascular
        disease 90
erosion of plaque 5, 14, 16, *16*, 18
E-selectin 30, 41, 46, 70, 135, 235, 248, 392, 402
    soluble (sE-selectin) 135
European Carotid Surgery Trial (ECST) 80
extracellular matrix turnover 33-5
extracellular SOD (ecSOD) 69

factor VII (FVII) 35
factor Xa activity 35
fat-derived stem cells 406
fibrinogen 36, 77-8
fibroatheromas 18
fibrous cap 15-16, 34
    atheroma 14
    disruption 35
    vulnerability of 42-3
flagellin 31
flow influence factor (FIF) 271, 272
FLU Vaccination Acute Coronary Syndromes (FLUVACS)
        trial 367-8

fluorescence-activated cell sorter (FACS) analysis 400
fluorescein isothiocyanate-labeled PGMC (PGMC-FITC)
        318-19
^{18}F-fluorodeoxyglucose (FDG) 79
FLUVACS trial 367-8
foam cells 31
Food and Drug Administration (US) 461-9
FOSS NIRSystems probe 204, *204*
four-dimensional ultrasound 80
fractalkine 235
free tissue factors pathway inhibitor (f-TFPI) 135
frequency of vulnerable plaques 8-10
FRISC II trial 145
fullerenes 290
FUTURE I trial 451
FUTURE II trial 451

gadofluorine 296
gamma-aminobutyric acid 405
gamma-interferon 17
gene therapy 7
glistening yellow plaque 6
glutathione 69
glutathione peroxidase 69
glutathione S-transferase 234
glycophorin A 22
glycoprotein (GP) 40
GP1b 40
GPIb/IX complex 40
GPIIb/IIIa 40, 45, 46
gp91phox 71
granulocyte-macrophage colony-stimulating factor
        (GM-CSF) 30

hazard ratio (HR) 78
healthcare expenditure 471-4
Heart Outcomes Prevention Evaluation (HOPE) trial 81
heat shock proteins 363-4
    HSP60 33, 364
    HSP65 78
hematopoietic stem cells (HSCs) 400
hemoxygenase I (HO-I) 234
heparan sulfate 60
heparin 60
high-density lipoprotein (HDL) 7, 41-3, 153, 290
high-performance liquid chromatography (HPLC) 323
high-risk plaque (vulnerable plaque) 3, 10
high-sensitivity CRP (hsCRP) 78
history 3-4
HIV 33
HMG-CoA reductase inhibitors 36, 70, 438
HOPE trial 81
hyaluronan 15, 18
hydrazino-nicotinamide (HYNIC) bifunctional agent 305-6
3-hydroxy-3-methylglytaryl enzyme A reductase inhibitors
        see HMG-CoA reductase inhibitors
hypercholesterolemia 22, 39, 41, 68
hyperlipidemia 43
hypertension 39
hypoxia inducible factor 1 α (HIF-1 α) 247

^{123}I-HO-CGS 27023A 307
ICAM-1 *see* intercellular adhesion molecule (ICAM-1)
immune system, actions in induction of plaque
        vulnerability 31-2
immunohistochemistry 245
immunomodulation 371-9
    antibodies and risk assessment 379
    antibody-based therapy 377-9
    development of therapy for atherosclerosis 376-7

immunomodulation *(Continued)*
  innate and adaptive immunity in atherosclerosis 371-3
  interactions between oxLDL and the immune
      system 373-4, *374-5*
  modulating the immune response against oxLDL 375-6
inducible nitric oxide synthase (iNOS) 268
Infiltrator catheter 110-11
inflammation, immune systems and 30-3
influenza vaccination 353-7
  cardiovascular disease and 354-5
  clinical implications 357
  coverage in cardiac patients 356
  effect of systemic infections on coronary
      artery pathology 356
  influenza as trigger of acute myocardial infarction 353-4
  trigger mechanisms of cardiovascular events 355-6
innate immune system in atherosclerosis 31-2, *31*
insulin-like growth factor 1 (IGF-1) 149
integrated backscatter (IBS) 181
integrin-αIIbβ3 3 44, 146
α$_v$β$_3$ integrin 294, 295, 296
intercellular adhesion molecule (ICAM) 30, 142, 188, 248
intercellular adhesion molecule (ICAM-1) 30, 41, 46, 70, 78,
      82, 188, 234, 235, 293, 385
  soluble (sICAM-1) 33, 391
interferon-α (IFN-α) 366
interferon-γ (IFN-γ) 30, 32, 33, 34, 35, 60, 77, 373
  interferon-γ-inducible protein-10 (IP-10) 235
INTERHEART study 89, 91
interleukin-1 (IL-1) 17, 30, 32, 33, 34, 35, 45, 56, 77
interleukin-1 receptor 78
interleukin-1α 35
interleukin-1β 17, 30
interleukin-2 33
interleukin-4 33, 366
interleukin-5 33, 366
interleukin-6 (IL-6) 30, 33, 46, 78, 80, 143, 144-5
interleukin-8 30, 46, 107, 235
interleukin-10 33, 145, 366, 373
interleukin-12 33
interleukin-18 30, 33, 107, 125, 136
intimal xanthoma 13
intracoronary thermography (ICT) 267-77, 279-84
  clinical studies 274-5
  cooling effect 281
  heat detection 276
  heat generation 267, 275-6
  heat selection 270
  heat transfer 268-70, 276
    conduction 269
    convection 269
    radiation and absorption 269-70
  in-vivo temperature measurement 280-1
  macrophage metabolism 267-8
    enzymatic extracellular matrix degradation 268
    lipid metabolism 268
    uncoupling proteins 268
  nitinol catheters 275
  polyurethane catheters 275
  simulations 270-4
    catheter 272-4
    convection 271-2
    heat source 272
    heat source production 274
  widespread inflammation 281-3
intracoronary ultrasound 6
intravascular elastography 141
intravascular palpography 141, 191-7
  clinical studies 194-5
  in-vivo validation 194

intravascular palpography *(Continued)*
  plaque characterization 192-3
  principle 191-2, *192*
  three-dimensional 195-7
  vulnerable plaque detection 193-4
intravascular ultrasound (IVUS) 9, 141, 172, 179, 180-1, 191,
      211, 223, 293
  intravascular ultrasound radiofrequency (IVUS-RF) data
      analysis 223
  see also intravascular ultrasound, virtual histology of
      (IVUS-VH)
intravascular ultrasound, virtual histology of (IVUS-VH) 223
  combining optical coherence tomography and IVUS-VH 228
  combining palpography and IVUS-VH 229
  positive remodeling detection 227-8
  technical aspects 223
  validation of the technique 223-4
intravascular ultrasound-derived thin-cap fibroatheroma
      (IDTCFA) 225-7
investigational device exemption (IDE) 462
investment in vulnerable plaque technology 471-82
  acceptance curves 481-2
  market nature 474-5
  market size 475-8
  risk 479-81
  timelines 478-9
iron oxide nanoparticles 290

KDR/FLK-1 402
Ki-67 406

LDLR$^-$/ApoB$^-$ mice 107
LDLR−/− mice 32
lectin-like oxLDL receptor (LOX-1) 126, 136, 234
leukocyte adhesion molecules 30
LightLab OCT system 213-14, *214*
  balloon-delivery catheter 213-14
  catheter system 213-14
  computer controller 213
  OCT imaging engine 213
  probe interface unit 213
lipid-lowering therapy in acute risk prevention 94
lipid pools 13-14, 15
lipopolyassociated molecular patterns (PAMPs) 31
lipopolysaccharide (LPS) 31
lipoprotein (a) 153
lipoprotein-associated phospholipase A$_2$ 147-8, **155-6**
  atherosclerosis and **158-9**
  Atherosclerosis Risk in Communities (ARIC) 148, 154-7
  coronary atherosclerosis and 157-61
  epidemiology 153-63
  extracoronary atherosclerosis and 161
  genetic polymorphisms affecting 161-2
  incident cardiovascular events in patients with CAD 157
  MONICA study 148, 157
  Rotterdam study 157
  West of Scotland Coronary Prevention Study (WOSCOP)
      147, 154, 162
  Women's Health Study (WHS) 148, 154
liposomes 289
low-density lipoprotein (LDL) 43, 67, 70, 153, 290
LOX-1 (lectin-like oxidized LDL) receptors 126, 303
luminal endothelial apoptosis 18

macrophage colony-stimulating factor (M-CSF) 34, 307
macrophages 30
  content in atherosclerotic plaques 215
  in-vivo concentration and distribution 219
  metabolism 267-8
  nuclear imaging 303-7

MAGIC trial 414
magnetic resonance angiography (MRA) 6
magnetic resonance imaging (MRI) 141, 177, 335-47
    3D free-breathing magnetic resonance coronary vessel
        wall imaging 337
    3D fluid structure interactions models 341
    3T MRI 336
    aortic atherosclerosis and risk factors 344
    as biomarker 342-6
    carotid artery 78, 79, 342
    contrast enhancement MRI (CEMRI) 338-9
    future challenges 346-7
    hardware 336-7
    in hemodynamic and tissue mechanical property studies
        341-2
    histologic validation of plaque imaging 336
    intracoronary 6
    intraplaque hemorrhage and carotid atherosclerosis 343-4
    intravascular 336-7
    longitudinal structural determinant of atherosclerotic
        plaque vulnerability 341-2
    nanoparticle contrast agents and 292, 293-4
    prediction of ischemic events 345-6
    pulse sequence design 337-8
    quadruple inversion-recovery (QIR) 337-8
    quantification of plaque composition by 343
    shear stress and in the thoracic aorta plaque 342
    statin-induced cholesterol lowering and plaque
        regression 345
    thoracic aorta, carotid intima–media thickness 344-5
    see also magnetic resonance imaging, intravascular
magnetic resonance imaging, intravascular 255-64
    preliminary experiments 261-4
    clinical studies 262-4
    ex-vivo human studies 261-2
    in-vivo animal studies 261
    principles 255-6
    technical properties of the IVMRI catheter 256-61, 256-60
    use 255
magnetic resonance thermography 270
magnetic resonance tomography (MRT) 252
major histocompatibility complex class II (MHCII) 32, 35
malondialdehyde (MDA)-modified peptide sequences 367
manganese SOD 69
markers
    of cellular activation and plaque destabilization 145-9
    of inflammation 143-5
    see also biomarkers
mast cells 30
matrix metalloproteinases (MMPs) 5, 76-7, 267, 289
    activated inflammatory cells and 43
    activation by ROS 70
    as biomarkers 57
    contribution to fibrous gap growth and stability 57-8
    expression 55, 56-7
    extracellular matrix (ECM) substrates 54
    genetic epidemiology 57
    genetic manipulation in mice and 58-60
    inhibitors 7, 60-1, 95
    levels of regulation 56
    membrane-type (MT-MMPs) 53
    non-traditional substrates 55
    MMP-1 (collagenase-1) 17, 34, 53, 55, 56, 57, 60,
        61, 77, 82, 238, 307
    MMP-1 genes 57, 58
    MMP-2 (gelatinase-A) 17, 34, 53, 55, 56, 57, 60,
        61, 238, 241, 307
    MMP-3 (stromelysin-1) 17, 34, 53, 55, 56, 57, 58,
        60, 61, 136, 238, 307
    deficiency in ApoE⁻/⁻ mice 59

matrix metalloproteinases (Continued)
    gene 57
    MMP-7 34, 53, 56, 57, 60
    MMP-8 17, 34, 53, 56, 77, 238
    MMP-9 (gelatinase-B) 17, 34, 53, 55, 56, 57, 60,
        61, 77, 82,107, 234, 238, 241, 268, 307
    deficiency in ApoE⁻/⁻ mice 59
    MMP-11 56, 58
    MMP-12 17, 34, 53, 56, 57, 58, 60, 77
    deficiency in ApoE⁻/⁻ mice 59-60
    MMP-13 17, 53, 56, 58, 238
    MMP-14 17, 34, 53, 56
    MMP-16 34, 56
    see also tissue inhibitors of MMPs (TIMPs) 53
mesenchymal stem cells 401-2
5,10-methylene tetrahydrofolate reductase 677
MGH OCT system 213
micro CT 245, 250
MILIS study 88, 95
molecular imaging 36
MONICA study 148, 157, 162
monocrystalline iron oxide nanoparticles (MIONs) 290
monocyte chemoattractant protein 1 (MCP-1)
    30, 46, 142, 143, 148, 235, 307
mouse models 105-8
    ApoB100/LDLR⁻ transgenic mice 107
    ApoE−/− mice 32, 34, 35, 44, 58-60, 106, 296
    LDL receptor-deficient 106-7
    LDLR−/− mice 32
    LDLR⁻/ApoB⁻ mice 107
    nu/nu 32
    RAG−/− mice 32
    severe combined immunodeficiency (SCID)
        mice 32, 373
    TIMP-1 deficient mice 60
MT-MMPI 34
Multicenter Investigation of Limitation of Infarct Size
    (MILIS) study 88, 95
multidetector computed tomography (MDCT),
    contrast-enhanced 6
multifocal coronary plaque instability 383-94
    coronary inflammation is widespread 388-90
    multifocal and pancoronary 385-8
    multifocal complex lesions, plaque progression and
        clinical outcomes 390-1
    panvascular multifocal plaque instability 393
    pathophysiologic role of inflammation in 384-5
    systemic inflammation multifocal plaque instability 391-4
multislice computed tomography (MSCT) 327-32
    contrast-enhanced CT coronary imaging 329-31
    coronary angiography 329
    coronary calcification 327-8
    coronary plaque imaging 329-31
    identification of high-risk plaques 331-2
muscle satellite cells (skeletal myoblasts) 404-5
MV0611 429, 431-2
MV0611-PDT 431-2
myeloperoxidase (MPO) 147, 147
myeloperoxidase (MPO)-positive cells 17
myocardial infarction (MI) see acute myocardial infarction
Myocardial Regeneration and Angiogeneisis in MI with
    G-CSF and Intracoronray Stem Cell Infusion
    (MAGIC) trial 414
Myostar catheter 409, 410, 411

NAD(P)H oxidase 70, 71
NAD(P)H:quinone oxidoreductase (NQO-1) 234
nanotechnology 289, 293-8, 3`6-`9
    imaging 293-7
    therapeutics 297-8

NASCET 80
natural killer cells 30
n-CoDeR 377
near-infrared (NIR) spectroscopy 199-209
　atherosclerotic plaque characterization 202-8
　definition of spectroscopy 199-200
　future of 208-9
　high-risk atherosclerotic plaques 203
　in-vivo catheter-based valuable plaque system 207-8
　light/tissue interactions and 200-2
　simulating in-vivo detection of vulnerable plaques 203-6
necrotic cores 15, 21-2, **21, 22**
　hemorrhage and angiogenesis in 22-3
neopterin 385
neuroimaging 79-80
nifedipine 94
nitrates in acute risk prevention 94-5
nitric oxide 39, 41, 60, 67, 135, 141
nitric oxide synthase 69
nitroglycerin 95
nitrotyrosine 268
NOGA catheter 416
NOGA electromechanical map 410
non-contact thermography 270
non-Hodgkin's lymphoma 379
non-ST-elevation myocardial infarction (NSTEMI) 316
non-vulnerable plaque 7
North American Symptomatic Carotid Endarterectomy
　Trial (NASCET) 80
nox 1 71
nox 4 71
nu/nu mice 32
nuclear factor κB (NF-κB) 31, 41, 82, 145, 234, 235
nuclear imaging 303-11
　18-fluorodeoxyglucose with PET 304-5
　annexin 305-7
　chemokines 307
　metalloproteinases 307
　OCLDL 307-9
　oxidized lipid targets 307-9
　targeting macrophages 303-7
　thrombus imaging 310-11

optical coherence tomography (OCT) 6, 141, 211-20
　fibrous cap 214-15
　future role 220
　human coronary arteries 214, 217-20
　clinical syndrome and 217-18
　comparison with IVUS 217
　in-vivo macrophage concentration and
　　distribution 219
　mechanical properties of the coronary artery
　　wall 219-20
　intravascular 212-14
　limitations 220
　macrophage content in atherosclerotic plaques 215
　for plaque characterization 214-15
　principle 211-12
　safety 220
　swine coronary arteries 215-17
optical coherence-domain reflectometry (OCDR) 211
optical frequency domain imaging (OFDI) 220
oxidized low-density lipoprotein (oxLDL) 17, 31, 33,
　　70, 126, 142, 234, 247, 303, 364, 366

p22^{phox} 70
paclitaxel 298, 314, 319, 320, 324
PAI-1 35, 36
palpography 7
pancoronary plaque 385-8

PAPP-A *150*
partial least-squares discriminate analysis (PLS-DA) 206
Pathobiological Determinants of Atherosclerosis in Youth
　(PDAY) study 235
pathogen-associated molecular patterns (PAMPs) 31, 371
pattern recognition receptors 31
PECAM 295
peptidoglycan 31
percutaneous coronary intervention (PCI) 146
percutaneous transluminal coronary angioplasty (PTCA)
　194, 313-14, 251
　cardiovascular disease and vulnerable plaque 315-16
　nanoparticle vehicles 316-19
perfluorobutane gas microbubble carriers (PGMCs),
　albumin/dextran 317-19
perfluorocarbon (PFC)-based nanoparticles 297
perfluorocarbon core emulsions 290
peroxisome proliferator-activated receptor
　(PPAR) γ-responsive elements 235
peroxynitrite 70, 241
PFOB 297
phosphatidylserine 35
phosphoesterase 4D gene 78
photodynamic therapy 7, 427-33
　atherosclerotic plaque and 430-3
　clinical trials for restenosis prevention 429-30
　mechanism of action 427-8
　photosensitizers and 428-9
　regional, with LS11, for vulnerable plaque 433
　for restenosis prevention 429
PhotoPoint PDT 428-9
placental-derived stem cells 406
placental growth factor 148-9
plasminogen activator inhibitor (PAI) 35
platelet-activating factor acetylhydrolase (PAF-AH)
　　see lipoprotein-associated phospholipase A$_2$
platelet aggregation inhibitors 36
platelet-derived growth factor (PDGF) 44, 56, 76, 234
platelet receptors and ligands *47*
platelets
　clinical implications 47-8
　inflammatory role 45-7
　role of 39-40
poly (D,L-lactide-*co*-glycolide (PLGA) 290
poly (lactic acid) (PLA) 290
polyamidoamine (PAMAM) dendrimers 290
polymorphonuclear cells (PMNs) 30
population stressors as trigger of acute cardiovascular
　disease 89-90
porcine model 43, 110-11, *110, 111-12*, 112-13, *113*
positron emission tomography (PET) 79, 290-1
positron emission tomography (PET)-MRI 347
pravastatin 82
pregnancy-associated plasma protein A (PAPP-A) 149
PREVAIL study 441, *442*, 447-57, *455-7*, *456*, **456**
　clinical events related to non-target lesion 447
　complex vs simple plaque; ruptured vs stable 447-9
　C-reactive protein levels and 450
　impact of drug-eluting stents 450-1
　intermediated coronary lesion 449
　rationale for study design 455-7
　risk stratification in coronary artery disease 451-5
PRISMA study 368
propranolol 94
prostacyclin 39
prostaglandin E$_2$ 17
protein C 68
protein kinase C 234
prothrombin 35
PROVE IT-TIMI 22 trial 144, 438

P-selectin (CD62P) 30, 33, 40, 44, 45-6, 70, 392
P-selectin glycoprotein ligand-1 (PSGL-1) 45
psychological triggers
    of acute cardiovascular disease 88-90
    acute risk factor 87
    characterization of triggers 95
    chronic stress and progression of
        atherosclerosis 90-1
    definition 87
    evidence for 87-8
    hazard period 87
    multiple triggers 95
    pathophysiology 91-2
    progression of atherosclerosis 95-6
    relationship between plaque vulnerability and 96
    strategy for acute risk prevention 92-5
    therapeutic approach 96
    triggered acute risk prevention (TARP) 88

quadruple inversion-recovery (QIR) 337-8
quantitative angiography 6
quantitative coronary assessment (QCA) 223
quantum dots 290, 291

rabbit models 108-10
    New Zealand white 108-9
    Watanabe heritable hyperlipidemic (WHHL)
        109, 109, 295
radiation therapy 7
RAG-/- mice 32
Raman near-infrared spectroscopy 6
ramipril 81
rapamycin 314, 320-3
reactive oxygen species (ROS) 67
    antioxidant mechanisms 96
    in atherosclerosis 67-8
    sources in atherosclerotic plaque 68-9
    targets 69-70
    after vascular injury 71
    in vulnerable plaque 70-1
regulatory T (Treg) cells 33
resident cardiac stem cells 406
rheumatoid arthritis 33, 379
rituximab 379
Rotterdam study 157, 162
roxithromycin in non-Q-wave coronary
        syndromes (ROXIS) 362
rupture of plaque 14, 16
    history 3-4
    inflammation–matrix interactions 17
    mechanical factors and shear stress 17-18
    mechanisms 17-18
    pathology 16-17
    regional factors 4

SADHART (Sertraline Antidepressant
        Heart Attack Randomized Trial)
        study 95
scavenger receptors 31
seasonal variations as trigger of acute cardiovascular
        disease 90
selective serotonin reuptake inhibitors (SSRIs) in acute risk
        prevention 95
serine proteases 76
serotonin (5-hydroxytryptamine; 5HT) 48
sertraline 95
Sertraline Antidepressant Heart Attack Randomized Trial
        (SADHART 95
severe combined immunodeficiency (SCID)
        mice 32, 373

shear stress
    definition 233
    destabilization of vulnerable plaque 238-41
    role of inflammation 238
    role of shear stress 238-41
    role in generation of vulnerable plaque 235-7
    in humans 235-6
    in mouse models 236-7
    role in vascular biology 233-5
shear stress responsive elements (SSREs) 235
SIRIUS trial 451
sirolimus 314, 319, 320
skeletal myoblasts 404-5
small particles of iron oxide (SPIOs) 290
SmartProbe™ 204
smooth muscle cells (SMCs) 5, 15, 42
soluble CD40 ligand (sCD40L) 33, 145-7
soluble E-selectin (sE-selectin) 391
soluble ICAM-1 (sICAM-1) 33, 391
soluble thrombomodulin (sTM) 135
soluble VCAM-1 (sVCAM-1) 391
SPECT 290, 306
statins 22, 70, 81-2, 93, 94, 160
    MMP expression and 60
ST-elevation myocardial infarction (STEM1) 170-1, 173, 316
stem cell therapy 399-420
    atherosclerosis and 401
    cardiac repair and 400-1
    clinical trials 411-20, 412
    AMI 411-14
    chronic ischemic heart disease 414-20
    stem cell mobilization 414
    delivery methods 408=11
    comparisons 410-11
    intracoronary infusion 409
    intramyocardial injection 409
    intravenous infusion 408
    retrograde coronary venous delivery 408-9
    stem cell mobilization 414
    transendocardial injection 409-10
    transepicardial injection 409
    stem cell identification 399-400
    stem cell types 401-7
stenting 7, 437-43
    dedicated stents 442
    mechanical stabilization of vulnerable plaque 439-40
    in non-obstructive plaque 440-1
    proposed clinical trials 441
    rationale 437-9
Stiletto catheter 409-10
Stockholm Heart Epidemiology Program (SHEEP) 88, 89
Streptococcus pneumoniae 376
stress reduction training 93
stromelysins 34
Study to Evaluation Carotid Ultrasound Changes in Patients
        Treated with Ramipril and Vitamin E
        (SECURE) 81
superoxide 67
superoxide dismutases (SODs) 69, 239-41
sVCAM 33
systemic lupus erythematosus (SLE) 33

T allele 79
T lymphocytes 30, 32-3
TACTICS-TIMI-18 trial 451-2
Takotsubo cardiomyopathy 90
targeted nanoparticle contrast agents 289-99
TAXUS IV trial 451
T-cell receptors (TCRs) 32
tetracyclines, MMP expression and 60-1

tetrahydrobiopterin 69, 70
Th1 33
Th2 33
thermal leakage 275
thermogenin 268
thermography 6, 141
thin cap atheroma 14
    calcification in detection of 23-4
    incidence in acute coronary syndromes 23
thin-cap fibroatheroma (TCFA) 3, 5, 9, 19-20,
        19, 104, 173
    detection 224-7
    morphologic variants 20, *20*
    non-hemodynamically *21*
    OCT analysis 218, *218*
three-dimension IVUS with integrated backscatter
        (3D-IBS-IVUS) 182, *183-4*
thrombin 17
Thrombolysis In Myocardial infarction (TIMI) risk score
        451-2, **452**
thrombomodulin/protein C anticoagulant system 68
thrombosed plaques 7
thrombosis-prone plaque (vulnerable plaque) 3, 10
thromboxane A$_2$ (TXA$_2$) 4, 43, 48
tissue factor (TF) 4, 35, 36, 39, 46
tissue factor pathway inhibitor (TFPI) 35, 43, 368
tissue inhibitors of MMPs (TIMPs) 34, 53, 76, 307
    TIMP-1 55, 56, 57
    TIMP-1 deficient mice 60
    TIMP-1 expression 60
    TIMP-1 genes 57
    TIMP-2 55, 56, 82
    TIMP-2 genes 57
tissue-type plasminogen activator (tPA) 35
α-tocopherol 69
Toll-like receptors (TLRs) 31, 366, 371
    TLR4 32, 78
TOPCARE-AMI (Transplantation of Progenitor Cells and
        Regeneration Enhancement in AMI) trial 411-13
tPA 36
transcranial Doppler (TCD) 77
transforming growth factor-β, (TGF-β)
        17, 33, 34, 56, 60, 373
    TGF-β$_1$ 234
transient ischemic attacks (TIAs) 78
    FDG-PET/CT scans 304, *305*
    SPECT *306*
transient left ventricular apical ballooning syndrome 90
Transplantation of Progenitor Cells and Regeneration
        Enhancement in AMI) (TOPCARE-AMI) trial 411-13
transthoracic echocardiography 179
treatment of vulnerable plaques 7
triggered acute risk prevention (TARP) 88
troponin 1 135
troponin T 145
tumor necrosis factor (TNF) 45, 248
    TNF-α 17, 30, 33, 34, 35, 56, 77, 148, 238, 364, 372

ultrasound 79-80, 179-88
    intravascular, plaque characterization by 181-7
    with integrated backscatter 182

ultrasound *(Continued)*
    optical coherence tomography 187
    virtual histology 185-7
    wavelet analysis 182-4
    intravascular and transthoracic, with targeted
            contrast agents 187-8
    surface, plaque characterization by 181
uncoupling proteins 268
    UCP-1 268
    UCP-2 268
unstable plaques 7-8

V protein 34
vaccination 361-9
    influenza 353-7
    mimicry and 362-7, *363*
vasa vasorum
    anatomy and physiology 245-6, *246*
    role in atherosclerosis 247-52
    animal models of plaque rupturing 251
    in-vivo imaging 251-2
    neovascularization 247-9
    plaque instability and 249-51
vascular cell adhesion molecules (VCAM) 30,
        142, 248
    VCAM-1 41, 46, 70, 78, 82, 135, 234, 235, 385
    nanotechnology 293, *294*, 294
    soluble (sVCAM-1) 391
vascular remodeling 236
VEGF 234, 247
VEGF receptor 2 (VEGFR-2) 402
very low density lipoprotein (VLDL) 153
verapamil 94
versican 15, 18
virtual histology (IVUS-VH) 141, 223-30
vitamin E 81
von Willebrand factor (vWF) 36, 40, 44, 77, 135
VSMC apoptosis, mediated by nitric oxide 239
vulnerable blood 3, 15, 75
vulnerable myocardium 3
vulnerable patient 3, 75
vulnerable period 87
vulnerable plaque detection 466-9

Watanabe heritable hyperlipidemic rabbit
        (WHHL rabbit) 109, *109*, 295
West of Scotland Coronary Prevention Study
        (WOSCOP) 147, 154, 162
Western blotting 245
Women's Health Initiative Observational Study 91
Women's Health Study (WHS) 148, 154
Women's Ischemia Syndrome Evaluation (WISE)
        study 455
work-related stress as trigger of acute cardiovascular
        disease 89

xanthine oxidase 69

yellow plaques, glistening 9-10

Printed and bound by CPI Group (UK) Ltd, Croydon, CR0 4YY

23/10/2024

01777711-0002